South-East Asia Eye Health

Taraprasad Das • Patanjali Dev Nayar
Editors

South-East Asia Eye Health

Systems, Practices, and Challenges

Springer

Editors

Taraprasad Das
L V Prasad Eye Institute
Hyderabad
India

Patanjali Dev Nayar
Regional office for South East Asia
World Health Organization - India
New Delhi
India

ISBN 978-981-16-3786-5   ISBN 978-981-16-3787-2 (eBook)
https://doi.org/10.1007/978-981-16-3787-2

This Springer imprint is published by the registered company Springer Nature Singapore Pte Ltd.
The registered company address is: 152 Beach Road, #21-01/04 Gateway East, Singapore 189721, Singapore

(Late) Dr. APJ Abdul Kalam

Former President of India

(Late) Professor G Venkataswamy

Founder, Aravind Eye Hospital, Madurai, India

Dr. Gullapalli N Rao

Founder, L V Prasad Eye Institute, Hyderabad India

who inspired generations of ophthalmologists
to the systemic practice of public health ophthalmology

Foreword

As per the World Report on Vision 2019, the South-East Asia Region was home to 12.049 million (30%) blind people and 78.482 million (32%) people with vision impairment in the year 2010. This amounts to 30% of global blindness and 32% of global visual impairment. Refractive error and cataract continue to be the principal causes of moderate visual impairment. The outcome of cataract surgery is suboptimal in some countries of the region. The current global data suggests that blindness and visual impairment have decreased over the past three decades by 28.5% due to sustained effort by all Member States and many non-government organizations. But the absolute number of blind and visually impaired people has increased due to two important factors: population aging and increased longevity. Moreover, aging, growth in population, and lifestyle factors are projected to cause a further increase in the number of people with vision impairment; thus, the need and demand for eye health care are projected to surge in the coming decades.

There are several prevalent challenges and gaps. Despite the majority of causes of vision impairment are preventable or addressable through early detection and timely management, yet eyecare is not an integral part of universal health coverage, and the "Targeted approach" is almost absent. Coverage rates of cataract surgery—an indicator of eye care service provision within populations—show marked variations by income level. Inequities also exist within countries: the prevalence of vision impairment tends to be higher in underserved populations. A shortage of trained human resources in low- and middle-income countries is one of the greatest challenges. Vast inequities exist in the prevalence of vision impairment which is not distributed equally. High-risk groups often include people residing in rural areas, those with low income; women; older people; indigenous persons; ethnic minorities; and people with disabilities, among others. Access to eye care for an increasing number of school-age children is critically important. Targets for the above need to be set by the Member States for prioritized outcomes, e.g. Cataract coverage that will also strengthen monitoring and equity.

Good eye health is essential for a better quality of life, economic growth, and sustainable development. The world is working for universal health coverage (UHC), but it cannot be "universal" without universal eye health coverage. The World Report on Vision reports that the disease burden is more in low- and middle-income countries, in older people, in the marginalized community, and the rural population. It has suggested adopting integrated people-centered eye care (IPEC) to address the significant eye care challenges that many countries face. The World Health Organization recognizes good eye health care as a fundamental human right which is also in line with its "triple billion" approach for "No one Left Behind." However, this is only possible when the challenges and gaps are met and eye health care delivered with equity and active engagement of the community without causing catastrophic expenditure. Thus, looking at eye health care through the public health framework is crucial.

In this context, the book *"South-East Asia Eye Health: The Systems, Practices, and Challenges,"* edited by Dr. Taraprasad Das and Dr. Patanjali Dev Nayar with contributions from some best-known professionals in the field, assumes great importance. Dr. Das is globally recognized for his dedication to improving eye health care at all levels and is the regional chair of the IAPB (International Agency for the Prevention of Blindness). My team and I have been working with him for quite some time to ensure better eye care in the region.

This book is not only a compilation of figures and facts, but also outlines doable strategies to deal with the gaps from a public health perspective. It includes the current practices and challenges in major eye disorders, the participatory roles of international organizations working in the region, and the status of the ophthalmic industry. There is no doubt that this book will serve as a good resource for eye care providers, and the data from the book could help frame the new strategies and policies in the region.

WHO is committed to good health and good eye care in the world and the region, and in its capacity, will execute all that is required to promote universal eye health and integrated people-centered eye care. We also hope that the ophthalmologists and the public eye health experts of this region will meet periodically and update the contents of this book in the future. I am sure that the policymakers, professionals, and public health experts will find the book useful.

World Health Organization,
Regional office for South-East Asia
New Delhi, India

Poonam Khetrapal Singh

Foreword

The data published by the Vision Loss Expert Group last year had some sobering numbers for us all. Not only do we know that all categories of vision loss are set to grow in the next 30 years, but also we know that nearly 1.7 billion people will be living with vision loss come 2050. Due to larger population sizes in constituent countries and several related factors, a significant portion of this figure will fall in the South-East Asia region. This is undoubtedly a cause for major concern. Yet, we know that this region is an engine of eye care innovation and practice. One can only expect that they will rise to the challenge, establishing a model for others around the world for the mobilization needed to tackle this looming disaster.

South-East Asia Eye Health: The Systems, Practices, and Challenges, expertly put together by Doctors Das and Nayar, brings together the promise and the challenge of delivering eye health in the South-East Asia region. Dr. Das, who has been the International Agency for the Prevention of Blindness' (IAPB) South-East Asia Regional Chair for a decade now, has worked closely with Dr. Nayar, a regional advisor with WHO SEARO, to implement change in the region. Together, they organized the first South-East Asia regional workshop in 2014, bringing together policy and clinical stakeholders from across the region. The workshop set a precedent, and from there, regular meetings were held across the region, bringing together an ever-growing and diverse group of eye care professionals. Since then, many countries in the region have published new RAABs and ECSATs, while a few have updated their national health plans to explicitly include eye care.

These policy and survey successes have been built through various IAPB regional workshops, Council and General Assembly meetings over the last decade. Together, armed with a robust eye care sector across the region, South-East Asia has developed many successful models of care to showcase and share with the world. Be it a health systems approach that delivers WHO's "Integrated people-eye care" (IPEC); tackling the many eye conditions, especially those slated to explode in the coming decades like uncorrected refractive errors or chronic conditions that affect the elderly in the region; the many stakeholders whose robust relationships are the bed-rock of success; and the many opportunities for private enterprise to join hands and support the health and well-being of the peoples of this region—*South-East Asia Eye Health* is a critical resource to help understand eye care in South-East Asia.

This book showcases the editors' extensive network of partnerships and relationships in the region, alongside their expertise in ophthalmology and eye health practice. I am also pleased to see many IAPB members among the contributors to this highly anticipated and much-needed book. This mix of fascinating topics and erudite authors with international expertise marks this book as a landmark study in understanding the promise and challenge of delivering eye health at a regional level.

International Agency for the Prevention of Blindness Bob McMullan
Canberra, Australia

Preface

Vision is the most dominant of human senses. Eye health touches all lives—directly or indirectly—from individuals and families to whole communities. The Lancet Global Health Commission (2021) defines eye health as "the state in which vision, ocular health, and functional ability are maximized, thereby contributing to overall health and wellbeing, social inclusion, and quality of life." In 2020, an estimated 596 million people had distance vision impairment worldwide; 43 million of them were blind. Another 510 million people had uncorrected near-vision impairment (Global Burden of Disease, The Vision Loss Expert Group). The annual global productivity loss from vision impairment is approximately over USD 410 billion purchasing power parity (The Lancet Global Health Commission). A large proportion of those affected live in low- and middle-income countries (LMICs). Improving eye health and reducing vision impairment are directly related to many Sustainable Development Goals (SDG), such as zero hunger, no poverty, economic growth, gender equity, reduced inequalities, quality education, and sustainable community (SDGs 2, 1, 8, 5, 10, 4, and 11, respectively).

The South-East Asia region has been bearing a disproportionate burden of vision impairment and blindness compared to the developed regions of the world. The common causes of vision impairment in adults are uncorrected refractive error, cataract, glaucoma, age-related macular degeneration, diabetic retinopathy, corneal scarring, and trachoma. In children, the common causes of vision impairment are uncorrected refractive error, cataract, retinopathy of prematurity, congenital ocular anomalies, corneal scarring, and cerebral visual impairment. However, public health approaches can prevent or treat many of these common eye diseases.

Eye health services of today in South-East Asia are very different from those in the yesteryears. Huge strides have been made in managing cataract loads and refractive errors; two countries in this region are trachoma-free. However, the numbers of visually impaired people in the region are still unacceptably high, and a "business as usual" attitude to this will not do. Global efforts are continuing to develop suitable strategies for tackling this problem in the South-East Asia region. The global movement for improved and equitable eye care began with the World Health Organization (WHO) Trachoma committee (1952); the World Vision Report (2019) release is their latest document to address the eye health issues globally. The 73rd World Health

Assembly (WHA 73.4) in 2020 adopted a resolution that calls for the advancement of eye health as an integral part of universal health coverage by implementing integrated people-centered eye care in a broader health services framework.

Efforts at the global level also include many international organizations. The International Agency for the Prevention of Blindness (IAPB) was formed in 1975, and VISION 2020 was formed in 1999. Both organizations work globally with the Member States and many partners to design and implement strategies to reduce avoidable blindness and visual impairment. Consequent to these efforts, the age-standardized global prevalence of blindness has decreased by 28.5% in the past three decades. However, population aging, growth, and urbanization may result in an estimated 895 million people with distance vision impairment by 2050, including 61 million of them blind.

Universal health coverage (UHC) is a global aspiration. It means that all people have access to the health services they need, when and where they need them, without financial hardship. The UHC includes the full range of essential health services, from health promotion to prevention, treatment, rehabilitation, and palliative care. But the UHC is *not* universal without universal eye health coverage. A pyramidal system of eye care, from the village (primary care) to cities (tertiary care), has been advocated to implement universal eye health coverage; it is both structural in population coverage and functional in service delivery.

The IAPB South-East Asia consists of 11 countries. This region is home to over 25% of the world population. It bears a disproportionately high percentage of the global eye disease burden—roughly 30% of the world's blind and the vision-impaired population lives in this region. Inequity exists not only between the countries in the South-East Asia region but also between communities within the countries. Nearly all countries of the region are middle-income countries. In 2017, the world ranking by GDP per capita in this region ranged from 74 (Thailand) to 159 (Nepal), and the combined share of world GDP in this region was only 5.63% (www.worldmeter.info). The problem in the region is not one of economy alone, but also those of suboptimal infrastructure, inadequate health workforce, low priority given to eye care, poor health-seeking behavior, and higher out-of-pocket spending for medical treatment.

Two dissimilar systems of medical care operate in the South-East Asia region. One is an entirely public-funded system (funded directly or through third-party insurance, such as in Bhutan and the Maldives, respectively), while the other is a hybrid system consisting of both public and private funding. Traditionally, several international and non-government organizations have played a significant role in data generation, service delivery, and capacity building. However, as recently as 2015, there were no data on blindness and visual impairment for the Maldives and Timor-Leste until the IAPB conducted these surveys. The lack of research exploring solutions to eye health problems does not provide the decision-makers sufficient and contextually relevant evidence.

Given these backgrounds and challenges, one needs to document the status of eye care available in this region, highlight the achievements gained over the years, identify current challenges, and use global publications like the World Report on Vision to redefine the program and policies to reach the 2030 SDGs and attain universal eye health coverage. This book, "*South-East Asia Eye Health: The Systems, Practices, and Challenges*," addresses these questions and attempts to provide evidence-based solutions.

The book has 6 parts and 35 chapters. Part I introduces the public health indicators used in the population health of the region. Part II (Chaps. 2–8) explores health systems and approaches, which include health management and information systems, universal health coverage and primary eye health, the SDGs with particular emphasis on SDG 3 (Good Health and Wellbeing), Integrated People-Centered Eye Care (IPCEC), health financing, and sustainability, disease burden, and population-based studies. Part III (Chaps. 9–16) describes common eye disorders in this region from a public health perspective. These include cataract, refractive error, childhood blindness, non-communicable diseases (diabetic retinopathy), neglected tropical diseases (trachoma), glaucoma, corneal blindness, eye banking, and assistive devices for alleviating low vision. Part IV (Chaps. 17–19) analyzes the human resources for health, namely, ophthalmologists, optometrists, and allied ophthalmic personnel. Part V (Chaps. 20–32) documents the work of international organizations working in the region. Part VI (Chaps. 33–35) documents the regional status of the ophthalmic industry, which is critical for the supply of essential ophthalmic medicines and devices.

Over 100 authors have contributed to this resource book that contains 92 tables, 143 figures, and 26 illustrative case studies of eye care management in the South-East Asia region. Many others have significantly contributed to making this book; the notable ones are Ms. Neha Hassija and Mr. Yella Yedukondalu from the Communication department of the LV Prasad Eye Institute, Hyderabad (India), Mr. Kumar Athiappan and Ms. Jagjeet Kaur Saini from Springer India, and Ms.Vickrutha Sudarsan, Striave. A special thanks to the book editor, Dr. Anusha Krishanan, who painstakingly corrected all the manuscripts.

We owe special thanks to Dr. Poonam Khetrapal Singh, Regional Director, WHO SEARO, and Mr. Bob McMullan, President, IAPB, for writing the Forewords. We dedicate the book to three people: the late Professor G Venkataswamy, Founder of the Aravind Eye Care System, Madurai (India); the late Dr. APJ Abdul Kalam, Former President of India; and Professor Gullapalli N Rao, Founder of the LV Prasad Eye Institute, Hyderabad (India) for introducing and inspiring generations of ophthalmologists to the systematic practice of public health ophthalmology.

We sincerely believe that this book will serve as a practical compendium to all ophthalmologists, public health specialists, and health administrators for future health planning in each country of the region.

Hyderabad, India — Taraprasad Das
New Delhi, India — Patanjali Dev Nayar

Contents

Part III Common Disorders

Part IV Human Resource for Health

Contributors

Carmen Abesamos-Dichoso Asia Pacific Council of Optometry, Manila, Philippines

Asela Abeydeera Association of Community Ophthalmologists of Sri Lanka, Colombo, Sri Lanka

Srijana Adhikari Tilganga Institute of Ophthalmology, Kathmandu, Nepal

Munir Ahmed Orbis International, Dhaka, Bangladesh

Rahul Ali Orbis, NY, USA

Lynn Anderson International Joint Commission on Allied Health Personnel in Ophthalmology, St. Paul, MN, USA

Samara Andrade SightLife, New Delhi, India
SightLife Seattle, Seattle, WA, USA

Anitha Arvind Optometry Practitioner, Chennai, India

Rashima Asokan Occupational Optometry Services, Medical Research Foundation, Sankara Nethralaya, Chennai, India

Shrikant Ayyangar Mission for Vision, Mumbai, India

Saugata Banerjee Essilor, Singapore, Singapore

Rolika Bansal Centre for Sight, Hyderabad, India

M. Baskaran Smt Jadhavabai Nathmal Singhvee Glaucoma Services, Sankara Nethralaya, Chennai, India

Sahithya Bhaskaran Aravind Eye Care System, Madurai, India

Kashinath Bhoosnurmath OEU, Hyderabad, India

Rupert R. A. Bourne Vision and Eye Research Unit, Postgraduate Medical Institute, Anglia, Ruskin University, Cambridge, UK

Sandeep Buttan Sightsavers, New Delhi, India

Suresh R. Chandra Combat Blindness International, Madison, WI, USA

Sunee Chansangpetch Department of Ophthalmology, Faculty of Medicine, Chulalongkorn University and King Chulalongkorn Memorial Hospital, Thai Red Cross Society, Bangkok, Thailand

Heidi Chase Seva Foundation, Berkeley, CA, USA

Sunita Chaurasia The Cornea Institute, L V Prasad Eye Institute, Hyderabad, India

Beula Christy Institute for Vision Rehabilitation, L V Prasad Eye Institute, Hyderabad, India

Jon Crail The Fred Hollows, Sydney, Australia

Taraprasad Das International Agency for the Prevention of Blindness South-East Asia Region, Hyderabad, Telangana, India

L V Prasad Eye Institute, Hyderabad, India

Sunu Dulal Karnali Academy of Health Sciences, Jumla, Nepal

Patrick Emery SightLife, New Delhi, India

Timothy Fricke Brien Holden Foundation, Sydney, NSW, Australia

Ronnie George Smt Jadhavabai Nathmal Singhvee Glaucoma Services, Sankara Nethralaya, Chennai, India

Clare Gilbert International Centre for Eye Health, Department of Clinical Research, London School of Hygiene & Tropical Medicine, London, UK

Suzanne Gilbert Seva Foundation, Berkeley, CA, USA

Parikshit Gogate Community Eye Care Foundation, Dr. Gogate's Eye Clinic, Pune, Maharashtra, India

Pirindha Govender-Poonsamy AVRI: University of KwaZulu-Natal, Global Ophthalmic Institute, Durban, South Africa

Ella Gudwin VisionSpring, New York, NY, USA

Rishibha Gupta Sightsavers, New Delhi, India

Vivek Gupta Community Ophthalmology, Dr. Rajendra Prasad Centre for Ophthalmic Sciences, All India Institute of Medical Sciences, New Delhi, India

Reeta Gurung Tilganga Institute of Ophthalmology, Kathmandu, Nepal

Aldiana Halim Cicendo Eye Hospital, Bandung, Indonesia

Anurag Hans Essilor, Singapore, Singapore

Prut Hanutsaha Department of Ophthalmology, Ramathibodi Hospital, Mehidol University, Bangkok, Thailand

Peter Holland International Agency for the Prevention of Blindness, London, UK

Santosh G. Honavar Centre for Sight, Hyderabad, India

Lutful Husain Orbis International, Dhaka, Bangladesh

A. H. M. Enayet Hussain Directorate General of Medical Education, Ministry of Health and Family Welfare, Dhaka, Bangladesh

Khaleda Islam Directorate General of Health Services, Ministry of Health and Family Welfare, Dhaka, Bangladesh

Ram Prasad Kandel Seva Foundation, Nepal Hospital, Nepal Netra Bhavan, Tripureswore, Kathmandu, Nepal

Harpreet Kapoor Inclusive Eye Health—Asia, New Delhi, India

Sashipriya Karumanchi Lions Aravind Institute of Community Ophthalmology, Aravind Eye Care System, Madurai, Tamil Nadu, India

Jordan Kassalow VisionSpring, New York, NY, USA

Jill E. Keeffe L V Prasad Eye Institute, Hyderabad, Telangana, India

Rohit C. Khanna Allen Foster Community Eye Health Research Centre, Gullapalli Pratibha Rao International Centre for Advancement of Rural Eye Care, L V Prasad Eye Institute, Hyderabad, India

Alisha Kishore RP Center, New Delhi, India

Satyaprabha Kotha Helen Keller International, Jakarta Selatan, Indonesia

Nick Kourgialis Helen Keller International, New York, NY, USA

Trupti Kulkarni Inclusive Eye Health, CBM, Cambridge, UK

Harish Kumar OEU, Hyderabad, India

Elizabeth Kurian Mission for Vision, Mumbai, India

Nor Tshering Lepcha Department of Ophthalmology, JDW National Referral Hospital, Thimphu, Bhutan

Faculty of Postgraduate Medicine, Khesar Gyalpo University of Medical Science of Bhutan, Thimphu, Bhutan

Manoj Mahajan Sun Pharma, Mumbai, India

Srinivas Marmamula Allen Foster Community Eye Health Research Centre, Gullapalli Pratibha Rao International Centre for Advancement of Rural Eye Care, L V Prasad Eye Institute, Hyderabad, Telangana, India

Parvez Memon OEU, Hyderabad, India

Sailesh Kumar Mishra Nepal Netra Jyoti Sangh, Kathmandu, Nepal

Lorraine Misquith SightLife, New Delhi, India

Y. S. V. S. Naga Mohan Sun Pharma, Mumbai, India

Viswanathan Mohan Dr. Mohan's Diabetes Specialties Centre and Madras Diabetes Research Foundation, Chennai, India

Rudra N. Mohanty Sightsavers, New Delhi, India

Manfred Mörchen Inclusive Eye Health—Asia, New Delhi, India

Habibah S. Muhiddin South Sulawesi Indonesian Ophthalmologists Association, Makassar, South Sulawesi, Indonesia

G. V. S. Murthy Indian Institute of Public Health, Hyderabad, India

Kovin Naidoo African Vision Research Institute: UKZN, Durban, South Africa

School of Optometry, University of New South Wales, Sydney, Australia

Raja Narayanan L V Prasad Eye Institute, Hyderabad, India

Varsha Narayanan Sun Pharma, Mumbai, India

Patanjali Dev Nayar Regional office for South East Asia, World Health Organization - India, New Delhi, India

Josie Noah SightLife, New Delhi, India

SightLife Seattle, Seattle, WA, USA

Phanindra B. Nukella VISION 2020, India, New Delhi, Delhi, India

Radhika Upreti Oli Tilganga Institute of Ophthalmology, Kathmandu, Nepal

Idayani Panggalo South Sulawesi Indonesian Ophthalmologists Association, Makassar, South Sulawesi, Indonesia

Prakash Paudel Brien Holden Foundation, Sydney, NSW, Australia

Krupa Philip Brien Holden Vision Institute, Sydney, NSW, Australia

Rajendra Pradeepa Dr. Mohan's Diabetes Specialties Centre and Madras Diabetes Research Foundation, Chennai, India

Keerti Bhusan Pradhan Global Advisor-Vision Spring, New Delhi, India

Nampermulsamy Vishnu Prasad Aurolab, Madurai, India

Vijayaraghavan Prathiba Department of Ophthalmology, Dr. Mohan's Diabetes Specialties Centre and Madras Diabetes Research Foundation, Chennai, India

M. Babar Qureshi Inclusive Eye Health (IEH) and Neglected Tropical Diseases, CBM, Cambridge, UK

Ramachandran Rajalakshmi Department of Ophthalmology, Dr. Mohan's Diabetes Specialties Centre and Madras Diabetes Research Foundation, Chennai, India

Reena Chandra Rajpal Combat Blindness International, Madison, WI, USA

Rajiv Raman Shri Bhagwan Mahavir Vitreoretinal Services, Sankara Nethralaya, Chennai, India

Dhivya R. Ramasamy LAICO, Aravind Eye Care System, Madurai, India

Gullapalli N. Rao L V Prasad Eye Institute, Hyderabad, India

Mehal Rathore Elite School of Optometry, Chennai, India

Thulasiraj Ravilla Lions Aravind Institute of Community Ophthalmology, Aravind Eye Care System, Madurai, Tamil Nadu, India

Amrita R. Rozario Sightsavers, Dhaka, Bangladesh

Paisan Ruamviboonsuk Department of Ophthalmology, Rajavithi Hospital, Bangkok, Thailand

Kujulva Kannan Rubanbabu Aurolab, Madurai, India

Sanduk Ruit Tilganga Institute of Ophthalmology, Kathmandu, Nepal

Padmaja Sankaridurg Brien Holden Vision Institute, Sydney, NSW, Australia

Department of Optometry and Vision Sciences, University of New South Wales, Sydney, NSW, Australia

Yuddha D. Sapkota International Agency for the Prevention of Blindness South-East Asia Region, Hyderabad, Telangana, India

Suraj Singh Senjam Community Ophthalmology, Dr. Rajendra Prasad Centre for Ophthalmic Sciences, All India Institute of Medical Sciences, New Delhi, India

B. R. Shamanna School of Medical Sciences, University of Hyderabad, Hyderabad, India

Indra P. Sharma Department of Ophthalmology, JDW National Referral Hospital, Thimphu, Bhutan

Faculty of Postgraduate Medicine, Khesar Gyalpo University of Medical Science of Bhutan, Thimphu, Bhutan

Gyalyum Kesang Choeden Wangchuck National Eye Center, Jigme Dorji Wanchuck National Referral Hospital, Thimphu, Bhutan

Sandeep Sharma Sun Pharma, Mumbai, India

Shaifali Sharma SightLife, New Delhi, India

Kuldeep Singh Seva Foundation, Berkeley, CA, USA

Yashwant Sinha OEU, Hyderabad, India

Sobha Sivaprasad Moorfield's Eye Hospital, London, UK

Shubhi Sood SightLife, New Delhi, India

Alagarajan Soundarrajan Aurolab, Madurai, India

Ravilla D. Sriram Aurolab, Madurai, India

Syumarti Section of Cataract Blindness Elimination of Indonesian Ophthalmologist Association West Java, Bandung, West Java, Indonesia

Aildrene Tan The Fred Hollows, Sydney, Australia

Kah Ooi Tan Asia Optometric Congress, Hong Kong, Hong Kong

Anshu Taneja VisionSpring India, New Delhi, India

Anurag Taneja SightLife, New Delhi, India

Hugh R. Taylor Melbourne School of Population and Global Health, University of Melbourne, Melbourne, VIC, Australia

Wayne Tennent OneSight, New York, USA

Chundak Tenzing Seva Foundation, Berkeley, CA, USA

Thaksaphon Tharmarangsi International Health Policy Program, Thailand, Bangkok

Tavisha Udupihille Sirimavo Bandaranaike Specialized Children's Hospital, Peradeniya, Central Province, Sri Lanka

Murugesan Vanathi RP Center, New Delhi, India

Sara Varughese CBM India, New Delhi, India

Praveen Vashist Community Ophthalmology, Dr. Rajendra Prasad Centre for Ophthalmic Sciences, All India Institute of Medical Sciences, New Delhi, India

Lingam Vijaya Smt Jadhavabai Nathmal Singhvee Glaucoma Services, Sankara Nethralaya, Chennai, India

P. Vijayalakshmi Aravind Eye Care System, Madurai, India

Jerry Vincent Department of Optometry, Rangsit University, Bangkok, Thailand

Dyah Ayu Windy South Sulawesi Indonesian Ophthalmologists Association, Makassar, South Sulawesi, Indonesia

Anup Zimba OEU, Hyderabad, India

Part I

The Region

1 The South-East Asia Region and Health Indicators

Taraprasad Das and Patanjali Dev Nayar

Key Points

- The WHO South-East Asia Region (SEAR) consists of 11 countries.
- The combined population of the SEAR is over 25% of the world population.
- Three countries in this region, namely, India (second), Indonesia (fourth), and Bangladesh (eighth), are among the ten most populous countries of the world
- In this region:
  - Urban population is highest in the Democratic People's Republic of Korea (61.9%)
  - Poverty is highest in Timor-Leste (30.3%)
  - Human Development Index is highest in Sri Lanka (0.78)
  - Gender Inequality Index is lowest in Thailand (0.377)
  - Access to modern sanitation is highest in the Maldives (96%)
  - Access to essential medicine is highest in Bhutan (95%)
  - The expenditure on health as a percentage of GDP is highest in Maldives (10.6%)
  - Universal Health Coverage is highest in DPR Korea (77 %) in the region
- Incidence of blindness and visual impairment is high in this region (Fig. 1.1)

T. Das (✉)
L V Prasad Eye Institute,
Hyderabad, India
e-mail: tpd@lvpei.org

P. D. Nayar
Regional office for South East Asia
World Health Organization - India,
New Delhi, India
e-mail: nayarp@who.int

The World Health Organization (WHO) South-East Asia Region (SEAR) consists of 11 countries: Bangladesh, Bhutan, Democratic People's Republic of (DPR) Korea, India, Indonesia, Maldives, Myanmar, Nepal, Sri Lanka, Thailand, and Timor-Leste. These 11 countries' population is close to 2001 million; roughly a quarter of the world's population. The Global Burden of Disease (GBD) group places these 11 countries in 3 regions, East Asia (one country), South-East Asia (six countries), and South Asia (four countries) (Table 1.1).

The Vision Loss Expert Group (VLEG) of the GBD has estimated that in 2020, the number of blind people would be roughly 43.2 million (95% UI: 37.5–48.2 million; 55% female); of these, 295.3 (95% UI 267–325.5) million would have moderate to severe visual impairment (MSVI), 257.3 (95% UI 232.2–284.7) million would have mild visual impairment, and 507.4 (95% UI 369.3–663.8) million would have visual impairment from uncorrected presbyopia. Globally, between 2015 and 2020, there was a 1.5% decrease in blindness (14.2–12.7%) and 1.5% increase in MSVI (85.8–87.3%) [1, 2]. However, due to rising population numbers and increasing

T. Das, P. D. Nayar (eds.), *South-East Asia Eye Health*,
https://doi.org/10.1007/978-981-16-3787-2_1

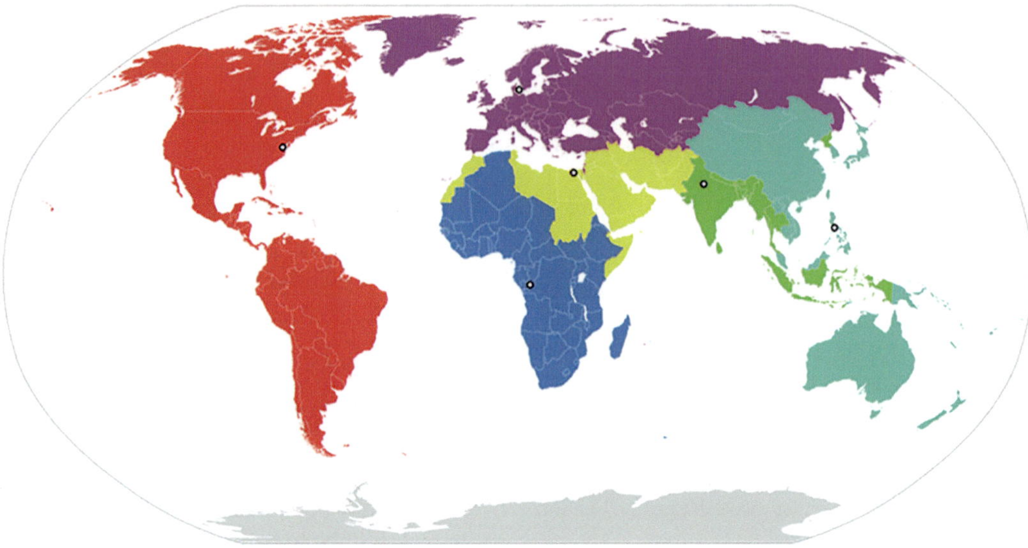

Fig. 1.1 The six WHO Regions. Source: World Health Organization. The World Health Organization (WHO) divides the world into six WHO Regions. These are (1) African Region (AFR), (2) Regions of the Americas (AMR), (3) South-East Asia Region (SEAR), (4) European Region (EUR), (5) Eastern Mediterranean Region (EMR), and (6) Western Pacific Region (WPR)

Table 1.1 Distribution of WHO South-East Asia Region (SEAR) countries within the Global Burden of Disease (GBD) regions

		GBD Countries	
WHO South-East Asia	GBD Region	Region	Country
Bangladesh	South Asia	East Asia 3 Countries	China, DPR Korea, Taiwan
Bhutan	South Asia		
DPR Korea	East Asia	South Asia 5 Countries	Bangladesh, Bhutan, India, Nepal, Pakistan,
India	South Asia		
Indonesia	South-East Asia	South-East Asia 13 Countries	Cambodia, Indonesia, Laos, Malaysia, Maldives, Mauritius, Myanmar, Philippines, Seychelles, Sri Lanka, Thailand, Timor-Leste, Vietnam
Maldives	South-East Asia		
Myanmar	South-East Asia		
Nepal	South Asia		
Sri Lanka	South-East Asia		
Thailand	South-East Asia		
Timor-Leste	South-East Asia		

lifespans, the actual numbers of the blind have increased by 19.4% (36 million to 43 million), and the numbers of people with MSVI have increased by 35.9% (217 million to 295 million). Near vision has been ignored for a long time in the estimation of visual impairment. However, with an increasingly higher number of people living for longer, uncorrected presbyopia is an important cause of vision impairment, and cannot be ignored any longer. The International Classification of Disease, 11th revision (ICD-11), which classifies both distance (9D-90) and near vision (9D-91) (Table 1.2) [3], states that for characterizing binocular vision impairment, vision acuity should be measured with both eyes open with presenting correction if any; for characterizing monocular visual impairment, visual acuity should be measured monocularly with presenting correction if any. The ICD-11 states that near vision refers to performing tasks that require detailed vision at a close distance. It should be measured with both eyes open at the subject's preferred viewing distance and with the subject's habitual near vision correction if any. Near vision impairment is characterized by near visual acuity worse than N6.

Vision loss that also includes near vision impairment is high in the WHO SEAR. The age-standardized prevalence of vision loss is highest in Nepal (27.2%) and lowest in DPR Korea (12.6%) [4]. In general, access to healthcare is relatively lower in rural areas than in urban areas, and poverty often accounts for healthcare affordability. Poverty is defined in two absolute terms by the World Bank: (1) extreme poverty is a condition where a person lives on less than USD1.90 (United States Dollars) per day; and (2) moderate poverty is a condition where a person lives on less than USD3.10 per day [5].

Table 1.2 The International Classification of Diseases 11 (ICD-11) (2018) classification for distance (9D-90) and near vision (9D-91) [3]

Level of vision impairment	Visual acuity scale		
	6 m	20 ft	Decimal
Mild	<6/12 but ≥6/18	<20/40 but ≥20/70	<0.5 but ≥0.3
Moderate	<6/18 but ≥6/60	<20/70 but ≥20/200	<0.3 but ≥0.1
Severe	<6/60 but ≥3/60	<20/200 but ≥20/400	<0.1 but ≥0.05
Blindness	<3/60	<20/400	<0.05
Near vision	Presenting near visual acuity worse than N6 at 40 cm (15 inches) with existing correction		

The WHO SEAR reports suggest that the numbers of people living in an urban area is highest in DPR Korea (61.9%) and lowest in Timor-Leste (30.6%); poverty is highest in Timor-Leste (30.3%) and lowest in the Maldives and Bhutan (1.5% each); the Gross Domestic Product (GDP) is highest in the Maldives, and lowest in Myanmar; health expenditure as a share of GDP is highest in the Maldives (10.6%) and lowest in Bangladesh and Timor-Leste (2.4% each) (Table 1.3) [6].

The United Nations (UN) and the WHO are advocating good health and well-being in the Member States through many World Health Assembly (WHA) and UN General Assembly (UNGA) resolutions. The notable ones connected to eye health in the last two decades are the Millennium Development Goals (MDG, 2000; UNGA 55/2–8 goals) [7], the Global Action Plan (WHA 66.4, 2013; 3 goals) [8], and the Sustainable Development Goals (SDG, 2015; UN GA/Res/70/1–17 goals) [9].

Health indicators are quantifiable characteristics of a population, and continuously monitoring them is required to document the progress of a health program. A good health indicator

Table 1.3 Essential parameters of the WHO South-East Asia Region (SEAR) countries [6]

Country	Population million	Urban Population %	Extreme Poverty %	GDP/ capita USD	Current health expenditure as part of GDP %
Bangladesh	163.04	37.4	1.8	1698.3	2.4
Bhutan	0.76	41.6	1.5	3360.3	2.5
DPR Korea	25.66	61.9	–	–	–
India	1366.41	34.0	21.2	2015.6	3.6
Indonesia	270.62	55.3	5.7	3893.6	3.1
Maldives	0.53	40.2	1.5	10 233.6	10.6
Myanmar	54.04	30.9	6.2	1326.0	5.1
Nepal	28.60	20.2	15.0	1025.8	6.3
Sri Lanka	21.32	18.5	0.8	4102.5	4.2
Thailand	69.62	49.9	0.0	7273.6	3.7
Timor-Leste	1.29	30.6	30.3	3893.6	2.4

should have four important characteristics [10]: (1) it should be easily measured/collected, (2) should have statistical validity, (3) can be measured uniformly across different countries, and (4) analysis of health indicator data should result in a recommendation on which people can make changes to improve health. Table 1.4 lists some of the important indicators that could qualify and quantify eye health in a given population.

A few other indices include the Human Development Index (HDI), the Inequality-adjusted Human Development Index (IHDI), and Gender Inequality Index (GII).

The Human Development Index or HDI is a summary measure of average achievement in three key dimensions of human development—long and healthy life, knowledge, and a decent living standard. The HDI is the geometric mean of normalized indices for each of the three dimensions (Fig. 1.2) [11].

Inequality-adjusted Human Development Index or IHDI [12] combines a country's average achievements in health, education, and income with how those achievements are distributed among the country's population by "discounting" each dimension's average value according to its level of inequality. Thus, the IHDI is a distribution-sensitive average level of human development. The difference between the IHDI and HDI is the human development cost of inequality (Fig. 1.3).

Table 1.4 Indicators used in population health

Domain	Indicator	Definition
Health	Crude death rate	The number of deaths in a particular population, scaled to the size of that population, per unit of time. Expressed in units of death per 1000 individuals per year
	Life expectancy at birth	The average number of years an individual is expected to live by birth year if the current mortality rates continue
	Infant mortality Rate	The number of deaths in children under 1 year of age per 1000 live births
	Maternal mortality rate	The number of maternal deaths per 100,000 live births in the population of a defined geographic area
	Proportional attributable risk	Incidence of a disease in a population that is attributed to exposure to a risk factor
Morbidity	Prevalence	Frequency of existing cases in a defined population at a given point of time
	Incidence	Frequency of new cases in a defined population at a given point of time
Health Status	Low birth weight	Birth weight less than 2499 gm (average: >2500 gm)
	Obesity	Body mass index is >30kg/m^2; a lower value is used in South-East Asia
	Diabetes	Fasting plasma glucose >126 mg/dL or HbA1c >7.0%
	Hypertension	Systolic blood pressure >140 mmHg; Diastolic blood pressure >90 mmHg.
Disability	Disability adjusted life years	The sum of years of potential life lost due to premature mortality and the years of productive life lost due to disability
Health Determinants	Smoking habits	Waiting less than 30 min from the time one wakes up until he/she lights the first cigarette
	Alcohol consumption habits	Volume of alcohol drunk over time; the pattern of drinking from occasional to regular drinking to intoxication; the drinking context if it increases the public health risks; and the quality or contamination of alcoholic beverages

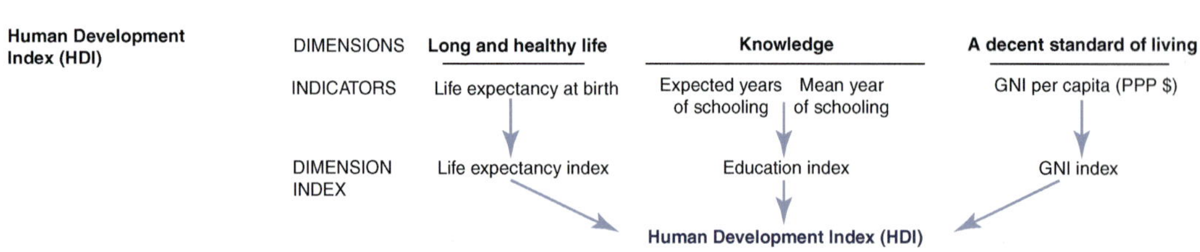

Fig. 1.2 Human development Index (HDI) [11]. *GNI* Gross national income

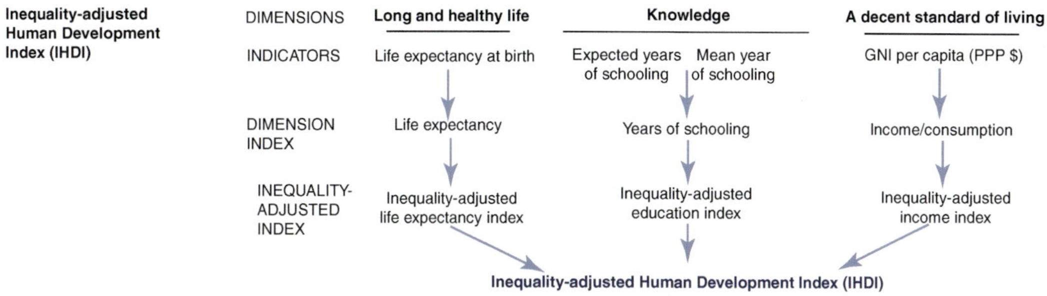

Fig. 1.3 Inequality-adjusted human development index (IHDI) [12]. *GNI* Gross national income

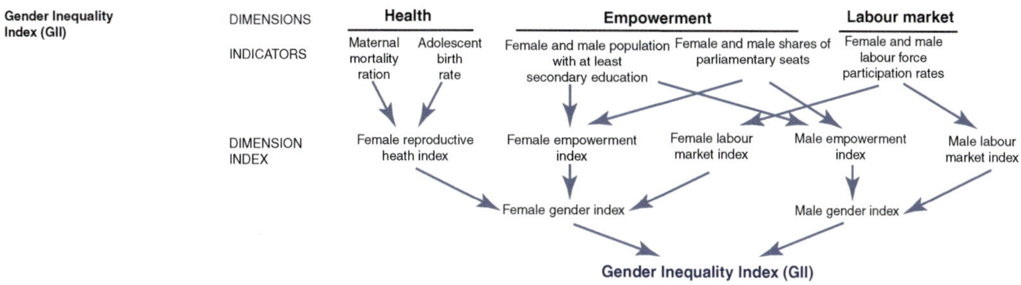

Fig. 1.4 Gender Inequality Index (GII) [14]

The Gender Inequality Index or GII is a composite measure reflecting inequality in achievements between women and men in three dimensions—reproductive health, empowerment, and the labor market (Fig. 1.4) [13, 14]. The GII varies between 0 (when women and men fare equally) and 1 (when men or women fare poorly compared to the other in all dimensions). Low status restricts women's opportunities and freedom, giving them less interaction with others, fewer opportunities for independent behavior, limiting the transmission of new knowledge, and damaging their self-esteem and self-expression [13, 14].

Several organizations such as the UNDP (www.undp.org), the World Bank (www.dataworldbank.org), and the WHO monitor the progress of all indicators globally; the WHO South-East Asia Region Office (WHO SEARO) monitors the progress towards universal health coverage and the SDGs in the South-East Asia region. The Vision Loss Expert Group (VLEG; www.globalvisiondata.org) of the GBD analyses the global, regional, and country-specific vision loss data. The International Agency for the Prevention of Blindness (IAPB; www.iapb.org) compiles eye health-related data from all available sources into the Vision Atlas. We have extracted essential health parameters and eye health data for all countries of the SEAR from these sources. The "total" category in the vision loss data is the sum of the blind, MSVI, mild vision impairment, and near vision loss (Fig. 1.5, Table 1.5; Fig. 1.6, Table 1.6; Fig. 1.7, Table 1.7; Fig. 1.8, Table 1.8; Fig. 1.9, Table 1.9; Fig. 1.10, Table 1.10; Fig. 1.11, Table 1.11; Fig. 1.12, Table 1.12; Fig. 1.13, Table 1.13; Fig. 1.14, Table 1.14; Fig. 1.15, Table 1.15)

Progress must be measured to close the gaps, make course corrections, and monitor progress. The WHO collects and publishes the world health statistics annually. These statistics for 2020 [15] show that the people of the world are getting healthier, with global increases in life expectancy and healthy life expectancy (HALE) of more than 8% between 2000 and 2016. There have also been increased in access to essential health services in the low- and lower middle-income countries (although these are still well below those of the wealthier countries). The UN Economic and

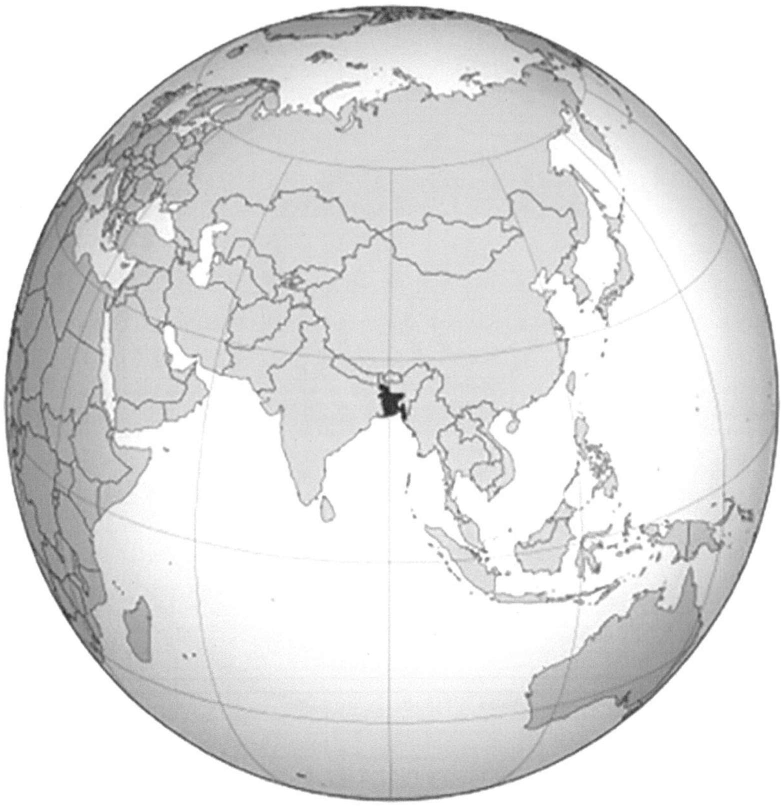

Fig. 1.5 Bangladesh. Source: Wikipedia. Magnitude of vision loss: Total—19.6%; Blind—0.8%; MSVI—5.5%; Mild—3.0%; and Near vision—10.1%

Table 1.5 Vital health-related parameters of Bangladesh

Parameters	Value
Human Development Index	0.614
World ranking	135
Inequality-adjusted Human Development Index	0.465
Gender Inequality Index	0.895
Employment to population ratio, %	57
Access to basic sanitation, %	47
Undiagnosed hypertension (2018), %	54.3
Undiagnosed diabetes (2018), %	70.5
Tobacco non-use, %	65
Health worker density per 10,000	19
Access to essential medicine, %	65
Health security, %	58
Universal Health Coverage Index	54
Impoverishment: People pushed to poverty (USD 1.90 level), %	7
Catastrophic expenditure (>10% of household expense), %	24.7

Social Commission for Asia and the Pacific (ESCAP) reports that the HALEs at 60 for many WHO SEAR countries are between 12 and 16 years (20 years in Japan). It also estimates that the proportion of people 60 and above, from 2016 to 2050, would increase by at least twofold in south and southwest Asia (8.7–19.3%) as well as in South Asia (9.6–21.1%) [16].

However, there is inadequate progress in preventing and controlling non-communicable diseases, with 85% of premature deaths due to non-communicable diseases occurring in low- and lower middle-income countries [15]. The WHO SEARO reports that access to essential health services remains below 60% in four countries (Nepal, Bangladesh, Myanmar, and Timor-Leste); universal health coverage is below 60% in three countries (Nepal, Myanmar,

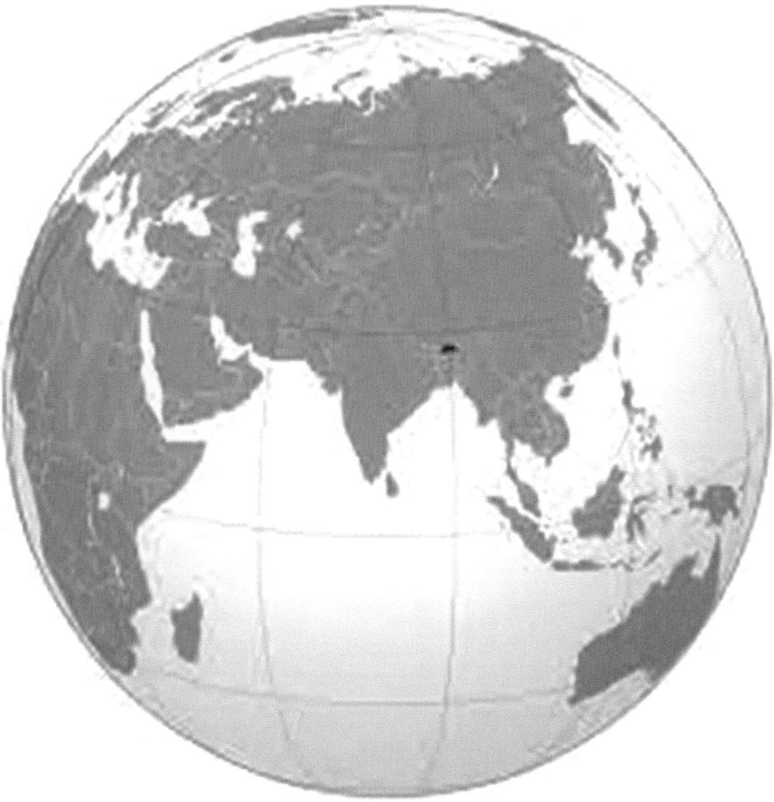

Fig. 1.6 Bhutan. Source: Wikipedia. Magnitude of vision loss: Total—17.0%; Blind—0.4%; MSVI—3.0%; Mild—3.3%; and Near vision—10.3%

Table 1.6 Vital health-related parameters of Bhutan

Parameters	Value
Human Development Index	0.617
World ranking	134
Inequality-adjusted Human Development Index	0.450
Gender Inequality Index	0.436
Employment to population ratio, %	65
Access to basic sanitation, %	63
Undiagnosed hypertension (2014), %	65.7
Undiagnosed diabetes (2014), %	85.8
Tobacco non-use, %	75
Health worker density per 10,000	44
Access to essential medicine, %	95
Health security, %	53
Universal Health Coverage Index	73
Impoverishment: People pushed to poverty (USD 1.90 level), %	0.6
Catastrophic expenditure (>10% of household expense), %	1.8

and Timor-Leste); and there is a large segment of undiagnosed hypertension (lowest: Thailand (44.7%); highest: Timor-Leste (93.5%)) and undiagnosed diabetes (lowest: Thailand (43.1%); highest: Timor-Leste (94.6%)) [6]. Hence, the WHO calls for acceleration of all programs and processes to achieve the SDGs by the year 2030.

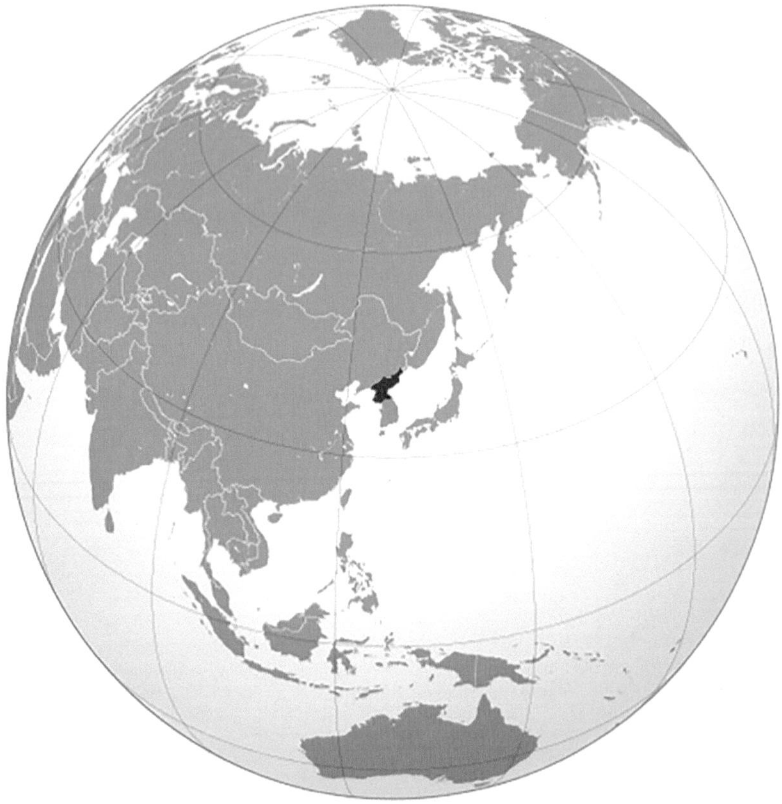

Fig. 1.7 DPR Korea. Source: Wikipedia. Magnitude of vision loss: Total—12.6%; Blind—0.1%; MSVI—1.8%; Mild—2.9%; and Near vision—7.8%

Table 1.7 Vital health-related parameters of DPR Korea

Parameters	Value
Human Development Index	–
World ranking	–
Inequality-adjusted HDI	–
Gender Inequality Index	–
Employment to population ratio, %	78
Access to basic sanitation, %	77
Undiagnosed hypertension, %	–
Undiagnosed diabetes, %	–
Tobacco non-use, %	80
Health worker density per 10,000	100
Access to essential medicine, %	–
Health security, %	63
Universal Health Coverage Index	77
Impoverishment: People pushed to poverty (US$ 1.90 level), %	–
Catastrophic expenditure (> 10% of household expense), %	–

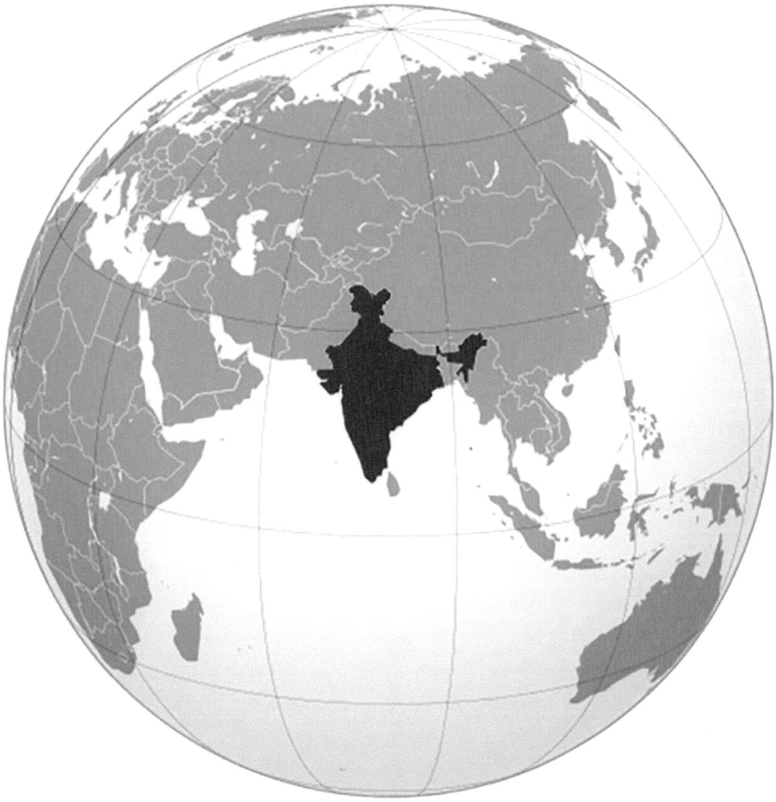

Fig. 1.8 India. Source: Wikipedia. Magnitude of vision loss: Total—22.8%; Blind—0.9%; MSVI—6.6%; Mild—4.0%; Near vision—11.3%

Table 1.8 Vital health-related parameters of India.

Parameters	Value
Human Development Index	0.647
World ranking	129
Inequality-adjusted HDI	0.477
Gender Inequality Index	0.501
Employment to population ratio, %	47
Access to basic sanitation, %	44
Undiagnosed hypertension (2017-18), %	72.3
Undiagnosed diabetes (2017-18), %	45.2
Tobacco non-use, %	71
Health worker density per 10,000	64
Access to essential medicine, %	–
Health security, %	75
Universal Health Coverage Index	61
Impoverishment: People pushed to poverty (USD 1.90 level), %	–
Catastrophic expenditure (>10% of household expense), %	–

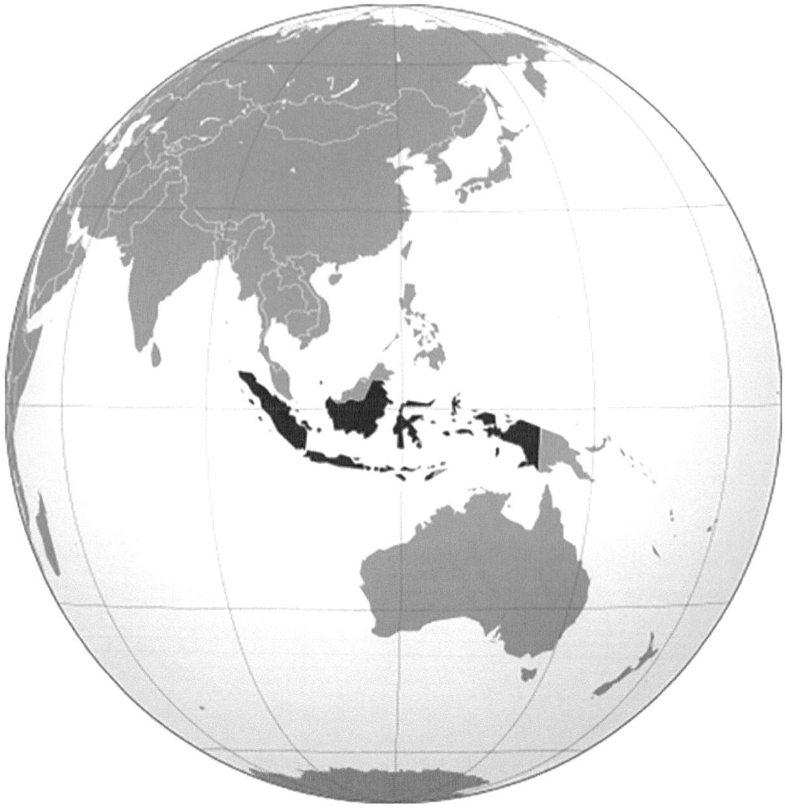

Fig. 1.9 Indonesia. Source: Wikipedia. Magnitude of vision loss: Total—15.4%; Blind—1.7%; MSVI—4.8%; Mild—4.8%; Near vision—4.1%

Table 1.9 Vital health-related parameters of Indonesia

Parameters	Value
Human Development Index	0.707
World ranking	111
Inequality-adjusted HDI	0.584
Gender Inequality Index	0.451
Employment to population ratio, %	64
Access to basic sanitation, %	68
Undiagnosed hypertension, %	–
Undiagnosed diabetes, %	–
Tobacco non-use, %	64
Health worker density per 10,000	55
Access to essential medicine, %	–
Health security, %	63
Universal Health Coverage Index	65
Impoverishment: People pushed to poverty (USD 1.90 level), %	0.2
Catastrophic expenditure (>10% of household expense), %	2.7

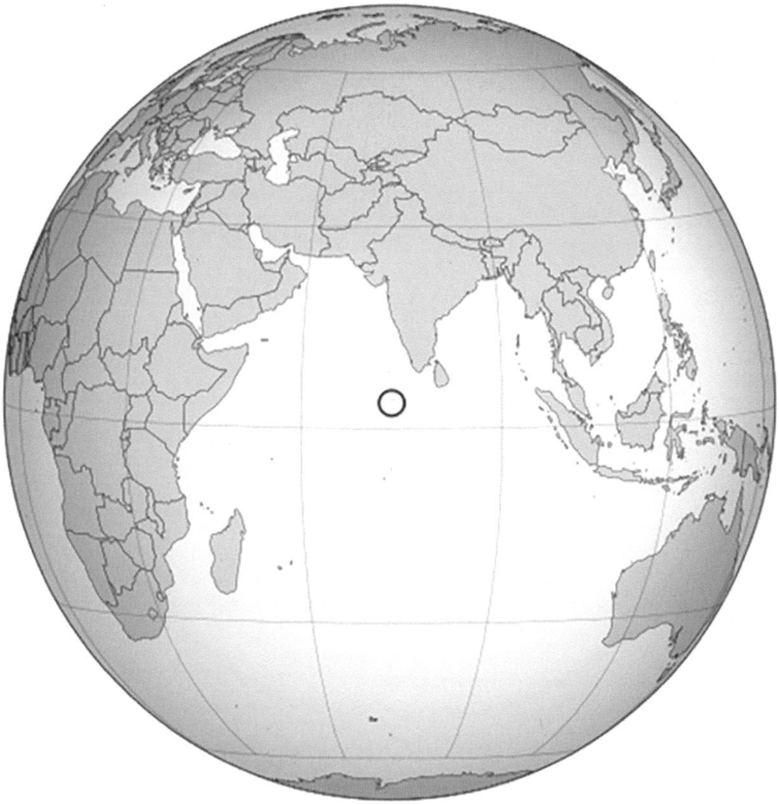

Fig. 1.10 Maldives. Source: Wikipedia. The magnitude of vision loss: Total—14.6%; Blind—0.4%; MSVI—4.0%; Mild—4.8%; and Near vision—5.4%

Table 1.10 Vital health-related parameters of the Maldives

Parameters	Value
Human Development Index	0.719
World ranking	104
Inequality-adjusted HDI	0.568
Gender Inequality Index	0.367
Employment to population ratio, %	66
Access to basic sanitation, %	96
Undiagnosed hypertension (2011), %	66.5
Undiagnosed diabetes (2011), %	50.0
Tobacco non-use, %	80
Health worker density per 10,000	100
Access to essential medicine, %	–
Health security, %	44
Universal Health Coverage Index	68
Impoverishment: People pushed to poverty (USD 1.90 level), %	0
Catastrophic expenditure (>10% of household expense), %	10.3

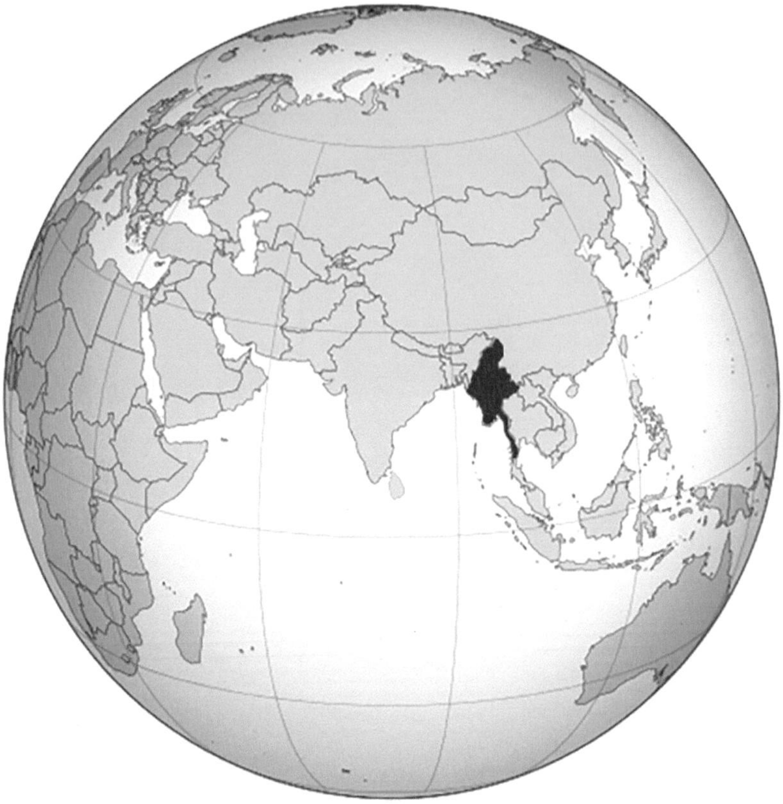

Fig. 1.11 Myanmar. Source: Wikipedia. Magnitude of vision loss: Total—16.6%; Blind—1.1%; MSVI—4.9%; Mild—4.9%; Near vision—5.7%

Table 1.11 Vital health-related parameters of Myanmar

Parameters	Value
Human Development Index	0.584
World ranking	145
Inequality-adjusted HDI	0.448
Gender Inequality Index	0.458
Employment to population ratio, %	60
Access to basic sanitation, %	65
Undiagnosed hypertension (2014), %	52.4
Undiagnosed diabetes (2014), %	68.1
Tobacco non-use, %	46
Health worker density per 10,000	40
Access to essential medicine, %	43
Health security, %	66
Universal Health Coverage Index	54
Impoverishment: People pushed to poverty (USD 1.90 level), %	0.6
Catastrophic expenditure (>10% of household expense), %	14.4

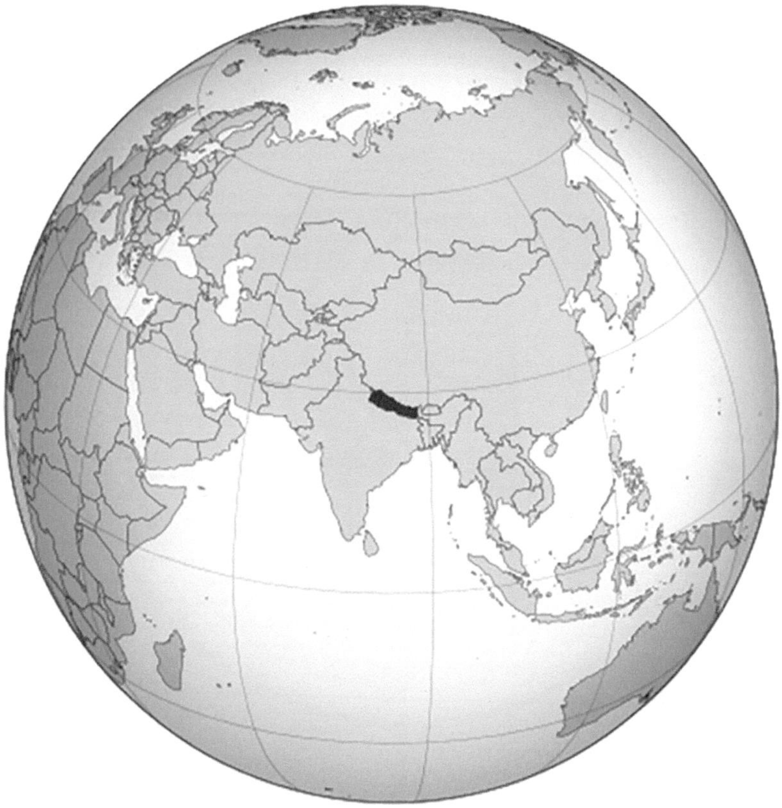

Fig. 1.12 Nepal. Source: Wikipedia. Magnitude of vision loss: Total—27.5%; Blind—0.5%; MSVI—5.4%; Mild—2.8%; Near vision—18.8%

Table 1.12 Vital health-related parameters of Nepal

Parameters	Value
Human Development Index	0.579
World ranking	147
Inequality-adjusted HDI	0.430
Gender Inequality Index	0.476
Employment to population ratio, %	83
Access to basic sanitation, %	46
Undiagnosed hypertension (2013), %	79.8
Undiagnosed diabetes (2013), %	75.5
Tobacco non-use, %	69
Health worker density per 10,000	75
Access to essential medicine, %	72
Health security, %	23
Universal Health Coverage Index	59
Impoverishment: People pushed to poverty (USD 1.90 level), %	1.7
Catastrophic expenditure (>10% of household expense), %	10.7

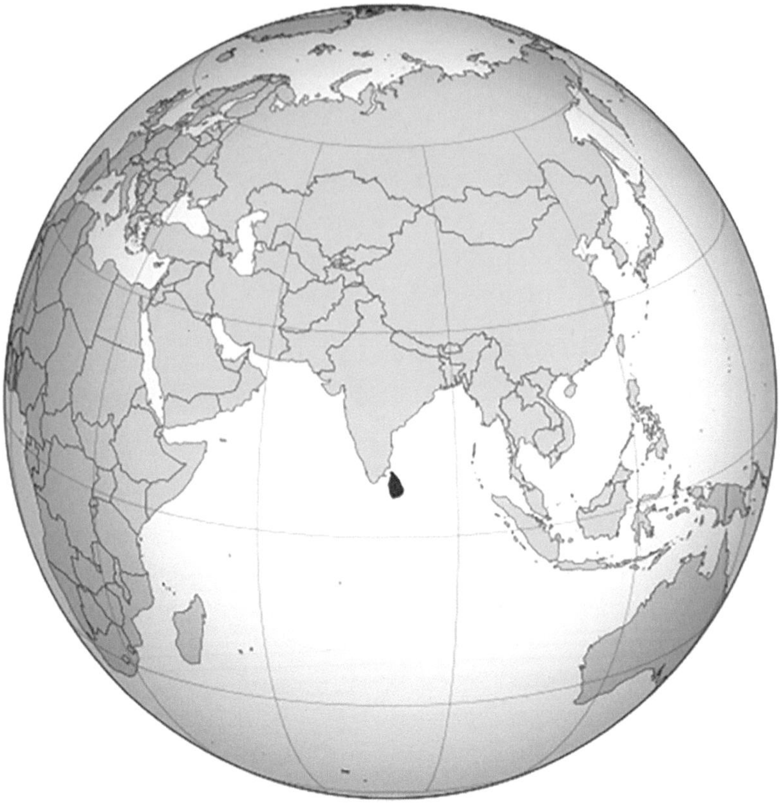

Fig. 1.13 Sri Lanka. Source: Wikipedia. Magnitude of vision loss: Total—15.4%; Blind—0.4%; MSVI—5.2%; Mild—4.6%; Near vision—5.2%

Table 1.13 Vital health-related parameters of Sri Lanka

Parameters	Value
Human Development Index	0.780
World ranking	71
Inequality-adjusted HDI	0.686
Gender Inequality Index	0.380
Employment to population ratio, %	51
Access to basic sanitation, %	94
Undiagnosed hypertension (2015), %	62.1
Undiagnosed diabetes (2015), %	42.9
Tobacco non-use, %	74
Health worker density per 10,000	71
Access to essential medicine, %	75
Health security, %	46
Universal Health Coverage Index	66
Impoverishment: People pushed to poverty (USD 1.90 level), %	0.7
Catastrophic expenditure (>10% of household expense), %	5.4

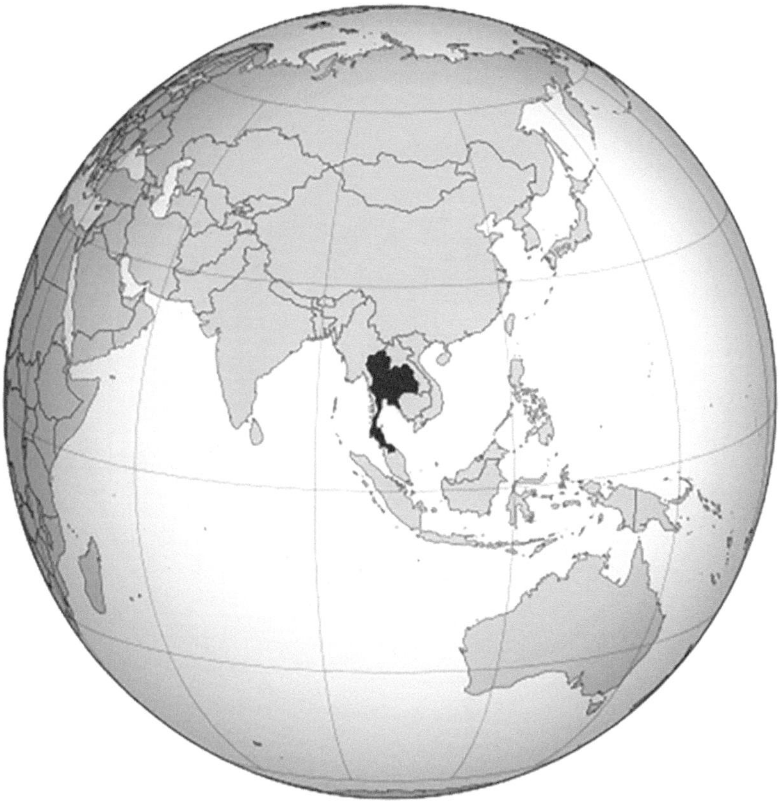

Fig. 1.14 Thailand. Source: Wikipedia. Magnitude of vision loss: Total—15.2%; Blind—0.4%; MSVI—5.0%; Mild—4.6%; Near vision—5.2%

Table 1.14 Vital health-related parameters of Thailand

Parameters	Value
Human Development Index	0.765
World ranking	77
Inequality-adjusted HDI	0.635
Gender Inequality Index	0.377
Employment to population ratio, %	66
Access to basic sanitation, %	95
Undiagnosed hypertension (2014), %	44.7
Undiagnosed diabetes (2014), %	43.1
Tobacco non-use, %	73
Health worker density per 10,000	86
Access to essential medicine, %	–
Health security, %	79
Universal Health Coverage Index	85
Impoverishment: People pushed to poverty (USD 1.90 level), %	0
Catastrophic expenditure (>10% of household expense), %	2.2

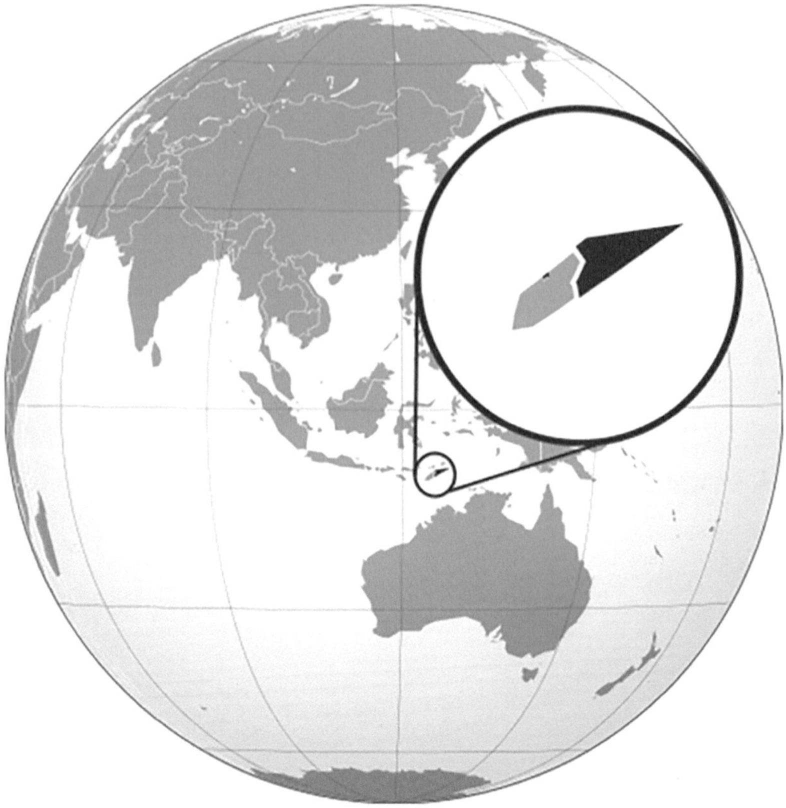

Fig. 1.15 Timor-Leste. Source: Wikipedia. Magnitude of vision loss: Total—17.5%; Blind—1.2%; MSVI—5.5%; Mild—5.0%; Near vision—5.8%

Table 1.15 Vital health-related parameters of Timor-Leste

Parameters	Value
Human Development Index	0.626
World ranking	131
Inequality-adjusted HDI	0.450
Gender Inequality Index	–
Employment to population ratio, %	64
Access to basic sanitation, %	0
Undiagnosed hypertension (2014), %	93.5
Undiagnosed diabetes (2014), %	94.6
Tobacco non-use, %	44
Health worker density per 10,000	56
Access to essential medicine, %	–
Health security, %	44
Universal Health Coverage Index	50
Impoverishment: People pushed to poverty (USD 1.90 level), %	1.0
Catastrophic expenditure (>10% of household expense), %	2.9

References

1. Bourne RRA, Flaxman SR, Braithwaite T, et al. Magnitude, temporal trends, and projections of the global prevalence of blindness and distance and near vision impairment: a systematic review and meta-analysis. Lancet Glob Health. 2017;5(9):e888–e97.
2. Bourne RRA, Jaimie J, Seth F, et al. Trends in prevalence of blindness and distance and near vision impairment over 30 years and contribution to the Global Burden of disease in 2020. Lancet Global Health. 2020. Advanced online publication; https://doi.org/10.2139/ssrn.3582742.
3. International classification of disease, 111th Revision. www.who.int. Accessed 14 Oct 2020.
4. Vision atlas 2020. www.iapb.org. Accessed 15 Oct 2020.
5. Poverty. www.worldbank.org. Accessed 16 Oct 2020.
6. Monitoring progress on universal health coverage and the health-related Sustainable Development Goals in the WHO South-East Asia Region: 2019 update. New Delhi: World Health Organization, Regional Office for South-East Asia; 2019.
7. UN millennium declaration. www.un.org. Accessed 16 Oct 2020.
8. Universal Eye health: a global action plan, 2014–2019. www.who.int. Accessed 15 Oct 2020.
9. Sustainable Development. www.un.org. Accessed 16 Oct 2020.
10. Larsen C, Mercer A. Global indicators: an overview. Canadian Medical Association J. 2004;171:1199–200. https://doi.org/10.1503/cmaj.1021409.
11. Human development index. www.hdr.undp.org. Accessed 14 Oct 2020.
12. Inequality-adjusted human development index. www.hdr.undp.org > content > inequality adjusted human development index. Accessed 13 Oct 2020.
13. Gender Inequality Index. www.who.int. Accessed 13 Oct 2020.
14. Gender Inequality Index. www.hdr.undp.org. Accessed 13 Oct 2020.
15. World Statistics 2020. Monitoring health for the SDGs. World Health Organization. 2000.
16. Ageing in Asia and Pacific. www.unescap.org. Accessed 17 Oct 2020.

Part II

The Health System

2 Health Management and Information: Key Principles and Enablers in Eye Health Program

Thulasiraj Ravilla, Sashipriya Karumanchi, and Taraprasad Das

Key Points

- Good health services are those, which deliver *effective, safe, quality, and personal and non-personal* health interventions to those that need them, when and where needed, with minimum waste of resources.
- A well-performing *health workforce* is one that works in ways that are responsive, fair, and effective in achieving the best health outcomes possible, given available resources and circumstances.
- A well-functioning *health information system* is one that ensures the production, analysis, dissemination, and use of reliable and timely information on health determinants, health system performance, and health status.
- A well-functioning supply-chain ensures *equitable access to essential medical products, devices, and technologies* that are of proven scientific benefit, assured quality, safety, and efficacy, and cost-effective.
- A good health financing system would ensure that people receive required healthcare services and will be protected from financial catastrophe or impoverishment associated with having to pay for such services. Such a system should also equally provide incentives for healthcare providers.
- *Leadership and governance* involve ensuring and enabling that strategic and policy frameworks exist for effective healthcare provision, and that these are combined with effective oversight, coalition-building, regulation, attention to system design, and accountability.

The World Health Organization (WHO) defines health as "a state of complete physical, mental and social well-being and not merely the absence of disease or infirmity," in its constitution (1946, adapted in 1948). It further states that good health is one of the "fundamental rights of every human being without distinction of race, religion, political belief, economic, or social condition" [1]. Despite these broad agreements, health outcomes are unacceptably low across much of the developing world, and the persistence of deep inequities in health status is a problem even within countries.

Health systems have multiple goals. The World Health Report 2000 defined overall health system goals as "improving health and health equity, in ways that are responsive, financially fair, and make the best, or most efficient, use of available resources."

The health system includes all the activities whose primary purpose is to promote, restore,

T. Ravilla (✉) · S. Karumanchi
Lions Aravind Institute of Community Ophthalmology, Aravind Eye Care System, Madurai, Tamil Nadu, India
e-mail: thulsi@aravind.org; sashi@aravind.org

T. Das
L V Prasad Eye Institute, Hyderabad, India
e-mail: tpd@lvpei.org

T. Das, P. D. Nayar (eds.), *South-East Asia Eye Health*,
https://doi.org/10.1007/978-981-16-3787-2_2

or maintain health [2]. The objective of a health system, however, extends beyond improving health—to instilling "goodness" and "fairness" in health [2]. *Goodness* in the health system is the "best attainable average level." *Fairness* in the health system is the "smallest feasible difference" among individuals and groups. Three fundamental objectives of a good health system are (1) improving the health of the population they serve, (2) responding to people's expectations, and (3) providing financial protection against the costs of ill-health. Generally, the government is ultimately answerable for a country's health system. However, the participation of private services and private financing is crucial for the overall effectiveness and sustainability of any health system. A continuous and systematic monitoring mechanism must be in place to ensure that all activities, including regulations and advocacy, are aligned with the stated goals of the community and the country. In a quest for greater efficiency, fairness, and people's expectations, three important health reforms in the past century have been brought about in different timeframes.

The first health reform (1940s–1950s) was the introduction of the national healthcare system and the social insurance system. However, in a couple of decades, this system was under stress because of rising costs as the volume and intensity of hospital-based care increased. In addition, this system could not reach economically underprivileged people. Ultimately, too many people continued to depend on their personal resources to pay for health and often received only ineffective or poor-quality care.

The second health reform (1970s–1980s) was the promotion of primary healthcare and universal coverage. There was an increasing commitment to assuring a minimum level of care for all health services, food and education, safe water, and basic sanitation. In 1978 the WHO/UNICEF adopted primary healthcare as the basis of the health system, "Health for All," at the 1978 International Conference on Primary Health (Alma-Ata Declaration). However, this system did not succeed because it was often provided by untrained personnel and was often delivered to the poor and marginalized community only. In many instances, the quality was too poor, and "primary" care became "primitive" care because the referral system, so vital for the success of this system, failed.

In general, the first two reforms were "supply" rather than "demand" oriented. The third reform in the late 1990s/early 2000s was the "new universalism" where high quality essential care, defined mostly by the criterion of cost-effectiveness, is delivered to everyone instead of all possible care for the whole population or only the simplest and most basic care for the poor. The health sector reforms now aim to reduce inequities in health, create conditions that promote health and self-reliance, and ensure basic health services to all while upholding and enforcing health ethics.

Effective eye care programs result from comprehensive planning using the right paradigm by having an inclusive design and flawless execution. Achieving this is a journey, and as with any journey, the paths and directions are determined by the destination. Thus, it becomes important to have clarity on the destination, and this has to be subscribed to and owned by all stakeholders. This chapter describes the key principles and enablers for an effective eye health program from a macro-level management perspective. Though presented at a macro level, it is equally applicable to national as well as institutional or hospital levels. It covers the broad areas of planning, advocacy, and creating an enabling environment using the WHO's health systems framework of six building blocks (Fig. 2.1).

The evidence presented in this chapter is either from published sources or collected and verified from those who have access to such information. This chapter is intended to guide or design a program for implementation at the hospital, regional, or national levels. This chapter is organized into two sections: (1) the first section is on the importance of developing a paradigm for effective planning and design of services and (2) the second section is on the implementation strategies to execute the developed plans.

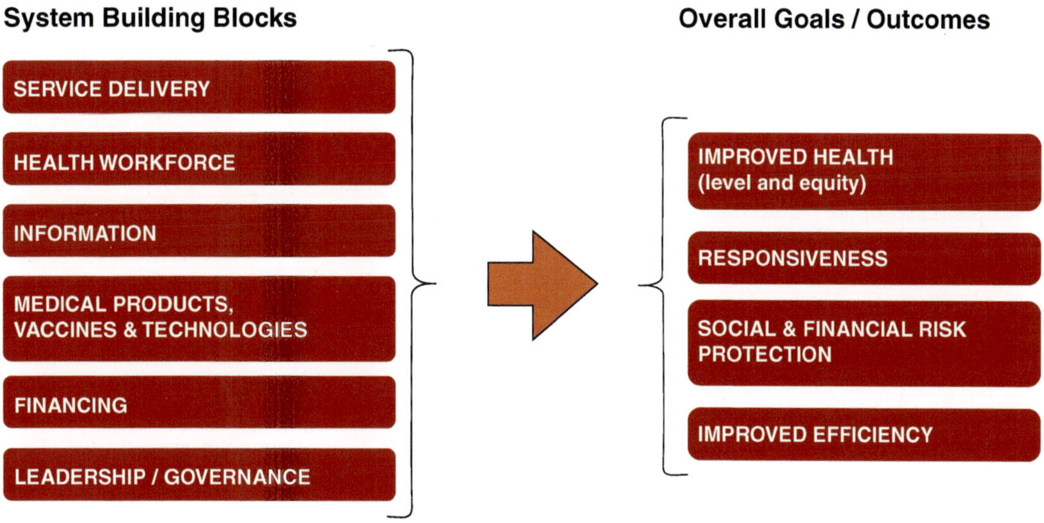

Fig. 2.1 Health system building blocks. Source: World Health Organization

2.1 Program Design to Address the Community's Eye Care Needs

2.1.1 Approach to Planning and Resource Allocation for Eye Care Delivery

Historically, eye care delivery did not enjoy a priority within the healthcare system in most countries and was often neglected. The joint launch of VISION 2020 "Right to Sight" by the WHO and International Agency for the Prevention of Blindness (IAPB) propelled several countries to develop or renew their focus on eye care, leading to the development of national plans. Several eye care-related resolutions adopted in the annual WHO's World Health Assembly meetings helped to focus on eye care at a national level and accelerate its development. Due to internal advocacy efforts, India was a forerunner in these efforts by (1) establishing a National Program for Control of Blindness as early as 1976 and (2) conducting a national survey to confirm the magnitude and causes of blindness that led to the development of a national plan. Most South-East Asia Region countries now have some form of a national plan that spells out goals, strategic directions, targets, and partnerships with different stakeholders to enhance eye care delivery.

Though all national planners would want to eliminate avoidable blindness, their plans and design of services do not necessarily reflect this aspiration.

Possible Versus Needed Most leaders and planners from national to institutional levels tend to be overly influenced by two factors while planning future eye care to eliminate avoidable blindness. These are (a) current resources and other factors that result in the current performance and (b) the desire to "succeed" in the public eye or from an accountability perspective. While these are compelling realities, they also limit the program to a short-term benefit and ignore long-term achievement. This self-imposed short-term goal-setting approach often becomes an impediment to developing the required visionary approach to planning. For example, consider a situation where the country has to perform at least 5000 cataract surgeries per million population in a year (defined as the cataract surgical rate or CSR), but is currently only performing 500. If a suggestion is made that the planners aim for a CSR of 5000, the immediate reaction would be, "that is impossible, we can never achieve that, we don't have the required human and other resources," and so on. So, they would end up setting their CSR goal as 600 or 1000, depending on their confidence in achieving such a goal. One can recognize that this is the result of the paradigm of limiting aspirations to what they think is practically possible, and potentially, fear of a failure. One can also realize that with this approach, the country will never build up capacity, resources, and determination to achieve the required goal, nor have in place enabling policies and processes to rid the country of blindness due to cataract. This applies to all eye care conditions.

Thus, the first step in the planning process is to determine the desired annual service levels (number of cataract surgeries, refractive error corrections, glaucoma or diabetic retinopathy management, etc.) to eliminate avoidable blindness. This should reflect the community's holistic eye care needs and not be limited by current resources, constraints, and policies. The next process would be one of determining what additional resources are required on all fronts—human resources, physical infrastructure, equipment, consumables, and finances. Clarity of the current situation and the aspirational destination is what will help create a comprehensive roadmap. This roadmap should include appropriate strategies, policies, timeframes, and resources required as well as processes to be followed. It must also be recognized that eye care services to eliminate avoidable blindness are not a one-time effort like smallpox or polio eradication, but one of building a robust, sustainable service delivery mechanism that will grow over time to meet increasing needs. There is a need to articulate targets for eliminating avoidable blindness in almost all countries in the South-East Asia region; in addition, there is also a need to carry out gap analyses against their current performance.

Table 2.1 provides some details of the estimated annual eye care needs for each country in the South-East Asia Region. The numbers mentioned are only indicative of the potential annual need. While these numbers may be debatable or need revision, what is essential to understand is the approach to estimating the yearly need. This assumes achieving universal eye care coverage as the ultimate goal.

Cataract Cataract occurs largely in the elderly. Hence the numbers are primarily driven by the population 50 years and older. But to eliminate blindness due to cataract, waiting till the person's vision reduces to less than 3/60 (blindness) is not advisable, interventions must begin much earlier. While "*when to intervene*" depends on an individual's visual needs, a threshold of vision < 6/12 is contemplated as the denominator for planning interventions for treating cataracts [3]. A few states in India have been posting an annual CSR of around 9000/million population for several years; as a result, blindness due to cataract has been steadily declining in these states. The desired CSR levels proposed in Table 2.1 are a combination of this benchmark and the revised threshold for cataract surgery.

Refractive Error The scale or need for treating refractive errors is driven by the need for presbyopic correction, which is required for almost all people 45 years or older (the proportion of this age group in the South-East Asia Region ranges from 17 to 39% of the general population) [4]. Some younger adults would also benefit from refractive error correction. While this combined percentage of those with refractive errors could vary from 25 to 40% across countries, the need to change glasses could occur once every 2–4 years. Factoring in all these requirements, it is subjectively estimated that 6–13% of the total population would need refractive services annually.

Glaucoma Several studies have indicated that roughly 1% of the population is estimated to be affected by glaucoma [5]. Since this is considered a "silent" disease, case detection would require different strategies and hence must be understood while planning. All persons likely to develop glaucoma would require at least one annual eye examination.

Diabetic Retinopathy All diabetic patients face the risk of developing retinopathy, and therefore,

Table 2.1 Estimated annual eye care needs in the South-East Asia Region

					% population and number of persons in need of specific eye care needs									
			CSR		Refractive errors		Glaucoma		Diabetes		Pediatric eye care		Low vision and Blind	
Countries	Population in Millions[a]	% 50+ years[a]	Desired	Current[b]	%	Numbers	%	Numbers	%[c]	Numbers	%	Numbers	%	Numbers
Bangladesh	161.1	18.7	9000	2625	8	13,153,471	1	1,610,629	5.9	9,483,384	4	1,733,037	0.2	322,126
Bhutan	0.8	17.0	7000	2107	7	57,564	1	7744	6.6	51,049	4	7682	0.2	1549
India	1311.6	19.6	9000	5050	9	112,794,092	1	13,115,592	6.7	7,297,381	4	14,007,452	0.2	2,623,118
Indonesia	267.0	22.5	9000	1410	10	25,634,531	1	2,670,264	4.0	10,766,503	4	2,595,496	0.2	534,053
Maldives	0.4	15.8	7000	1440	7	27,695	1	3919	5.9	23,075	4	3433	0.2	784
Myanmar	56.6	19.9	9000	1970	9	4,810,156	1	565,901	2.5	1,412,488	4	595,328	0.2	113,180
Nepal	30.3	16.5	7500	4360	7	2,153,279	1	303,279	4.6	1,397,509	4	350,590	0.2	60,656
Sri Lanka	22.9	26.9	9000	5380	11	2,502,553	1	228,892	6.8	1,567,452	4	214,243	0.2	45,778
Thailand	69.0	31.6	9000	3100	13	9,059,032	1	689,774	4.5	3,090,188	4	458,010	0.2	137,955
Timor-Leste	1.4	12.5	5000	780	6	76,566	1	13,837	4.3	59,334	4	22,140	0.2	2767

[a]Population data from https://www.census.gov/data-tools/demo/idb/informationGateway.php
[b]Current CSR for the countries, Bhutan, Indonesia, Maldives, Myanmar, Sri Lanka, Thailand, and Timor-Leste is from the IAPB Atlas, http://atlas.iapb.org/global-action-plan/gap-implementation/;
[c]Data from https://www.diabetesatlas.org/upload/resources/material/20200302_133351_IDFATLAS9e-final-web.pdf, page 150
CSR cataract surgical rate

all people with diabetes will need at least one annual examination. (www.diabetesatlas.org).

Pediatric Eye Care According to population-based studies, roughly (as a rule of thumb) 4% of all children in the age group 0–14 years in South-East Asian countries are likely required an annual eye examination for refractive errors or other conditions. The population proportion of children varies between 17% and 28% (except in Timor-Leste, where this number is estimated to be 40%) [4].

Low Vision and Blindness Roughly 1 in every 1000 person is estimated to be incurably blind; this is similar to the numbers of people with low vision problems that are incurable. Such people need appropriate rehabilitation services depending on their age; their individual needs—academic pursuit, employment, and daily living activities—must be addressed. There are emerging technologies that offer steadily increasing options for such individuals to lead a more normal life.

Backlog Is Not the Target or Workload Currently, most planning exercises are almost always built on data obtained from population-based prevalence studies, such as the RAAB (Rapid Assessment of Avoidable Blindness), which gives a cross-sectional estimate of blindness/visual impairment and their main causes. Typically, these surveys estimate the backlog or "what was not done." When repeated over time, such population surveys are useful in measuring changes or impacts of intervention programs. If several of these surveys are done in different parts of a country, their results could indicate variations in the magnitude of the problem across geographies. However, these surveys are not very useful in estimating the annual healthcare/eye care workload for a country or region. The backlog or magnitude of blindness and visual impairment is the proverbial tip of the iceberg, and it grossly underestimates the quantum of work required to eliminate avoidable blindness or vision impairment. For every person who falls into this category and gets measured as a statistic, several others are visually affected, but do not fall under this definition yet. This situation can be explained with the following example:

If a tap is open and there is a lot of water wasted, rather than employing all one's energy in draining the wastewater, every effort should be made to close the tap, which is the root cause of the problem. Similarly, not intervening early and at the right time are the main reasons why people with avoidable conditions become blind or visually impaired. Therefore, it is not only imperative that the blind and visually impaired be treated, but also equally imperative that strategies be put in place to prevent others from being similarly affected.

In recent times, several surveys have been done to estimate the magnitude of various ocular morbidities regardless of their severity; these include refractive errors to macular degeneration. However, even these surveys cannot gain insights into transient conditions like conjunctivitis, presence of a foreign body in the eye, minor trauma, etc., which also need ophthalmic attention. Thus, the current surveys, which are all cross-sectional by design, tend to underestimate the real workloads in eye care. Some conditions such as cataracts or the presence of a foreign body in the eye require one-time interventions. In contrast, many other conditions require periodic interventions, with the frequencies for these ranging from a few times a year to once in 2 or 3 years. Such an ongoing need for intervention applies to refractive errors too, which affect almost 25% of the global population [6]. This is further complicated by the health-seeking behavior of the community, with some seeking early intervention because of their functional needs and quality of life, while others do not seek care, even when the condition progresses to extremely poor vision. There are also conditions like glaucoma or diabetic retinopathy that does not cause any noticeable vision loss until the condition reaches a fairly advanced stage.

The *default caregiving* mode at most levels is reactive, that is, to provide care to those seeking it. This reactive mode of functioning, while necessary from a treatment perspective, does not contribute much to the prevention of blindness or

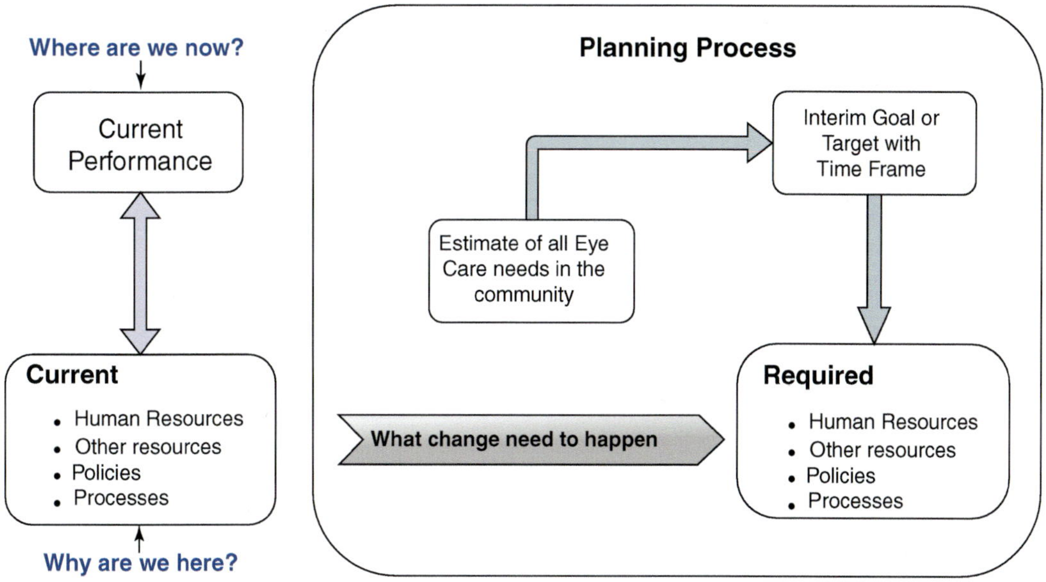

Fig. 2.2 Theory of change

visual impairment in people other than those who seek care. It is the *proactive mode* of reaching out to everyone that can reduce avoidable blindness. These requirements add on to the workload for eye care, which cannot be estimated by cross-sectional estimates of blindness and visual impairment.

Holistic Planning Process In order to tackle both the issues described above (that planning is driven by need, and that determining the actual workload is difficult) require a paradigm shift in thinking. This paradigm shift, in principle, will be applicable for both national- and institution-level planning. A good planning process must start by asking, "*where are we now?*" as well as "*why are we here?*" in order to identify an ultimate goal. This process must also clearly visualize the levels of service needed to reach the ultimate goal (which in this case is to truly eliminate avoidable blindness) without being constrained by thoughts of current resources and other realities. This assessment of holistic needs should then consider the current realities in order to set interim targets that should challenge the current status. In turn, this interim goal should dictate the resources required to reach the ultimate goal and the policies and processes that must change to achieve this. A good plan should also incorporate the "theory of change" (Fig. 2.2).

2.1.2 Advocacy

At a higher level, advocacy is a process of creating alignment among all stakeholders towards an ultimate purpose and interim goals. Such alignment has to happen internally among all those responsible for implementation, and externally with those who can create the enabling eco-system and address the resource requirements. Often, advocacy is aimed at the external cohort of senior bureaucrats, political leaders, and policymakers. This group can influence policies, but putting them to best use, enabling optimum productivity with good quality, is the direct responsibility of the implementing stakeholders. Similarly, the quantum of funding or budgetary allocation is often in the hands of the external stakeholders, but the policies and processes to put it to best use are in the hands of the implementers. Thus, advocacy is essentially centered around the question "*what changes need to happen?*" which requires the alignment of both external and internal stakeholders of eye care. Thus, a holistic plan is a foundation for mounting effective advocacy initiatives.

Case Study 1 The Nepal Blindness Survey and Nepal Netra Jyoti Sangh (Fig. 2.3)

Nepal then (in the 1970s)

Nepal had rudimentary eye care services primarily offered at Bir Hospital (government-run) that had not even had basic equipment like slit lamps and had a long waiting times for cataract surgeries. About 500 cataract surgeries were performed in a year. People with the means to do so traveled to India for their eye care needs. Eye care services started getting attention after Dr. Ram Prasad Pokharel (referred to as Dr. Pokharel henceforth), a young and ambitious ophthalmologist, returned from London. He mobilized local support, including the Ministry of Health (MoH) to set up the Nepal Eye Hospital in Kathmandu, the capital city, in 1974.

The key turning point came in 1978 when Dr. Pokharel attended a WHO meeting on "Curable Blindness" held in Delhi. His concerns and efforts were appreciated by many who participated in the meeting. Dr. Nicole Grasset, who was one amongst them, later played a key role in raising funds and supporting the Nepal eye care program. The "Prevention and Control of Blindness program" was created under the MoH with some financial support from the WHO. With limited eye care services in the country, the team agreed to the Seva Foundation's suggestion to conduct a national survey to assess the burden, causes, and distribution of blindness in the country as a first step towards planning eye care services for Nepal. The national survey was conducted in 1981, the first of its kind (in eye care) anywhere in the world, with technical support from the Seva Foundation and funding support from the Danish government through the WHO. The survey estimated the prevalence of blindness at 0.84%, with 72% of blindness due to cataract, followed by trachoma in the mid-west and far-west regions, and xerophthalmia in specific communities.

Dr. Pokharel convinced the MoH and several international agencies to develop a countrywide eye care program. This was not an easy task, but ultimately led to the formation of the Nepal Netra Jyoti Sangh (NNJS). The Government entrusted the development of Nepal's eye care services to NNJS, marking the beginning of eye care development in Nepal with Dr. Pokharel at the helm. His focus was on three key areas:

1. **Infrastructure development**: Recognizing the need to set up an eye hospital in each zone to ensure better access to eye care, Dr. Pokharel requested international agencies' support. The Seva Foundation, Fred Hollows Foundation, CBM, Swiss Red Cross, and Norwegian Association for the Blind and Partially Sighted supported the development of both secondary and primary eye care centers with assistance from local communities and district-level NNJS chapters. Today, several of these secondary eye hospitals have become tertiary eye hospitals. Dr. Pokharel was also able to motivate Dr. Henning from Germany and Dr. Kolstad from Norway to work in different regions of Nepal. They worked for almost three decades in the far east and far west regions of the country, respectively, and left a legacy of highly functional, high volume tertiary eye hospitals.
2. **Human resource development**
Ophthalmic assistants: With very few ophthalmologists available in the country, one of the first steps taken by the NNJS was the training of ophthalmic assistants. This was started with the first few batches being trained at Aravind Eye Hospital, Madurai. Subsequently, the hospitals in Nepal incorporated this

training as an integral part of their human resource development. The pipeline for training ophthalmic assistants also helped NNJS set up primary eye care centers in the country's rural and remote areas. In many ways, the allied ophthalmic personnel (AOP) cadre (as they are categorized now by the WHO) was pioneered by Nepal; the AOP are the backbone of the eye care services in Nepal.

Ophthalmologists: In the early days, doctors from Nepal underwent an ophthalmology residency mostly in India, typically at the Dr. RP Centre of Ophthalmic Sciences, AIIMS, New Delhi, under a special agreement. In subsequent years, an ophthalmology residency program was introduced in the government-run Tribhuvan University, Kathmandu, and later in many non-governmental eye hospitals and private medical colleges across the country.

3. **Technology**: The Nepal program attracted visionaries like Dr. Fred Hollows, who later founded the Fred Hollows Foundation. He helped set up an intraocular lens (IOL) manufacturing unit under the Tilganga Institute of Ophthalmology in 1992. This reduced the country's dependency on imported intraocular lenses (IOLs).

Nepal today

With an estimated 30 million people in 2020, Nepal has about 180 eye hospitals and primary eye care centers spread across all 77 districts in the country; 160 of these are under NNJS management. Today, there are at least four tertiary eye hospitals. For a country which had minimal eye care services four decades ago, Nepal has come a long way. Today, Nepal performs close to 400,000 eye surgeries annually, with 40% of them on Nepali patients and the rest on Indians from the bordering districts. Cataract surgery constitutes 80% of eye surgeries in Nepal, translating to a CSR of 4000. The 2012 survey indicated that the prevalence of blindness in Nepal has reduced to 0.35%. There is an increased drive to improve access to eye care for every citizen of the country. Annually, 320 ophthalmic assistants graduate from eight training institutes accredited by the Council of Technical Education and Vocational Training. Every year, 45–50 ophthalmologists graduate from Nepali institutes after completing a 3 year-long MD program; roughly 10–15% of these graduates are from neighboring countries including India.

Nepal is an inspiring example of a country that went from having almost no eye care to becoming a model nation for developing countries, all due to the leadership of Dr. Pokharel and the team. Dr. Pokharel's exemplary work also motivated his younger colleagues to pursue this path of continually enhancing eye care in Nepal, both in geographic coverage, and in the scope of eye care services.

Source: Nepal Netra Jyoti Sangh, Nepal

2.1.3 Designing to "Close the Loop"

In most instances, the actual delivery of eye care on the ground evolves organically over time. Eye care delivery programs are often designed in response to the demands of the patients seeking care, and not on a broader goal of reducing avoidable blindness in the community. Those who can comply with the intervention plan usually benefit by obtaining the required medicines and glasses or undergo surgeries or other procedures. There are two fundamental flaws in this mode of working if we recognize that the care pathway begins with identifying those in need of eye care in the community and culminates with follow-up after the prescribed intervention (Fig. 2.4).

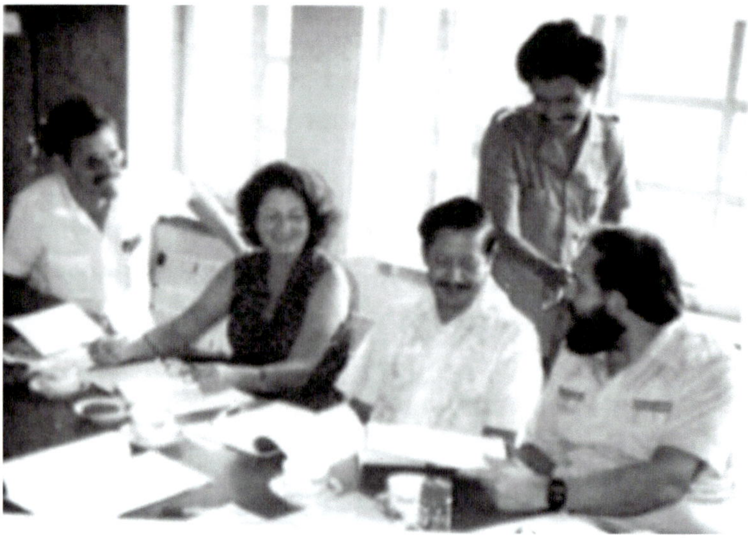

Fig. 2.3 Dr. Nichole Grasset and Dr Ram Prasad Pokharel (second and third from left) discussing the Nepal Blindness Survey data

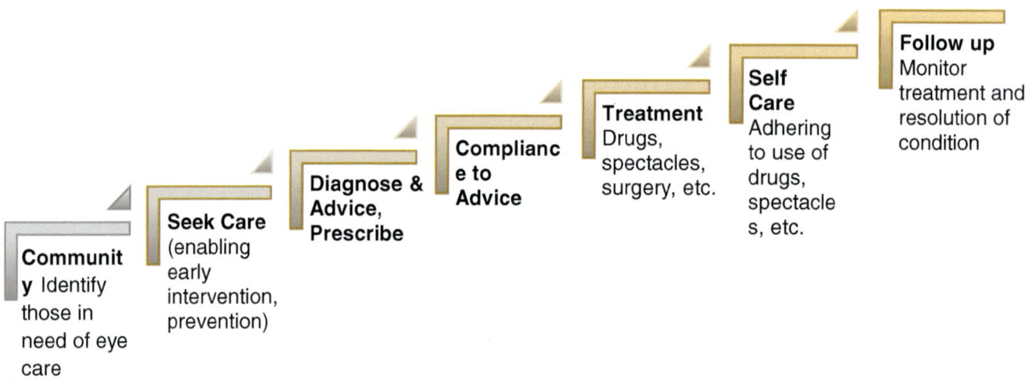

Fig. 2.4 The comprehensive care pathway

Of the several steps in the care cycle, the current caregiving design is optimized to address only a few, i.e., diagnose and prescribe to those who visit, treat those who decide to undergo the treatment, and follow-up those who return. The other steps are by and large ignored. A second lacuna in this system is the leakage that happens between each step. The irony is that this leakage is seldom measured. Most programs do not routinely monitor the denominator (the number of patients who need eye care) and concentrate only on the numerator (those who seek eye care). They do not routinely monitor if everyone is adequately diagnosed; whether all those prescribed bought the medicines or spectacles; whether those advised a surgery underwent the same; whether those treated were followed-up to ensure that their complaint was resolved. A study in south India estimated that less than 7% of those who felt the need for some eye care intervention presented themselves at an eye camp organized in their vicinity [7]. Whether in an eye camp or the hospital, among those advised to undergo cataract surgery, a very significant proportion, as high as 50%, do not get operated on, for various reasons.

Similarly, the post-intervention follow-up is limited to only those who return, which is usually only a small proportion of those who opted for the intervention. These leakages, especially between diagnosis and intervention, directly translate to resource wastage expended by the providers and the efforts and money spent by the patients, since diagnosis by itself does not improve the condition. This is a tremendous waste of the limited resources existing in many countries in the South-East Asia Region.

It is, therefore, critical for every program to actively seek and plug such leakages. Taking responsibility for preventing these leakages is a fundamental and ethical responsibility of the eye care service providers. This approach of "closing the care loop" will eventually result in a well-designed, effective eye care service delivery system. There are several good examples of this that one can learn from.

Case Study 2 Cataract Blindness Control Program by the National Program for Control of Blindness in India (Fig. 2.5)

India was one of the first countries to establish a National Program for Control of Blindness (NPCB) in 1976. Since then, it has regularly conducted national surveys and made a budgetary allocation for eye care. The successive surveys indicated that cataract was the leading cause of blindness, both in absolute numbers, and in proportion of blindness. This caused concern in the leadership at the national level, which decided to launch a targeted program for the control of blindness due to cataract. Towards this end, the Ministry of Health at the Government of India initiated a dialogue with the World Bank for a loan. The goal was to augment the country's capacity to provide cataract surgeries and finance this enhanced work, especially for the economically underprivileged. After an iterative and consultative process, India designed a comprehensive and well-thought-through proposal. The World Bank approved a loan of USD140 million to be spent over 7 years from 1995 to 2002; however, only USD117.8 million was drawn over the course of the program. Seven states, which accounted for over 70% of cataract blindness in India, were selected for the project. These were Andhra Pradesh (including Telangana then), Madhya Pradesh (including Chhattisgarh then), Maharashtra, Odisha (named Orissa then), Rajasthan, Tamil Nadu, and Uttar Pradesh (including Uttarakhand then). The 7-year project sought to eliminate the backlog of cataract cases by conducting more than 11 million surgeries. This project was completed successfully and in the World Bank's performance rating achieved the following comments:

Outcome: *Highly Satisfactory*; Sustainability: *Highly Likely*; and Institutional Development Impact: *Substantial.* These high ratings were a testimony to a well-conceived and executed project. Although the funding was sought for only seven districts, all the proposed activities were extended to the rest of the states as well, and were funded by internal national resources, thereby demonstrating the political will behind this project to address eye health care in the country.

This project was comprehensive in its design and included four major components: (1) *enhancing quality of eye care and expanding service delivery;* (2) *developing human resources for eye care;* (3) *promoting outreach activities and public awareness*; and (4) *building institutional capacity.* Other than the "human resource development" component, support for this project came from both the Government and non-government charitable sector. The project now accounts for over 50% of India's eye care. As a direct result of the project, a strong public–private partnership for implementation of projects was forged. Over 80% of the funds were budgeted towards "enhancing quality of eye care and expanding service delivery."

On the quality front, the project helped build the nation's capacity to shift from the traditional intracapsular cataract extraction (ICCE) surgery to the extracapsular cataract extraction with IOL (ECCE-IOL) surgery. This was no mean feat as it required equipping all hospitals across the country with surgical microscopes, ultrasound scans to perform biometry, and YAG (yttrium-aluminum-garnet) lasers; in addition, organize a supply-chain mechanism to ensure IOL availability. Besides this, thousands of ophthalmologists had to be trained in this new technique.

During the project period, the proportion of IOL surgeries increased from a low 3% to over 90%. In addition to this holistic approach for enhancing quality, the service delivery design mandated "closing the care loop." A scheme under this project provided a subsidy for each "free" cataract surgery. It mandated that such patients be identified in the community through outreach camps, transported to an eye hospital, and be provided with accommodation, food, surgery, and medications by the care provider. A follow-up after 4–6 weeks was also required to qualify for the subsidy. This scheme eliminated barriers that could potentially arise due to issues of access and affordability for those afflicted by cataract in the community. This exceptional design led to the success of the project (Fig. 2.6) and received high-performance ratings by the World Bank [8].

2.2 Enabling an Eco-system for and Implementing Policies for Effective Eye Care Delivery

The disaggregation of health systems into six building blocks (Fig. 2.1) by the WHO offers a practical framework towards building an enabling eco-system and policies for effective eye care delivery. This has to be done within the context of and understanding that eye care in each country is delivered by multiple stakeholders supplementing the efforts of the government eye care delivery system. Table 2.2 gives a very high-level national estimate of eye care delivery by various providers in South-East Asian countries.

2.2.1 Health System Building Blocks and Eye Care

2.2.1.1 Service Delivery

The keys to good service delivery are access, availability, utilization, and coverage of care. *Access* includes the physical, economic, and socio-psychological aspects of people's ability to use health services. *Availability* refers to the physical presence or delivery of services that meet a minimum standard. *Utilization* is the extent to which healthcare services are used. *The coverage* of interventions is the proportion of people who receive a specific intervention or service among those who need it. The effectiveness and coverage of service delivery systems depend on how well they adhere to and execute the holistic care pathway, as shown in Fig. 2.4. The design at the national level ought to cover the entire pathway. At the minimum, the design must close the loop in the caregiving process for at least those seeking eye care. A significant proportion of patients have barriers or challenges in complying with advised treatment. Some of these barriers are ignorance, undue fear of treatment, apprehension on the outcomes, lack of family/social support, challenges in access to medicines/spectacles, and affordability. A study in south India showed that only 25% of patients purchased a pair of spectacles when a prescription alone was given in an eye camp [9]. This number dramatically increased to 80% when the spectacles were available for sale at the eye camps. The same is true for medicines as well, especially when they are prescribed in rural settings, as ophthalmic drugs are unlikely to be readily available in local pharmacies. Sometimes, however, these measures are not possible due to restrictive regulations. These issues prevent the patient from receiving the prescribed intervention (ranging from surgery to purchasing medicines or a pair of glasses). This indirectly has a bearing on quality. Excellence in diagnosis or treat-

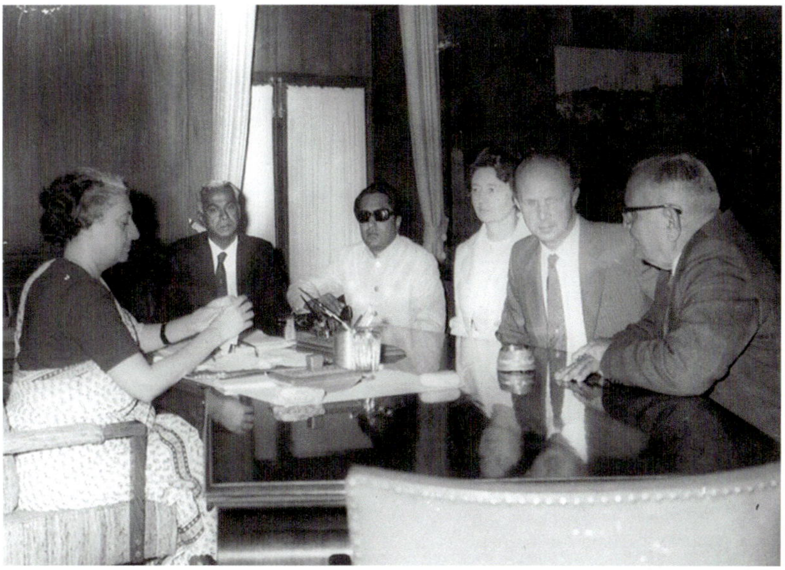

Fig. 2.5 The meeting that laid the National Program for Control of Blindness (NPCB) foundation in India in 1976. Dr. Govindappa Venkataswamy (Founder, Aravind Eye Hospital), Dr. Rajendra Vyas, Lady Wilson, Sir John Wilson (Founder, Royal Commonwealth Society for the Blind), and Dr. M. P. Mehra (Founder, Sitapur Eye Hospitals), meeting with Mrs. Indira Gandhi, the Prime Minister of India

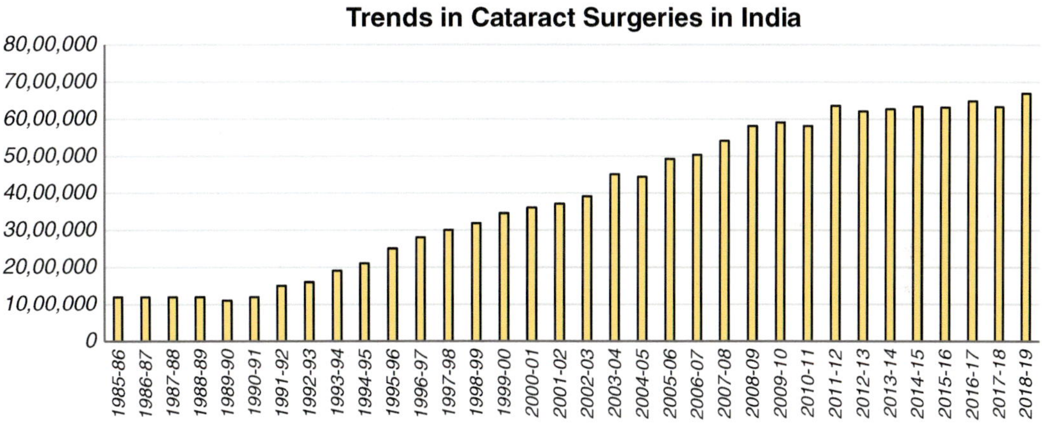

Fig. 2.6 Trends in cataract surgeries in India. (Source: NPCB)

ment advice, by themselves, does not improve a patient's condition. The ease of use of the service delivery system from the patient's perspective is an important determinant of good outcomes. With such high proportions of those entering the system not getting better, directly or indirectly, the demand for eye care becomes dampened as people become negative advocates. One could classify these quality issues as emerging from acts of omission, that is, not doing what should have been done, for whatever reason. There are also issues of quality in what was done, such as surgical complications or medical errors. Both of these problems are best addressed by improving patient monitoring. Compliance rates, complication rates, and estimations of visual outcomes are all measures that can help improve the service delivery process.

Table 2.2 Proportion of eye care delivery by various providers

Provider	Bangladesh (%)	Bhutan (%)	India (%)	Indonesia (%)	Maldives (%)	Myanmar (%)	Nepal (%)	Sri Lanka (%)	Thailand (%)	Timor-Leste (%)
Government	30	100	25	30	80	65	10	50	80	100
Private	30	–	25	60	20	15	20	20	20	–
Voluntary	40	–	50	10	–	20	70	30	–	–

2.2.1.2 Large Scale Programs to Improve Service Delivery

Large scale program interventions with specific goals implemented in a time-bound manner have helped leapfrog the development of eye care sustainably. These interventions most often (a) contribute to capacity building, human resources, and infrastructure at the regional/national level; (b) evolve innovative ideas to address the challenges of access and quality of care; and (c) bring together a variety of stakeholders with similar goals, such as policymakers, service providers, and community organizations to forge alliances for long-term collaborations. The following examples illustrate this:

(a) **India—***Long-term benefits*—The World Bank-funded cataract surgery program in India resulted in an additional 11.6 million cataract surgeries being performed; this led to a doubling of surgical volumes from 1.9 million in 1994–95 to 3.7 million in 2001–2002. The key outcome in addition to the increased surgical output was the enhanced capacity to (a) perform high volume cataract surgery; (b) building of infrastructure and availability of resources to train ophthalmologists and AOPs for sustainable development; and (c) proactive involvement of public and private sector organizations in addressing the issue of cataract blindness. A demonstration of the development and success of such a sustainable program enabled the Government of India to continue with the grant-in-aid program. In 2018–19, India performed 6.2 million cataract surgeries, which translates to a CSR of 5100. At this juncture, there is an urgent need to design a similar targeted effort to increase the surgical outputs in the under-performing states to achieve the desired CSR levels of 9000–10,000 to eliminate blindness due to cataract.

(b) **Bangladesh—***Targeted benefits*—The Bangladesh Childhood Cataract Campaign (2004–2009) was the outcome of the efforts made by Dr. Mohammad Abdul Muhit, the Executive Director of the Child Sight Foundation. He brought together Orbis, Sightsavers, and the Government of Bangladesh to eliminate the backlog of cataract blindness in children in a time-bound manner. Through this initiative, 12,000 cataract-blind children were identified across the country, and sight-restoring cataract surgeries were performed on over 10,000 blind children at no cost to the children's families. The program adopted the "key informant method" for case finding. Though a short-term initiative, this program built the country's capacity to deal with cataract in children, from point finding to surgery.

(c) **Orbis in South-East Asia—***Holistic approach to building sub-specialty services*—Pediatric eye care received a fillip with Orbis's capacity-building initiative to develop pediatric eye care in this region. In less than a decade, capabilities were developed (infrastructure and human resources, etc.) in over 50 eye hospitals in India, Bangladesh, and Nepal to provide comprehensive eye care services to children, both in the community and at the hospital level. This addressed the void in pediatric eye care services. The intervention ultimately resulted in the upskilling of 100+ pediatric ophthalmologists, anesthetists, 1000+ AOPs, outreach coordinators, etc. to handle pediatric eye care services. Taking a long-term view on human resource development, resource centers with training and research capacity were also developed. Some of these centers have since then started fellowship training programs in pediatric eye care. Building on this successful intervention, Orbis is now implementing a massive project to address refractive error in children across India and Nepal, aiming to screen five million+ school children in 15 districts and follow them over time. Findings from this pilot effort could provide crucial insights on the management of refractive errors and a blueprint for scaling up eye care services.

(d) **Technology Innovations—***Service design to address an eye problem*—The effective management of diabetic retinopathy, that could lead to blindness, depends on early detection and intervention. Programmatic intervention for diabetic retinopathy requires a multi-sectoral approach involving different stakeholders, from community-level partners and general physicians for effective case finding to technology companies for effective diagnosis.

(i) Concerted efforts by different international agencies, beginning in the late 1990s, brought a sharp focus on to the development of a community-centric comprehensive service delivery model for diabetic retinopathy.
(ii) Collaboration among eye care providers and technology companies have resulted in the development of technological solutions for easy access to detection services and early identification of diabetic retinopathy. Some of these technological examples include low-cost fundus cameras operated by non-physician personnel in primary care settings and tech giant Google's efforts to develop algorithms using artificial intelligence to grade fundus images. The ultimate aim of these innovations is to simplify and democratize eye care.

2.2.1.3 Achieving Operational Excellence for Better Service Delivery

The quality of eye care services, by and large, tends to be cataract-centric and mostly limited to factors such as post-operative visual acuity, complications, and infections. The WHO's benchmark for a successful intervention is achieving a best-corrected visual acuity of 6/18 and better vision post-operatively at 4 weeks in 85% of cataract surgeries. While these outcomes could be monitored at hospitals at the patient level, such outcomes in the community can only be measured through population-based surveys. At present, prevalence studies and RAAB surveys are the only sources of such outcome data at the population level. Given the cost and efforts involved in conducting these activities, surveys can neither be frequent nor cover all countries/regions. While cataract surgery constitutes a significant proportion of the total numbers of eye surgeries performed, one should redefine quality of care through a more holistic approach. Quality initiatives should cover all domains to improve eye care services to achieve universal coverage.

The National Academy of Medicine (formerly, the Institute of Medicine), USA, defined six aims of quality at the patient care delivery level—safety, patient-centeredness, effectiveness, efficiency, timelines, and equity (Fig. 2.7).

The holistic approach to quality of care at provider levels encompasses two core dimensions:

(a) *Improving what is currently done*—This includes adopting preferred clinical practices, ensuring patient safety, and adopting

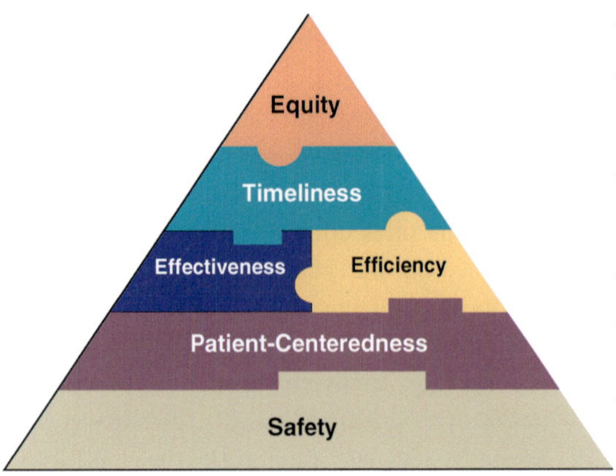

- ***Safety:*** *Avoiding injuries to patients from the care that is intended to help them*
- ***Patient centeredness:*** *Providing care that is respectful of and responsive to individual patient preferences, needs and values, and ensuring that patient values guide all clinical decisions*
- ***Effectiveness:*** *Providing services based on scientific knowledge to all who could benefit, and refraining from providing services to those not likely to benefit (avoiding underuse or overuse)*
- ***Efficiency:*** *Avoiding waste, in particular, -waste of equipment, supplies, ideas, and energy*
- ***Timelines:*** *Reducing waiting timesand sometimes harmful delays for both, those who receive and those who give care*
- ***Equitable:*** *Providing care that does not vary in quality because of personal characteristics such as gender, ethnicity, geographical location, and socio-economic status*

Fig. 2.7 The National Academy of Medicine's model for quality in healthcare

patient-centered care to achieve better outcomes and enhanced patient experience.

(b) *Addressing what is currently not done*—Achieving universal coverage in a true sense is possible only when the service design is proactively inclusive, in terms of pricing, access, reducing the cost of care for the patient, and eliminating "waste" by both providers and patients alike; most importantly, it also includes ensuring that the intervention is timely (diagnosis to treatment management). At a macro level, recent recommendations by the Lancet Commission and the WHO-World Bank-OECD (Organization of Economic Cooperation and Development) report [10] have placed quality at the center of universal health coverage, which can be achieved if the boundaries of multi-sectoral consultations are expanded beyond health systems and the ministries of health. Governments may need to focus on (1) developing an enabling ecosystem such as quality roads, transportation, sanitation, and education; (2) improving the training of nurses and doctors, since all of these affect the quality of care; and (3) put in place a monitoring and accountability mechanism to facilitate continuous improvement, that all quality systems need.

2.2.1.4 Measuring Quality

(a) *At the providers' level*

Quality of care is largely influenced by the processes in a hospital or caregiving setting. Quality is an ongoing process, which should be measured at periodical intervals, and every effort should be made to benchmark quality with the best global practices. Hence, there is a need to

- adapt workflow process and clinical protocols that ensure better clinical outcomes and patient satisfaction,
- develop metrics that will help assess the six aims of quality (Fig. 2.7),
- a system to generate correct and timely data followed by periodic reviews leading to continuous improvements.

With an increasing need for sub-specialty services, there has been an emerging need for the development of standards and metrics for specifically monitoring the clinical process and outcomes of these sub-specialties.

(b) *At the national level*

The World Report on Vision (WRV) [3], launched in October 2019, has reemphasized quality of care and suggested a people-centric approach revolving around patient experience, clinical outcomes, and its impact on the quality of life. As signatories to the World Health Assembly resolutions, most governments focus on establishing quality standards at a country level. For instance, the Quality Council of India launched the National Accreditation Board for Hospitals and Healthcare Providers (NABH) that accredit and benchmark services offered by healthcare providers in India. With lobbying at the national level, NABH has also developed standards specific to eye care. Similarly, the National Quality Improvement Committee, Bangladesh, has set up a Quality Improvement Secretariat (QIS) to develop quality standards, protocols, and measures.

There are now initiatives to develop common platforms to benchmark care quality at both individual provider and institutional levels. This is now made easier with the increasing usage of Electronic Medical Records (EMR) in hospitals. Eye care programs in the South-East Asia Region can learn from already available solutions and build on the existing ones, platforms relevant to local conditions. Over time, several quality benchmarking systems have evolved in the USA, Europe, and a few other countries. Table 2.3 lists some of these systems which have played a major role in enhancing outcomes. It is time that such initiatives are developed at the national level in all countries to drive quality. A beginning is being made in India by the "VISION 2020—The Right to Sight" program, which proposes to monitor cataract surgical outcomes.

2.2.1.5 Health Workforce

A knowledgeable, skilled, empowered, and motivated health workforce is essential for sound health delivery. Often there is a direct and

Table 2.3 List of initiatives for measuring clinical outcomes

Across health disciplines
The **ICHOM (International Consortium of Health Outcomes Measurement)** [11] was launched in 2012 to create standard measurement sets using a global consensus process by involving leading clinicians and patients. Its measurements are used by the OECD and the World Economic Forum's programs of value in healthcare. With hospitals from different countries adopting the standard sets, ICHOM plans to introduce international benchmarking of the outcomes. ICHOM has developed standard sets for cataract surgery in eye care
Across countries for eye care
EUREQUO (European Registry of Quality Outcomes for Cataract and Refractive Surgery) [12] provides the means by which surgical results may be audited and encourages surgeons to adjust their techniques and improve their outcomes. This platform, designed as a benchmarking tool, is funded by the European Society of Cataract and Refractive Surgeons (ESCRS) and co-financed by the European Union through a grant. Currently, this database has more than 2.9 million cataract surgeries recorded
Country/institutional level
The **American Academy of Ophthalmology (AAO)'s IRIS (Intelligent Research in Sight) Registry (within the USA)** [13] is a centralized data repository system. The IRIS registry is integrated into the electronic medical records system, allowing the compilation of a comprehensive eye disease and conditions registry. The benchmarking of clinical practices and outcomes through IRIS can validate ophthalmologists' quality of care and opportunities for improvement
National Eye Database, MoH, Malaysia [14] is a national registry of eye diseases for the assessment of distributions of eye disorders, evaluation of risk factors, and outcome measures of treatment for key eye conditions. This includes the assessment of cataract surgery outcomes also. This team has developed a monitoring tool using the CUSUM (Cumulative Sum) technique to measure and improve cataract surgeons' (especially trainees' performance)
The **Cataract Quality Assurance (CATQA) tool** developed by **Aravind Eye Care System, India** [15] measures key metrics of cataract surgery, namely, surgical outcomes, complication rates, infection rates, etc. Additionally, it can also provide performance patterns at any given time or measured over a specific period. This platform is designed to assess an individual's performance and benchmark it against the rest of the ophthalmologists within an eye unit or the entire network. The data for about 1.86 million cataract surgeries are archived within this system
VISION 2020: India's initiative for the member hospitals will show visual acuity outcomes following cataract surgery across participating hospitals and allow benchmarking of individual institutions with others
Mobile application capable of assessing essential outcome indicators
Better Operative Outcomes Software Tool (BOOST) [16] is a simplified mobile app tool that allows doctors to record the first-day post-operative visual acuity of 60 consecutive patients, and the results of 20 consecutive patients with poor vision at 6 weeks. The app is designed to provide specific recommendations. It also provides a benchmarked score of the individual or an eye hospital. There is ongoing research assessing this platform

positive link between the health workforce and population health outcomes [17]. Broadly, the health workforce includes all people engaged in actions whose primary intent is to enhance health. One of the major limitations in the delivery of eye care is the development and deployment of human resources for health (HRH). In several countries, this is a chronic problem as there is a disconnect between eye care needs and human resource planning. One ophthalmologist supported by a well-trained team of 4 to 5 clinical support staff to carry out all repetitive skill-based activities can achieve a high productivity level. The desired ratio of community-based, independent workers would be one per 30,000–40,000 people to address refractive errors, provide primary eye care, and organize referrals; currently, there is one ophthalmologist per 50,000 people, who performs all these functions. Against this need, the availability of ophthalmologists and other cadres and their annual output are grossly inadequate in most countries. The ideal numbers of eye health personnel per million people are shown in Table 2.4.

We examined the current availability and training possibilities of skilled eye care personnel in the South-East Asia Region countries (Tables 2.5 and 2.6).

Over the years, the roles and responsibilities of the two cadres of the eye care team, the ophthalmologists and optometrists, have become better defined, with structured training, accreditation, career paths, and employment opportunities. However, this has not been the case for other cadres of the eye care team, most notably, for the clinical support staff. It has long been recognized that the lack of well-trained clinical support staff is a significant barrier to eye care delivery. Not having them in adequate numbers within an eye hospital significantly compromises the efficiency of the ophthalmologists and, to some extent, compromises the quality of care and patient satisfaction. Likewise, without this cadre, providing primary eye care in the community is not feasible, as ophthalmologists and optometrists prefer to work in larger towns. Thus, clinical support staff are emerging as essential cadres in delivering eye care services. Where they are in sufficient numbers (example, Nepal), eye care delivery is very efficient, both, at the hospital and the national level. Yet, the development of this cadre continues to be neglected, with wide gaps and variations in their skills and capacities. A lot of this is attributable to the lack of a structured training curriculum, a paucity of training resources, and trainers.

The WHO has acknowledged the significance of this critical human resource in eye care and redefined this cadre as "allied ophthalmic personnel (AOPs)"; the AOP includes opticians, ophthalmic nurses, orthoptists, ophthalmic and

Table 2.4 Human resources (eye health personnel) needed for a million people

HR Cadre	Estimated requirement
Ophthalmologists	20
Hospital-based allied ophthalmic personnel	80–100
Community-based allied ophthalmic personnel	30–40
Rehabilitation workers and itinerant teachers	15–20
Eye care managers	2

Table 2.5 Availability and training capacity—ophthalmologists

Ophthalmologists					
Countries	Population (million)	Currently available	Per million	Degree and years in Residency	Annual intake
Bangladesh	161	1300	8	MS—5 years FCPS—4 years DO/DCO—2 years	60 per year
Bhutan	0.8	12	14	4 years	2
India	1312	25,000	19	MS/DNB—3 years	1983 MS (1660) + DNB (323)
Indonesia	267	2000	7	MD—4 years	120
Maldives	0.4	12	30	Undergo ophthalmology residency courses at other countries and are recognized by the Maldives Medical and Dental Council	
Myanmar	57	400	7	MS—3 years	Capacity: 40 Actual: 30
Nepal	30	350	12	MD—3 years	50[a]
Sri Lanka	23	200	9	MD 3 years + Board Certification 2 years	Need-based— Intake varies
Thailand	70	1600	23	MD—3 years	74
Timor-Leste	1.4	5	4	–	–

Note
Bangladesh: *MS* Master of Surgery, *FCPS* Fellow of College of Physicians and Surgeons, *DO* Diploma in Ophthalmology, *DCO* Diploma in Community Ophthalmology, *DNB* Diplomate of National Board, *MD* Doctor of Medicine
India: MS/MD annual capacity: https://www.mciindia.org/CMS/information-desk/college-and-course-search
Sri Lanka: MD Degree: https://pgim.cmb.ac.lk/wp-content/uploads/2016/07/Ophthalmology.pdf
[a]5–10% intake includes candidates from other countries

Table 2.6 Availability and training capacity—optometrists and allied ophthalmic personnel

	Optometrists			Allied ophthalmic personnel (AOP)		
Country	Currently available	Degree/Diploma	Annual intake	Currently available	Degree/Diploma	Annual intake
Bangladesh	700	B. Optom/Diploma/ Certificate		800	One-year Certificate course	30
Bhutan	9	Trained in India	Need-based	62	Dip. in Oph. Technology (3 years)	
				6	Ophthalmic nurses—Diploma in Nursing +6 months training in ophthalmic nursing	Need-based
India	4000+	M. Optom (2 years) B. Optom (4 years) Dip. Optom (2 years)			AOP certificate (2 years) Vision technician course—1 year	
Indonesia	8600 (Refractionists)	Dip. Optom (3 years)	600	4000	AOP certificate training (3 months)[a]	120
Maldives				Trained from other countries		
Myanmar	54	Refractionists and optometry (2 years)	20	221	Diploma in nursing (Eye & ENT) (9 months)	9
Nepal	1247	B. Optom (4 years)	67	1350	Certificate course by CTVET	320
		M. Optom (2 years)	12			
Sri Lanka	750[b]	Dip. Optom (2 years)	70–100	1200[c]	On-the-job training of general nurses	
Thailand	300	Doctor of Optometry (6 years)	80–100	5000–6000 (estimated)	Ophthalmic nurse practitioner (4 months)	120
Timor-Leste						

Sources:
Nepal: *CTVET* Council for Technical Education and Vocational Training, *AOPs* are called ophthalmic assistants; (https://www.eyehealthnepal.com/2020/06/optometry-in-nepal.html): in addition to in-country training, every year, at least 50 candidates and 10 candidates graduate in B. Optom and M. Optom from India
India: Optometrists availability—taken from the member list of the Optometry Council of India
[a]Eligibility: 3-year diploma degree in general nursing and at least 1-year experience in ophthalmology
[b]This includes Diploma and competency certificates
[c]In Sri Lanka, there is no separate cadre for ophthalmic nursing; general nurses with a 3 year degree are provided a short orientation and trained on the job
M. Optom Master of Optometry, B. Optom Bachelor of Optometry, *Dip. Optom* Diploma in Optometry, *Dip. in Oph. Technology* Diploma in Ophthalmic Technology

optometric assistants, ophthalmic and optometric technicians, vision therapists, ocularists, ophthalmic photographers/imagers, and ophthalmic administrators. In March 2015, international organizations such as the IAPB, International Council of Ophthalmology, and the International Joint Commission on Allied Health Personnel in Ophthalmology came together. They launched the "Cambridge Declaration" to ensure high quality capacity development and skills of eye care teams [18]. The declaration specifically states that "Allied Ophthalmic Personnel are committed members of eye health teams in every country globally and play an essential role in delivering high quality, efficient, comprehensive eye services, inclusive of all persons, and in achieving Universal Eye Health."

Human resource development requires a holistic approach starting with a comprehensive estimate of eye care needs at all levels, and thereby, an estimate of the human resource requirements in all cadres. This will help determine the gap in availability and the annual throughput required to bridge this gap. Alongside the improvement in training, there is a need for an enabling environment to perform optimally. An enabling environment includes the supply of required equipment, having them in good working condition, and effective retention strategies. Good professional development plans are equally important to keep pace with the rapid advancements in eye care techniques and technology. The government has a key role in creating such training pipelines and accrediting the various cadres of AOPs.

There are strong positive correlations between HRH density, service coverage, and health outcomes. An adequate health workforce is one that is available, competent, responsive, productive, and well distributed. A resource mapping, work-specific training, financing, and providing form of employment are the basic ingredients for success.

Case Study 3

Within the last decade, the government of India has taken effective steps to alleviate shortages of human resources in the health sector. Based on the estimates of future needs for specialists, the annual intake of students in this sector was doubled a few years ago. To enhance the pipeline of doctors who can then be trained in various specialties and to ensure distribution across the country, a policy decision was taken to have a government medical college in every district of the country. Therefore, new medical colleges have been established all over the country. The intake capacity of several existing medical colleges was also significantly increased; in many instances, even doubling. An allied health professionals council is on the anvil to give impetus to this cadre of health staff. Governments need to be forward-looking and proactive to ensure adequacy of human health resources. They also need to have the courage and wisdom to overcome forces of protectionism of professional groups where it exists.

2.2.1.6 Health Information Systems

Information is the core foundation for planning, design, and monitoring implementation. The key functions of a health information system include: (a) data generation, (b) compilation, (c) analysis and synthesis, and (d) communication and use. Additionally, this system also serves the broader objectives of providing an early warning in case of epidemics or other major health emergencies, supporting patient and health facility, enabling planning, and stimulating health system research. Very seldom is there a reporting requirement to a national or a regional level. As a consequence, there is very little information available at an aggregated level, whether at the national or subnational levels. Amongst institutions, there is a wide variation in what information is collected, its sources, how current is it, and how is it used. Overall, there is a lot of scope for enhancing management of health information systems.

Achieving excellence in eye health or moving towards universal eye health is a journey, and it hinges on, amongst other things, having a robust information system. Against this background, a generic framework for an information system is proposed. For an information system to be effective, it must first recognize the logical linkages and dependencies between inputs, activities or processes, outputs, outcomes, and impacts (Fig. 2.8).

A well-functioning health information system is one that ensures the production, analysis, dissemination, and use of reliable and timely health information by decision-makers at different levels of the health system, both on a regular basis, as well as in emergencies. The "output" and "outcome," as well as the ensuing "impact," are consequences of "input" and "process" (Fig. 2.8). Hence a robust information system has to consider all these elements to ensure that the desired outcomes are achieved. However, quite often, information systems are built to mainly monitor output. As a result, under-performance is often explained away as being due to inadequate inputs or due to issues relating to the process. This shifting of accountability does not help the overall program. Timely and frequent monitoring of inputs and processes results in appropriate remedial action to keep programs on track and on time (Table 2.7).

Under input, items like human resource, infrastructure, equipment, supplies, and finance are easily understood. However, it is equally important to also recognize "community and patients" as inputs. A community is the source of many inputs and can effectively facilitate many activities relating to demand generation, such as outreach. Good community engagement and a mutual buildup of trust and confidence between the community and program partners help with both staffing and patient demand. Similarly, it is the number of patients treated, that ultimately drive output and impact. Hence, it is important to have structured processes for community engagement and appropriate strategies for bringing patients into the system.

The "process" phase is where the inputs are transformed into outputs. An inefficient process

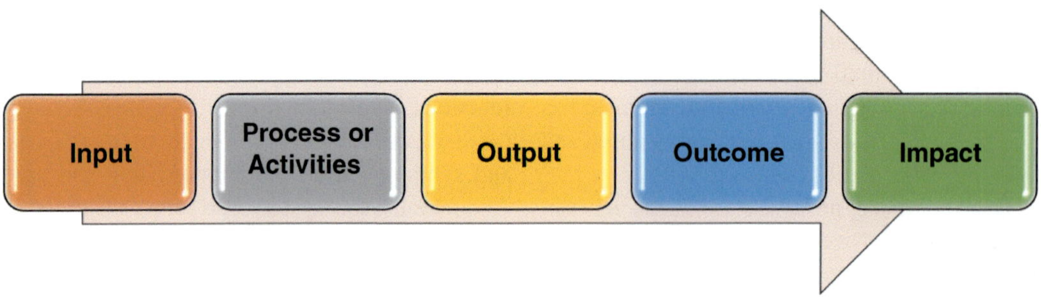

Fig. 2.8 Input–output framework

Table 2.7 Elements in the eye care delivery pathway that needs to be monitored

Input	Process	Output	Outcome	Impact
Community Patients Human resource Infrastructure Equipment Supplies Finance	Procedures Activities Patient care Outreach Training	Number of patients – Examined – Treated – Operated	Vision restored Vision improved Rehabilitated Quality of Life (QoL)	Blindness levels Economic growth

adversely impacts the output; improper processes result in poor quality and affect both outcomes and impacts. A good information system monitors the systems and protocols and recognizes quality issues early enough to make appropriate remedial measures. Continuous monitoring and review enable continuous improvement of the process.

Both inputs and processes have a very direct bearing on the rest of the stages and thus benefit from continuous monitoring. At caregiving facilities, such as hospitals, the inputs and processes are managed transactionally at an operational level. Since real-time management at the point of care is possible today using digital technology, a well-designed information system could highlight the exceptions or deviations as they occur.

At a national level, input monitoring would include monitoring the availability of resources, their distribution, and gaps in supply, or issues in adopting best practice protocols or quality initiatives.

These three elements—input, process, and output—are largely in the institutional domain; therefore, information systems for these are usually institution or program-based. This is relatively easy to do, since all institutions have information systems in place to some extent.

The three domains of health information are health determinants, health systems performance, and health status. To achieve this, a health information system must generate population and facility-based data, investigate and communicate events that impact public health security, and finally synthesize and apply the newly acquired knowledge.

These are never easy. Ultimately what matters are the outcomes and impacts on blindness and visual impairment. These two measures—outcomes and impact—occur largely in the community or population domain. Population-based surveys are expensive in terms of time, finance, and human resources. Rapid surveys such as the Rapid Assessment of Avoidable Blindness (RAAB) or Rapid Assessment of Refractive Error (RARE) are, however, relatively quick and inexpensive. These surveys influence planning at the national level. A stellar example is the national eye care survey in Nepal, which was conducted in the early 1980s, that essentially laid the foundation for Nepal's successful eye care program (see case story 1). Successive national surveys in India highlighted the need to significantly increase the numbers of cataract surgeries and reduce cataract blindness. The World Bank-financed cataract intervention program was born out of such population-based surveys (see case story 2). Several RAABs carried out in the last decade in several countries in the South-East Asia Region have significantly contributed to national eye health program planning [19–21]. Table 2.8 has brief details of several current outcomes and impact metrics used in these surveys.

Studies on the impacts of sight restoration or reduction in blindness on individuals, communities, or countries have been rare in general, and very sparse in the South-East Asia Region countries. In India, there has been only one study on the impact of refractive error correction on the productivity of tea plantation workers in Assam, India [23]. Similarly, a multi-country (Bangladesh, the Philippines, and Kenya) study has been conducted to assess the economic impact of cataract surgery over the long term [24]. In Nepal, the NNJS has developed a centralized and granular information system of both resources and outputs. Similar information grids that aggregate information from individual caregivers in all sectors are required at the national and subnational levels. It is also important to ensure that information flow is always bi-directional with the delivery units receiving regular feedback by way of benchmarking reports.

2.2.1.7 Medical Products and Technologies

Management decisions in eye care are often dependent on the images obtained from various segments of the eye. Hence, these investigational devices should be accessible to patients and affordable to care providers. From the patients' perspective, it is equally important that glasses and medicines be easily available. Many factors, such as the country's eco-system and capacity to produce the supplies locally, and the country's regulatory practices for importing such supplies

Table 2.8 List of key metrics to assess the outcomes and impact of eye care delivery

Cataract Surgical Rate (CSR)	Number of cataract surgeries done in a year in one million population $\mathbf{CSR} = \frac{\text{No of cataract surgeries done in a year}}{\text{Population in millions}}$
Cataract Surgical Coverage (CSC)	Of those requiring cataract surgery, the proportion (%) operated $\mathbf{CSC} = \left\{\frac{\text{Number operated for cataract}}{\text{Number operated} + \text{Number needing cataract operation}}\right\} \times 100$
Effective Cataract Surgical Coverage (eCSC) [22]	Of those requiring cataract surgery the proportion (%) operated with a threshold vision or better (e.g. post-operative vision ≥6/12) $\boldsymbol{eCSC} = \left\{\frac{\text{Number operated for cataract achieving threshold vision}\left(\text{Post op vision} \geq 6/12\right)}{\text{Number operated} + \text{Number needing cataract operation}\left(\text{with visual acuity} < 6/12 \text{ due to cataract}\right)}\right\} \times 100$
Refractive Error Coverage (REC)	Of those requiring refractive error (RE) correction, the proportion (%) corrected with glasses or other methods $\mathbf{REC} = \left\{\frac{\text{Number of people with RE correction}}{\text{Number people RE correction} + \text{Number of people not corrected}}\right\} \times 100$
Effective Refractive Error Coverage (eREC) [22]	Of those requiring RE correction, the proportion (%) corrected with glasses or other methods with a threshold vision or better (e.g. corrected vision ≥6/12) $\mathbf{eREC} = \left\{\frac{\text{Number of people with RE correction}\left(\text{with a vision} \geq 6/12\right)}{\text{Number of people with RE correction} + \text{Number of people with RE below a threshold vision}\left(\text{e.g. } 6/12 \text{ uncorrected}\right)}\right\} \times 100$

influence the availability of equitable, accessible, safe, and affordable care. These are essential for achieving universal eye health coverage in the country. Current trends in managing ophthalmic equipment, supplies, and spectacles in the South-East Asia Region are shown in Tables 2.9 and 2.10.

Markets in the South-East Asia Region countries are open and not restrictive, allowing multiple brands to sell their products. Local production of ophthalmic devices and high demand for them create good competition, and have resulted in better quality and reduced costs of such devices as compared to other WHO regions. Considerations in addressing some regulatory policies can further help to bring down the cost of eye care services in the South-East Asia Region. These include: (a) revisiting import taxes on ophthalmic equipment and supplies, particularly in countries that do not have domestic production and (b) a single window registration of equipment and devices in recognized blocks such as the SAARC (South Asian Association for Regional Cooperation), and the BIMSTEC (Bay of Bengal Initiative for Multi-Sectoral Technical and Economic Cooperation) could further reduce costs and improve supply. This practice is already in vogue in some groups of countries in Africa.

Table 2.9 Ophthalmic supplies

Ophthalmic equipment: diagnostic and surgical instruments	• All of the South-East Asia Region countries import some or all of the equipment and instruments; India manufactures most of the ophthalmic equipment and supplies it requires • All countries require permits or permissions to import equipment/instruments while few countries require product registration which may take 3–6 months • Imports attract import duties or local taxes that range from 2.5 to 50%; Bhutan and Maldives do not have import duty or taxes
Pharmaceuticals	• Ophthalmic medicines and topical medications are available through imports; India, Indonesia, Myanmar, and Thailand also have domestic production • Product registration/approvals by a competent authority are mandatory • Imports attract import duty/local taxes that range from 2.5 to 40%; Bhutan and Maldives do not have import duty or taxes
Consumables (IOLs, sutures & blades)	• Consumables are available through imports; India has significant production of consumables. Nepal has a local IOL factory • With the advent of phacoemulsification and manual small incision cataract surgery, the use of ophthalmic sutures is on the decline • Product registration/approvals by a competent authority are a must except in the Maldives and Timor-Leste • Import duty/local taxes vary from 2.5 to 30%

Note
1. Import of supplies are normally not impacted by FOREX reserves among the WHO South-East Asia Region countries
2. *Indonesia–for products that are also locally produced, import duties could be as high as 50%

Table 2.10 Spectacles

Lenses	• India, Indonesia, the Maldives, and Thailand have manufacturing units locally, in addition to importing specific brands of lenses. The rest of the countries in the South-East Asia Region import all types of lenses • Import duties range from 5 to 30%; in Thailand, they can go up to 60%
Frames	• India and Thailand have manufacturing units locally in addition to importing frames. Some countries in the South-East Asia Region import all types of frames • Import duties range from 8 to 30%; they can go up to 60% in Thailand and 76% in Bangladesh
Surfacing labs	Surfacing labs to make spectacles as per individual prescriptions are available in most countries except Bhutan, the Maldives, and Timor-Leste (due to low scale)

Note: Import duties depend on the following factors: country of origin of the product; type of frames imported (e.g. acetate/ shell/supra/rimless); sunglasses vs. a spectacle frame; trade agreement between the countries

2.2.1.8 Health System Financing

Financing needs can be broadly grouped into three categories:

- *Investment*: for infrastructure, equipment, etc., both for patient caregiving and training of human resources.
- *Recurring or operating costs*: for salaries, consumables, electricity, and other overheads related to running a health facility and providing care.
- *Financing*: to essentially cover the above two (investments and ongoing recurring costs), government services are financed through a budgetary allocation from tax revenues, whereas other sectors address this through user fees. Such fees are usually covered by out-of-pocket spending by patients, insurance, payment agreements with different agencies, government subsidies, etc. In recent times, the National Health Insurance scheme and other mechanisms are emerging to make healthcare more inclusive and affordable to all economic strata.

Government financing of eye care in the country happens through budgetary allocation. The quantum of this allocation depends on national plans and on advocacy capabilities of the national eye care leadership. The third element is about the actual cost of care, which in government hospitals, tends to be free or subsidized. Costs of care delivery in private and other non-government sectors are met by personal insurance or out-of-pocket spending so as to recoup the investment and recurring costs, as well as generate a surplus for future investments. Out-of-pocket spending becomes a barrier for people at the bottom of the pyramid. To address this, many governments are now launching national or social health insurance schemes. This is largely to address catastrophic health expenses and pre-empt situations where financially marginal communities get pushed into irretrievable poverty. In some instances, a significant amount of funding for eye care for all the three areas is provided by international development agencies. Table 2.11 summarizes the availability of inclusive national insurance policies to provide financial protection to various populations.

2.2.1.9 Leadership and Governance

Leadership and governance in building a health system involve ensuring that strategic policy frameworks exist and are combined with effective oversight, coalition-building, regulation, attention to system design, accountability for implementation, and achieving desired outcomes. There are two indicators of effective health system leadership/governance: (1) rules-based and (2) outcome-based. *Rules-based indicators* measure whether countries have appropriate policies, strategies, and codified approaches for health system governance. *Outcome-based indicators* measure whether rules and procedures are effectively implemented or enforced, based on the experience of relevant stakeholders. Intrinsic to good leadership and governance is accountability—for outcomes and appropriate use of resources. Thus, under good leadership, one sees good plans and

Table 2.11 National/Social Health Insurance schemes

Country	National/Social Health Insurance
Bangladesh	NA
Bhutan	Free universal healthcare for all citizens (1970)
India	Rashtriya Swasthiya Bima Yojana (2008) and Ayushman Bharat (2018)
Indonesia	Jaminan Kesehatan National (JKN), National Health Insurance scheme
Maldives	Universal health insurance scheme, "Aasandha" (2012)
Myanmar	NA
Nepal	National Health Insurance Program (2016)
Sri Lanka	Plans to set up a National Health Insurance Scheme
Thailand	National Health Insurance under three different Schemes (2002)
Timor-Leste	NA

NA not available

clear direction, which in turns help in mobilizing required resources, shaping policies, and becoming accountable for stated outcomes. This form of leadership/governance requires both political and technical action because it involves reconciling competing demands for limited resources in changing circumstances.

While leadership has proven to be the most important element in the health systems, we are yet to see systematic processes that nurture and grow leadership, both at the institution and national levels.

2.3 Future Directions

In conclusion, effective eye care (to eliminate avoidable blindness and visual impairment) can be achieved at sub-national or national levels. However, this requires planning for the true eye care needs of the community, developing an enabling eco-system, and designing service delivery to be inclusive by addressing key barriers such as access and affordability. The delivery system should also own the entire care process until the care loop is closed. The first step towards this is to ensure that all those who will benefit from an eye care intervention, seek it, and receive a comprehensive eye examination, appropriate diagnosis, and intervention advice. The next step is to ensure that they can comply with the intervention advised, regardless of whether it is medicines, glasses, surgery, or a routine follow-up visit to keep the condition under control as required in glaucoma or diabetic retinopathy. To achieve all of this, a good plan, an involved leadership, appropriate resources, enabling policies, and a robust contemporary information system both at the hospital and program levels are required to attain "Health for All."

References

1. World Health Organization. Constitution. www.who.int. Accessed 17 Aug 2020.
2. The World health report 2000: health systems: improving performance. https://www.who.int/whr/2000/en/. Accessed 28 Oct 2020.
3. World Report on Vision. Geneva: World Health Organization. 2019. www.who.int. Accessed 22 Oct 2020.
4. https://www.census.gov/data-tools/demo/idb/informationGateway.php. Accessed 28 Sept 2020.
5. Tham YC, Li X, Wong TY, et al. Global prevalence of glaucoma and projections of glaucoma burden through 2040. A systematic review and meta-analysis. Ophthalmology. 2014;121:2081–90.
6. https://population.un.org/wpp/Download/Standard/Population/. Accessed 29 Oct 2020.
7. Fletcher AE, Donoghue M, Devavaram J, et al. Low uptake of eye services in rural India: a challenge for programs of blindness prevention. Arch Ophthalmol. 1999;117:1393–9.
8. India—Cataract blindness control project. Washington, DC: World Bank Group. http://documents.worldbank.org/curated/en/238341468752788935/India-Cataract-Blindness-Control-Project. Accessed 26 Sept 2020.
9. Ramasamy D, Joseph S, Valaguru V, et al. Cluster randomized trial to compare spectacle delivery systems at outreach eye camps in South India. Ophthalmic Epidemiol. 2013;20:308–14.
10. Delivering quality health services: a global imperative for universal health coverage, Geneva: World Health Organization, Organisation for Economic Co-operation and Development, and The World Bank; 2018. https://www.who.int/servicedeliverysafety/quality-report/en/. Accessed 24 Aug 2020.
11. https://ichom.org/files/medical-conditions/cataracts/cataracts-reference-guide.pdf. Accessed 5 Oct 2020.
12. https://www.eurequo.org/. Accessed 5 Oct 2020.
13. https://www.aao.org/iris-registry. Accessed 5 Oct 2020.
14. http://www.acrm.org.my/ned/cataractSurgeryRegistry.html. Accessed 5 Oct 2020.
15. Ravindran RD, Gupta S, Haripriya A, et al. Seven-year trends in cataract surgery indications and quality of outcomes at Aravind Eye Hospitals, India. Eye. 2020; https://doi.org/10.1038/s41433-020-0954-5.
16. Congdon N, Dodson S, Chan VF, et al. Improving the practice of cataract surgical outcome measurement. Community Eye Health. 2019;31(104):91–2.
17. The World Health Report 2006—working together for health. Geneva: World Health Organization. 2006, https://www.who.int/whr/2006/en/. Accessed 22 Mar 2010.
18. Cambridge declaration 2015. www.icoph.org. Accessed 5 Oct 2020.
19. Foster A. Cataract and "Vision 2020- the right to sight" initiative. Br J Ophthalmol. 2001;85:635–9.
20. Ramke J, Gilbert CE, Lee AC, et al. Effective cataract surgical coverage: An indicator for measuring quality-of-care in the context of Universal Health Coverage. PLoS One 2017; https://doi.org/10.1371/journal.pone.0172342. Accessed 5 Oct 2020.
21. McCormick I, Mactaggart I, Bastawrous A, et al. Effective refractive error coverage: an eye health indicator to measure programs towards universal health coverage. Ophthalmic Physiol Optics. 2019; https://doi.org/10.1111/opo.12662.

22. Web-based consultation on the development of feasible global targets for 2030 on integrated people-centred eye care. WHO. 13 Oct 2020. Geneva: Call for Consultation. Accessed 5 Oct 2020.
23. Reddy PA, Congdon N, MacKenzie G, et al. Effect of providing near glasses on productivity among rural Indian tea workers with presbyopia (PROSPER): a randomised trial. Lancet Glob Health. 2018; https://doi.org/10.1016/S2214-109X(18)30329-2.
24. Danquah L, Kuper H, Eusebio C, et al. The long term impact of cataract surgery on quality of life, activities and poverty: Results from a six- year longitudinal study in Bangladesh and the Philippines. PLoS One. 2014; https://doi.org/10.1371/journal.pone.0094140.

Universal Health Coverage and Primary Eye Care

3

Khaleda Islam, A. H. M. Enayet Hussain, Taraprasad Das, Lutful Husain, and Munir Ahmed

Key Points

- Universal health coverage (UHC) is defined as the availability of the full range of essential health services and means that all people must have access to the health services they need, when and where they need them, without financial hardship.
- UHC is one of the targets of sustainable development goals (SDG; goal 3, target—3.8).
- At the Alma-Ata Declaration of 1978, all countries belonging to the World Health Organization (WHO) committed to primary healthcare; this commitment was reconfirmed in 2018 Astana Declaration.
- Primary Health Care is the provision of appropriate, accessible, and affordable healthcare that also meets patients' primary eye care (PEC) needs in a comprehensive and competent manner to identify diseases before they become serious medical issues.
- The essential health services index for the UHC in the WHO South-East Asia Region is less than 61%.
- SDG promotes multisectoral engagement and integration of PEC with general health.
- The WHO South-East Asia Region needs an increase in the eye health workforce; training and deploying a large number of allied ophthalmic personnel.
- Effective public–private partnerships and engagement with non-government organizations are required to accomplish this (Fig. 3.1).

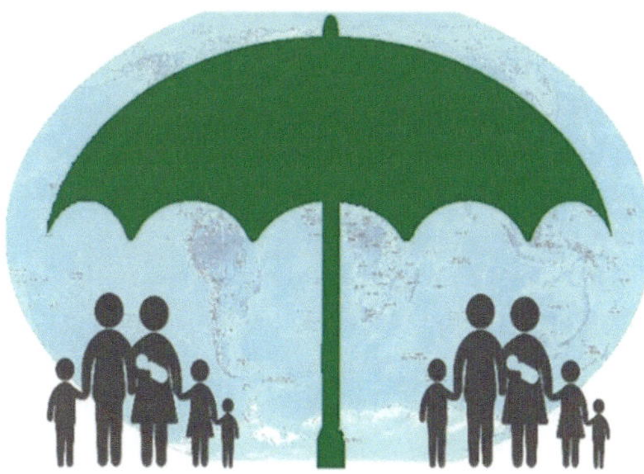

Fig. 3.1 Source: World Health Organization

K. Islam
Directorate General of Health Services, Ministry of Health and Family Welfare, Dhaka, Bangladesh

A. H. M. Enayet Hussain (✉)
Directorate General of Medical Education, Ministry of Health and Family Welfare, Dhaka, Bangladesh

T. Das
L V Prasad Eye Institute, Hyderabad, India
e-mail: tpd@lvpei.org

L. Husain · M. Ahmed
Orbis International, Dhaka, Bangladesh
e-mail: Lutful.husain@orbis.org; Munir.Ahmed@orbis.org

T. Das, P. D. Nayar (eds.), *South-East Asia Eye Health*, https://doi.org/10.1007/978-981-16-3787-2_3

3.1 Universal Health Coverage (UHC)

UHC is defined as the availability of health services to people when and where they are required, without causing financial hardship. It includes the full range of essential health services, from health promotion to disease prevention, treatment, rehabilitation, and palliative care [1]. For sound health policies, the two main dimensions of UHC are access to essential healthcare and financial protection.

Achieving UHC is one of the targets of sustainable development goals (SDG; goal 3, target 3.8). This target addresses issues of financial risk protection during a health crisis, access to essential healthcare services of good quality, and access to safe, effective, and affordable essential medicines and vaccines of good quality for all. The UHC works best when it is contextualized against every country's social, political, and cultural backgrounds. SDG 3.8 has two indicators: (1) SDG 3.8.1, which covers essential health services (reproductive, maternal, newborn and child health, infectious diseases, non-communicable diseases) and service capacity and access among the general and most disadvantaged population; and (2) SDG 3.8.2, which focuses on health expenditures and indicates the proportion of families with large household expenditures on health as a share of total household expenditure. Monitored together, these two indicators can capture all dimensions of healthcare service coverage and financial protection [2].

The service coverage index (SCI) of UHC is an indicator of the service capacity of and access to essential health services (defined as the average coverage of essential services based on tracer interventions) among the general and most disadvantaged populations. The UHC SCI monitoring report of 2019 on SDG indicator 3.8.1 emphasizes that although service coverage has increased from a global average of 45% in 2000 to 66% in 2017, this increase is not happening fast enough. The increase in SCI has been greatest in lower-income countries and was mainly driven by infectious disease interventions. The increase was also due to interventions for improving reproductive, maternal, newborn, and child health services, though this was to a much lower extent. However, the poorest countries and those affected by conflict generally lag far behind the global average; besides, the middle-income countries that account for the largest populations usually lack coverage for essential health services [3].

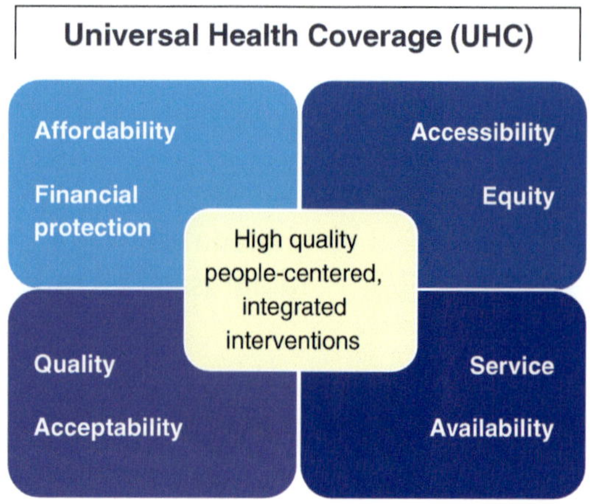

Fig. 3.2 Essential qualities of universal health coverage (UHC) [5]

Ideally, UHC should provide for good quality care integrated with other health systems; also, this care must be 'people-centered' rather than 'disease-centered' [4]. The four essential components of UHC are (1) affordability (financial protection), (2) accessibility (equity), (3) quality (acceptability), and (4) service (availability) (Fig. 3.2) [5].

3.1.1 Health Financing for Universal Health Coverage

Health financing is a critical component of UHC. Every country has its unique financial systems of collection (such as government budget, general tax, and insurance) and distribution [6]. In 2017, the national health expenditure measured by gross domestic product (GDP) was highest in the Maldives and lowest in Bangladesh in the South-East Asia region (Fig. 3.3) [7]. Out-of-pocket spending is currently lowest in the Maldives (18%) and highest in Bangladesh (67%) [8].

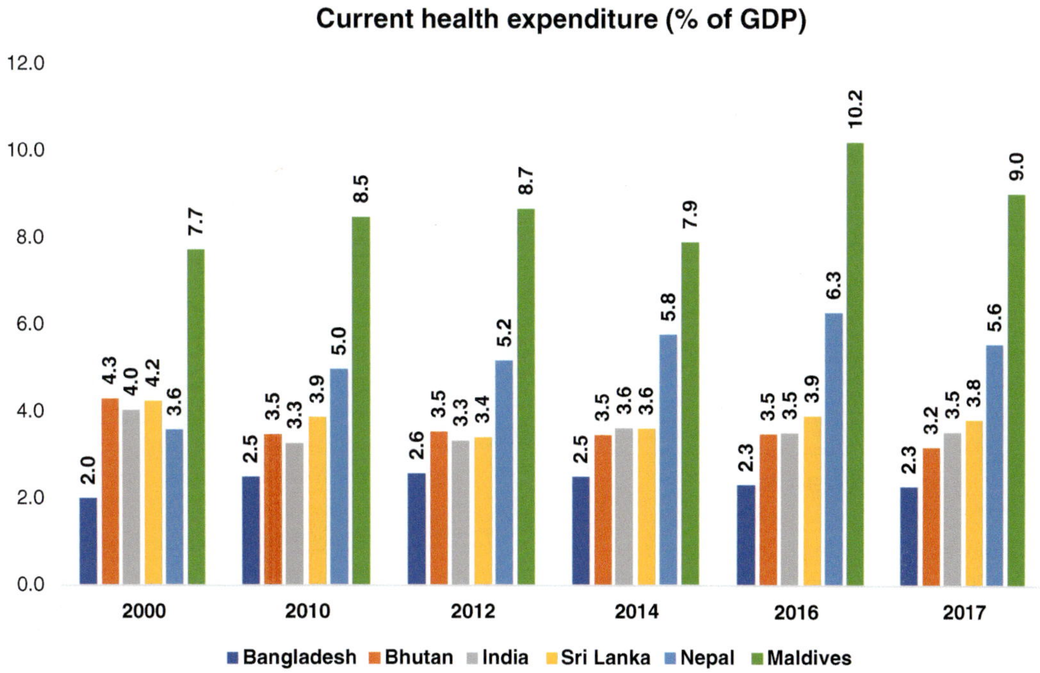

Fig. 3.3 Current health expenditure in GDP of selected South-East Asian countries in 2017 [7]

3.1.2 Global and Regional Policies and Programs Related to UHC

The countries in the WHO South-East Asia Region are at different stages of developing their UHC policies. The regional average for essential SCI is at 57%, and the expenditure for healthcare from pre-paid mechanisms is at 42%. West Africa's free healthcare system [9] is not practiced in the South-East Asian region, and policies vary widely between different countries. For example, eye health in Bhutan is mostly free, while it is entirely insurance covered (third party engaged by the government) in the Maldives; in other countries in this region, eye health operates on a hybrid system of government-supported free care, government or private insurance, and out-of-pocket spending. With the global commitment to UHC for 1 billion more people by 2023, the WHO South-East Asia Region will need to provide UHC for at least 300 million people by 2023 [10].

The WHO South-East Asia Regional Committee is tracking UHC's progress with particular emphasis on the human resource for health (HRH) and access to medicines [10]. As of now, there is a shortage of eye care HRH in all countries in the region [11]. Although global efforts have reduced the age-standardized prevalence of blindness and visual impairment, over the next 30 years, aging and growth of the global population will lead to a tripling in the numbers of people affected with eye problems; this is likely lead to 700 million visually impaired people including 115 million blind people [12]. Global estimates of annual costs for medical treatment and management of these patients are likely to exceed USD3 trillion and will have substantial economic implications for affected individuals, families, and communities [13]. The good news is that ~80% of the projected numbers of vision loss is preventable or treatable. The bad news is that 90% of the disease burden will occur in low- and middle-income countries (LMICs) [13]. The added challenge of weak healthcare systems in this region, particularly, essential primary eye care, remains a concern [8]. The private sectors, including non-governmental organizations (NGOs), contribute to a large portion of eye care finance in many South-East Asian countries, mostly secondary and tertiary eye care. At the primary level, however, governments are usually the principal service providers.

Many countries in South-East Asia have adopted several innovative approaches to eye care delivery, including mobile eye care (outreach services, 'eye camps') for cataract surgery and pilot projects for trachoma control. In general, eye care programs tend to be more successful in countries with well-developed central healthcare that has a robust functioning primary health care system [8].

> **Box 3.1 Levels of healthcare** [18]
>
> **Primary healthcare**
>
> Primary health care denotes the first level of contact between individuals and families with the health system. Primary health care should include care for mother and child (which provides for family planning and immunization), prevention of locally endemic diseases, treatment of common diseases or injuries, provision of essential facilities, health education, provision of food and nutrition, and ensuring an adequate supply of safe drinking water.
>
> **Secondary healthcare**
>
> Secondary healthcare refers to the second level of the health system, in which patients from the primary care centers are referred to specialists in higher tier hospitals for treatment.
>
> **Tertiary healthcare**
>
> Tertiary healthcare refers to the third level of the health system, in which specialized consultative care is usually provided on referral from primary and secondary medical care. Specialized intensive care units, advanced diagnostic support services, and specialized medical personnel are the key features of tertiary healthcare.

3.2 Primary Healthcare

In October 2018, health policymakers from more than 120 countries met in Astana, Kazakhstan, and renewed their commitment to ensuring comprehensive primary health care for all; this came to be known as the Astana declaration. This declaration reconfirmed the earlier Alma-Ata declaration (1978) that 'the enjoyment of the highest attainable standard of health without distinction of any kind is the fundamental right of every human being' [14].

The Alma-Ata Declaration had an ambitious goal of achieving 'health for all by the year 2000' [15]. The Alma-Ata declaration also changed healthcare interpretation to include universal access, equity, intersectoral collaboration, and continuity of care; it encouraged all member states to offer a full spectrum of healthcare from households to hospitals, where prevention is as important as the cure [16]. The Astana declaration recognizes that remaining healthy is challenging for 'particularly poor' people and that inequity in health delivery and disparities in health outcomes are 'unacceptable' [14]. The fundamental concepts of 'health for all' are: (1) health is a fundamental human right, and attainment of the highest possible level of health is the most critical social goal; (2) unacceptable inequality in the health status of people is the common concern of all countries; (3) active engagement of people to take responsibility of own health is the main objective; (4) Primary health care should provide universally accessible essential service packages at an affordable cost; (5) Primary health care should bring healthcare to the doorstep of the community and must create the first level of contact for individuals with the national health system; (6) countries must allocate finances for primary health care [17].

3.2.1 Primary Eye Care (PEC)

PEC is providing care for and identifying diseases of the eyes before they become serious medical issues. It is the provision of appropriate, accessible, and affordable care that meets patients' eye care needs in a comprehensive and competent manner [18]. Competent management and decision-making are critical in promoting the quality and efficiency of PEC. PEC usually covers (1) eye health education, (2) symptom identification, (3) visual acuity measurements, (3) basic eye examinations, (4) diagnosis, and (5) timely referrals (Table 3.1) [19].

3.2.2 Current Status of UHC in South-East Asia

The essential health services index for UHC in the WHO South-East Asia Region has increased from an average of 46% in 2010 to an average of 61% in 2019; however, over 65 million people are still pushed into poverty because of healthcare expenditure. In the South-East Asian region, the WHO is focusing on supporting countries in improving their health workforce and access to medicines [20] (Fig. 3.4).

3.2.2.1 PEC in Bangladesh

The 2003, published data reported that in people aged 30 years or more in Bangladesh, 13.8% had low vision in both eyes and that the age-standardized prevalence of blindness was 1.53%. The leading causes of visual impairment were cataract (74.2%), refractive error (18.7%), and macular degeneration (1.9%). Cataract was the

Table 3.1 Primary eye care services at the local level through a vision center approach [19]

	Diagnosis	Referral	Intervention			
Eye health concerns			Preventive	Curative	Rehab	Compliance and follow-up
Refractive error	X	X	–	X	–	X
Cataract	X	X	–	–	–	X
Diabetic retinopathy	X	X	–	–	–	X
Glaucoma	X	X	–	–	–	X
Corneal injury/infection	X	X	X	–	–	X
Children eyecare	X	–	X	–	X	X
Low vision	X	–	–	–	X	X
Visually challenged	X	–	–	–	X	X

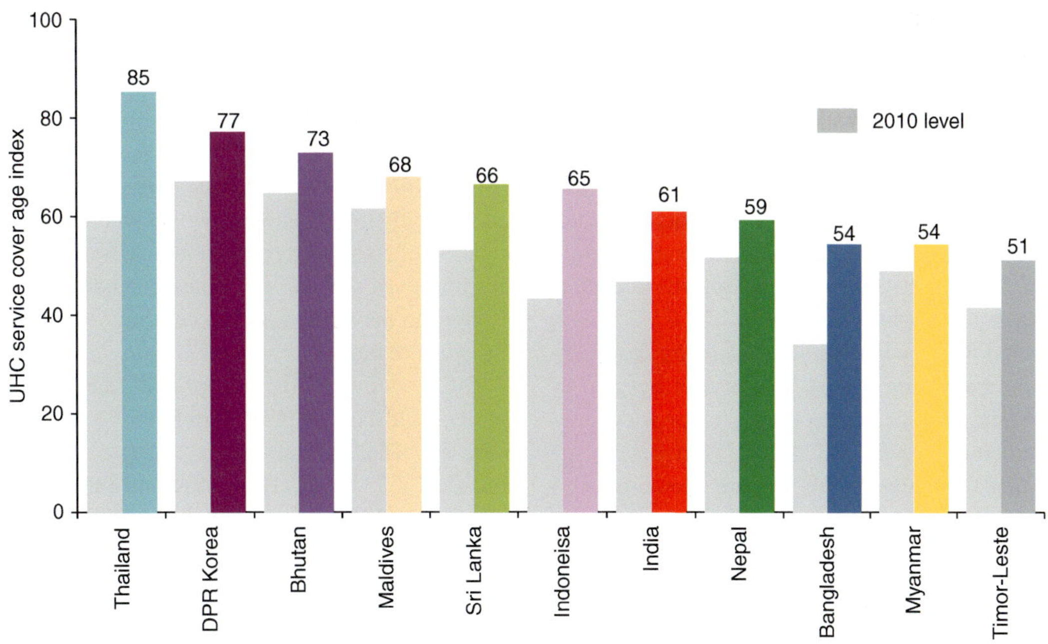

Fig. 3.4 Changes in the coverage of essential health services in the WHO South-East Asia Region between 2010 and 2019 [20]

predominant cause (79.6%) of bilateral blindness, followed by uncorrected aphakia (6.2%) and macular degeneration (3.1%). The study recommended the need for implementation of a national PEC plan to deliver effective eye care services, resolve the cataract backlog, and reduce the burden of refractive error [21]. The current prevalence of diabetes in Bangladesh is 8.4% [22] and is increasing, as are the prevalence of other noncommunicable diseases such as retinopathy of prematurity (ROP) and glaucoma. In Dhaka slums, the prevalence of vision impairment is 16.4%; the usual causes are refractive error (63.2%) and conjunctivitis (17.1%), both of which can be managed effectively with the PEC [23].

In 2017, Bangladesh spent ~2.3% of the GDP on healthcare services [7]. To establish and maintain PEC, the country needs to increase the efficiency of revenue collection by reprioritizing government budgets, designing an innovative financing strategy, or managing development assistance [24]. The 4th Health Population Nutrition Sector Program (HPNSP; January 2017 to June 2022) in Bangladesh addressed UHC and healthcare financing strategy [25, 26]. It recommended customized and context-specific policy adjustments for progress towards UHC and achieving the SDGs [27]. The program further suggested a collaborative partnership between for-profit and not-for-profit private sectors, development partners, and the community to resolve the financing challenges. Bangladesh also has a National Eye Care (NEC) operation plan that advised establishing Community Vision Center (CVC) at the Upazila (sub-district) Health Complex (UzHC) and populating these centers with trained ophthalmic nurses. The CVC is connected with the base center (secondary or tertiary eye care facility located at a district hospital or medical college, respectively) to provide telemedicine support and referral services to the patients. Currently, 70 CVCs are operating in 24 districts in Bangladesh, against a plan to establish 200 CVCs by the end of June 2022 [28]. Several NGOs working on eye care are complementing the government effort to establish CVCs in Bangladesh. Bangladesh has demonstrated a successful model of public–private/NGO partnership in eye care and reaching communities, especially poor, women, and children. This approach could be leveraged to faster the process in achieving universal eye health coverage.

3.2.2.2 PEC in Bhutan

Bhutan faces a twin challenge an inadequate health workforce and a hilly terrain in providing PEC. Currently, Bhutan has only 8 ophthalmologists, the majority of whom work in the capital city. Bhutan relies on a network of over 50 allied ophthalmic personnel (AOP) in remote locations to provide appropriate and essential PEC, and much of its population depends on 'eye camps' for eye care. With technical assistance from development partners, Bhutan is strengthening the PEC system in its primary health care facilities [29].

3.2.2.3 PEC in India

In 1976, India transformed the National Trachoma Control Program into a more comprehensive National Program for Control of Blindness (and Visual Impairment) to address national eye health priorities. The country introduced self-monitoring and institutional monitoring records for cataract surgery. India also developed and validated rapid assessment tools for blindness and cataract surgical services between 1992 and 1996. In the 1980s and 1990s, India developed and promoted cataract surgery protocols, encouraged manual small-incision cataract surgery (MSICS), and used intraocular lenses (IOL), which led to reduced cost and better visual outcomes after cataract surgery. This initiative improved access to cataract surgery for economically disadvantaged people, and discontinuation of cataract surgery in improvised facilities improved surgical outcomes. Many LMICs in Asia and the world have successfully adopted this eye care model.

PHC is delivered through primary and community health centers (CHCs) in India. Currently, India has 160,713 sub-centers, 30,045 PHCs, 5685 CHCs, 734 district hospitals, and 542 medical colleges [30, 31]. In the recent past, the Indian Government has planned to convert sub-centers into "Health and Wellness Centers." However, eye care service is not available in many publicly funded primary and community health centers. In addition, although several not-for-profit eye hospitals provide primary eye care, these are not integrated into the general healthcare system.

3.2.2.4 PEC in the Maldives

The provision of primary eye care in the Maldives faces similar problems to those faced by Bhutan, namely, an inadequate healthcare workforce that is unequally distributed (most of the healthcare workforce is concentrated in the capital city). Studies have shown that nearly half of the patients in the Maldives travel outside the country for cataract surgeries. In addition, despite good cataract surgical coverage, the outcomes of cataract surgeries are below the WHO standard. The country needs a robust regional and primary eye care plan [32].

3.2.2.5 PEC in Thailand and Myanmar

Thailand contextualized the WHO guideline for emphasizing the prevailing eye conditions of the country and initiated a PEC model in 1981. In the same year, Myanmar also started its own PEC model and prioritized specific eye problems that seemed most prevalent or important in the country [33].

3.3 Integration

The SDGs promote multisectoral engagement and envisage the maximum benefits of universal health coverage only when it is integrated into general healthcare systems. Globally, 3.46% of people are blind or visually impaired; this roughly translates to 253 million people of the world's 7.3 billion population. Of these, 36 million (0.49%) are blind and 217 million (2.97%) are visually impaired [34]. Although it may seem difficult to sustain an entire program around vision problems, this can be achieved by integrating primary eye care with primary health care; such integration could make eye care more cost-effective. For example, cataract screening can be combined with healthy aging, refractive error testing can be integrated with healthy school life, testing for ROP can be integrated with maternal and child health, and screening for diabetic retinopathy can be integrated with management of non-communicable diseases [19]. When the primary eye care is combined with a robust referral system, the setup works well for complete and comprehensive eye care. With the availability of technology today, such integration is very much possible (Fig. 3.5). By aligning current technology and available resources, every country can improve its health policies by focusing on capacity building, task sharing, public–private partnerships, digitization of health records, and cross-learning of best practices across the region.

Box 3.2 Programs to Address: Refractive Error and Diabetic Retinopathy in Bangladesh

DRESTI (District Refractive Error and Eye Care Search and Treat Initiative)

VisionSpring with the Ministry of Health and Family Welfare (MOH&FW) of Bangladesh initiated the DRESTI project in the Sherpur district (Fig. 3.6) under the Clear Vision Collective (CVC) consortium. CVC is formed by VisionSpring and ten other NGOs and is being implemented from January 2019 to December 2020. DRESTI is focused on addressing refractive error at the primary eye care level. The initiative is driven by existing or newly established vision centers, training rural medical providers to dispense reading glasses, supporting optical outlets, and training health workers to conduct community vision camps. CVC is also operating eye care programs in schools. The project is creating a model to encourage the availability of affordable glasses at people's doorsteps, at the school and community levels. It is also establishing a robust referral system linking the community-level primary care with secondary and tertiary care services.

In 2019, a total of 78,994 people of all ages were screened, 31,294 (40%) were diagnosed with presbyopia/refractive error, and 12,750 (41% of those diagnosed) received spectacles at an affordable cost. In the same year, 2806 cataract surgeries (for 6014 diagnosed patients) were performed in the Sherpur district in public and/or

NGO eye care facilities. The DRESTI project has now been extended to benefit other urban, rural, and ethnic minorities [35].

Diabetic Retinopathy (DR) Referral Network

Based on the Diabetic Retinopathy National Strategy, Orbis International in collaboration with The National Eye Care (NEC), Non-Communicable Disease Control (NCDC) under the MOH&FW and the Bangladesh Diabetic Society (BADAS) have created a diabetic retinopathy referral network in the Gopalganj district (Fig. 3.6), centered on the Sheikh Fazilatunnesa Mujib Eye Hospital and Training Institute (SFMEHTI), a tertiary eye hospital. Eyecare is provided in the district at different levels—at the Community Clinic (CC) of Community Based Health care (CBHC), Community Vision Center (CVC) at the Upzila Health Complex, the district diabetic hospital of BADAS, and SFMEHTI. Comprehensive eye care is provided at the CVC; people with diabetes are referred to SFMEHTI for further management of retinopathy. The district diabetes hospital provides training of midlevel ophthalmic personnel (DR grader and Fundus Photographer), and SFMEHTI trains physicians, including the ophthalmologists.

In 2019, the project identified 1476 people with diabetes (after screening 5664 people) at the community level and detected diabetic retinopathy in 580 people (after screening 3728 people with diabetes) at the hospital level [36].

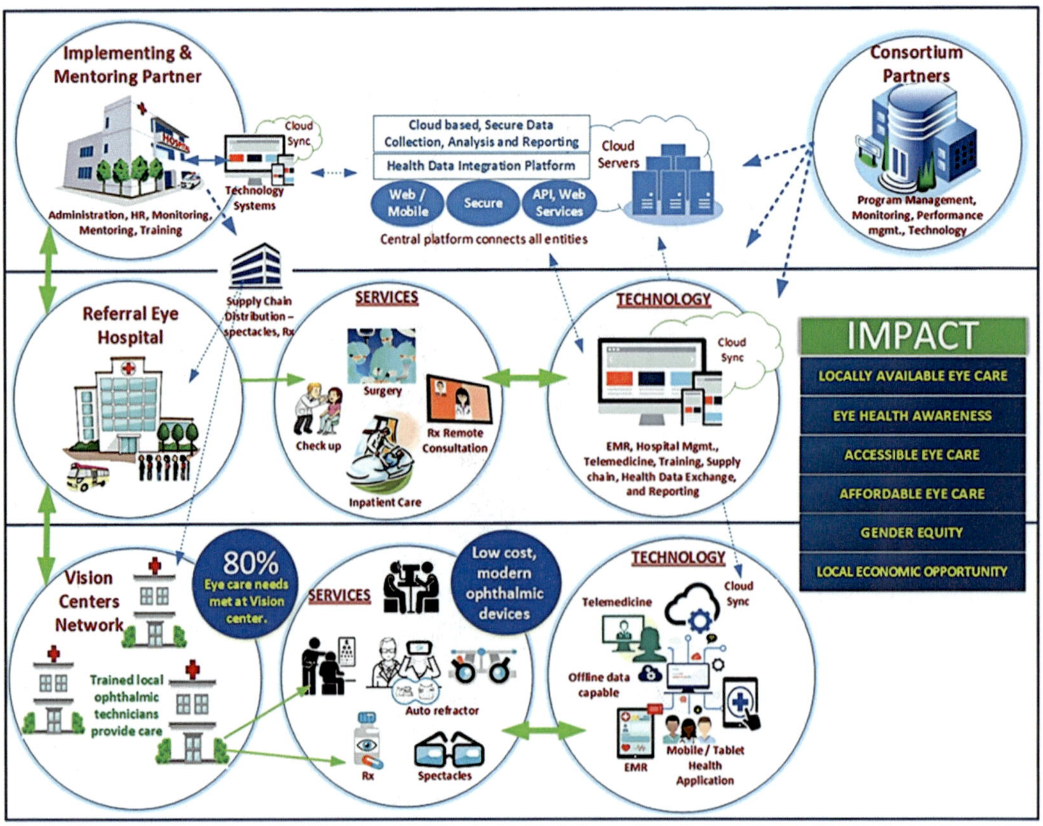

Fig. 3.5 Leveraging technology for universal eye health

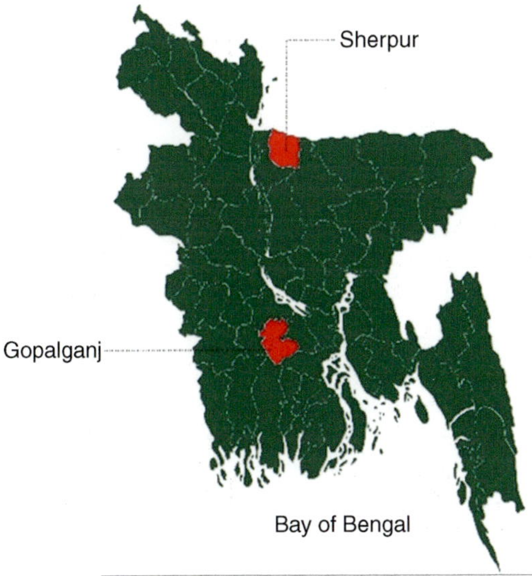

Fig. 3.6 Project locations in Bangladesh

3.4 Conclusion and Recommendations

- The integration of primary eye care into essential healthcare service packages is necessary. This must include an assured and regular supply of spectacles and eye care medicines. The system should encompass all sectors of the population, including women and children and the poor, vulnerable, disabled, and remote rural and hard-to-reach sections of the population.
- Recognition of ophthalmic allied personnel, with appropriate training for different cadres, such as vision technicians, refractionists, etc. and their fair distribution in all health posts is important.
- An innovative pro-poor and pro-disadvantaged primary eye care program uniquely designed for each country can reduce/prevent out-of-pocket spending and ease the burden of medical bills in poor households.
- Establishing a responsive referral system from the community level to the district and tertiary eye hospitals is essential to ensure the entire spectrum of eye care.
- Public and private partnerships, including NGOs with innovative approaches to exploring cost-effective primary eye care models, can improve health financing.

References

1. World Health Organization. Universal health coverage (UHC), Key facts; What is UHC? Available: www.who.int. Accessed 22 Aug 2020.
2. World Health Organization. UHC service coverage index, Associated Indicators, UHC Index of service coverage (SCI). www.who.int. Accessed 22 Aug 2020.
3. Global Monitoring Report. Primary health care on the road to universal health coverage. 2019. www.who.int. Accessed 22 Aug 2020.
4. World report on vision. www.who.int. Accessed 22 Aug 2020.
5. Universal health coverage. Key facts. www.who.int. Accessed 22 Aug 2020.
6. Bump JB. The long road to universal health coverage: historical analysis of early decisions in Germany, the United Kingdom, and the United States. Health Syst Reform. 2015;1(1):28–38. https://doi.org/10.4161/23288604.2014.991211.
7. The World Bank. Current health expenditure (% of GDP)—Bangladesh, Nepal, Bhutan, India, Maldives, Sri Lanka. www.worldbank.org. Accessed 22 Aug 2020.
8. Murthy GV. Eye care in South Asia, 1988–2018: developments, achievements and future challenges. Community Eye Health. 2017;30(100):99–101.
9. World Health Organization. Free health care policies; Key facts, 3 May 2020. Available: https://www.who.int/news-room/fact-sheets/detail/free-health-care-policies. Data retrieved on 23 Aug 2020.
10. WHO. Universal Health Coverage: everyone, everywhere. www.who.int. Accessed 23 Aug 2020.
11. Das T, Keeffe J, Sivaprasad S, Rao GN. Capacity building for universal eye health coverage in South East Asia beyond 2020. Eye. 2020;34:1262–70. https://doi.org/10.1038/s41433-020-0801-8.
12. Bourne RRA, Flaxman SR, Braithwaite T, et al. Magnitude, temporal trends, and projections of the global prevalence of blindness and distance and near vision impairment: a systematic review and meta-analysis. Lancet Glob Health. 2017;5:e888–97.
13. Gordois A, Cutler H, Pezzullo L, et al. An estimation of the worldwide economic and health burden of visual impairment. Glob Public Health. 2012;7:465–81.
14. World Health Organization. Declaration of Astana. Geneva: World Health Organization. www.who.int. Accessed 26 Aug 2020.
15. World Health Organization. Declaration of Alma Ata. Geneva: World Health Organization. www.who.int. Accessed 26 Aug 2020.
16. World Health Organization. 2008 World Health Report. Primary health care: now more than ever. Geneva: World Health Organization. www.who.int/whr. Accessed 26 Aug 2020.
17. Social determinants of health: WHO called to return to the Declaration of Alma-Ata; International conference on primary health care. www.who.int/social_determinants/tools. Accessed 22 Aug 2020.

18. Primary Eye Care. www.aao.org/clinical-statement/defintion-of- primary-eye-care-policy-statement. Accessed 27 Aug 2020.
19. Murthy GVS, Raman U. Perspectives on primary eye care Community Eye Health. 2009;22:10–11. PMID: 19506714
20. Monitoring progress on universal health coverage and the health-related Sustainable Development Goals in the WHO South-East Asia Region: 2019 update. www.who.int]soutjesastasia/health-topics/universal-health-coverage. Accessed 24 Aug 2020.
21. Dineen BP, Bourne RR, Ali SM, et al. Prevalence and causes of blindness and visual impairment in Bangladeshi adults: results of the National Blindness and Low Vision Survey of Bangladesh. Br J Ophthalmol. 2003;87(7):820–8. https://doi.org/10.1136/bjo.87.7.820.
22. Ministry of Health and Family Welfare Bangladesh. Bangladesh NCD risk factor survey 2018. Fact sheet.
23. Sutradhar I, Gayen P, Hasan M, et al. Eye diseases: the neglected health condition among urban slum population of Dhaka, Bangladesh. BMC Ophthalmol. 2019;19:38. https://doi.org/10.1186/s12886-019-1043-z.
24. World Health Organization. The world health report 2010: health systems financing: the path to universal coverage. Geneva. 2010. www.who.int. Accessed 22 Aug 2020.
25. The 4th Health, Nutrition and Population Sector Program (HNPSP) (January 2017–June 22), Program Implementation Plan (PIP), Volume-1, January 2017, Ministry of Health and Family Welfare, Government of People's Republic of Bangladesh.
26. Government of Bangladesh, Expanding Social Protection for Health Towards Universal Coverage: Health Care Financing Strategy 2012–2032, Dhaka, Bangladesh, 2012. www.socialprotection.gov.bd. Accessed 24 Aug 2020.
27. Joarder T, Chaudhury TZ, Mannan I. Universal health coverage in Bangladesh: activities, challenges, and suggestions. Adv Public Health. 2019; https://doi.org/10.1155/2019/4954095.
28. 4th Health Population Nutrition Sector program (HNPSP), National Eye Care (NEC) Operation Plan (OP). Ministry of Health and Family Welfare, Government of People's Republic of Bangladesh.
29. Bhutan: Strengthening Eye Care Services and Training. Cure Blindness; Himalayan Cataract Project. www.ngoaidmap.org/projects/18673. Accessed 25 Aug 2020.
30. www.mohfw.gov.in. Accessed 16 Jul 2020.
31. www.niti.gov.in. Accessed 16 Jul 2020.
32. Thoufeeq U, Das T, Limburg H, et al. First rapid assessment of avoidable blindness survey in the Maldives: prevalence and causes of blindness and cataract surgery. Asia Pac J Ophthalmol (Phila). 2018;7:316–20. https://doi.org/10.22608/APO.2017332.
33. Konyama K. Essential components of primary eye care. Community Eye Health. 1998;11:19–21.
34. IAPB. Vision atlas. www.atlas.iapb.org. Accessed 20 Aug 2020.
35. OneSight helps launch multi-year eyecare initiative in Bangladesh. 24 Jan 2019. www.onesight.org. Accessed 25 Aug 2020.
36. Project report of BADAS ICOM database, and Orbis Bangladesh (Unpublished). Data retrieved on 30 Aug 2020.

Sustainable Development Goal 3: Good Health and Well-being

4

Taraprasad Das, Peter Holland, Munir Ahmed, and Lutful Husain

Key Points

- In 2015, the United Nations adopted Sustainable Development Goals (SDG).
- The broad agenda of SDG are to end poverty, combat climate change, and fight injustice and inequality over the next 15 years (2030).
- The UN resolution on the SDGs often refers to the five "P"s—People, Planet, Prosperity, Peace, and Partnerships.
- SDG has 17 inter-connected goals and 169 targets.
- SDG 3 is "Good Health and Well-being." It has 13 targets and 26 indicators.
- There has been variable achievement of SDG 3 goals in the South-East Asia region.
- Many infectious diseases have reduced. This includes two countries with zero trachoma and two countries malaria-free.
- Substantial resource commitment and policy-planning are required to accelerate the process to achieve universal health coverage by 2030.
- Concurrent development of connected SDG goals are required to meet the targets of SDG 3 goals.

In September 2015, the United Nations (UN) proposed Agenda 2030, an ambitious initiative to end poverty, combat climate change, and fight injustice and inequality over the next 15 years. Agenda 2030 promises a better future for all by setting out 17 sustainable development goals (SDGs) that the Member States of countries all over the world have committed to achieving. These goals cover a range of different topics—from ending poverty, improving healthcare, and building more inclusive and sustainable cities, to reducing the impacts of climate change (Fig. 4.1). The goals were adopted by all Member States of the UN formally in 2015 (September 25–27, 2015; at the 70th anniversary of the UN), and were effective from 1st January 2016 for the period 2016–2030.

These 17 goals, which are intimately interconnected with each other (Table 4.1), have 169 targets [1]. The practical and political importance of the SDGs, and the associated challenges follow the Millennium Development Goals (MDG, 2000–2015). The MDGs consisted of 8 international development goals: (1) eradicate extreme poverty; (2) achieve universal primary education; (3) promote gender equity and empower women; (4) reduce child mortality; (5) improve maternal health; (6) combat human immunodeficiency

T. Das (✉)
L V Prasad Eye Institute, Hyderabad, India
e-mail: tpd@lvpei.org

P. Holland
International Agency for the Prevention of Blindness, London, UK
e-mail: pholland@iapb.org

M. Ahmed · L. Husain
Orbis International, Dhaka, Bangladesh
e-mail: Munir.Ahmed@orbis.org; Lutful.husain@orbis.org

T. Das, P. D. Nayar (eds.), *South-East Asia Eye Health*,
https://doi.org/10.1007/978-981-16-3787-2_4

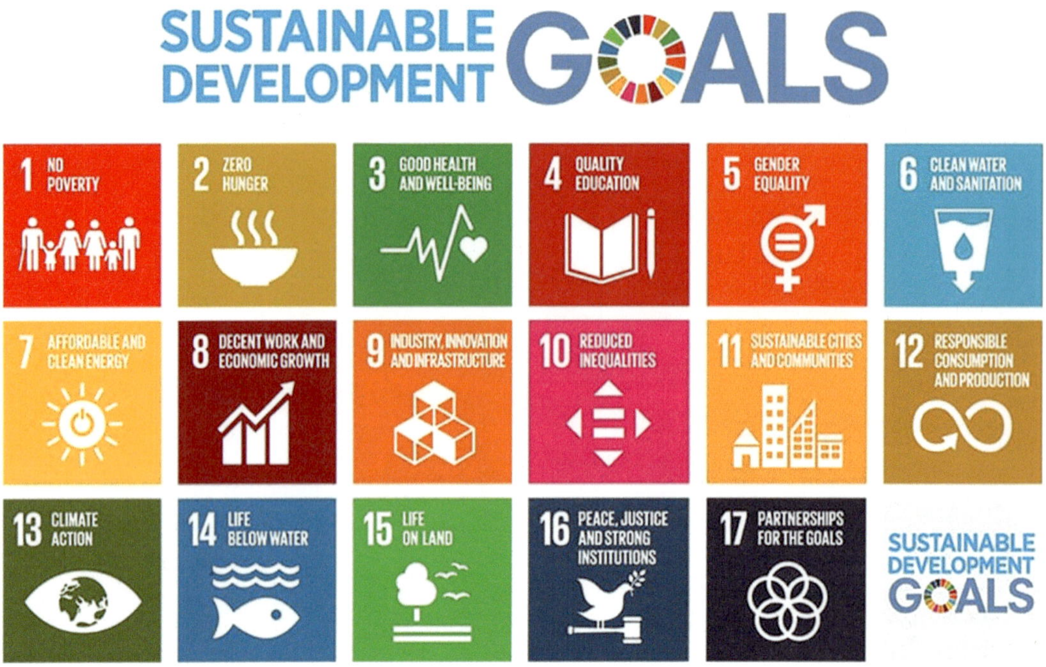
SUSTAINABLE DEVELOPMENT GOALS
1 NO POVERTY
2 ZERO HUNGER
3 GOOD HEALTH AND WELL-BEING
4 QUALITY EDUCATION
5 GENDER EQUALITY
6 CLEAN WATER AND SANITATION
7 AFFORDABLE AND CLEAN ENERGY
8 DECENT WORK AND ECONOMIC GROWTH
9 INDUSTRY, INNOVATION AND INFRASTRUCTURE
10 REDUCED INEQUALITIES
11 SUSTAINABLE CITIES AND COMMUNITIES
12 RESPONSIBLE CONSUMPTION AND PRODUCTION
13 CLIMATE ACTION
14 LIFE BELOW WATER
15 LIFE ON LAND
16 PEACE, JUSTICE AND STRONG INSTITUTIONS
17 PARTNERSHIPS FOR THE GOALS
SUSTAINABLE DEVELOPMENT GOALS

Fig. 4.1 The 17 Sustainable Development Goals (Source: WHO) [1]

virus (HIV)/acquired immunodeficiency syndrome (AIDS), malaria, and other diseases; (7) ensure environmental sustainability; and (8) develop global partnerships for development. The MDG focused primarily on the needs of developing countries.

The SDGs are broader in scope, collective in action, detailed in content, and are applicable to both developed and developing countries. The SDGs also required a political commitment (SDG goal 17) from developed countries to support less developed countries in finance, technology transfer, capacity building, increased trade, public–private partnership, and data management. The UN encouraged developed countries to commit an official development assistance (ODA) of 0.7% of their gross national income (GNI), and ODA of 0.15–0.2% of GNI for developing and least developed countries (LDCs) [2]. Achieving the SDGs will require an estimated collective investment of USD5–7 trillion (United States Dollars) annually by all member countries in the world. Up to 2017, the ODA share of the richer countries has reached USD147.2 billion [3].

The UN resolution on the SDGs often refers to the five "P"s which are five areas of critical importance, namely, People, Planet, Prosperity, Peace, and Partnerships.

- *People*—to end poverty and hunger and to ensure that all human beings can fulfill their potential in dignity and equality and in a healthy environment;
- *Planet*—to protect the planet from degradation; this includes steps to encourage sustainable consumption, production, and management of our planet's natural resources, and taking urgent action on climate change;
- *Prosperity*—to ensure that all human beings can enjoy prosperous and fulfilling lives and that economic, social, and technological progress occur in harmony with nature.
- *Peace*—to foster peaceful, just, and inclusive societies, which are free from fear and violence.
- *Partnership*—to mobilize the means required to implement the agenda through a revitalized global partnership for sustainable development, based on a spirit of strengthened global

Table 4.1 Sustainable Development Goals (17 targets and 169 indicators) [1]

Goal	Target	Indicators
1	End poverty in all its forms everywhere	7
2	End hunger, achieve food security and improved nutrition, and promote sustainable agriculture	8
3	Ensure healthy lives and promote well-being for all at all ages	13
4	Ensure inclusive an equitable quality education and promote lifelong learning opportunities for all	10
5	Achieve gender equality and empower all women and girls	9
6	Ensure availability and sustainable management of water and sanitation for all	8
7	Ensure access to affordable, reliable, sustainable, and modern energy for all	5
8	Promote sustained, inclusive, and sustainable economic growth; full and productive employment and decent work for all	12
9	Build resilient infrastructure, promote inclusive and sustainable industrialization, and foster innovation	8
10	Reduce inequality within and among countries	10
11	Make cities and human settlements inclusive, safe, resilient, and sustainable	10
12	Ensure sustainable consumption and production patterns	11
13	Take urgent action to combat climate change and its impacts	5
14	Conserve and sustainably use the oceans, seas, and marine resources for sustainable development	10
15	Protect, restore, and promote sustainable use of terrestrial ecosystems; sustainably manage forests, combat desertification, halt and reverse land degradation, and halt biodiversity loss	12
16	Promote peaceful and inclusive societies for sustainable development, provide access to justice for all, and build effective, accountable, and inclusive institutions at all levels	12
17	Strengthen the means of implementation and revitalize the Global Partnership for Sustainable Development	19

solidarity and particularly focused on the needs of the poorest and most vulnerable; this must be done with the participation of all countries, stakeholders, and people of the world [4].

The SDG has 17 goals and 169 targets (Table 4.1). The goals are interconnected. SDG 3 is "Good Health and Well-being." It is intimately connected with "Quality Education" (SDG 4), "Gender Equity" (SDG 5), "Clean water and Sanitation" (SDG 6), "Reduce Inequalities" (SDG 10), "Sustainable Cities and Communities" (SDG 11), and "Climate Action" (SDG 13).

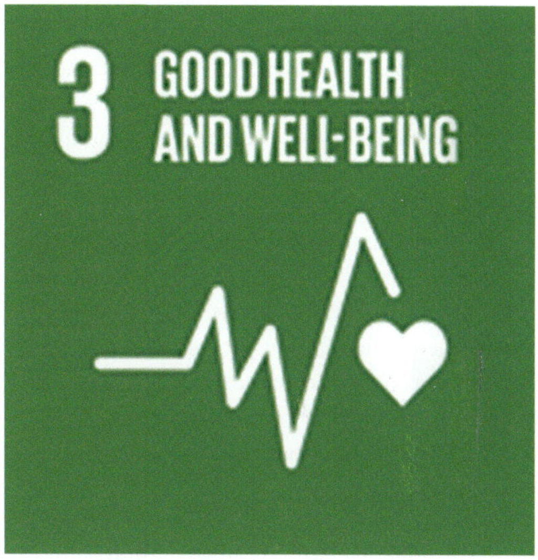

Good Health and Well-being: Ensure healthy lives and promote well-being for all at all ages

The World Health Organization (WHO) founding constitution (proposed at the International Health Conference, on 22 July 1946, and entered into force on 7 April 1948) defined health as "a state of complete physical, mental, and social well-being and not merely the absence of disease or infirmity" [5]. The WHO further clarified health as a "resource for everyday life, not the objective of living" at the Ottawa Charter for Health Promotion (21 November 1986) [6]. Health combines social and personal resources and physical capabilities. In 2009, a new dimension was added to health—the "ability of the body to adapt to new threats and infirmities" [7]. This was based on two important factors: (1) that human health cannot be separated from the health of the planetary biodiversity; and (2) our daily interaction with the inanimate world. Both physical and mental health are important components of good health. Physical well-being is pursuing a healthy lifestyle to decrease the risk of disease, and mental well-being is pursing emotional and social stability to decrease the risk of psychological breakdown.

The SDG 3 agenda takes into account widening economic and social inequalities, rapid urbanization, threats to the climate and environment, the continuing burden of infectious diseases, and emerging challenges of non-communicable diseases. Universal health coverage (UHC) is integral to achieving SDG 3, ending poverty, and reducing inequalities. Another new and emerging global health priority is to fight antimicrobial resistance.

The world has made tremendous progress in the last century. Globally, at least one dreaded disease such as smallpox has been eliminated, and another, poliomyelitis, is close to elimination. But progress has been uneven, both between and within countries [8]. In South-East Asia, two countries are malaria-free and two countries are zero trachoma.

However, inequalities in access to medicine do exist. One essentially needs multisectoral, rights-based, and gender-sensitive approaches to address such inequalities within and outside countries. In 2017, an estimated 400 million people did not have access to basic healthcare, 40% lacked social protection; and every 2 s, someone aged 30–70 years died prematurely from a non-communicable disease [9].

SDG 3 has 13 targets and 26 indicators interconnected to many other SDG goals (Table 4.2). Table 4.2 also includes the target values where available.

The following is a detailed description of the specific targets and their relevance to South-East Asia.

SDG 3.1. By 2030, reduce the global maternal mortality ratio to less than 70 per 100,000 live births.

Maternal mortality refers to maternal deaths due to complications of pregnancy (includes death within 42 days of pregnancy termination) and childbirth. It is considered a primary indicator of overall health status and quality of life of a given geographic area. Two regions, sub-Saharan Africa (533 maternal deaths per 100,000 live births and 68% of all maternal deaths worldwide) and South Asia (163 maternal deaths per 100,000 live births, and 19% of all maternal deaths worldwide) account for 85% of global maternal mortality. From 2000 to 2017, the global maternal mortality rate (MMR) declined by 38%—from 342 to 211 maternal deaths per 100,000 live births. But this annual rate of reduction (averaging 2.9%) is still less than half of the required annual reduction rate of 6.4% to achieve the SDG 3 goal of 70 maternal deaths per 100,000 live births by 2030. Between 2000 and 2017, the reduction in MMR in South-East Asia was 59%, from 395 to 163 maternal deaths per 100,000 live births [10]. In 2017, of all the South-East Asian countries, Myanmar reported the highest MMR (250 maternal deaths per 100,000 live births) and Sri Lanka recorded the lowest (36 maternal deaths per 100,000 live births) (Table 4.3).

SDG 3.2. By 2030, end preventable deaths of newborns and children under 5 years of age, with all countries aiming to reduce neonatal mortality to at least as low as 12 per 1000 live births and under-5 mortality to at least as low as 25 per 1000 live births.

The neonatal (life up to 28 days) mortality rate (NMR) is a key outcome indicator for newborn care, and directly reflects prenatal, intrapartum, and neonatal care. Globally, this was halved between 1990 (36.7 neonatal deaths per 1000 live births) and 2018 (17.7 neonatal deaths per 1000 live births). In 2017, the annual NMR was 26.9 neonatal deaths per 1000 live births in South Asia. SDG 3 aims at reducing the NMR to 12 neonatal deaths per 1000 live births by 2030. At the current NMR, it is estimated that 27.8 million babies could die in their first month of life between 2018 and 2030; if the SDG 3 target of reducing this rate can be achieved, only 22.7 million neonatal deaths would occur by 2030 [11].

Table 4.2 SDG 3. Targets indicators and selected target values

Target	Indicator	Description	Target value
3.1	3.1.1	Maternal mortality. Death/100,000 live births	70
	3.1.2	Births attended by skilled health personnel % of live births	100
3.2	3.2.1	Under-5 mortality. Deaths/1000 live births	25
	3.2.2	Neonatal mortality. Deaths/1000 live births	12
3.3	3.3.1	New HIV infections/100,000 population	0
	3.3.2	Tuberculosis incidence/100,000 population	0
	3.3.3	Malaria incidence/1000 population at risk	0
	3.3.4	Hepatitis B incidence/100,000 population	
	3.3.5	Number of people requiring interventions against neglected tropical diseases	
3.4	3.4.1	Mortality rate attributed to cardiovascular disease, cancer, diabetes, or chronic respiratory disease. Probability %	18.5
	3.4.2	Suicide mortality/100,000 population	4.3
3.5	3.5.1	Coverage of treatment interventions (pharmacological, psychosocial and rehabilitation and aftercare services) for substance use disorders	
	3.5.2	Alcohol per capita consumption. Liters/annum	2.1
3.6	3.6.1	Road traffic injuries. Death/100,000 population	7.8
3.7	3.7.1	Proportion of women of reproductive age (15–49 years) who have their need for family planning satisfied with modern methods	100
	3.7.2	Adolescent fertility rate. Live births/1000 women (15–49 years) in that age group	13
3.8	3.8.1	Coverage of essential health services (reproductive, maternal, newborn and child health, infectious diseases, and non-communicable diseases; service capacity and access among the general and most disadvantaged populations)	
	3.8.2	Household expenditures on health. % of population	>10% = 5.4 >25% = 0.7
3.9	3.9.1	Mortality rate attributed to household and ambient air pollution	
	3.9.2	Mortality rate attributed to lack of safe water, sanitation, and hygiene (WASH)	
	3.9.3	Mortality rate attributed to unintentional poisoning/100,000 population	0.3
3.A	3.A.1	Age-standardized prevalence of current tobacco use among persons aged 15 years and older	
3.B	3.B.1	Proportion of the population with access to affordable medicines and vaccines on a sustainable basis [this includes three doses vaccination against diphtheria-tetanus-pertussis (DPT3); Pneumococcal conjugate 3rd dose vaccination (PCV3); Measles (MCv2)]. % of population	100
	3.B.2	Total net official development assistance to medical research and basic health sectors	
3.C	3.C.1	Health worker density/1000 population	
		Dentistry	1
		Nurse/Midwife	10.5
		Pharmacist	1
		Physician	4.1
3.D	3.D.1	International Health Regulations (IHR) capacity and health emergency preparedness. Index	100

Infant (life up to 1 year) mortality rate (IMR) indicates the overall physical health of a community. High IMRs are generally indicative of unmet human health needs in sanitation, medical care, nutrition, and education. In the last two decades, the global IMR has reduced from 65 infant deaths per 1000 live births in 1990 to 29 infant deaths per 1000 live births in 2018 [12]. In 2017, the world registered 4.1 million infant deaths as compared to the 8.8 million deaths in 1990 [13]. SDG 3 has not set any target for infant mortality rate, probably because IMR is clubbed with child mortality.

The global child (under 5) mortality rate has reduced from 93.2 child deaths per 1000 live

Table 4.3 Important health indices in South-East Asian countries

Country	NMR[a] 2018	IMR[a] 2018	Children (under 5) mortality[a] 2018	MMR[a] 2017	Life expectancy[a] (years) 2018
Bangladesh	17	25	30	173	72
Bhutan	16	25	30	183	71
India	23	30	37	145	69
Indonesia	13	21	25	177	72
Maldives	5	7	9	53	79
Myanmar	23	37	46	250	67
Nepal	20	27	32	186	70
Sri Lanka	5	6	7	36	77
Thailand	5	8	9	37	77
Timor Leste	20	39	46	142	69
SDG 3 goal	12	–	25	70	–

[a]Source: World Bank www.data.worldbank.org

IMR infant mortality rate (per 1000 live births), *NMR* neonatal mortality rate (per 1000 live births), *MMR* maternal mortality rates (per 100,000 live births)

births to 38.6 child deaths per 1000 live births between 1990 and 2018; in absolute numbers, this translates to a reduction of child mortality from 12.6 million children in 1990 (1 in 11 children) to 5.3 million children (1 in 26 children) in 2018 [14]. Two regions, sub-Saharan Africa and Central and Southern Asia, that account for 52% of the global population of under-5 children also accounted for more than 80% of deaths in children under five in 2018. Five countries, namely, the Democratic Republic of Congo, Ethiopia, India, Nigeria, and Pakistan accounted for half of all deaths in children under five in 2018 [15]. Diarrhea, and acute respiratory diseases such as pneumonia were the major causes of such deaths, and the major risk factors for such deaths were low birth weight, malnutrition, non-breastfeeding, overcrowding, and unsafe drinking water [15]. The SDG 3 target aims to reduce mortality in children under five to 25 per 1000 live births by 2030.

Life expectancy, a key metric for assessing population health, refers to the number of years a person is expected to live. Increased life expectancy is usually linked to good diet and public health. Between 1960 and 2018, there has been a steady increase in life expectancy from 52.6 years (1960) to 72.5 years (2018) [16]. The global average in life expectancy increased by 5.5 years between 2000 and 2016 [17].

Table 4.3 lists the values of various health indices in South-East Asian countries. Three countries (Maldives, Sri Lanka, and Thailand) have already achieved the SDG 3 goals in these indices and must continue to consolidate their positions. The remaining seven countries are required to design appropriate policies and execute specific programs to improve their health indices.

Despite global increases in average life expectancy, years of life lost (YLL), which is an estimate of the years of potential life lost due to premature death is also expected to rise. Compared to 2016, several non-communicable diseases (NCD) in many high- and middle-income countries (which account for 67.3% of YLLs) and communicable, maternal, neonatal, and nutritional (CMNN) diseases in many lower-income countries (which cause 53.5% of YLLs in sub-Saharan Africa) are likely to account for a large share of YLLs in 2040 [18]. In South Asia and the South-East Asia–Oceania regions, NCDs are expected to increase and CMNNs are expected to decrease (Table 4.4) [18].

SDG 3.3. By 2030, end the epidemics of AIDS, tuberculosis, malaria, and neglected tropical diseases, and combat hepatitis, water-borne diseases, and other communicable diseases.

Tuberculosis (TB) is one of the top 10 causes of death worldwide and the leading cause of

Table 4.4 Comparison of important health disorders in South Asia and the South-East Asia–Oceania region between 1980 and 2040 [18]

Year	Category	Global	HIC	South Asia	SEA & Oceania
1980	NCD %	29.8	76.1	17.6	36.3
	CMNN %	58.9	9.4	75.0	47.7
	Injuries %	11.3	14.5	7.3	16.0
2040	NCD %	67.3	85.7	67.8	83.2
	CMNNs%	21.4	5.9	18.4	8.0
	Injuries%	11.2	8.4	13.8	8.8

CMNN communicable, maternal, neonatal, nutritional, *HIC* high-income country, *NCD* non-communicable disease, *SEA* South-East Asia

death due to a single infectious agent. In 2018, an estimated 10 million people fell ill with tuberculosis and 1.5 million people died. Thirty high TB burden countries accounted for 87% of new cases and eight countries (Bangladesh, China, India, Indonesia, Nigeria, Pakistan, the Philippines, and South Africa), which includes three from the South-East Asian region that account for two-thirds of the total new cases of TB every year [19]. In September 2018, the UN held its first high-level meeting on epidemic TB, where a re-commitment was made to meet SDG target 3.3 (end TB strategy milestones for 2020–2025 and targets for 2030–2035) for reduction in TB cases and deaths. The targets for 2030 are a 90% reduction in the number of TB deaths and an 80% reduction in the TB incidence rate (new cases per 100,000 population per year) levels in 2015. This meeting noted that the current reduction in TB incidence at 2% per year must be accelerated to 4–5% per year to meet the 2030 targets. There was also a financial commitment to mobilize at least USD13 billion annually for universal access to TB diagnosis, treatment, and care by 2022, as well as to mobilize at least USD2 billion annually for TB research [19].

Malaria accounted for an estimated 228 million cases and 405,000 deaths in the world in 2018 [20]. While the African region has a disproportionately high share of the global malaria burden (93% of malaria cases and 94% of malaria deaths in 2018), there were eight million cases and 11,600 deaths related to malaria in the WHO South-East Asia Region. The WHO global technical strategy for malaria 2016–2030 (World Health Assembly (WHA), 2015) has 2030 aims to reduce incidence of malaria and malaria-related mortality by at least 90% by the year 2030. The strategy also aims to eliminate malaria in at least 35 countries and prevent the disease resurgence in all malaria-free countries [20]. The WHO has certified two South-East Asian countries, the Maldives (2015) and Sri Lanka (2016), malaria-free, and two more countries, Bhutan and Timor Leste are close to being malaria-free; in addition, Bangladesh, India, and Thailand have also reported substantial declines in reported malaria cases.

Water-borne diseases spread through contaminated water. Important water-borne diseases include diarrheal diseases, cholera, shigella, typhoid, hepatitis A and E, and poliomyelitis. In 2016, diarrheal diseases were the eighth leading cause of death in all age groups (1.65 million deaths), the fifth leading cause of death for under-5 children (446,000 deaths) and an increasing burden on people aged 70 and above [21]. Childhood wasting (low weight-for-height score), unsafe water, and unsafe sanitation were the leading risk factors. In 2018, the average numbers of diarrheal episodes in South-East Asia and South Asia were 22.8 and 64.4 per 100,000 people, respectively, against the global average of 7.06 per 100,000 people. In both these areas, the numbers of episodes per person-year was 1.60 and 1.49, respectively, against the global average of 1.75 episodes per person-year [22]. While safe drinking water and improved sanitation are important global goals (SDG 6) and many organism-specific vaccines are currently available to combat water-borne diseases, oral rehydration therapy (ORT) is an inexpensive and effective treatment that has saved many lives (approximately 70 million), since its introduction in the late 1970s in Bangladesh [23].

Poliomyelitis is a highly infectious disease that invades the nervous system. It is transmitted mainly through the fecal–oral route, and often causes irreversible paralysis (usually in the legs). In 1988, the 48th WHA (41.28) adopted a resolution for the worldwide eradication of polio. It marked the launch of the Global Polio

Eradication Initiative (GPEI), which followed the smallpox eradication strategy of the 1980s. By 2018, the occurrence of poliovirus infections reduced from an annual incidence of 350,000 cases in 125 countries to only 33 cases identified in two countries, Afghanistan and Pakistan [24]. The WHO launched the Polio Eradication & Endgame Strategic Plan (PEESP) in 2013 that followed the GPEI program period from 2013 to 2018 [25]. The net gain of the program is that over 18 million children have been saved from polio-affected paralysis. However, this effort must continue; because discontinuation will lead to a global rise of 200,000 cases per year in polio-related morbidities. With these factors in mind, the Polio Endgame Strategy 2019–2023 was launched to face the final challenges of polio eradication and lay the groundwork for a sustainable future free of polio [26]. In September 2018, the Polio Oversight Board (POB) approved a multiyear budget and recognized the resource requirements of the GPEI to an overall cost of USD5.1 billion [26].

Neglected tropical diseases (NTDs) are a diverse group of communicable diseases in tropical and subtropical areas in 149 countries. Populations living in poverty, without adequate sanitation, and in close contact with infectious vectors, domestic animals, and livestock are worst affected by NTDs. There are 17 common NTDs and between 1978 and 2011, the WHA has passed 10 resolutions to end or substantially reduce these 10 NTDs: treponematoses (WHA 31.58 in 1978), lymphatic filariasis (WHA 50.29 in 1997), trachoma (WHA 51.11 in 1998), leprosy (WHA 51.15 in 1998), schistosomiasis (bilharziasis) and soil-transmitted helminthiases (intestinal worms) (WHA 54.19 in 2001), African trypanosomiasis (sleeping sickness) (WHA 57.2 in 2004), leishmaniasis (WHA 60.13 in 2007), onchocerciasis (river blindness) (WHA 62.1 in 2009), Chagas disease (WHA 63.20 in 2010), and dracunculiasis (guinea-worm disease) (WHA 64.16 in 2011) [27].

Worldwide, ~2 billion people are at risk of one or more NTDs and more than 1 billion people are affected by these diseases. Annually, up to half a million deaths and 57 million disability-adjusted life years (DALY) are attributed to NTDs [28]. The London declaration on NTDs (30 January 2012) is the first joint effort of the WHO, the World Bank, the Bill & Melinda Gates Foundation, and 13 leading pharmaceutical companies to commit to an NTD eradication program at a global level. Since then, much progress has been made to eradicate guinea-worm disease, lymphatic filariasis, leprosy, sleeping sickness (African trypanosomiasis), and blinding trachoma. The incidences of diseases such as schistosomiasis, soil-transmitted helminths, Chagas disease, visceral leishmaniasis, and river blindness (onchocerciasis) have also reduced [28].

SDG 3.4. By 2030, reduce by one-third, all cases of premature mortality due to NCDs through prevention and treatment; also promote mental health and well-being.

Globally, the principal NCDs are cardiovascular diseases (CVDs), cancers, chronic respiratory diseases, and diabetes. The numbers of NCD deaths worldwide are expected to increase by 15% between 2010 and 2020 (to 44 million deaths) with an estimated 10.4 million deaths in South-East Asia [29]. Modifiable risk behaviors for NCDs include tobacco use, physical inactivity, unhealthy diets, and harmful use of alcohol. The metabolic risk factors include high blood pressure, overweight/obesity, hyperglycemia, and hyperlipidemia. A global Non-Communicable Disease Alliance (NCDA) was formed in 2009 with a vision of "a world where everyone has the opportunity for a healthy life, free from the preventable suffering, stigma, disability, and death caused by non-communicable diseases." The NCDA partners with civil societies, governments, and the UN to jointly work towards reducing NCD-related morbidity and mortality. Today, the global NCDA is a 2000-strong member organization from 170 countries. The global NCDA has successfully influenced political commitments (such as the resolution to reduce overall NCD-related mortality by 25% by the year 2025; the "25 by 25" target), created multisectoral partnerships, positioned NCDs in the 2030 SDG, and cultivated national and regional NCDAs. As a part of this movement, the South-East Asia Region

NCDA (SEAR-NCDA) was formed in February 2020 [30]. Chapter 12 has further details of NCDs and diabetic retinopathy in the WHO South-East Asia Region.

SDG 3.5. Strengthen systems for the prevention and treatment of substance abuse, including narcotic drug abuse and harmful use of alcohol.

Substance abuse refers to the harmful or hazardous use of psychoactive substances, including alcohol and illicit drugs. It can have negative consequences on health, economy, productivity, and social aspects of communities [31]. In 2016, the most common substance and drug disorders worldwide were alcohol (an estimated 100.4 million people have alcohol addiction-related issues; the age-standardized prevalence of alcohol addiction is 1320.8 cases per 100,000 people) and cannabis (22.1 million cases of cannabis addiction; the age-standardized prevalence of cannabis addiction is 289.7 cases per 100,000 people) [32]. The 2019 report of the United Nations Office on Drugs and Crime (UNODC) indicates that an estimated 35 million people suffer from drug use disorders; of those who require deaddiction services, only 1 in 7 receive treatment [33].

SDG 3.6. By 2020, halve the number of global deaths and injuries caused by road traffic accidents.

The United Nations Conference on Trade and Development (UNCTAD) in 2017 reported that each year, over 1.35 million people die, and an additional 50 million are injured or permanently disabled in road accidents [34]. Death due to road traffic injury is the 8th leading cause of all deaths and the first cause of death in the 5–29 years age group in the world. Most (90%) of road traffic deaths occur in low- and middle-income countries, although these countries only have 54% of the world's vehicles. In the WHO South-East Asia Region, deaths due to road traffic injuries increased by 1% between 2013 and 2016 (from 19.8 to 20.7 per 100,000 population); furthermore, most deaths (43%) occurred due to 2- or 3-wheeler drivers/riders [35]. In addition to SDG 3.6, road traffic injury is interconnected with SDG 11 (make cities and human settlements inclusive, safe, resilient, and sustainable by 2030) through specific indicator 11.2, which calls for access to safe, affordable, accessible, and sustainable transport systems for all, and to improve road safety for vulnerable populations.

SDG 3.7. By 2030, ensure universal access to sexual and reproductive healthcare services, including family planning, information, and education; reproductive health must also be integrated into national strategies and programs.

Widening access to contraception and ensuring that demands for family planning are satisfied using elective contraceptive methods are essential for achieving universal access to reproductive healthcare services. The 2030 agenda reaffirms the commitments made in the Program of Action of the International Conference on Population and Development (ICPD, 1994), adopted by 179 Member States. Among the 1.9 billion women of reproductive age (15–49 years) living in the world in 2019, as many as 1.1 billion women have a need for family planning, and 10% of these women's needs are unmet [36]. Significant disparities exist across countries and regions in the use of modern family planning methods. Approximately 1 in 10 women of reproductive age use traditional methods in 21 countries including 7 countries in Asia [36]. Among the countries in the WHO South-East Asia Region, as per the UN report in 2019, the prevalence of modern contraceptive use was highest in Thailand and Bangladesh (median percentile 46.6% and 45.5%, respectively) and very low in Timor Leste (median percentile 12.9%). The unmet needs for family planning methods was low in Thailand and Sri Lanka (median percentile 3.7% and 5.9%, respectively) [37]. In addition to SDG 3.7, the WHO has a very specific goal targeted to achieve gender equality and empowerment of all women and girls (SDG 5) to promote healthy lives and well-being for all by 2030.

SDG 3.8. Achieve universal health coverage, including financial risk protection, access to quality essential healthcare services, and access to safe, effective, quality, and affordable essential medicines and vaccines for all.

UHC means that all individuals and communities receive the health services they need without suffering financial hardship [38]. It includes the full spectrum of essential, quality health services, from health promotion to prevention, treatment, rehabilitation, and palliative care. The UHC encompasses all components of the health system, including service delivery, workforce, facilities, communications networks, technologies, information systems, quality assurance mechanisms, governance, and policy legislation. The degree to which UHC has been achieved can be measured by the proportion of a population that can access essential quality health services as well as the proportion of the population that spends a large amount of household income on health [38].

Currently, at least half of the world's population does not have full coverage for essential health services. About 100 million people are still being pushed into extreme poverty (defined as living on USD1.90 or less a day) because they have to pay for healthcare. Over 930 million people (around 12% of the world's population) spend at least 10% of their household budgets to pay for healthcare. Approximately 800 million people do not have full health coverage and 65 million people are pushed to extreme poverty when they pay for their healthcare in the WHO South-East Asia Region, which has 26% of the world's population [38].

SDG 3.9. By 2030, substantially reduce the number of deaths and illnesses from hazardous chemicals, and air, water, and soil pollution and contamination.

Pollution is the largest environmental cause of disease and premature death in the world today. Diseases caused by pollution were responsible for an estimated nine million premature deaths in 2015, and nearly 92% of pollution-related deaths occurred in low- and middle-income countries. The Lancet Commission on Pollution and Health estimated that pollution-related diseases cause productivity losses equivalent to 2% of the gross domestic product (GDP) in low- and middle-income countries. Pollution-related diseases also result in increased healthcare costs; up to 1.7% of annual health spending in high-income countries and up to 7% of health spending in middle-income countries [39]. While the household air and water pollution (usually associated with profound poverty and traditional lifestyles) are on a decline, the ambient air, chemical, and soil pollution—produced by industry, mining, electricity generation, and petroleum-powered vehicles—are on the rise, especially in the developing and industrializing low- and middle-income countries. In addition to SDG 3.9, the WHO has a very specific goal targeted towards achieving climate and environmental control through affordable and clean energy (SDG 7), sustainable cities and communities (SDG 11), and climate action (SDG 13).

SDG 3.A. Strengthen the implementation of the WHO framework convention on tobacco control in all countries, as appropriate.

Tobacco smoking is one of the world's largest health problems. The Global Burden of Disease (GBD) reported that more than 8.2 million people died prematurely as a result of smoking in 2017; this included 7 million primary and 1.2 million secondary smokers [40]. The mean annual death rate due to smoking-related issues in ten South-East Asian countries was 93.04 deaths per 100,000 population in 2017; the highest mean annual death rate was in Myanmar (175.06 deaths per 100,000 population) and lowest was in Bhutan (54.19 deaths per 100,000 population) [41]. Of these deaths, 93% occurred in people 59 years or older, and 51.3% occurred in people aged 70 years or older. Between 1990 and 2017, smoking-related death rates have fallen (146 deaths per 100,000 population in 1990 to 90 deaths per 100,000 population in 2017); however, this decline has occurred mostly in the rich countries [41].

SDG 3.B. Support the research and development of vaccines and medicines for those communicable and non-communicable diseases that primarily affect developing countries, provide access to affordable essential medicines and vaccines, and provide access to medicines for all.

There are many reasons why people do not get the healthcare they need; this includes problems such as under-resourced health systems, a lack of sufficiently qualified and skilled healthcare workers, inequalities between and within countries, exclusion, stigma, discrimination, and exclusive marketing rights [42]. Often times, it is related to unaffordability, poor quality, inappropriate use, and procurement of medicines, and problems with supply chains and regulatory obstacles to obtaining such medicines in the least developed countries. One of the main objectives under SDG 3 is to ensure access to affordable medicines for all. Following the adoption of the SDGs in September 2015, the WTO's Council for TRIPS (Trade-Related aspects of Intellectual Property Rights) in November 2015, extended its scope to promote access to medicines for all [42].

SDG 3.C. Substantially increase health financing and recruitment, development, training, and retention of health workforce in developing countries, especially in the least developed countries and small island developing states.

Human Resource for Health (HRH) is a key enabler for the attainment of UHC, and achievement of SDG 3. This requires a knowledgeable, skilled, and motivated health workforce. The health workforce includes those people who provide health services directly (physicians, nurses, and paramedics) and indirectly (hospital managers and administrators). As a result of chronic under-investment in education and training of health workers, the WHO estimates a projected global shortfall of 18 million health workers, including 9 million nurses or midwives by 2030; it is likely that this shortage would mostly occur in low- and lower-middle income countries. This is despite the fact that the global economy is projected to create around 40 million new health sector jobs by 2030 [43]. The WHO Global Health Observatory estimates that South-East Asia would need 10.9-million health workers by 2030; this translates to an increase of 75% from the 6.2 million health workers in active service in 2013. This health workforce includes 1.9 million physicians, 5.2 million nurses, and 3.7 million other health workers [44]. The eye health personnel directly involved in patient care (ophthalmologists, optometrists, and allied ophthalmic personnel) in 2019 and their densities are shown in Table 4.5.

In 2015, there were 232,866 ophthalmologists in the world according to a survey by the International Council of Ophthalmology (ICO) [45]. Although there has been a 2.6% annual growth in the number of ophthalmologists worldwide, these ophthalmologists were unequally distributed; there were fewer ophthalmologists in low-income countries (3.7 per million population) than in high-income countries (76.2 per million population). In addition, within the low-middle income countries, most ophthalmologists were located in urban areas than in rural localities [45]. The current numbers of allied ophthalmic personnel (AOP), who form the backbone of eye care in the community and primary eye care level as recommended in the World Report on Vision (WRV), are not enough to meet demands [46]. It is estimated that in order to develop a patient-centered eye care system from community to tertiary care, the 10 South-East Asian countries would need more than 164,000 AOPs [47]. At the current level (Table 4.5), there is an acute

Table 4.5 Eye health workforce in SEAR member states (2019 data)

		Ophthalmologist density			Optometrist density		AOP density	
Country	Population (Million)	n	Per population	Per million population	n	Per population	n	Per population
Bangladesh	163.0	1200	1/135,883	7.36	1485	1/109,764	500	1/326,000
Bhutan	0.75	10	1/75,000	13.33	9	1/83,333	56	1/13,393
India	1366.0	23,567	1/56,689	17.64	12,000	1/113,833	30,000	1/44,433
Indonesia	267.6	2712	1/98,672	10.13	2470	1/108,340	6250	1/42,816
Maldives	0.53	26	1/20,384	49.05	13	1/40,769	0	–
Myanmar	54.0	390	1/138,461	7.22	95	1/568,421	0	–
Nepal	29.1	335	1/86,865	11.51	857	1/33,955	1246	1/23,354
Sri Lanka	21.3	130	1/163,000	6.13	670	1/31.800	1355	1/15,700
Thailand	69.6	1700	1/40,941	24.42	320	1/217,500	1200	1/55 ,500
Timor Leste	1.3	4	1/325,000	3.07	2	1/650,000	24	1/52,000

AOP allied ophthalmic personnel

imbalance in the density of ophthalmologists and an acute shortage of AOPs.

3.D. Strengthen the capacity of all countries, in particular, developing countries, for early warning, risk reduction, and management of national and global health risks.

People across the world are faced with a wide and diverse range of risks associated with health emergencies and disasters. These comprise of infectious disease outbreaks, natural hazards, conflicts, unsafe food and water, chemical and radiation and other accidents, lack of water and power supply, air pollution, antimicrobial resistance, etc. The health, economic, political, and societal consequences of these events can be devastating, both in the acute phase and in the longer term. Sound risk management is essential for development and implementation of the SDG goals. The Health Emergency and Disaster Risk Management (EDRM) framework of the WHO provides the framework for management of unforeseen health emergencies [48]. Health EDRM is a continuum of measures, and not merely a response to a health event or crisis. Globally, approximately 190 million people are directly affected annually by emergencies due to natural and technological hazards, which cause over 77,000 deaths [49]. A further 172 million are affected by conflict [50]. From 2010 to 2019, WHO recorded more than 2000 outbreaks of infectious diseases in 168 countries, including those due to new or re-emerging infectious diseases, including the recent epidemic caused by the Zika virus (2015), Ebola virus (2014–2016), and novel Corona virus (2019) [51].

Between 1990 and 2015, unsafe sanitation, household air pollution, childhood underweight, childhood stunting, and smoking have decreased by more than 25%. However, high body-mass index (BMI), and drug use have increased by more than 25% [52]. Together, all these health risks in 2015 accounted for 57.8% of global deaths and 41.2% of DALY. In 2015, the ten largest contributors to global DALYs were high systolic blood pressure (211.8 million), smoking (148.6 million), high fasting plasma glucose (143.1 million), high BMI (120.1 million), childhood under-nutrition (113.3 million), ambient particulate matter (103.1 million), high total cholesterol (88.7 million), household air pollution (85.6 million), alcohol use (85 million), and high-sodium diets (83 million) [52]. Although eye conditions were not in this list, it is known that high blood pressure, high plasma sugar, high total cholesterol, high BMI, and childhood under-nutrition can cause several eye disorders, reduce vision, and even lead to early blindness. All these conditions adversely impact the quality of life.

In 2017, there were 56 million deaths in the world; the most common cause of these were NCDs (73.4%; 41.1 million), followed by CMNN diseases/disorders (18.6%; 10.4 million), and injuries (8.0%, 4.5 million). These diseases accounted for 1.65 billion years of life lost caused by NCDs, CMNN diseases/disorders, and injuries by 53.0%, 35.1%, and 11.9%, respectively [53]. Between 1990 and 2017, there has been a substantial change in these patterns (Fig. 4.2). While there the numbers of deaths due to injury have not changed much, there has been a significant change in the numbers of deaths caused by NCDs (which has increased by 26.73%) and CMNN diseases/disorders (which has reduced by 43.93%). The age-specific mortality and the most common causes of death are shown in Table 4.6 [54].

The UN has developed a mechanism to track the progress of SDGs. The Economic and Social Commission for Asia and the Pacific (ESCAP) monitors this progress in the Asia Pacific region. The 2018 ESCAP report indicates that South-

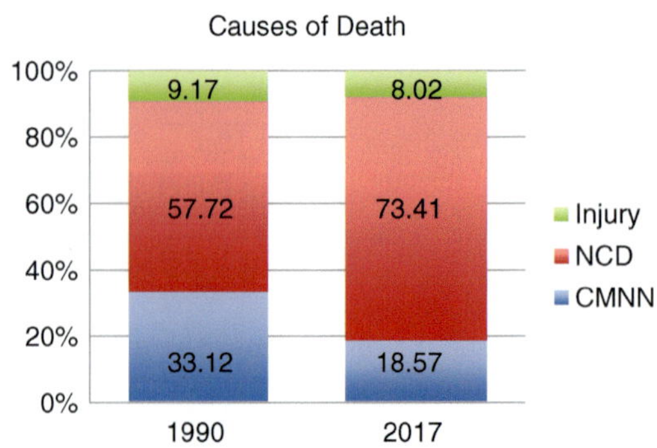

Fig. 4.2 Comparison of the percentages of causes of death due to CMNN diseases/disorders, NCDs, and injuries between 1990 and 2017 [53]

Table 4.6 Age-specific causes of death between 1990 and 2017 [54]

Year	70+	50–69	15–49	5–14	<5
1990 in percentage	33.46	23.31	15.06	2.84	25.32
2017 in percentage	48.64	26.81	13.61	1.31	9.64
Most common cause in 2017	CVD	CVD	CVD	Road accidents	Lower respiratory infections

East Asia is ahead of other sub-regions in quality education (Goal 4), affordable and clean energy (Goal 7) and industry, and innovation and infrastructure (Goal 9); but this region has regressed on economic growth (Goal 8), climate action (Goal 13), and peace and justice (Goal 16). Areas requiring immediate action to reverse these trends include harmful use of alcohol (SDG 3.5.2) and shrinking above-ground forest biomass (SDG 15.2.P1) (Fig. 4.3) [55].

Health is affected by multitude of factors inherent to each individual, though many societal factors also influence it. Eye health is an important component for overall human development and well-being. The SDG 3 is connected to many other SDGs [56]. The 73rd WHA (2020), while adopting the resolution (73.12) on "integrated people-centered eye care, including preventable vision impairment and blindness" has mentioned these interconnections. More specifically these are Goal 1 (end poverty in all its forms everywhere), Goal 4 (ensure inclusive and equitable quality education and promote lifelong learning opportunities for all), Goal 5 (achieve gender equality and empower all women and girls), Goal 6 (ensure availability and sustainable management of water and sanitation for all), Goal 8 (promote sustained, inclusive and sustainable economic growth, full and productive employment and decent work for all), and Goal 10 (reduce inequality within and among countries) [1].

Despite many remarkable gains in health over the past few decades, the world will need to significantly increase its efforts to achieve the SDGs by 2030. In response to these needs, 11 global health, development, and humanitarian agencies aligned with the WHO committed to closer collaboration and alignment in October 2018 to help accelerate the progress towards attaining the SDGs [57]. These 11 agencies include Gavi (the vaccine alliance for equitable use of vaccines in lower-income countries); GFF (Global Finance Facility for women, children and adolescents, currently working in 36 countries); Global Fund to Fight AIDS, TB and Malaria (invests over USD4 billion a year to support programs); UNAIDS (UN Program on HIV/AIDS), UNDP (UN Development Program, supports over 100 counties in addressing health determinants and developments); UNFPA (UN Population Fund, working to deliver universal access to sexual and reproductive health); UNICEF (United Nations Children's Fund, partners in 190 countries to promote the rights and well-being of children); Unitaid (working to fill the gap between late-stage development of heath products and their adoption); UN Women (dedicated to gender equality and empowerment of women); World Bank (with a global strategy to improve health, nutrition and population (HNP) parameters, with an commitment of USD3 billion annually); and WFP (World Food Program, delivering food assistance during emergencies) [58].

These agencies have adopted the following four strategies: *Engage* with countries to identify priorities and implement plans together; *Accelerate* progress in countries through joint actions under seven accelerator themes; *Align* by harmonizing operational and financial strategies and country-specific policies; *Account* by reviewing progress and enhance shared accountability [58]. The seven *accelerators* are (1) primary health; (2) sustainable financing; (3) community and civil society engagement; (4) determinants of health; (5) innovative programs for handling fragile and vulnerable settings and for disease outbreak responses; (6) research, development, innovation, and access; and (7) data and digital health [58].

2023 is the mid-point to 2030. By 2023, these 11 agencies along with the WHO plan to achieve better coordination among the different agencies

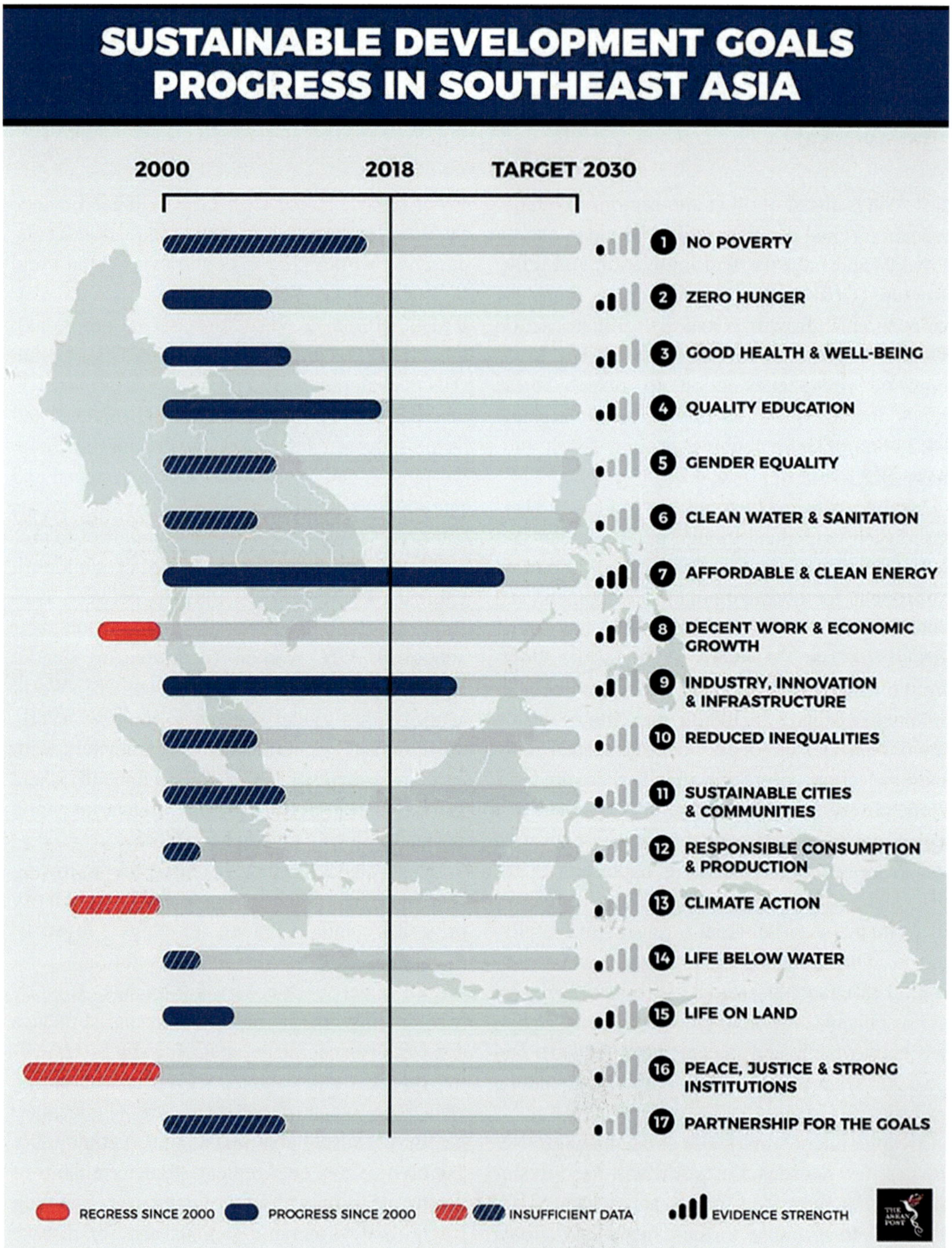

Fig. 4.3 Snapshot of SDG progress in 2018: South-East Asia [56]

in their global, regional, and in-country processes; superior operational and financial policies; and focus on purpose-driven collaboration [59]. This is aimed at providing the required momentum in the final push to achieve "good health and well-being" to all by 2030.

Case Story

Medical Mission for Refugees in South-East Asia (FDMN in Bangladesh)

Munir Ahmed and Lutful Husain

Since August 2017, over 700,000 Myanmar nationals (Rohingyas) have migrated from the northern Rakhine state of Myanmar to Teknaf and Ukhyia sub-districts of the Cox's Bazar district of Bangladesh (Fig. 4.4). The United Nations High Commission for Refugees (UNHCR) estimates this migrated population of 'forcibly displaced Myanmar nationals (FDMN)' to be 1.2 million people, including all earlier arrivals. This sudden and massive influx overwhelmed existing health services in Bangladesh. In response, the Government of Bangladesh, with a number of international non-government organizations (INGOs) set up 74 health centers, including health posts in and around the resettled migrant population. This was in accordance with the WHA resolution 70.15 of 2017 (promoting the health of refugees and migrants) that urges member states to oversee safe and orderly migration, address health needs, strengthen international cooperation on the health of refugees, and provide health-related assistance through bilateral/international cooperation [60].

The Bangladesh government accepted the Orbis International proposal to make provisions for primary eye care, integrated with general healthcare in this region, both for the host community, and the migrant population (Fig. 4.5). The systematic planning for this included a rapid assessment of avoidable blindness (RAAB) for people 50 years and older, establishing provisions for basic eye care, and engaging the Cox's Bazar Baitush Sharaf Hospital (CBBSH, 34 km

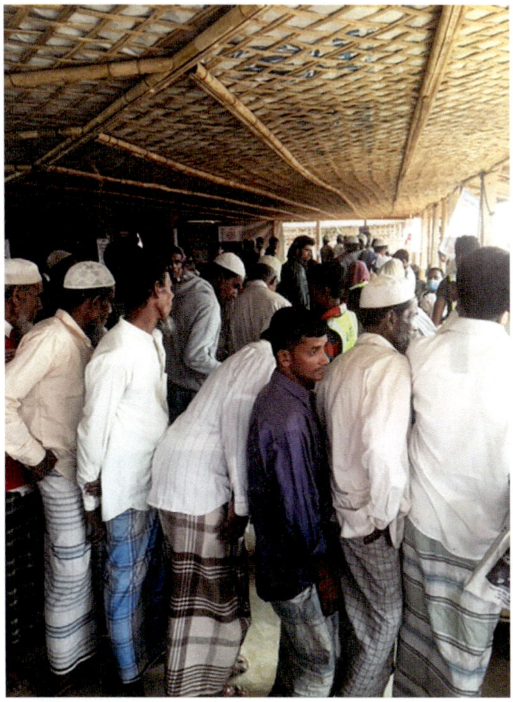

Fig. 4.5 FDMNs at the improvised eye screening facility at Kutupalong (camp # 4), Ukhyia, Cox's Bazar, Bangladesh (Source: Orbis, Bangladesh)

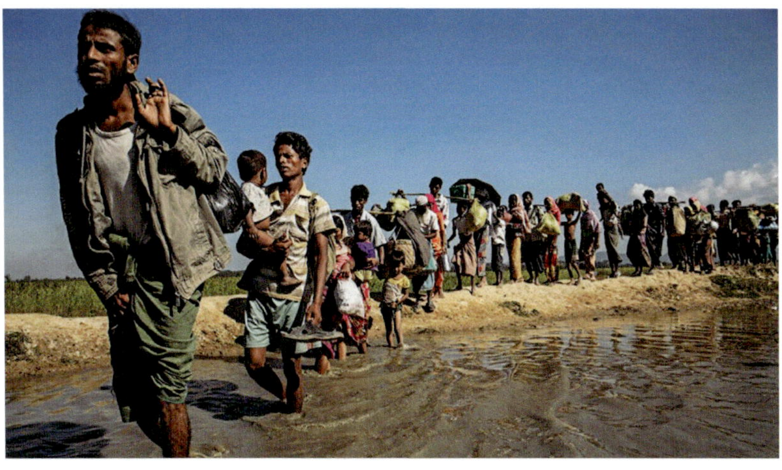

Fig. 4.4 FDMN on way to southern Cox's Bazar district I Bangladesh (Source: UNHCR)

from the migrant population) for referrals and ophthalmic surgery. A study recorded the high burden of untreated eyes of young adults [61] and the RAAB study showed prevalences of blindness (vision < 3/60) and severe visual impairment (vision < 6/60) at 2.1% and 2.4%, respectively, in the elderly people of this population.

Orbis International also addressed issues of system strengthening through the following measures: improving eye health infrastructure and service delivery at primary and secondary levels; skill development of primary eye care personnel; defining the referral pathway; building efficient data management and patient information systems; and identifying and engaging leaders from both, the host and migrant communities. Orbis International spearheaded the collaborative platform for this migrant population health crisis and formed the 'Eye Health Forum of Cox's Bazar' that included the government, various UN agencies (UNHCR, WHO, IOM (International Organization for Migration), and UNICEF), and INGOs (Orbis, Seva, International Agency for the Prevention of Blindness (IAPB), the Fred Hollows Foundation, and the CBM). When this article was being written (July 2020), the Eye Health Forum had trained 800 medical and other professionals in eye health, screened 160,000 people, provided spectacles to 8370 people, and facilitated 3389 eye surgeries.

Globally, an estimated 65 million people are forcibly displaced from their homes. Developing countries host 86% of such displaced populations [60]. While this is a global tragedy calling for a political solution, experience in dealing with FDMNs in Bangladesh suggests that humanitarian efforts could be maximized by good collaboration and linkage between the Government, community, and INGOs. Additionally, an effective health model that basically consists of three phases: emergency phase, settlement phase, and (long-term) engagement phase must be put in place. Activities in the *Emergency phase,* include provision of emergency services when the displaced population is still moving and is dispersed; it is possibly the time for eye health scoping and positioning. In the *Settlement phase,* the moving population is mostly contained and settled in specific locations with a supply system of basic needs; this could be the right time for health intervention. Once this is done, a strategic, integrated, comprehensive, sustainable, inclusive eye care system could be planned for the *Engagement phase*. The lessons learned and evidence generated from this instance could guide policy makers in eye care and healthcare during similar human disasters.

References

1. The United Nations. 17 Sustainable Development Goals (SDGs). www.un.org. Accessed 29 June 2020.
2. Mainstreaming trade to attain the Sustainable Development. 2018. www.wto.org english> res_e> publications_e> sdg> e. Accessed 28 June 2020.
3. UNDP. Goal 17. Partnerships for goals. www.undp.org > Home> Sustainable Development Goals. Accessed 28 June 2020.
4. United Nations Conference on Trade and Development (UNCTAD). Trading into sustainable development: trade, market access, and the sustainable development goals. Developing countries in international trade studies. 2016. UNCTAD/DITC/TAB/2015/3
5. WHO constitution. www.who.int. Accessed 29 June 2020.
6. WHO. The Ottawa Charter for health promotion. www.who.int. Accessed 29 June 2020.
7. What is health? The ability to adapt. Lancet Published: March 07, 2009. https://doi.org/10.1016/S0140-6736(09)60456-6.
8. Roser M, Ortiz-Ospina E, Ritchie H. Life expectancy. https://ourworldindata.org/life-expectancy. Accessed 19 June 2020.
9. UNDP. Goal 3: Good health and well-being. www.undp.org Home> Sustainable Development Goals. Accessed 29 June 2020.
10. Maternal mortality- Unicef data. www.data.unicef.org topic>maternal-health. Accessed 21 June 2020.
11. Hug L, Alexander M, Yiu D, et al. National, regional, and global levels and trends in neonatal mortality between 1990 and 2017, with scenario-based projections to 2030: a systematic analysis. Lancet Global Health. 2019;7:E710–20. https://doi.org/10.1016/S2214-109X(19)301639.
12. Mortality rate, Infant. www.data.worldbank.org. Accessed 28 June 2020.
13. World Health Organization. Global health observatory. www.who.int >gho. Accessed 21 June 2020.
14. Mortality rate, under 5. www.data.worldbank.org. Accessed 29 June 2020.
15. World Health Organization. Reducing childhood mortality. www.who.int. Accessed 21 June 2020.
16. Life expectancy at birth. www.data.worldbank.org. Accessed 29 June 2020.
17. Life expectancy. www.who.int >gho. Accessed 29 June 2020.

18. Foreman KJ, Marquez N, Dolgert A, et al. Forecasting life expectancy, years of life lost, and all-cause and cause-specific mortality for 250 causes of death: reference and alternative scenarios for 2016–40 for 195 countries and territories. Lancet. 2018;392:2052–90.
19. Global Tuberculosis Report 2019. Geneva: World Health Organization. 2019.
20. WHO Malaria. www.who.int > malaria. Accessed 29 June 2020.
21. Silva KT. Decolonization, development and disease: a social history of malaria in Sri Lanka. Asian J Social Sci. 2015;43:527–8. https://doi.org/10.1163/15685314-04304013.
22. Dadonaite B, Ritchie H. Diarrheal diseases. 2018.; https://ourworldindata.org/diarrheal-diseases. Accessed 23 June 2020.
23. GBD 2016 Diarrhoeal Disease Colaborators. Estimates of the global, regional, and national morbidity, mortality, and aetiologies of diarrhoea in 195 countries: a systematic analysis for the Global Burden of Disease Study 2016. Lancet Infect Dis. 2018;18:1211–28.
24. Fontaine O, Paul Garner P, Bhan MK. Oral rehydration therapy: the simple solution saving lives. Br Med J. 2007;334:S1. https://doi.org/10.1136/bmj.39044.725949.94.
25. World Health Organization. Poliomyelitis. www.who.int. Accessed 29 June 2020.
26. Global Polio Eradication Initiative. Polio Eradication and Endgame Strategy 2013-2018. Geneva, WHO 2013. www.polioeradication.org /wp-content/uploads/2016/07/PEESP
27. Polio Endgame Strategy 2019–2023: eradication, integration, certification and containment. Geneva: World Health Organization; 2019 (WHO/Polio/19.04).
28. Hotez PJ, Alvarado M, Basáñez M-G, et al. The global burden of disease study 2010: interpretation and implications for the neglected tropical diseases. PLoS Negl Trop Dis. 2014;8:e2865. https://doi.org/10.1371/journal.pntd.0002865. PMID: 25058013
29. London declaration on neglected tropical diseases. www.who.int > neglected diseases > London_ Declaration. Accessed 27 June 2020.
30. WHO. Non-communicable diseases in the South East Asia. www.who.int. Accessed 29 June 2020.
31. Global NCD Alliance Forum 2020. www.ncdallinace.org NCDAF2020. Accessed 29 June 2020.
32. WHO. Substance abuse. www.who.int > topics> substance _ abuse. Accessed 23 June 2020.
33. GBD 2016 Alcohol and Drug Use Collaborators. The global burden of disease attributable to alcohol and drug use in 195 countries and territories, 1990–2016: a systematic analysis for the Global Burden of Disease Study 2016. Lancet Psychiatry. 2018;5:987–1012. https://doi.org/10.1016/S2215-0366(18)30337-7.
34. World drug report 2019. www.unodc.org. Accessed 23 June 2020.
35. United Nations Conference on Trade and Development. 2017. UNCTAD/DTL/TLB/2017/4.
36. Global status report on road safety. The South East Asia story. 2019. www.itf.org. Accessed 23 June 2020.
37. United Nations, Department of Economic and Social Affairs, Population Division. Family Planning and the 2030 Agenda for Sustainable Development: Data Booklet. (ST/ESA/SER.A/429). 2019.
38. United Nations, Department of Economic and Social Affairs, Population Division. Contraceptive Use by Method 2019: Data Booklet (ST/ESA/SER.A/435). 2019.
39. www.who.int > universal _coverage. Accessed 24 June 2020.
40. Landrigan PJ, Fuller R, Acosta NJR. The Lancet Commission on pollution and health. Lancet. 2018;391:462–512.
41. Stanaway JD, Afshin A, Gakidou E, et al. Global, regional, and national comparative risk assessment of 84 behavioral, environmental and occupational and metabolic risk or clusters of risks for 195 countries and territories, 1990–2017: a systematic analysis for the Global Burden of Disease Study 2017. Lancet. 2018;392(10159):1923–94.
42. Hannah Ritchie and Max Roser (2019 revised)—"Smoking" www.ourworldindata.org /smoking. Accessed 25 June 2020.
43. Mainstreaming trade to attain the Sustainable Goals. www.wto.org. Accessed 26 June 2020.
44. Global strategy on human resources for health: workforce 2030. www.who.int/hrh/resources/globstrathrh-2030/en. Accessed 26 June 2020.
45. Buchan J, Dhillon IS, Campbell J, editors. Health employment and economic growth: an evidence base. Geneva: World Health Organization; 2017.
46. Resnikoff S, Lansingh VC, Washburn L, et al. Estimated number of ophthalmologists worldwide (International Council of Ophthalmology update): will we meet the needs? Br J Ophthalmol. 2020;104:588–92.
47. World Report on Vision. www.who.int. Accessed 30 June 2020.
48. Das T, Keeffe J, Sivaprasad S, Rao GN. Capacity building for universal eye health coverage in South East Asia beyond 2020. Eye. 2020;34:1262–70. https://doi.org/10.1038/s41433-020-0801-8.
49. Health emergency and disaster risk management framework. 2019. Geneva: World Health Organization.
50. World disasters report 2016. Resilience: saving lives today, investing for tomorrow. Geneva: International Federation of Red Cross and Red Crescent Societies. 2016. www.ifrc.org. Accessed 31 March 2019.
51. People affected by conflict—humanitarian needs in numbers, 2013. Brussels: Centre for Research on the Epidemiology of Disasters; 2013. www.reliefweb.int report/world/people-affected-conflict-humanitarian-needs-numbers-2013. Accessed 31 March 2019.
52. WHO. Disease outbreaks by year. www.int/csr/don/archive/year/en. Accessed 26 June 2020.
53. GBD 2015 Risk Factors Collaborators. Global, regional, and national comparative risk assessment

of 79 behavioural, environmental and occupational, and metabolic risks or clusters of risks, 1990–2015: a systematic analysis for the Global Burden of Disease Study 2015. Lancet. 2016;388(10053):1659–724.

54. Roth GA, Abate D, Abate KH, et al. Global, regional, and national age-sex-specific mortality for 282 causes of death in 195 countries and territories, 1980–2017: a systematic analysis for the Global Burden of Disease Study 2017. Lancet. 2018;392(10159):1736–88.
55. Causes of death—our world in data. www.ourworld-data.org. Accessed 1 July2020.
56. Fernandez RM. SDG 3 good health and well-being: integration and connection with other SDGs. In Filho WL, et al (eds) Good health and well-being. Springer Nature, Switzerland 2020. Pg 629-636.
57. South East Asia SDG progress; Asia Pacific progress report. The Economic and Social Commission for Asia and the Pacific (ESCAP). 2019. UN Publication.
58. Towards a global action plan for healthy lives and well-being for all: uniting to accelerate progress toward the health-related SDGs. Geneva: World Health Organization. 2018. https://apps.who.int/iris/bitstream/handle/10665/311667/WHO-DCO-2018.3-eng.pdf. Accessed 5 July 2020.
59. Stronger collaboration, better health: global action plan for healthy lives and well-being for all. Strengthening collaboration among multilateral organizations to accelerate country progress on the health-related Sustainable Development Goals. Geneva: World Health Organization; 2019.
60. World Health Organization. Refugee and migrant health. www.who.int >migrants. Accessed 2 July 2020.
61. Ahmed M, Whitestone N, Patnaik JL, Hossain MA, Husain L, Alauddin M, et al. Burden of eye disease and demand for care in the Bangladesh Rohingya displaced population and host community: a cohort study. PLoS Med. 2020;17(3):e1003096. https://doi.org/10.1371/journal.pmed.1003096.

5 Integrated People-Centered Eye Care: The Game Changer

Taraprasad Das, Thaksaphon Tharmarangsi, Sobha Sivaprasad, and Srinivas Marmamula

Key Points

- The World Report on Vision (2019) recommended integrated people-centered eye care (IPCEC).
- In 2020, the World Health Assembly adopted by resolution—WHA 73.4.
- The IPCEC was based on the World Health Organization's global strategy recommendation for People-Centered and Integrated Health Services in 2016.
- IPCEC covers four-tier service delivery from the community to tertiary levels and includes all four dimensions, promotion, prevention, treatment, and rehabilitation.
- IPCEC has four cardinal strategies: engage and empower people and community, reorient service delivery, coordinate within and between services, and create an enabling environment.
- Multisectoral consultation and a good referral system are keys to success of IPCEC.
- In populous countries, an addition of the fifth layer, advanced tertiary care, is suggested.
- Political commitment, engagement of patients and community, governance for the coordinated system, multisectoral collaboration, and investment in eye healthcare infrastructure, especially in eye health workforces, are urgently needed.

On the 2019 World Sight Day (observed on the second Thursday of October every year), the World Health Organization (WHO) released the first-ever World Report on Vision (WRV) [1]. The WRV describes the prevailing magnitude of eye disorders, as well as the success of global efforts, current challenges, and strategies for universal health coverage through eye care. One of the most important recommendations for the future of eye care is the Integrated People-Centered Eye Care (IPCEC). The IPCEC is built on the WHO global strategy on people-centered and integrated health services, endorsed at the 69th World Health Assembly in 2016 (Resolution WHA 69.24) [2]. This is a call for a fundamental paradigm shift in the delivery and financing of health services. This well thought-through strategy is to help people access high-quality health services, while also allowing the providers to

T. Das (✉)
L V Prasad Eye Institute, Hyderabad, India
e-mail: tpd@lvpei.org

T. Tharmarangsi
International Health Policy Program, Thailand, Bangkok

S. Sivaprasad
Moorfield's Eye Hospital, London, UK
e-mail: Sobha.Sivaprasad@moorfields.nhs.uk

S. Marmamula
Allen Foster Community Eye Health Research Centre, Gullapalli Pratibha Rao International Centre for Advancement of Rural Eye Care, L V Prasad Eye Institute, Hyderabad, Telangana, India
e-mail: sri.marmamula@lvpei.org

T. Das, P. D. Nayar (eds.), *South-East Asia Eye Health*,
https://doi.org/10.1007/978-981-16-3787-2_5

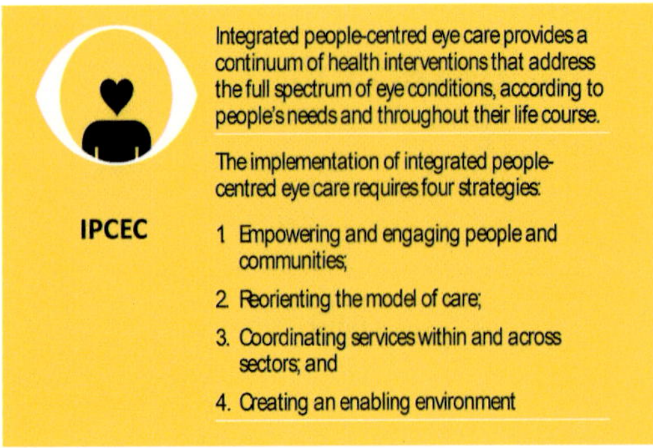
IPCEC
Integrated people-centred eye care provides a continuum of health interventions that address the full spectrum of eye conditions, according to people's needs and throughout their life course.
The implementation of integrated people-centred eye care requires four strategies:
1 Empowering and engaging people and communities;
2 Reorienting the model of care;
3. Coordinating services within and across sectors; and
4. Creating an enabling environment

Fig. 5.1 Integrated people-centered eye care (IPCEC). (Source: World Report on Vision)

Table 5.1 Benefits of people-centered integrated health services

Beneficiaries	Benefits
Individual/ family	Increased satisfaction; improved access; shared decision making
Community	Care of marginalized people; a healthier and more engaged community
Health professionals	Job satisfaction; shared responsibilities; career growth
Health system	Equitable resource distribution; enhanced patient safety; reduced duplication of health investment
Government/ society	Control over total health expenditure; healthier citizens; more productive labor workforce

maintain financial sustainability so that healthcare becomes more responsive to individual and community needs (Fig. 5.1). The compelling reasons behind this strategic shift are the aging population, increasing longevity, increasing urbanization, unhealthy lifestyles, and the gradual shift of the disease spectrum to non-communicable diseases. While hospital-based "curative" treatment is still required for more advanced stages of diseases or when complex procedures and surgery are necessary, "preventive" care is equally imperative and health "promotion" is critical to bring about behavioral changes in the population.

5.1 New Paradigm of Healthcare

5.1.1 What Is People-Centered Health Service?

The WRV states the people-centered health service as an "approach where the individuals, families, and communities are both participants and beneficiaries of the health system that responds to their needs and preferences in humane and holistic ways" [2]. People make their own choices according to preferences in people-centered healthcare.

5.1.2 What Is an Integrated Health Service?

The WHO defines integrated health service as "health service where people receive a continuum of care including health promotion and disease prevention according to their needs at the different levels and sites of care within the health system" [2].

The guiding principles of integrated people-centered health services are comprehensive, equitable, sustainable, continuous, holistic, and evidence-based care that empowers people to make a choice, respects people's dignity, is ethical in practice, and is transparent in delivery. Besides, the health service should focus equally on preventive and rehabilitative care. The system benefits individuals and families, the community, health professionals, and the overall health system (Table 5.1).

5.2 Patient–Physician Relationship

Four models of the patient–physician relationship have been described [3]. These are: (1) paternalistic: where the physician acts as a guardian and dictates the treatment; (2) informative: where physicians share information and respect the patient's choice of care; (3) interpretive: where the physician takes on the role of a counselor to resolve a patient's dilemma in treatment decisions; and (4) deliberative: where the physician acts as a friend/ teacher to arrive at a consensus treatment decision (Table 5.2).

Each model could be considered by its own merits, though the deliberative model upholds the patient's shared values and morals [4]. Patient-centric healthcare emphasizes the deliberative model of the patient–physician relationship.

5.3 Universal Health Coverage and Primary Healthcare

Central to IPCEC is universal health coverage (UHC) and primary healthcare. The UHC aims to bridge gaps in uncovered services, populations, and financial protection as per the *UHC cube* described in the 2010 World Health Report (Fig. 5.2) [5].

The right care at the right place with the right resources, while also meeting the expenses for all of these is possible only when healthcare is integrated and people-centered. Since the Alma Ata declaration in 1978 [6], primary care has remained the cornerstone of health reform. That 40 years later, in 2018, it was required to be reconfirmed at the Astana meeting [7] clearly suggests that primary care is not yet fully or uniformly realized in all countries in the world. One of the stated reasons for incomplete realization was the lack of complete guidelines. It has been suggested that the assignment of disease-centric goals and time-bound programs may help countries to realize the goals of primary care. This was the origin of the selective primary healthcare (SPHC) system [8] as different from comprehensive primary healthcare (CPHC) system [9]. The basic differences between SPHC and CPHC are shown in Table 5.3. As a practical approach for the system development, programs may begin as SPHC systems, focused on a disease with the

Table 5.2 Four models of the patient–physician relationship [3]

	Paternalistic	Informative	Interpretive	Deliberative
Patient values	Objective: shared by physician and patient	Defined: fixed and known to the patient	Inchoate and conflicting, requiring elucidation	Open to development and revision through discussion
Physician's obligation	Promoting patient's well-being independent of the patient's current preferences	Providing relevant facts and implementing patient's selected intervention	Elucidating and interpreting relevant patient values; informing and implementing the patient's selected intervention	Articulating and persuading the patient of the most admirable values; informing and implementing the patient's selected intervention
Patient's autonomy	Assenting to objective values	Choice of and control over medical care	Self-understanding; relevant to medical care	Moral self-development relevant to medical care
Physician's role	Guardian	Competent technical expert	Counselor or advisor	Friend or coach
Best time to adopt	Emergency; saves precious time	Respect patient's second-order desires	Conflicting patient values	Improve the moral values of the patient

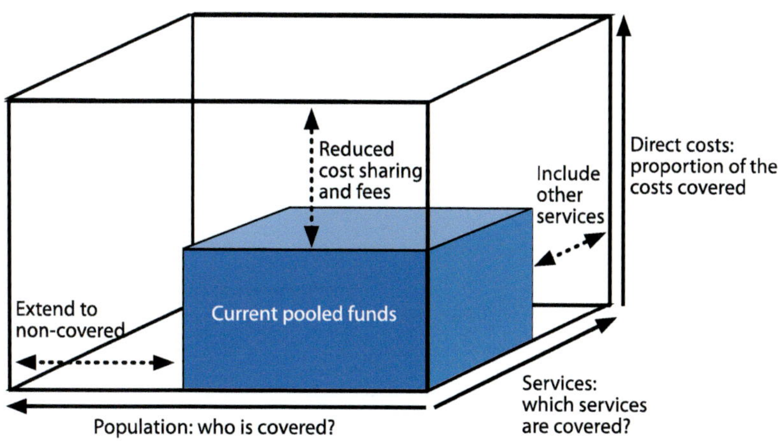

Fig. 5.2 The universal health coverage (UHC) cube (Source: World Health Report, 2010)

Table 5.3 Differences between selective and comprehensive primary healthcare [10]

Approach	Selective primary healthcare (SPHC)	Comprehensive primary healthcare (CPHC)
Values	Effective, efficient, cost-effective	Equity, community participation, inter-sectoral collaboration
Concepts	Health as an absence of disease	Health as well-being
Orientation and accountability	Vertical: Success depends on vertical management and support	Horizontal: Success depends on multisectoral links, community support, and capacity building
Time scope	Short term: Dependent on donors and program managers	Long term: Dependent on population and public health

highest morbidity and mortality, but must move toward the CPHC system.

Both approaches, SPHC and CPHC, have advantages and disadvantages. The disease-specific programs are usually time-bound, and it is relatively easy to measure the outcomes in such programs, and many donors prefer to support such programs, particularly in low- and middle-income countries. Long-term and sustainable benefits are derived when the vertical and horizontal programs are combined for equitable care and community ownership.

5.4 Inequity Versus Inequality

Inequity is not the same as inequality.

Inequality is "the state of not being equal in status, rights, and opportunities" (United Nations, [11]).

Inequity is unfair social justice—systematic differences in the health status of different population groups that have significant social and economic costs both to individuals and societies. Health inequity arises due to the "differences in health that are unnecessary, avoidable, unfair, and unjust" (WHO) [12, 13].

People-centered and integrated health services are the right approach to strengthening health systems in all countries irrespective of their economic status because both, inequity and inequality, exist between various groups and sections of society. Most countries in the WHO South-East Asia Region are middle-income countries. This region has two unique characteristics, the rapid urbanization, and a growing economy. In general, urbanization disrupts social structures, making it harder to engage communities in decision making and maintain a close patient-provider relationship. Being an emerging market with recent significant economic growth allows for greater private investment, with many sunrise technologies, thereby attracting a larger number of patients; however, this often entails greater out-of-pocket spending.

5.5 Five Directions to People-Centered Integrated Healthcare

The WHO's five proposed inter-dependent strategic directions towards people-centered and integrated healthcare are: (1) empowering and engaging people; (2) strengthening governance and accountability; (3) reorienting the model of care; (4) coordinating services; and (5) creating an enabling environment (Fig. 5.3) [14].

People and the community are empowered when they receive the right opportunity to enhance their skills and resources to become equal partners in healthcare decision making. These include advocacy, health education, and care of disadvantaged or marginalized people. Good governance, stewardship, and accountability are the keys to any growth, including the health services. These improve policy dialogue on national health policies, strategies, and plans with citizens and communities. The requirement is adequate information on the accountability of service providers and empowerment of people. Participatory deficit and lack of transparency are

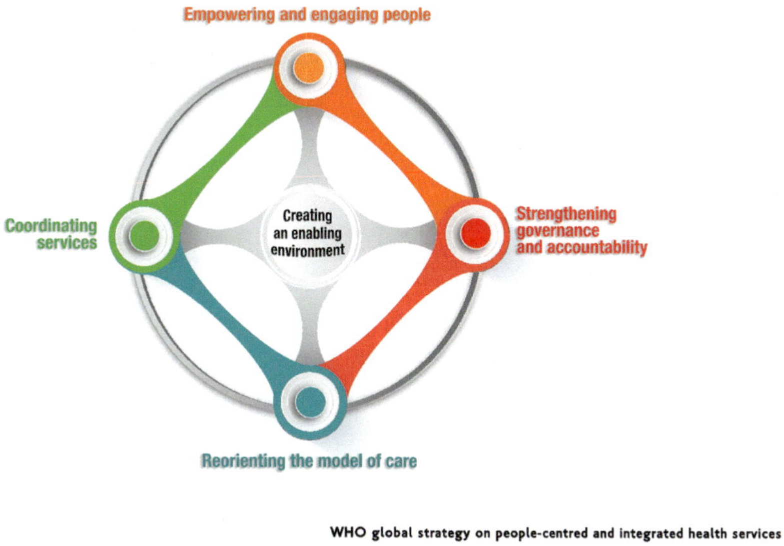

Fig. 5.3 Five strategic directions of people-centered and integrated health services (Source: WHO)

more common in countries with lower than higher incomes. A good model of people-centered healthcare builds on primary and preventive care as much as tertiary and curative care. Preventive care should assume a greater significance, given the increasing prevalence of non-communicable diseases. These activities create new multisectoral engagements and opportunities in the community. However, people-centered healthcare does not discount hospital-based care, but makes it a part of the continuum of care.

There is a greater demand for change in the model of care. With new technologies and health information systems, it is more than possible today to meet this demand. Health and well-being are integrated as per the WHO definition (health is a state of complete physical, mental, and social well-being, and not merely the absence of disease or infirmity) [15]. Coordination of services of health and related sectors and overcoming fragmentation in healthcare are needed to achieve these goals. Coordination of services and workflow is different from merging; coordination focuses more on improving the continuity of care and relationship with people.

The four strategies of people-centered and integrated healthcare would function well only when there is an enabling environment to bring together all stakeholders to make these transformational changes in health policy, behavior, and delivery. There has been a constant dialogue on reorienting the health system and service delivery as far back as 1986 with the first international conference on Health Promotion (Ottawa Charter) [16]. The Ottawa charter identified "reorienting healthcare services" as one of five "Pillars" action items (the others were: (1) building healthy public policy, (2) creating supportive environments, (3) strengthening community action, and (4) developing personal skills) [16]. Despite this commitment three decades ago, the reorienting of the service model has not met with considerable success. It is principally because medical service primarily revolves around qualified medical personnel (usually the physician) and medical infrastructure (usually the hospital). There is a need for significant behavioral change at the individual level, task sharing by professional bodies, and above all, a strong political will to empower individuals and the community.

5.6 Integrated People-Centered Eye Care (IPCEC)

The WHO 2019 recommendation on IPCEC is built on the framework of the integrated people-centered health services (2016 WHA 69.24). Similar to the integrated health services, the four strategies of IPCEC are: (1) empowering and engaging people and communities; (2) reorienting the model of care; (3) coordinating services within and across sectors; and (4) creating an enabling environment.

5.6.1 Empowering and Engaging People and Communities

Empowering people and the community begin with understanding population needs and opinions. A population consultation is a necessary step for policymaking and policy implementation. Population consultation could happen at any stage of the national planning process, from subnational to supranational, on varying themes from preventive to curative, and with all parts of the population. The methods include face-to-face invited participations and surveys which create a continuous dialogue between the policymakers and other stakeholders. Such consultation increases the population's ownership of policies and plans.

Some eye conditions, such as, glaucoma and diabetic retinopathy, do not cause visual impairment till an advanced stage of the disease. Additionally, unlike cataract surgery or correction of refractive error, glaucoma and diabetic retinopathy require early detection and life-long treatment. Referral of and use of low vision devices and access to currently available assistive devices need good advocacy and health literacy for both, care providers and affected individuals. Finally, all outreach activities, either through direct (mass eye camps popular in certain countries and communities) or remote (teleophthalmology) methods, need both community involvement and a robust referral system.

5.6.2 Reorienting the Model of Care

Reorienting the model of care ensures that appropriate and accessible care is available to all people when and where they need it. An effective modality is strong primary eye care with a good referral system. At the primary level, refractive errors, cataract, corneal injuries, and low vision can be diagnosed; if glaucoma and diabetic retinopathy are suspected, the patient can be referred for further care. While correcting spectacles can be dispensed in most cases (except for very difficult situation, such as keratoconus), an appropriate referral could be made for other ophthalmic disorders. With little extra training, simple low vision devices could also be prescribed at the primary care level. School eye health, community outreach, and community-based rehabilitation are best performed through the primary eye care level.

Three critical but interrelated components of a well-functioning IPCEC are the healthcare delivery infrastructures, human resources for health, and health financing. The WRV suggested a 4-tier model for IPCEC (Fig. 5.4). These are: (1) community care—eye care delivered at the community, school, and home level; (2) primary care—eye care for treatment of simple disorders (refractive error) and referral of common eye disorders (cataract, glaucoma, diabetic retinopathy); (3) secondary care—eye care with surgery for common disorders such as cataract, and nonsurgical care for common ophthalmic disorders (laser therapy for diabetic retinopathy and angle-closure glaucoma); (4) tertiary care—medical and surgical eye care for more complex eye disorders. Effective execution of the four-tier model concept requires robust system governance and coordination across levels.

The 4-tier model of integrated eye care is an excellent model of comprehensive eye care with the involvement of the community and spreading beyond curative to promotive and rehabilitative care. The model proposed by the WRV, however, did not specify the number of people it could serve. The L V Prasad Eye Institute (Hyderabad, India) had proposed a 5-tier model (the eye health pyramid) with a suggestion for the population numbers that each tier can serve and the level of eye care that each tier can deliver (Fig. 5.4; Table 5.4) [17–19]. The 5-tier model is applicable to countries with large populations in the South-East Asia Region such as Bangladesh, India, Indonesia, Myanmar, and Thailand.

In India, the Government has demonstrated the intention of delivering universal health cover-

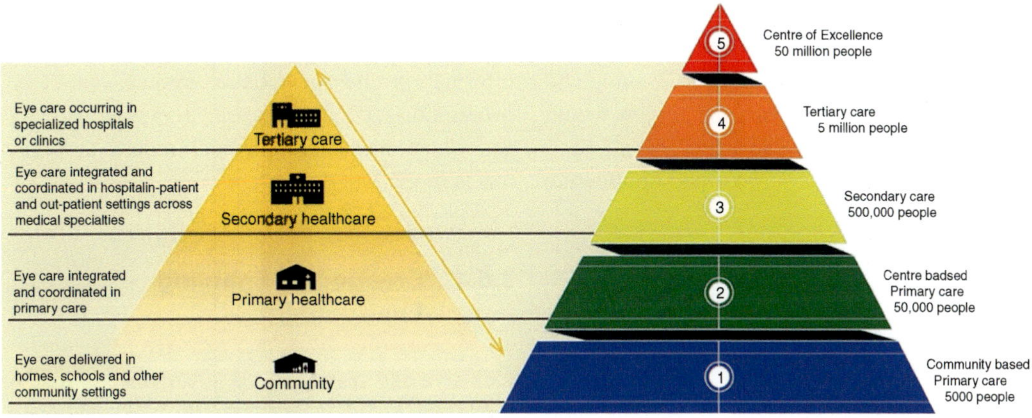

Fig. 5.4 The alignment of 4-tier and 5-tier eye care delivery model [17]

Table 5.4 The structure and function of the 5-level integrated eye care system [18]

Structure	Suggested population coverage	Technical personnel	Level of care	Quantum of care
Community	5000	Vision guardian	Advocacy; health promotion; prescription of simple near vision glasses	10% of visual impairment (simple single-vision reading glasses)
Primary	50,000	Vision technician	Eye screening; refraction; dispensing spectacles; referral	49% of visual impairment cases (URE)
Secondary	500,000	Ophthalmologists; vision technicians; surgery assistants	Comprehensive eye exam; community care; surgery for common disorders	75% of visual impairment cases (URE + cataract surgery)
Tertiary	5 million	Ophthalmologists; optometrists; nurses; rehabilitation personnel; microbiology; pathology; eye banking	Secondary level care + all eye surgeries; corneal transplants; rehabilitation for low vision and blindness; training; clinical research	90% of visual impairment cases (URE + surgery + care for glaucoma and DR)
Advanced tertiary	50 million	Tertiary level personnel + basic scientists; policymakers	Tertiary level care + translational research; policy and planning	100% of visual impairment cases; policy execution

DR diabetic retinopathy, *URE* uncorrected refractive error

age and primary care through the Health and Wellness Center (HWC) system which is designed to cover 3000 to 5000 people. The HWC system, as designed by the Government of India, has all the components of IPCEC at the community level, including the referral system and continuum of care. The ophthalmic care at the community level includes screening for blindness and refractive errors in adults, counseling, and support for care for neonates and infants through mobile health teams [20].

To ensure that community and primary eye care systems meet the targets of the sustainable development goals (SDGs) in 2030, for an estimated population of 3879 million people (the population in the South-East Asia Region in 2030 without counting those in the Democratic People's Republic of Korea), the region would need 429,802 community eye centers, 43,374 primary eye centers, and 164,784 allied ophthalmic personnel [17].

5.6.3 Coordinating Services Within and Across Sectors

A successful health program thrives on good coordination between the individuals seeking service and the healthcare providers, between the programs in the same service, and between different health sectors. This makes eye care more comprehensive, less repetitive, and improves the quality, equity, and continuity of care. At the infrastructural level, good coordination helps in meaningful referrals and reduces the cost of care.

The world is committed to the 17 goals of the SDGs and is working to resolve, by 2030, "end poverty and hunger everywhere; combat inequalities within and among countries; build peaceful, just and inclusive societies; protect human rights and promote gender equality and the empowerment of women and girls; and ensure the lasting protection of the planet and its natural resources" [21]. SDG 3, on good health and well-being, pledges to "ensure healthy lives and promote well-being for all ages" [22]. To progress towards all 13 targets, SDG 3 has to work with many other interconnected targets. While all the other targets are important for the success of SDG 3, the more evident ones are SDG 6 (clean water and sanitation), SDG 2 (zero hunger), SDG 4 (quality education), SDG 5 (gender equality), SDG 10 (reduced inequality), and SDG 1 (no poverty).

In many countries in the South-East Asian region, private and non-government organizations (NGOs) play equal roles within the public system for eye care. Also, in many countries of the region, more than one international NGO supports eye care delivery. Good coordination is required between public and private supporters (including civil society organizations, philanthropic agencies, and NGOs) and international agencies. Finally, the role of a robust health information and surveillance system cannot be overemphasized. Today, with digital technology and electronic health/medical record systems, this is more than possible.

5.6.4 Creating an Enabling Environment

Inclusive and participatory governance is essential in any health system reform. Leadership and governance are one of the WHO's six health system building blocks (the other five are service delivery, workforce, information system, access to essential medicine, and finance) Good governance involves transparent leadership that is inclusive, participatory, and makes the best use of available resources and information to ensure the best possible results [1]. The national government makes strategic health and eye health plans for health priority and resource allocation in all countries. It also oversees the implementation and monitors the progress of these plans.

One of the important elements of health finance is strategic health service purchasing [23]. Purchasing refers to the allocation of pooled funds to healthcare providers to deliver health services on behalf of certain groups or the entire population. Strategic purchasing transforms budgets into benefits, intending to distribute resources equitably and improve the quality [23].

In most countries, eye care is not included in national health strategic plans. Globally, less than 5% of people are blind or visually impaired (338 million people are visually impaired amongst the 7.8 billion people globally; as of 2020, 0.55% (43 million people) are blind and 3.78% (295 million people) have moderate to severe visual impairment [24]) It may seem difficult to sustain an entire program of work around vision problems. Besides, visual impairment does not always occur in isolation. Some examples of associations between biological and environmental factors with common eye disorders are cataract and aging, reduced out-door activity and myopia progression, diabetes mellitus and retinopathy, poor hygiene and trachoma, and premature birth/low birth weight and retinopathy of prematurity. Hence, integration of primary eye care with primary health could be a more cost-effective method of eye healthcare delivery, such as cataract being integrated with healthy aging, refractive error being integrated with healthy school-age life, retinopathy of prematurity being integrated with maternal and child health, and diabetic retinopathy being integrated with non-communicable diseases [25].

There is an epidemiological transition in all countries in the WHO South-East Asia Region along with economic and demographic changes. The epidemiologic transition describes the changes in mortality and morbidity patterns (from infectious to chronic diseases) as the demographic, economic, and social structures of a society change [26]. The four phases of epidemiologic transition are: (1) age of pestilence and famine (mid-eighteenth century) with high fertility and high mortality resulting in low population growth; (2) age of receding pandemics (nineteenth and early twentieth century) with high fertility and decreased mortality, resulting in high population growth; (3) age of degenerative and man-made disease (twentieth century) with controlled fertility and low mortality resulting in higher longevity; and (4) age of delayed degenerative diseases (twenty-first century) with slow and fluctuating mortality and advances in medical technology resulting in reduced community risk [27].

Health transition is a dynamic process, one where the health and disease patterns of a society evolve in response to broader demographic, socioeconomic, technological, political, cultural, and biological changes [28]. In many countries of the region, there is a decline in communicable diseases (two countries each in the region have been declared as trachoma- and malaria-free); but increased longevity, cases of myopia and diabetes mellitus, and usage of neonatal intensive care units would add to numbers of cataract, presbyopia, myopia, diabetic retinopathy and retinopathy of prematurity cases. Along with this shifting spectrum of eye disorders and lifestyle changes, particularly among the young population, the region, now more than ever, needs functioning intra- and inter-sectoral collaborations and integration.

In addition to political commitment and leadership, the success of the IPCEC system would depend on two other important factors: (1) human resource for health (HRH) workforce and (2) health technology [29]. The World Health Assembly (WHA 60.29 in 2007) defined health technology as "the application of organized knowledge and skills in the form of devices, medicines, vaccines, procedures, and systems developed to solve a health problem and improve quality of life." The World Health Assembly also requests WHO member states to work on the following five actions: (1) collect, verify, update, and exchange information on health technologies; (2) formulate, as appropriate, national strategies and plans for the establishment of systems for the assessment, planning, procurement, and management of health technologies; (3) formulate national or regional guidelines for good manufacturing and regulatory practices; (4) establish, where necessary, regional and national institutions of health technology; and (5) collect information that interrelates medical devices which deal with priority public health conditions at different levels of care. Recognizing the importance of the HRH workforce in realizing universal health coverage and SDG 3, the WHO, in 2016, has suggested four objectives and set 13 milestones for 2020 and 2030 [30]. The emphasis has been on capacity building with local talent, accreditation of different medial courses, and the creation of mechanisms to retain the workforce.

We describe here, two models of the IPCEC system, one used in England and supported by public funding and the other used in India by major not-for-profit eye care organizations.

5.7 National Health Service and Eye Care in England

The National Health Service (NHS) in England, initiated on fifth July 1948, is an exemplar public-funded health system that provides universal health coverage and is, therefore, free at the point of care for those seeking healthcare. The NHS has a good network of general practices around the country that provide primary care, and patients who need specialist care are referred to secondary care centers. Some of these secondary care centers also have tertiary care facilities. The health system works as follows:

1. Primary eye care: Contracted optometrists in England provide general ophthalmic services (GOSs). They are funded at the national level by NHS England. Certain categories of the population are provided NHS-funded sight tests at no cost, but need to purchase their own spectacles. Examples of people eligible for free eyesight tests are those under 16 and above 60 years, those diagnosed with diabetes or glaucoma, and those registered as visually impaired.
2. There are several protocol-based screenings as part of primary care. These include screening of neonates for retinopathy of prematurity, pre-school screening for uncorrected refractive errors, and annual diabetic retinopathy screening for people with diabetes.
3. Secondary care: All eye abnormalities detected by optometrists or at screening are referred to secondary care. There are key performance indicators. National audits are carried out on cataract surgery centers to ensure consistency in the provision of high-quality care. The secondary care center facilities are well equipped with state-of-art diagnostic equipment and offer advanced eye care.

There are several national guidelines, such as those developed by the Royal College of Ophthalmologists, that are also used in many other countries. Quality standards issued by the national screening program for diabetic retinopathy have helped reduce the rate of blindness due to diabetic retinopathy in England.

5.7.1 Challenges

The NHS was initiated in 1948 when the population of England was 49.4 million, and today, it is serving a population of 61.4 million. The life expectancy in England has also increased from 68.4 years in 1948 to 80.8 in 2018. Lack of capacity is a major issue. Currently, the numbers of ophthalmologists are insufficient to cater to the required provision of eye services. Allied healthcare professionals and nurses are employed to delegate some of the services. The aging population and the cost of new technologies have put the NHS system under strain. Diabetic retinopathy, glaucoma, cataract, and age-related macular degeneration are projected to increase exponentially over the next decade. The use of anti-vascular endothelial growth factor agents in many retinal vascular disorders, including diabetic retinopathy and age-related macular degeneration, requires patients to return several times to the hospital for several years, which will also place a great strain upon the system.

Despite these challenges, eye care services in England are considered one of the world's better models. Under this model, ophthalmology has the highest number of outpatient appointments and attendances in the NHS. A total of 7.8 million people attended ophthalmology appointments in hospital eye services in the NHS in 2018–19, out of a total of 96.4 million out-patients attendances in the NHS (https://files.digital.nhs.uk).

5.8 Eye Health Pyramid Model: Adopted by Major Not-For-Profit Eye Care Organizations in India

India has pioneered multitier eye care models for service delivery, covering the entire gamut of care from basic screening at the community level to managing complex cases at the tertiary and quaternary levels of care. These models had encapsulated the core elements of IPCEC.

The government has adopted the eye health pyramid model in its policy planning. Some of the not-for-profit eye care organizations in India's private sector are already using this model for the delivery of comprehensive eye care. Under this model, 9 large organizations serve 14 states and 2 union territories in India (Fig. 5.5). Together, these organizations have established 425 primary, 38 secondary, and 26 tertiary level eye care facili-

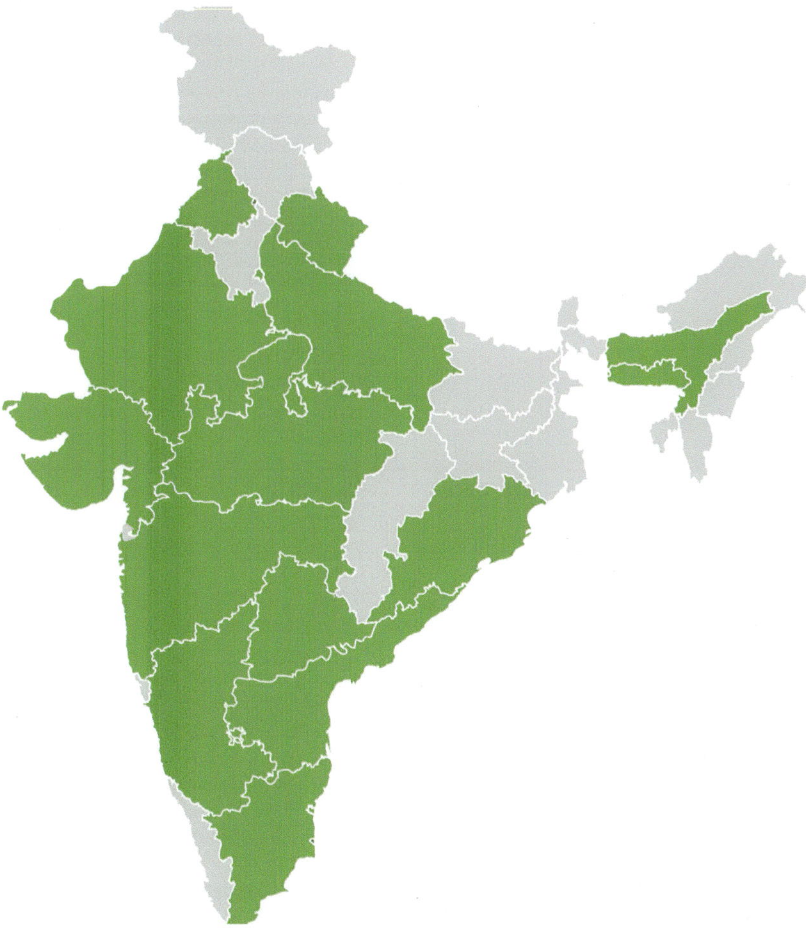

Fig. 5.5 Major not-for-profit eye care organizational operations (green-shaded) in India, using the eye health pyramid model to deliver eye care

ties. In 2019, these organizations provided consultation to over 12.25 million people (22.5% of them outreach) and eye surgery to over 1.17 million people.

In appreciation of the effort made by its Member States and international partners, the World Health Assembly adopted a resolution in support of the IPCEC in 2020 (WHA.73.4) as recommended in the World Report on Vision [31]. The resolution urged member states to also "make eye care an integral part of universal health coverage and promote high-quality health systems research complementing existing evidence for effective eye care interventions" [31]. The resolution also urged the member states to focus on two common avoidable eye disorders, namely, refractive error and cataract surgery. It is hoped that all member states will work to meet the goals and targets for universal health coverage by the year 2030 and offer integrated people-centered eye care as per the 2030 Sustainable Development Goals.

References

1. WHO. World report on vision. Geneva: World Health Organization; 2019.
2. WHO. Framework on integrated people-centered health services. 2016. www.who.int. Accessed 26 Oct 2020.
3. Emanuel EJ, Emanuel LL. Four models of physician-patient relationship. JAMA. 1992;267:2221–6.
4. Das T. Anatomy of medicine with compassion (Alim Memorial lecture 2018). J Ophthalmological Soc Bangladesh. 2019;47:5–10.

5. WHO. World health report: the road to universal coverage. Geneva: World Health Organization; 2010.
6. Declaration of Alma-Ata. International conference on primary health care, Alma-Ata, USSR, 6–12 September 1978. http://www.who.int/publications/almaata_declaration_en.pdf. Accessed 24 Oct 2020.
7. Astana Declaration on Primary Health Care. www.who.int. primary-health. Accessed 24 Oct 2020.
8. Walsh J, Warren K. Selective primary health care. N Engl J Med. 1979;301:967–74.
9. Rifkin SB, Walt G. How health improves: defining the issues concerning "comprehensive primary health care" and "selective primary health care". Soc Sci Med. 1986;23:559–66.
10. Rifkin SB. Health for all and primary health care, 1978–2018: a historical perspective on policies and programs over 40 years. 2018; https://doi.org/10.1093/acrefore/9780190632366.013.55.
11. The United Nations. Concept of inequality. www.un.org. Accessed 25 Oct 2020.
12. Whitehead M. The concepts and principles of equity in health. Int J Health Serv. 1992;22:429–45.
13. WHO. Ten facts on health inequities and their causes. www.who.int. Accessed 25 Oct 2020.
14. WHO. Global strategy on people-centered and integrated health services. Interim report. Geneva: WHO; 2015.
15. World Health Organization. Constitution. www.who.int. Accessed 17 Aug 2020.
16. WHO. The Ottawa charter for health promotion. www.who.int. Accessed 26 Oct 2020.
17. Das T, Keeffe J, Sivaprasad S, Rao GN. Capacity building for universal eye health coverage in South East Asia beyond 2020. Eye (London). 2020;34:1262–70.
18. Rao GN. The Barrie jones lecture-eye care for the neglected population: challenges and solutions. Eye (London). 2015;29:30–45.
19. Das T. Reaching the last mile in eye care. Indian J Ophthalmol. 2020;68:s3–5.
20. Comprehensive primary healthcare through health and wellness centre. http://www.nhsrcindia.org. Last accessed 2019 Dec 20.
21. Transforming our world: the 2030 agenda for sustainable development. Resolution adopted by the General Assembly on 25 September 2015. www.sustainabledevelopment.un.org. Accessed 15 Nov 2020.
22. The United Nations. 17 sustainable development goals (SDGs). www.un.org. Accessed 29 June 2020.
23. Mathauer I, Dale E, Jowett M, et al. Purchasing health services for universal health coverage: how to make it more strategic? Geneva: World Health Organization; 2019.
24. Bourne RRA, Jaimie J, Seth F, et al. Trends in prevalence of blindness and distance and near vision impairment over 30 years and contribution to the Global Burden of disease in 2020. Lancet Glob Health. 2020. Advanced online publication. https://doi.org/10.2139/ssrn.3582742
25. Murthy GVS, Raman U. Perspectives on primary eye care. Community Eye Health. 2009;22:10–1.
26. Omran AR. The epidemiologic transition. A theory of the epidemiology of population change. Milbank Mem Fund Q. 1971;49:509–38.
27. Olshansky SJ, Ault AB. The fourth stage of the epidemiologic transition: the age of delayed degenerative diseases. Milbank Q. 1986;64:355–91.
28. Frenk J, Bobadilla JL, Stern C, Frjka T, Lozano R. Elements for a theory of the health transition. Health Transit Rev. 1991;1:21–38.
29. Das T, Panda L. Imagining eye care in India (2018 Lalit Prakash Agarwal lecture). Indian J Ophthalmol. 2018;66:1532–8.
30. WHO. Global strategy on human resources for health: workforce 2030. Geneva: WHO; 2016.
31. Integrated people-centered eye care. www.who.int. Accessed 30 Oct 2020.

Health Financing and Sustainability

6

Taraprasad Das, Raja Narayanan, and Gullapalli N. Rao

Key Points

- The World Health Organization defines good health financing as raising adequate funds for health so that people who use the needed services can be protected from financial catastrophe or impoverishment associated with having to pay for the health services.
- It is estimated that an increment of USD274–371 billion funding is required per year till 2030 to make satisfactory progress towards the sustainable development goals.
- The three main sources of financing in the healthcare system are: public funding, out-of-pocket spending, and developmental assistance for health.
- In 2016, among the South-East Asia Region countries, the spending on health per gross domestic product (GDP) was highest in the Maldives; the proportion of public health spending out of the total spent on health was highest in Thailand; the proportion of out-of-pocket spending out of the total spent on health was highest in Myanmar; and the amount invested in developmental assistance for health as a proportion of total health spending was highest in Timor-Leste.
- Health for all without causing impoverishment due to health expenditure is one of the primary goals of universal health coverage.
- Globally, 808 million people (12% of the world's population) in 2010 became impoverished due to catastrophic health expenditures at the 10% threshold. Aging and new medical technology impact catastrophic health expenditure.
- Responsible investment is critical for allocating resources that would also complement the Environmental, Social, and corporate Governance (ESG) initiatives, as developed by the United Nations Principles for Responsible Investment.
- Global spending on health is increasing (USD7.8 trillion; 10% of GDP in 2017) though, it is insufficient in low-income countries. In 2017, the average amount spent on health was only USD41 per person in low-income countries and USD2937 per person in high-income countries.

Sustainable Development Goal 3 (SDG 3) 2030 calls for healthy lives and promoting well-being for all ages. Healthcare refers to the entire range of curative, preventive, promotive, and rehabilitative care delivered at all care levels, from the primary (often in the community) to the tertiary level (hospitals). Health financing refers to the sourcing of funds from all sources that can be used to pay for the entire range of health-

T. Das (✉) · R. Narayanan · G. N. Rao
L V Prasad Eye Institute, Hyderabad, India
e-mail: tpd@lvpei.org; narayanan@lvpei.org; gnr@lvpei.org

T. Das, P. D. Nayar (eds.), *South-East Asia Eye Health*,
https://doi.org/10.1007/978-981-16-3787-2_6

care services. It is one of the six World Health Organization (WHO) health system building blocks. The overall goal of health financing is to protect healthcare users from social and financial risks and also to build a sustainable health system for healthcare providers to continue providing care. In 2000, the WHO defined health finance as a function of "a health system concerned with the mobilization, accumulation, and allocation of money to cover the health needs of the people, individually and collectively" [1]. In 2007, the definition of good health financing was expanded to include "raising adequate funds for health, so that people can use the needed services protected from financial catastrophe or impoverishment associated with having to pay for them" [2]. Health financing today must be prepared for additional expenditures to accommodate increasing healthcare costs related to increased longevity and improved quality of life in the elderly. It is estimated that an increment of USD274–371 billion in funding is required per year till 2030 to make satisfactory progress towards the SDGs. Three-quarters of this financial resource would be required for health system strengthening (health workforce, infrastructure, and medical equipment). With an additional annual funding of USD20–54 billion, one could save 97 million lives globally and increase life expectancy by 3.1–8.4 years [3]. Low- and middle-income countries (most South-East Asia Region countries belong to this category) receive health financing of approximately USD141–183 billion per year. This chapter will deal with three broad subjects: (1) health financing, (2) health system sustainability, and (3) health financing sustainability with reference to the SEAR countries.

6.1 Health Financing

The three main sources of financing in the healthcare system are: (1) public funding (includes tax and compulsory health insurance), (2) out-of-pocket spending (includes private health insurance), and (3) developmental assistance for health. In 2016, among the South-East Asia region (SEAR) countries, the amount spent on health per gross domestic product (GDP) was highest in the Maldives and lowest in Timor-Leste (10% and 2%, respectively); the proportion of public health spending out of the total amount spent on health was highest in Thailand and lowest in Nepal (77.3% and 18.5%, respectively); the proportion of out-of-pocket spending out of the total amount spent on health was highest in Myanmar and lowest in Timor-Leste (71% and 10.6% respectively); and the proportion of developmental assistance for health of total health spending was highest in Timor-Leste and lowest in the Maldives (22.9% and 0.2% respectively) (Fig. 6.1; Table 6.1) [4].

Public finance is usually tax-based funding. It includes all forms of general government revenue, such as income tax, sales tax, special taxes, and different levies. This is an important component of health financing. The *compulsory health insurance* system, either mandatory social health insurance or a stand-alone government health insurance, mandates a certain percentage of income be deducted from every working individual and deposited into a central insurance fund; this is then utilized, in full or in part, in the event of illness. With an aging population and a shrinking working population, the revenue from direct taxation or compulsory health insurance is likely to decline gradually. *Voluntary private health insurance* is an option, but has the problem of adverse selection (people with higher disease probabilities of using the services are enrolled more often than the younger, healthier population) and risk-based premium (higher premiums for older and less healthy people). Elderly and retired people without regular incomes could find the insurance premium unaffordable. Hence, this system may not be an effective financing mechanism for countries with a growing elderly population.

Out-of-pocket spending (OOPS) refers to user fees charged to the patient, either in part or full. High OOPS creates hardship for the individual and family. OOPS is usually incurred due to outpatient care (outpatient—76%; inpatient—24%)

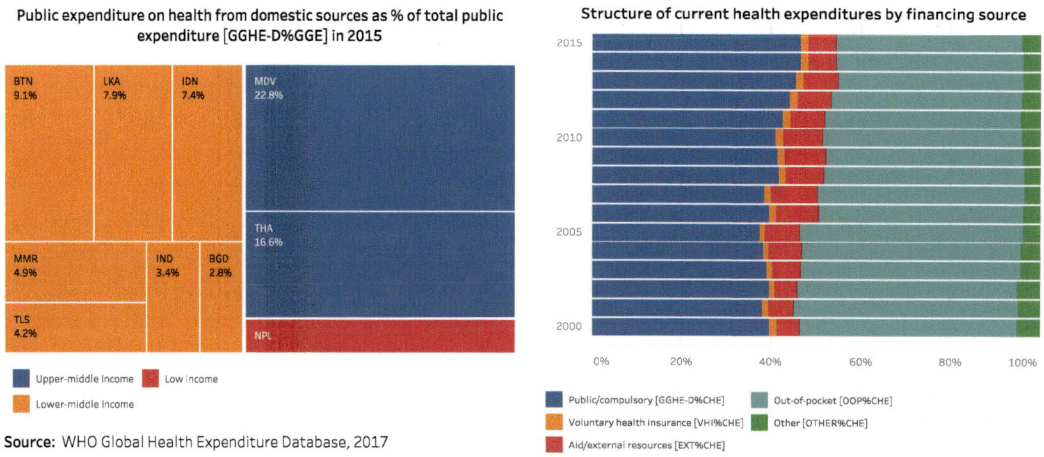

Fig. 6.1 Health expenditure in the World Health Organization (WHO) South-East Asia Region (SEAR). Left: Public expenditure on health in WHO-SEAR. *BGD* Bangladesh, *BTN* Bhutan, *IDN* Indonesia, *IND* India, *MDV* Maldives, *MMR* Myanmar, *NPL* Nepal, *LKA* Sri Lanka, *THA* Thailand, *TLS* Timor-Leste. Right: Structure of current health expenditure according to financing source

Table 6.1 Health expenditure in the South-East Asia Region in 2016 [4]

Country	Health spending per GDP	Public health spending per total health spending	OOPS per total health spending	DAH per total health spending
Bangladesh	3.1	19.2	71.4	6.7
Bhutan	2.5	72.7	20.0	6.1
India	3.0	25.4	64.2	0.9
Indonesia	2.3	40.3	40.1	0.7
Maldives	10.0	70.5	20.1	0.2
Myanmar	4.6	19.5	71.0	9.4
Nepal	5.4	18.5	60.1	8.2
Sri Lanka	3.5	43.6	48.9	1.4
Thailand	3.2	77.3	12.3	0.3
Timor-Leste	2.0	65.2	10.6	0.3
World	8.6	74.0	18.6	22.9

DAH developmental assistance for health, *GDP* gross domestic product, *OOPS* out-of-pocket spending

and from expenditure on medicines (medicine—72%; others—28%) [5]. Development assistance for health (DAH) is the financial and in-kind support from major development agencies.

6.2 Universal Health Coverage and Health Financing

The primary goals of universal health coverage (UHC) are the availability of health services to people when and where these are required, without causing financial hardship and catastrophic health expenditure. Catastrophic health expenditure of a household's income leads to the entire household suffering from the economic burden of disease [6]. A household is impoverished by medical expenses when the healthcare expenditure has caused it to drop below the poverty line [7]. There is no consensus on the catastrophic health expenditure threshold; it could be from medical costs exceeding 10% of the monthly household income to 40% of a household's non-subsistence income (the income available after basic needs have been met) [7, 8].

6.2.1 Catastrophic Health Expenditure

Catastrophic health expenditure (CHE) can occur in all countries at all stages of development. It does not automatically disappear with rising income. National health financing systems with a robust prepayment mechanism supported by a combination of the several health financing channels mentioned earlier could reduce CHE. However, there cannot be a blanket rule. It has to be contextual based on the country's need or desire for population coverage through prepayment mechanisms, and protection of the poor and disadvantaged along with a design of benefits package, and the level of cost-sharing by the patients [9].

CHE is measured by the percentage of people in households whose OOPS is large relative to their income. A study covering 133 countries showed that the global estimated incidence of CHE at the 10% threshold has increased over a period of time; it was 9.7% in 2000, 11.4% in 2005, and 11.7% in 2010. Globally, 808 million people (12% of the world's population) in 2010 incurred catastrophic health expenditure at the 10% threshold. This was higher than in 2000 (599 million people; 10% of the world's population) and 2005 (741 million people; 11% of the world's population) [10]. Catastrophic health expenditure is an indicator of financial protection. Poverty, type of illness, mode of treatment (out or in patient), location (rural versus urban), and lack of health insurance contribute to CHE [11]. Two other factors that also impact the CHE, are population aging and medical technology.

6.2.1.1 Aging

Improved health technology has helped people live longer and with a better quality of life. Increasing longevity and rising elderly populations are a global phenomenon. In 2010, an estimated 8% of the world's population (524 million people) were 65 years or older. By 2050, this number is expected to increase to 16% of the world's population (1.5 billion people). While older people are likely to live in more developed countries, the proportionate growth of older people in less developed countries, between 2010 and 2050, is estimated to be nearly 3.5 times higher (250% in less developed countries compared to 71% in developed countries) [12]. The number of people 65 years or older in India, the most populous country in the SEAR (and the second most populous in the world after China), is estimated to exceed 227 million in 2050 (in China, this number will exceed 300 million). It is expected that over the next two decades, people in every region of the world will suffer more death and disability from non-communicable diseases than from infectious and parasitic diseases. There is always a higher probability of adverse health outcomes when the aging population is exposed to more health risks [13].

The *S*tudy on Global *AGE*ing (SAGE) and adult health is a WHO's ongoing longitudinal study for more than a decade and a half. The SAGE is collecting data on six health risk factors on adults aged 50 years and older; in addition, the study also collects data on a smaller comparison sample of adults aged 18–49 years. The data are collected from nationally representative samples in six countries, China, Ghana, India, Mexico, Russia, and South Africa. The six health risk factors being studied are: (1) physical inactivity (responsible for 6% of global death), (2) current tobacco use (responsible for 9% of global death), (3) heavy alcohol consumption (responsible for 5.3% of global death), (4) high-risk waist-hip ratio (responsible for myocardial infarction), (5) hypertension (responsible for 13% of global death), and (6) obesity (responsible for 5% of global death) [14]. The study has shown a decline in the overall health status score (range: 0—worst health and 100—best health) in all the studied populations. The study has also reported a rise in at least 3 of 6 risk factors with age [14]. Smaller family sizes and declining co-residence by multiple generations are further likely to introduce additional challenges in caring for older relatives by families in developing countries.

6.2.1.2 Medical Technology

There is a proliferation of more precise medical technology. However, unlike most other industries, higher use of technology in healthcare does not necessarily result in lowering the cost of care [15]. In fact, many new technologies and therapy result in higher costs with only marginal improvements in health outcomes. The classic example in eye care is in the technological advances in cataract surgery. Studies from India have shown a clear benefit of extracapsular cataract extraction and intraocular lens (IOL) implantation over intracapsular cataract extraction and aphakic spectacles correction [16]. However, the advantages of phacoemulsification cataract surgery (technologically more advanced and more expensive) over manual small incision cataract surgery (MSICS) or a foldable IOL (more expensive) than a rigid IOL are quite small [17]. Therefore, an objective evaluation of medical technology should be a regular exercise in every country before that technology is adopted into either public or private healthcare sectors.

6.3 Health System Sustainability

Sustainability refers to achieving a target outcome and maintaining this achievement over a long period. The key in sustainability lies in good strategic planning that, in turn, depends on available resources, community participation, partnership with all stakeholders, workload distribution, effective monitoring, reduced donor dependency, and friendly policy [18]. From the above analyses, it is clear that healthcare financing systems in most countries are not efficient enough to maintain quality and/or quantity of care in the face of population aging.

Generally, there are two kinds of efficiencies, the "allocative" and "technical." *Allocative efficiency* is a state of the economy in which production represents consumer preferences. It concerns allocating resources in such a way as to produce the maximum benefits to society. Under allocative efficiency, all goods, services, and capital are allocated and distributed to their very best use. Allocative efficiency occurs at the intersection of the supply and demand curves. At this equilibrium point, the price offered for a given supply exactly matches the demand for that supply at that price, and so all products are sold [19]. *Technical efficiency* is the effectiveness with which a given set of inputs are used to produce an output [20]. The two systems do not necessarily work together always. Despite evidence of better health of the population at a lower cost, there is invariably less public funding allocation for primary and preventive care. The pay-for-service for the use of high-end diagnostic services when private healthcare is paid for often ends in the most expensive rather most cost-effective care.

Medical savings account (MSA) is another healthcare financing system that could be sustainable even with population aging. In the MSA system, individuals save and pay for their own medical needs. Under this system, working adults are required to contribute a percentage of their income to a medical savings account. Upon reaching a certain age, decided by the country, the balance can be used to pay for healthcare expenses. MSAs purport to address some of the main inefficiencies of private health insurance—moral hazard, escalating costs, adverse selection, and gaps in private insurance coverage [21]. In general, health insurance provides incentives to over-consume and over-supply. The full cost of care is not evident when the healthcare payments are borne by a third party, even partially. As a result, consumers may engage in riskier behavior, increasing the likelihood of needing more healthcare and/or merely purchasing more healthcare than medically required. Besides, the providers may also supply more care than necessary. Such behavioral changes lead to the overuse of a society's resources without proportionate community welfare. Cost-sharing, on the other hand, creates conscious consumption choices for quality and cost-benefit. MSA is more of a self-responsible healthcare financing system. Four countries—Singapore, China, South Africa, and the USA—have been using the MSA system for some time now [21]. Limited experience suggests that MSA may not create a sustainable health finance environment without consumer responsibility and some form of government stewardship. Besides, the system needs strong political will and commitment.

Strategic purchasing of services is one of the health financing models proposed by the WHO as a way to progress towards UHC. Strategic purchasing is an active system that involves the transfer of funds to the providers, at least in part, based on their performance or the health needs of the population they serve. This is in contrast to passive purchasing, where the providers automatically receive funds (budgeted allocations) independent of performance. In strategic purchasing, the payment is often linked to the health outcome of the individual or the population. The objectives of strategic purchasing are to enhance equity in the distribution of resources, increase efficiency ("more health for the money"), manage expenditure growth, and promote quality in the health service delivery [22]. The factors that influence healthcare efficiency are: (1) good governance and multi-sectoral coordination; (2) precise information on diseases, demands, and people (performance and population health); (3) appropriate choice of benefits package (clear delineation of what is covered and not covered); (4) a mixed provider payment system (aligned with other forms of health financing); and (5) dynamic alignment with other health reforms (health system stewardship and continuous assessment of benefit packages). Strategic purchasing works well when one has defined the priority (of service and population), and the providers (good and cost-effective service) and aligned them with incentives (which promote efficiency, equity, and access) and accountability (which promotes good performance and effective use of funds).

6.4 Health Financing Sustainability

A sustainable health finance system is essential for a stable health system. Two essential components are: economic evaluation of health and responsible investment in healthcare.

6.4.1 Economic Evaluation of Health

An economic evaluation of health (EEH) is the "comparative analysis of alternative courses of action in terms of costs and consequences" [23]. It aims to answer two main questions: (1) is a health procedure beneficial with the available resources? and (2) is the spending for such a procedure justified? The benefits may be direct (personal gain in health status) or indirect (societal gain in production). Costs may also be direct (medical costs to the provider and individual/family) or indirect (loss of productivity).

Two terms repeatedly used in EEH are "opportunity cost" and "return on investment." *Opportunity cost* is the loss of potential gain from other alternative investments when one particular investment is chosen over others. It is the loss of the benefit that *could* have been enjoyed had a given choice not been made. *Return on investment* (ROI) is a performance measure to evaluate or compare the efficiency of an investment. ROI is traditionally used in finance; however, in healthcare, there are returns beyond what money can count, such as quality of life, social status of an individual, and independent living. These returns are termed as *social return on investment* (SROI).

Methods of measuring the EEH include cost-minimization analysis, cost-effectiveness analysis, cost–benefit analysis, and cost–utility analysis [24]. The *cost-minimization analysis* (CMA) compares programs and identifies those with the lowest cost but comparable benefits. *Cost-effective analysis* (CEA) identifies the most efficient program vis-à-vis the cost per program. *Cost–benefit analysis* (CBA) measures the cost of care and the benefits derived from such care. *Cost–utility analysis* (CUA) refers to the value of a particular health state or an improvement in that health state. Utility values lie between 0 and 1, where 0 is equivalent to death and 1 is equivalent to perfect health. CUA is best expressed by the gain of quality-adjusted life years (QALYs).

The EEH has often been described as a nested structure, where the different segments are layered in concentric rings around the core value of effectiveness. The innermost circle is the "effectiveness," and the progressive outer circles are the healthcare cost, CEA, CBA, and the CUA (Table 6.2) [25]. These are not silos, but are intimately connected.

Table 6.2 Zones of the economic evaluation of health

Economic evaluation of health	Zone	Parameter	Description
4 3 2 1 0	0	Effectiveness	The quantity of health gains resulting from the intervention
	1	Cost	The investment required for the intervention
	2	Cost-effective	The quantity of health gains resulting from the intervention compared to the cost of the intervention
	3	Cost-benefit	The value of the outcomes compared to the cost of the investment
	4	Cost-utility	The improvement in health state compared to the cost of intervention and investment

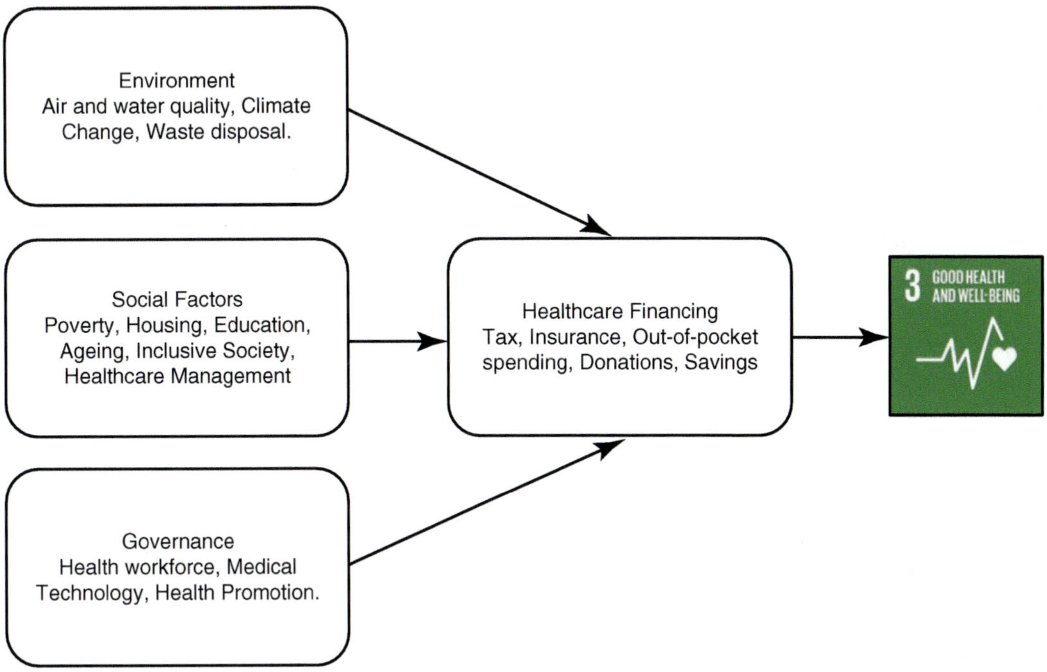

Fig. 6.2 A framework for health financing based on ESG (environmental, social, and corporate governance). Adapted from Yuen PP, et al. "Good Health and Well-Being" (2020; Springer Nature Switzerland)

6.4.2 Responsible Investment in Healthcare

Responsible investment is critical for allocating resources that would also complement environmental, social, and corporate governance (ESG) initiatives, as developed by the UNPRI (United Nations Principles for Responsible Investment, launched in 2006) [26]. The environmental factors include air and water quality, climate change, and waste disposal; the social factors include poverty, housing, education, aging, inclusive society, and healthcare system; the governance includes the human resource for health, medical technology, and health promotion (Fig. 6.2).

Some of these areas have been investigated; these include cities, energy, water-sanitation, healthy food, and agriculture [27]. Unplanned urban growth causes the expansion of slums and substandard housing. This imposes undue stress on safe drinking water, sewage, and solid-waste management, that exacerbates the burdens of water-borne and vector-borne communicable diseases as well as those of non-communicable diseases from risks related to outdoor air pollution, physical inactivity, and injuries from exposure to extreme weather. The urban slum population in the world has decreased from 35.4% in 2005 to 29.5% in 2018; however, the urban slum population in South-East Asia is higher than the global average in seven of eight countries where data was available. Urban slum populations are highest in Myanmar (56%) and lowest in Thailand (24%) (Table 6.3) [28].

Inability to access clean energy sources results in high levels exposure to domestic and ambient fine particulate air pollution. In 2017, an estimated 3.4 million premature deaths amounting to 6% of all deaths were due to air pollution [29]. In four of the SEAR countries, death due to air pollution was higher than the global average; this was highest in Nepal (8.7%) and lowest in Timor-Leste (2.8%) (Table 6.3).

Unsafe water causes a host of diseases in children and adults. In 2017, 1.2 million people died due to unsafe water, accounting for 2.2% of all deaths worldwide [30]. In the SEAR countries, death due to unsafe water was higher than the global average in four of ten countries; it was highest in Nepal (4.89%) and lowest in the Maldives (0.24%) (Table 6.3). In addition, in 2017, two of five people in the world did not have basic handwashing facilities with soap and water at home, and 673 million (9% of the world's population) still practiced open defecation [33].

Present patterns of unsustainable food production and distribution are linked to hunger and undernutrition on one hand and overweight and obesity on the other. In 2018, 8.9% of people in the world were undernourished [31]. In the SEAR, undernutrition was higher than the global average in six of eight countries; it was highest in Timor-Leste (31%) and lowest in Nepal (6%). In 2016, 13% of the world's population was obese (Body Mass Index, BMI > 30) [32]. In the SEAR, incidence of obesity in adults was lower than the global average (highest the Maldives: 8.6%; lowest Bangladesh: 3.6%) (Table 6.3).

6.5 Lessons from Developed Systems and the Way Forward

The Canadian health system has significantly lower costs with overall better health outcomes than the system in the USA. Health insurance in Canada is a publicly funded national health insurance system, whereas that in the USA is largely private (though Medicare and Medicaid provide substantial government funding). Under the Canadian Health Act (1984), the Canadian health system is publicly administered, comprehensive, universal, portable across provinces,

Table 6.3 Percentage of people living in urban slums and death due to outdoor air pollution and unsafe water, percentage of people undernourished or obese in SEAR countries against global average [28, 29, 30, 31, 32]

Country	% people living in urban slums Estimate year 2018	% death due to outdoor air pollution Estimate year 2017	% death due to unsafe water Estimate year 2017	% adult undernutrition Estimate year 2018	% adult obesity Estimate year 2016
Bangladesh	47	6.32	2.86	13	3.6
Bhutan	–	6.75	2.03	–	6.4
India	35	8.26	5.75	14	3.9
Indonesia	31	3.46	3.01	9	6.9
Maldives	30	3.56	0.24	–	8.6
Myanmar	56	4.63	1.60	14	5.8
Nepal	49	8.70	4.89	6	4.1
Sri Lanka	–	2.37	0.40	8	5.2
Thailand	24	5.26	0.73	9	10.0
Timor-Leste	33	2.08	1.88	31	3.8
World	29.3	6.00	2.2	8.9	13.0

and accessible, without user fees, and offers free choice to patients. There is no extra billing (balance billing). A centralized system of health insurance results in significantly lower administrative costs than the cost of multiple systems as in the USA [34]. In Canada's National Health Systems, the government constitutes a monopsony (single buyer) of physician labor, which reduces the overall cost of healthcare [34].

A single provider system has multiple benefits which include: (1) negotiation with local medical societies for physician services; (2) reduced administrative costs; [35] (3) limited capital costs associated with expensive new technologies; and (4) regulated drug prices, even for branded prescription drugs [36].

To be more effective, a combination of private and public health insurance may be required, as rationed healthcare cannot always meet patient demands in a timely basis. In the absence of the safety valve provided by additional private insurance, patients who are willing to pay more for high value care may be denied the opportunity. It could be assumed that primary healthcare and health outcomes for those of lower socioeconomic status could improve in a predominantly public insurance system, the wait time for services may be too long for certain needs [37]. Patient satisfaction levels would be lower due to longer wait times in a non-competitive, public health system. Use of technology and purchase of capital equipment may be restricted, depending on the budgetary allocations.

Although policies that capitate demand through rationing and fixed budgets are effective in lowering health costs, they also reduce patient choice for value-based care. Policies that focus more on the cost–benefit ratio and efficiency, such as greater use of health technology and activity-based funding with administratively set prices, are more likely to succeed. Patient choice of providers with additional service options could be increased by the optional purchase of private insurance with limited providers. This would lead to provider competition, reduced wait times for services, and higher-value care.

6.6 Conclusion

Sustainable health financing has to be a part of universal health coverage. The three common challenges in healthcare financing and sustainability are: the aging population, new technologies, and rising consumer expectations on quality of care. Concurrently, these challenges raise three common questions on public health policy: (1) how much should the government (the country) spend on healthcare?; this will require weighing benefits of healthcare spending against other public expenditure; (2) what level of coverage should one provide?; this will require specifying the distribution of benefits between population groups; and, (3) how does one increase the value of the existing health system resources?; this will require maximizing performance on a limited budget [38]. The decisions taken on the health budget of any country must be context specific. While good health contributes directly to societal well-being and wealth creation, individuals' benefit is closely linked to access and affordability. The challenges in health financing lie in exploring the means to deliver more with fewer resources and to gain more with additional spending by reducing opportunity costs.

In 2017, the global spending on health was USD7.8 trillion (10% of GDP). However, there is a large disparity in health expenditure between low- and high-income countries. The average health spending was only USD41 per person in low-income countries, and USD2937 per person in high-income countries in 2017. This situation is improving as the social health insurance (SHI) is gradually increasing (from 113 countries in 2000 to 126 countries in 2017). Despite increase in global spending on health, public spending on health is still low in low-income countries.

In general, the healthcare industry and market have adapted quickly to the growing demands, but the public policies to address these growing needs especially to the most vulnerable population has been slow to catch up. Large inequities remain between and within countries. Progress in healthcare, particularly technological advances, has come at a cost, with increasing levels of global out-of-pocket-spending. However, new technologies could be profitably harnessed to help non-physician healthcare providers perform many technology-enabled primary eye care functions. This will significantly reduce the health workforce scarcity and human resources cost. The goals of universal health coverage could be achieved with robust primary care. Re-orienting the health system and finance towards primary healthcare requires prioritizing health sector resource allocation.

References

1. World Health Organization (WHO). The world health report, 2000. Health systems: improving performance. Geneva: WHO; 2000. www.who.int/whr/2000/en
2. World Health Organization (WHO). Everybody's business-strengthening health systems to improve health outcomes: WHO's framework for action. Geneva: WHO; 2007. www.who.int/healthsystems/Strategy
3. Stenberg K, Hanssen O, Edejer TT, et al. Financing transformative health systems towards achievement of the health Sustainable Development Goals: a model for projected resource needs in 67 low-income and middle-income countries. Lancet Glob Health. 2017;5:875–87. https://doi.org/10.1016/S2214-109X(17)30263-2.
4. Global Burden of Disease Health Financing Collaborator Network. Past, present, and future of global health financing: a review of development assistance, government, out-of-pocket, and other private spending on health for 195 countries, 1995–2050. Lancet. 2019;393:2233–60. https://doi.org/10.1016/S0140-6736(19)30841-4.
5. Reddy KS. Health assurance: giving shape to a slogan. Current Med Res Prac. 2015;5:e9. https://doi.org/10.1016/j.cmrp.2015.02.003.
6. Ekman B. Catastrophic health payments and health insurance: some counterintuitive evidence from one low-income country. Health Policy. 2007;83:304–13. https://doi.org/10.1016/j.healthpol.2007.02.004.
7. Xu K. Distribution of health payments and catastrophic expenditures methodology. Geneva: Department of Health System Financing, World Health Organization; 2005.
8. O'Donnell O, Doorslaer EV, Wagstaff A, et al. Analysing health equity using household survey data: a guide to techniques and their implementation: the World Bank. Washington, DC: World Bank; 2008.
9. Xu K, Evans DB, Carrin G, et al. Designing health financing systems to reduce catastrophic health expenditure. Geneva: World Health Organization; 2005.
10. Wagstaff AW, Flores G, Hsu J, et al. Progress on catastrophic health spending in 133 countries: a retrospective observational study. Lancet Global Health. 2018;6:e169–79. https://doi.org/10.1016/s2214-109x(17)30429-1.
11. Puteh SEW, Almaualm Y. Catastrophic health expenditure among developing countries. Health Syst Policy Res. 2017;4:1. https://doi.org/10.21767/2254-9137.100069.
12. World Health Organization and National Institute on Aging (National Institute of Health). Global health and aging. 2011. NIH-11-7737.
13. World Health Organization (WHO). Global health risks: mortality and burden of disease attributable to selected major risks. 2009. https://www.who.int/healthinfo/global_burden_disease/GlobalHealthRisks_report_full.pdf
14. World Health Organization. Study on global AGEing and adult health. Sage. http://www.who.int/healthinfo/systems/sage/en/
15. Yuen PP, Ng AW. Health care financing and sustainability. In: Filho WL, et al., editors. Good health and well-being. Switzerland: Springer; 2020. p. 364–73.
16. Fletcher A, Vijaykumar V, Selvaraj S, et al. The Madurai intraocular lens study. III. Visual functioning and quality of life outcomes. Am J Ophthalmol. 1998;125:26–35.
17. Jain S, Chauhan A, Rajshekar K, et al. Generic and vision related quality of life associated with different types of cataract surgeries and different types of intraocular lens implantation. PLoS One. 2020;15(10):e0240036. https://doi.org/10.1371/journal.pone.0240036.
18. Umar I. Health system, sustainability of. In: Filho WL, et al., editors. Good health and well-being. Switzerland: Springer; 2020. p. 356–64.
19. www.investopedia.com›Investing›Markets. Accessed 25 Dec 2020.
20. www.economicshelp.org. Accessed 25 Dec 2020.
21. Hsu J. Medical savings accounts: what is at risk. Geneva: World Health Organization; 2010.
22. Mathauer I, Dale E, Meessen B. Strategic purchasing for Universal Health Coverage: key policy issues and questions. A summary from expert and practitioners' discussions. Geneva: World Health Organization; 2017.
23. Drummond MF, Sculpher MJ, Claxton K, et al. Methods for the economic evaluation of health care programmes. Oxford: Oxford University Press; 2015.
24. Cunningham S. Economic evaluation of healthcare—is it important to us? Br Dent J. 2000;188:250–4. https://doi.org/10.1038/sj.bdj.4800444.
25. Lauer JA, Morton A, Culyer AJ, Chalkidou K. What counts in economic evaluations in health? Benefit-cost analysis compared to other forms of economic evaluations. Geneva: World Health Organization; 2020.
26. www.unpri.org. Accessed 26 Dec 2020.
27. Dora C, Haines A, Balbus J, et al. Indicators linking health and sustainability in the post-2015 devel-

opment agenda. Lancet. 2015;385(9965):380–91. https://doi.org/10.1016/S0140-6736(14)60.
28. People living in slums (% urban population). www.worldbank.org. Accessed 27 Dec 2020.
29. Outdoor air pollution. www.ourworldindata.org. Accessed 27 Dec 2020.
30. Clean water. www.ourworldindata.org. Accessed 27 Dec 2020.
31. Prevalence of undernourished. www.data.worldbank.org. Accessed 27 Dec 2020.
32. Obesity. www.ourworldin.data.org. Accessed 27 Dec 2020.
33. Water and sanitation. www.unicef.org. Accessed 27 Dec 2020.
34. Folland S, Goodman AC, Stano M. The economics of health and health care. 8th ed. New York: Taylor and Francis; 2017.
35. https://www.aarp.org/health/drugs-supplements/
36. https://www.nber.org/papers/w13429
37. Willcox S, Seddon M, Dunn S, et al. Measuring and reducing waiting times: a cross-national comparison of strategies. Health Aff (Millwood). 2007;26:1078–87.
38. Thomson S, Foubister T, Figueras J, et al. Addressing financial sustainability in health systems. Denmark: World Health Organization, WHO Regional Office for Europe; 2009.

7 Disease Burden: Blindness and Vision Impairment in South-East Asia

Jill E. Keeffe, Hugh R. Taylor, and Rupert R. A. Bourne

Key Points

- The Global Burden of Disease (GBD) was initiated at the Institute for Health Metrics and Evaluation at the University of Washington. Data have been collected from 190 countries for 291 diseases and injuries to assess mortality and disability patterns starting with data for 1990, followed by 2010, 2015, and 2018.
- As part of the GBD, a Vision Loss Expert Group (VLEG) was formed to provide global and regional data on vision impairment and blindness. The VLEG collected data from 188 countries in all 21 global regions, which were grouped into seven GBD world super regions (Fig. 7.1).
- In 2020, the estimated prevalence of blindness was 0.85% and 1.12% in South-East Asia men and women, respectively; and 0.85% and 0.94% in South Asia men and women, respectively.
- In 2020, the estimated prevalence of moderate to severe visual loss (MSVI) was 4.51% and 4.77% in South-East Asia men and women, respectively; and 6.11% and 6.78% in South Asia men and women, respectively.
- The estimated number of people blind and with MSVI in 2020 are 3.68 million and 22.46 million respectively in South-East Asia, and 12.94 million and 68.27 million respectively in South Asia.
- Cataract and uncorrected refractive errors are the leading causes of blindness and visual impairment.
- The World Health Organization has declared Nepal and Myanmar as trachoma zero countries.

J. E. Keeffe (✉)
L V Prasad Eye Institute, Hyderabad, Telangana, India
e-mail: jillkeeffe@lvpei.org

H. R. Taylor
Melbourne School of Population and Global Health, University of Melbourne, Melbourne, VIC, Australia
e-mail: h.taylor@unimelb.edu.au

R. R. A. Bourne
Vision and Eye Research Unit, Postgraduate Medical Institute, Anglia, Ruskin University, Cambridge, UK
e-mail: rb@rupertbourne.co.uk

To ensure universal eye care coverage of a country's population, good evidence of the need for services is required. This evidence comes from quality data on the prevalence and causes of vision impairment and blindness. These data are used to plan eye care services and to monitor and evaluate the outcomes of services and coverage of the needs.

The World Health Organization (WHO) Global Action Plan 2014–2019 [1] was built on the goals and processes laid out in the global initiative "VISION 2020—The Right to Sight." The Global Action Plan aimed to reduce avoidable vision impairment as a global public health problem and secure access to rehabilitation services

T. Das, P. D. Nayar (eds.), *South-East Asia Eye Health*,
https://doi.org/10.1007/978-981-16-3787-2_7

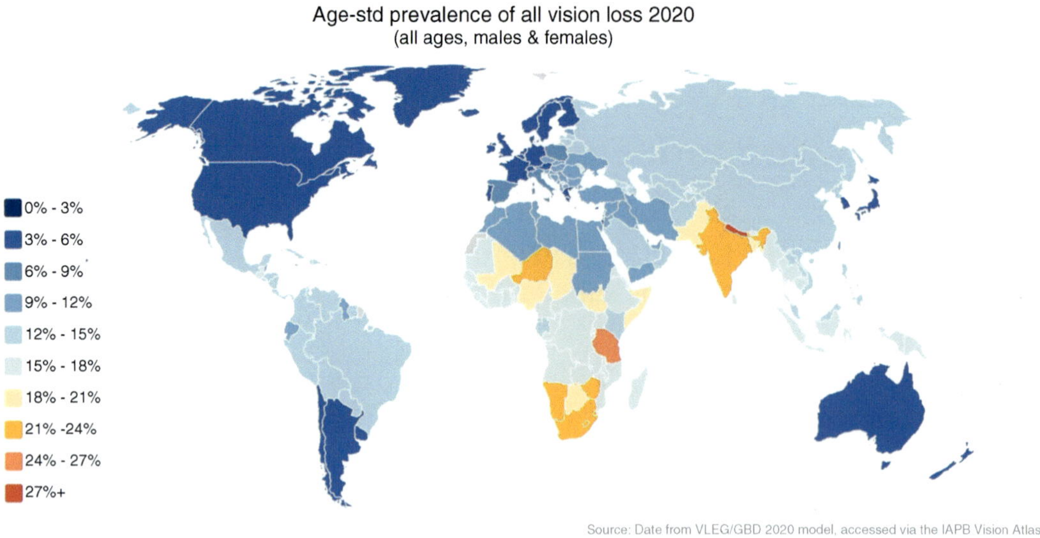

Fig. 7.1 Age-standardized prevalence of vision loss in 2020 (Source: Vision Atlas 2020)

for those people who are vision impaired. The first of the three objectives addressed the need to generate evidence on the magnitude and causes of vision impairment and eye care services and to monitor progress, identify priorities, and advocate for commitment to eye health by national governments. The need for all countries to assess and monitor the magnitude and causes of vision impairment and effectiveness of services over time was an important lesson from the earlier 2009–2013 Action Plan. The World Report on Vision (WRV) [2] also states that collecting and reporting information on met and unmet eye care needs are key for planning and improving services as part of universal health coverage (UHC).

7.1 The Global Burden of Disease: Vision Impairment and Blindness

The Global Burden of Disease (GBD) was initiated at the Institute for Health Metrics and Evaluation at the University of Washington [3]. Data have been collected from 190 countries for 291 diseases and injuries to assess mortality and disability patterns starting with data for 1990, followed by 2010, 2015, and 2018. As part of the GBD, a Vision Loss Expert Group (VLEG) was formed to provide global and regional data on vision impairment and blindness. The VLEG collected data from 188 countries in all 21 global regions, which were grouped into seven GBD world super regions [4, 5]. The 11 countries in the WHO South-East Asia Region were clustered in the South-East Asia and South Asia regions of the GBD data (Table 7.1) [6, 7].

Table 7.1 Countries in the WHO South-East Asia Region and their regional allocations in the GBD regions

Global Burden of Disease (GBD) regions	Countries
South-East Asia	Indonesia, Maldives, Myanmar, Sri Lanka, Thailand, Timor-Leste
South Asia	Bangladesh, Bhutan, India, Nepal

Data were obtained by members of the VLEG from a review of published and unpublished publications of population-based studies, but not those from clinical settings [4, 5]. Data from the publications were included if they reported the prevalence of blindness, vision impairment, or both, from population-based studies where participants were randomly selected to be representative of the population of a region. Criteria for inclusion also included publications that reported the prevalence of blindness, mild visual impairment, and moderate to severe vision impairment (MSVI). Both corrected and uncorrected visual acuity was included. Blindness was defined as visual acuity <3/60 and MSVI was defined as visual acuity <6/18. The papers published with data for 2015 and 2018 also included mild vision impairment (visual acuity >6/18 but <6/12) and near vision impairment (defined as visual acuity worse than N6 or N8 at 40 cm with best-corrected visual acuity ≥6/12). A clear statement of the procedures used for visual acuity testing was an important criterion for inclusion in the VLEG analysis.

7.2 Prevalence Rate of Blindness and MSVI

The stated aim of VISION 2020 was to eliminate avoidable blindness. Although this was not achieved, the global prevalence of blindness and MSVI have decreased. From 1990, the global prevalence of blindness decreased from 0.75 to 0.52% in 2010 and to 0.48% in 2015 [8]. The global prevalence of MSVI also reduced from 3.83% in 1990 to 2.9% in 2015. Between 2015 and 2020, the prevalence was similar in the South-East Asia and South Asia regions (Table 7.2). In both regions, the prevalence of MSVI was high. In the GBD South Asian region, two countries India (Blindness: 0.9%; MSVI: 5.1%; Mild VI: 4.0%; Near vision loss: 11.3%) and Nepal (Blind: 0.5%; MSVI: 5.1%; Mild VI: 2.8%, Near vision loss: 18.8%) are in the ten countries listed to having the highest age-standardized prevalence rates of vision loss across all ages and both genders in 2020 [9].

In the South-East Asia Region, the age-standardized prevalences of blindness for men and women were 0.57% and 0.83%, respectively. The differences in prevalence of MSVI between men (4.64%) and women (5.09%) were narrow [5]. A similar pattern was seen in the South Asia region, with women having a higher rate of blindness (0.99%) than men (0.92%) [7].

7.3 Numbers of People with Blindness and MSVI

While there has been a small decrease in the prevalences of blindness and MSVI, the numbers of people suffering from the two conditions have seen a global increase from 191 million in 1990 to 253 million in 2015. This change has been seen in the South Asian and South-East Asian regions also [6, 7]. Although these numbers also increased between 2015 and 2020, the differences were not significant (Table 7.3). The International Agency for the Prevention of Blindness (IAPB) Vision Atlas lists the 20 countries with the highest numbers of people with blindness and MSVI combined. From the South Asia region, India (56,555,033 people), Indonesia (8,878,452 people), Bangladesh (5,715,518 people), Thailand (3,200,470 people), and Myanmar (2,802,753 people) are included in the list [9]. India was ranked second, after China, as having the greatest number of people with blindness or MSVI.

Globally, women suffer more from blindness and MSVI (55%) than men [2, 9]. This gender difference is greater for people with blindness and MSVI, and lower for those with mild VI. The increases in both blindness and MSVI increased between 1990 and 2015 for both genders; however, the differences are not significant.

Table 7.2 Age-standardized prevalence of blindness and MSVI in men and women in the WHO South-East Asia and South Asia Regions in 2015 and 2020

		Blindness, %, (95% CI)		MSVI; %, (95% CI)	
Year	Region	Men	Women	Men	Women
2015	South-East Asia	0.57 (0.2–1.06)	0.83 (0.31–1.49)	4.64 (1.46–8.79)	5.1 (1.65–9.57)
	South Asia	0.94 (0.35–1.72)	1.03 (0.36–1.91)	4.53 (2.29–7.18)	4.98 (2.45–7.92)
2020	South-East Asia	0.85 (0.74–0.95)	1.12 (0.97–1.26)	4.51 (4.16–4.86)	4.77 (4.42–5.13)
	South Asia	0.85 (0.74–0.95)	0.94 (0.81–1,06)	6.11 (5.50–6.78)	6.78 (6.10–7.51)

MSVI moderate and severe visual impairment, *CI* confidence interval

Table 7.3 Numbers of people in millions (with 80% uncertainty intervals) who are blind or have MSVI in 2015, and the projections for 2020

Region	Blind, %, (95% CI) (millions)		MSVI, %, (95% CI) (millions)	
	2015	2020	2015	2020
South Asia	11.76 (4.14–21.72)	12.94 (4.37–24.2)	61.19 (29.65–98.57)	68.27 (31.3–110.79)
South-East Asia	3.54 (1.3–6.33)	3.68 (1.29–6.69)	20.8 (9.77–38.87)	22.46 (9.8–37.34)

Table 7.4 Life expectancy from birth in 1990, 2015, and 2020

Country	1990	2015	2020
Bangladesh	65.5	72.2	73.57
Bhutan	61.1	70.2	72.77
India	62.5	68.5	70.42
Indonesia	66.1	69.1	72.32
Maldives	69.7	78.1	79.89
Myanmar	61.8	65.5	67.78
Nepal	62.2	69.0	71.74
Sri Lanka	71.6	75.2	77.56
Thailand	70.6	75.3	77.74
Timor-Leste	59.1	68.3	70.18

A major reason for these increases in numbers is the increase in life expectancy. Essentially these numbers reflect the increase in older age-group people, where blindness and vision impairment are more common. In the WHO-compiled data on life expectancy by country, [10] all ten countries in the WHO South-East Asia Region have had an increase in life expectancy between 1990 and 2015, with six countries having an increase of >5 years across the two decades (Table 7.4). The number of countries with life expectancy >70 years increased from two countries in 1990 to five countries in 2015 and nine countries in 2020. This increase in life expectancy has contributed to the increase in numbers of people with blindness and MSVI.

7.4 Causes of Blindness and MSVI

The proportions of populations with blindness or MSVI due to cataract and refractive errors in the South-East Asian and South Asian regions have changed very little over the last three decades (from 1990 to 2020) (Tables 7.5 and 7.6). Cataract causes approximately one-third of all MSVI cases in the South Asian region [6, 7].

From 1990 to 2020, refractive error was the main cause of MSVI across all South Asian countries. In the GBD South Asian region, two-thirds of all MSVI cases were due to refractive error (Table 7.5) [7]. In the South-East Asian countries, refractive error was also one of the main causes of MSVI, ranging from 44.1% in 1990 to 46.6% in 2020.

Cataracts have been the most common cause of blindness in the South-East Asian countries from 1990 to 2020; however, in the South Asian countries, the percentage of blindness due to cataract is similar to that of blindness due to refractive error (Table 7.6).

The aim of VISION 2020 was to eliminate avoidable blindness and MSVI; however, the percentage of the population suffering from avoidable blindness has changed very little over the last three decades. The lower rates of blindness caused by unavoidable causes have a similar trend over the same period of time. Trachoma is the one exception (as one of the causes of avoidable blindness and MSVI) as it has been almost wiped out during this period (Tables 7.5 and 7.6).

Percentages of the other causes of blindness and MSVI such as glaucoma, age-related macular degeneration, diabetic retinopathy, and cornea are generally lower in the South Asian countries than of those in the South-East Asian countries. Although the prevalence of diabetes is relatively high in this region, blindness and MSVI due to diabetic retinopathy affect only a small proportion of those with diabetes.

The prevalence of trachoma has decreased over the last two decades and this disease has been eliminated in Nepal and Myanmar.

7.5 Blindness and Vision Impairment in Children

Prior to 2000, there were very few population-based studies of the prevalences of vision impairment and blindness in children. The only such studies were conducted in schools for blind chil-

Table 7.5 Percentages of MSVI cases (at 80% uncertainty intervals) caused due to different conditions in 1990, 2015, and 2020 in the South-East Asian and South Asian regions according to GBD data

Region, year	RE, % (95% CI)	Cataract, % (95% CI)	Glaucoma, % (95% CI)	AMD, % (95% CI)	DR, % (95% CI)	Cornea, % (95% CI)	Trachoma % (95% CI)	Other % (95% CI)
South-East Asia								
1990	44.14 (38.96–48.67)	37.59 (31.31–43.79)	1.58 (0.58–2.87)	4.06 (0.89–8.7)	0.33 (0.06–0.68)	2.52 (0.41–5.48)	0.34 (0.33–0.35)	9.41 (2.8–18.53)
2015	46.41 (42.19–49.51)	33.95 (26.09–42.07)	1.57 (0.56–2.94)	3.46 (0.79–7.33)	0.71 (0.12–1.48)	1.63 (9.26–3.53)	0.07 (0.05–0.08)	12.48 (3.71–24.59)
2020	46.55 (42.14–49.89)	32.65 (24.0–41.77)	1.6 (0.52–3.11)	3.56 (0.73–7.74)	0.97 (0.44–2.09)	1.56 (0.21–3.45)	0 (0–0)	13.1 (3.89–24.85)
South Asia								
1990	66.08 (61.8–69.66)	24.2 (19.5–28.8)	1.07 (0.38–1.97)	1.35 (0.39–2.67)	0.13 (0.03–0.26)	0.79 (0.16–1.63)	0.06 (0.04–0.08)	6.3 (1.89–12.5)
2015	66.5 (62.19–70.14)	23.37 (17.5–29.26)	1.09 (0.34–2.09)	1.18 (0.3–2.14)	0.15 (0.03–0.35)	0.71 (0.11–1.53)	0 (0–0)	7.0 (2.09–13.9)
2020	64.59 (58.92–69.42)	25.8 (21.67–29.77)	1.12 (0.37–2.09)	1.76 (0.41–3.7)	0.1 (0.02–0.2)	1.28 (0.21–2.75)	0.14 (0.12–0.16)	5.21 (1.57–10.32)

AMD age-related macular degeneration, *CI* confidence interval, *DR* diabetic retinopathy, *RE* refractive error

Table 7.6 Percentage of blindness (at 80% uncertainty intervals) caused by various conditions in 1990, 2015, and 2020 in the South-East Asia and South Asia regions according to GBD data

Region, year	Cataract, % (95% CI)	RE, % (95% CI)	Glaucoma, % (95% CI)	AMD, % (95% CI)	DR, % (95% CI)	Cornea, % (95% CI)	Trachoma % (95% CI)	Other % (95% CI)
South-East Asia								
1990	36.67 (30.11–43.22)	12.21 (10.29–14.08)	7.15 (2.72–19.94)	6.13 (1.47–12.91)	0.29 (0.05–0.60)	6.49 (1.25–13.89)	0.67 (0.65–0.68)	18.81 (6.52–34.21)
2015	45.00 (34.22–55.54)	12.57 (10.79–14.33)	6.99 (2.69–12.56)	5.24 (1.27–10.81)	0.59 (0.09–1.26)	4.39 (0.73–9.72)	0.13 (0.11–0.15)	25.09 (8.66–45.62)
2020	43.59 (31.74–55.37)	12.64 (10.87–14.40)	7.04 (2/50–13.01)	5.29 (1.16–11.14)	0.79 (0.11–1.72)	4.21 (0.61–9.52)	0.00 (0.00–0.00)	26.43 (9.11–48.08)
South Asia								
1990	37.39 (30.16–44.61)	36.29 (33.63–38.73)	5.77 (2.27–10.26)	2.52 (0.76–4.88)	0.14 (0.03–0.29)	2.58 (0.53–5.54)	0.09 (0.06–0.12)	15.24 (5.41–28.01)
2015	36.17 (27.11–45.30)	36.5 (33.89–38.90)	5.76 (2.02–10.64)	2.21 (0.58–4.41)	0.16 (0.02–0.36)	2.32 (0.38–5.25)	0.00 (0.00–0.00)	16.88 (5.97–31.02)
2020	38.79 (32.99–44.43)	35.54 (32.29–38.41)	5.93 (2.20–10.85)	3.10 (0.83–6.32)	0.10 (0.02–0.21)	3.91 (0.73–8.47)	0.20 (0.18–0.23)	12.42 (4.42–22.80)

AMD age-related macular degeneration, *CI* confidence interval, *DR* diabetic retinopathy, *RE* refractive error

dren, and so had information on a very limited number of cases. Recently, there have been more population-based studies to assess the prevalences and numbers of children who are blind or have low vision [11–15]. These studies have obtained very useful data on the prevalences of vision impairment and blindness, and the causes of vision loss. Before such population-based studies on all causes of vision loss, the Refractive Error Studies in Children (RESC) were conducted in many countries, including this region [12–15]. The children included in the RESC were of school age and attending regular schools.

Recommendations

- Continue to monitor the prevalence of blindness and MSVI, including regional differences within countries to evaluate service impact and continuing needs.
- Support women's access to eye care services to eliminate gender differences in blindness and MSVI, and monitor changes.
- Focus on services to reduce the prevalence of avoidable causes of blindness and MSVI.
- Obtain data on prevalence and causes of blindness, and vision impairment in children to plan services and monitor outcomes.

7.6 Conclusion

The countries in the WHO South-East Asia Region have seen positive changes in the reduction of the prevalence of blindness and VI from 1990 to 2020. While this is in line with the aims of VISION 2020, the original objective of elimination or even significantly reducing the prevalence of avoidable blindness has not been achieved. Cataract and uncorrected refractive error remain the main causes of blindness and MSVI in this region.

References

1. World Health Organization. Universal eye health: a global action plan 2014–2019. http://www.who.int/blindness/actionplan/en/
2. World Health Organization. World report on vision. 2019. www.who.int.org
3. Institute for Health Metrics and Evaluation. www.healthdata.org
4. Bourne RRA, Flaxman SR, Braithwaite T, et al. Magnitude, temporal trends, and projections of the global prevalence of blindness and distance and near vision impairment: a systematic review and meta-analysis. Lancet Glob Health. 2017;5(9):888–97.
5. Bourne RRA, Jaimie J, Seth F, et al. Trends in prevalence of blindness and distance and near vision impairment over 30 years and contribution to the Global Burden of disease in 2020. The Lancet Global Health. 2020. Advanced online publication. https://doi.org/10.2139/ssrn.3582742
6. Keeffe JE, Casson RJ, Presudovs K, et al. Prevalence and causes of vision loss in South-east Asia and Oceania 2015: magnitude, temporal trends and projections. Br J Ophthalmol. 2018;103(7):878–84.
7. Nangia V, Jonas J, George R, et al. Prevalence and causes of vision impairment: magnitude, temporal trends and projections in South and Central Asia. Br J Ophthalmol. 2018;103(7):871–7.
8. Flaxman SR, Bourne RRA, Resnikoff S, et al. Global causes of blindness and distance vision impairment 1990–2020: a systematic review and meta-analysis. Lancet Glob Health. 2017;5(12):e1221–e34.
9. IAPB. Vision atlas. http://atlas.iapb.org. Accessed 18 Oct 2020.
10. World Health Organization. Life expectancy https://www.who.int/gho/countries/en/
11. Negrel AD, Maul E, Pokharel GP, et al. Refractive error study in children; sampling and measurement methods for a multi-country survey. Am J Ophthalmol. 2000;129:421–6.
12. Pokharel GP, Negrel AD, Munoz SR, et al. Refractive error study in children: results from Mechi Zone, Nepal. Am J Ophthalmol. 2000;129:436–44.
13. Dandona R, Dandona L, Srinivas M, et al. Refractive error in children in a rural population in India. Invest Ophthalmol Vis Sci. 2002;43:615–22.
14. Murthy GVS, Gupta SK, Ellwein LB, et al. Refractive error in children in an urban population in New Delhi. Invest Ophthalmol Vis Sci. 2002;43:623–31.
15. Sharma IP, Lepcha NT, Lhamo T, et al. Visual impairment and refractive error in school children in Bhutan: the findings from the Bhutan School Sight Survey (BSSS 2019). PLoS One. 2020;15(9):e0239117. https://doi.org/10.1371/journal.pone.0239117.

Population-Based Eye Disease Studies

8

Yuddha D. Sapkota, Srinivas Marmamula, and Taraprasad Das

Key Points

- Epidemiological data is a prerequisite for the planning and monitoring of eye care services.
- Classical epidemiological studies and rapid assessments methods are commonly used tools for providing valuable data on vision loss.
- Classical epidemiological study methods provide extensive and comprehensive data though these are often expensive and resource intensive.
- Rapid assessments are quick and relatively low-cost study methods that provide baseline data for planning eye care services. Repeating these studies can help in assessing trends in the prevalence of vision loss and impacts of ongoing eye care services in a given region.
- In South-East Asia, many countries have conducted population-based studies on vision loss and some countries have conducted their first such vision survey only in the last 5 years.
- A repeat survey in a few countries has shown a reduction in the prevalence of blindness and increased access to cataract surgery (Fig. 8.1).

Vision loss is a global challenge affecting over 253 million people worldwide [1]. Effective planning of healthcare systems are an essential step for building healthy communities. These factors apply to eye health as well. Changing demographics associated with decreasing birth rates and rapidly increasing life expectancy in developing countries means that healthcare systems should be prepared to adapt to rising and continually changing needs. Healthcare planning depends on reliable, measurable, and repeatable information to assess the impact of programs. Classical large-scale epidemiological survey methods, which can provide baseline data on prevalence and risk factors, are seen as a luxury that not many economically fragile developing countries can afford, given the limited resources of both, expertise of personnel and required finances. There is a real need for an evidence base that can emerge from survey methods undertaken with sufficient scientific rigor to make informed policy and programmatic decisions. Rapid assessment methods are indispensable tools in situations where data are needed

Y. D. Sapkota (✉)
International Agency for the Prevention of Blindness South-East Asia Region, Hyderabad, Telangana, India
e-mail: ysapkota@iapb.org

S. Marmamula
Allen Foster Community Eye Health Research Centre, Gullapalli Pratibha Rao International Centre for Advancement of Rural Eye Care, L V Prasad Eye Institute, Hyderabad, Telangana, India
e-mail: sri.marmamula@lvpei.org

T. Das
International Agency for the Prevention of Blindness South-East Asia Region, Hyderabad, Telangana, India

L V Prasad Eye Institute, Hyderabad, India
e-mail: tpd@lvpei.org

T. Das, P. D. Nayar (eds.), *South-East Asia Eye Health*,
https://doi.org/10.1007/978-981-16-3787-2_8

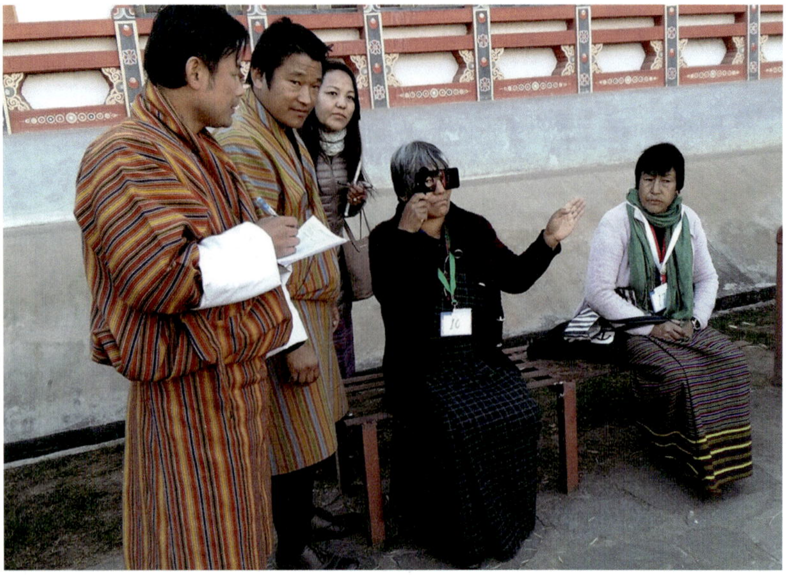

Fig. 8.1 Vision testing in a Rapid Assessment of Avoidable Blindness (RAAB) in a repeat survey in Bhutan (Source: Ministry of Health, Bhutan)

quickly, and where time or cost-related factors prohibit the use of classical epidemiological surveys [2]. While these are not a substitute for conventional epidemiological study methods, rapid assessment methods have a wide range of public health applications for analysis and monitoring interventions.

8.1 Classical Epidemiological Studies

Classical epidemiological studies can achieve multiple objectives and provide comprehensive data on several aspects of public health importance, including risk factors and associations. The study designs for these are complex and require experts using high-end technological devices for clinical examinations. The sampling methodologies are often complex and may involve multiple stages. The sample sizes are calculated based on the least prevalent disease under study. Hence, the sample sizes are usually large to achieve the desired objectives. For example, the sample size for the Andhra Pradesh Eye Disease Study (APEDS) was calculated based on the anticipated prevalence of age-related macular degeneration [3]. Data collection is exhaustive and data entry is time-consuming. Data analysis and reporting of results can take several months. Due to their complexity and enormity, classical surveys are prohibitively expensive and can significantly burden the healthcare system. Therefore, these cannot be repeated at short intervals.

Despite their drawbacks, large studies provide comprehensive information on prevalence, incidence, risk factors, and associations that can be used for planning, advocacy, and policymaking. With accurate sampling, the results can represent large populations and, in some cases, also be applicable to an entire state or country. Several classical studies like the APEDS have provided significant information and helped bring about changes in service delivery [3].

8.2 Rapid Assessment Studies

Rapid assessment methods prioritize the most affected regions, identify high-risk groups, and help develop a targeted intervention for those who can benefit the most [2]. The important features of rapid assessment methods include the use of local resources, simplified survey methodology, and a quick examination protocol/data collection method that can be performed by locally available personnel without the need of an expert. The analysis is quick and easy to interpret. Due to these attributes, rapid assessment methods can be repeated at regular intervals to understand trends in the prevalence and causes of vision loss, and the impact of any ongoing interventions in a given region.

Additionally, in countries such as India, which have marked diversities and regional variations in the prevalence of vision loss, and large populations (as large as two million people in each district, planning unit for most studies/interventions), programmatic decisions based on nation-wide surveys may not always be applicable. For example, the prevalence of blindness in the APEDS ranged from 1.6% in one district (Mahbubnagar) to 2.4% in another district (West Godavari), a distance of 328 km [4]. In such cases, the regional or district level planning for interventions should be based on locally relevant and rapidly obtained information.

The sample selection for rapid assessment studies is often based on a two-stage cluster random sampling design with a sample size proportionate to the population. Unlike conventional epidemiological designs, rapid assessment methods have only one or two related objectives, and sample size estimation is based on the single leading factor under consideration. Because the sampling approach targets risk groups with a relatively high prevalence of the disease/disorder/condition, the required sample sizes are usually smaller than those required for classical epidemiological studies and have dramatically lower expenses. Data analysis is simpler and results are available within a few days of completion of data collection; in most cases, results can be obtained without any assistance from an expert statistician. Automated software programs are now available for two rapid assessment methods in eye care: (1) Rapid Assessment of Cataract Surgical Services (RACSS) and (2) Rapid Assessment of Avoidable Blindness, (RAAB) [5, 6]. Use of a standardized methodology combined with automated analysis makes it possible to compare the results of repeated surveys over time, allowing one to monitor trends and assess the impact of an intervention without calling upon an expert. However, some rapid assessments (such as RAAB) require experts to plan and conduct the survey. Rapid assessments should never be done where no intervention is planned, following the dictum "*No surveys without service.*" The RAAB survey method has also been improved in recent years; for example, the RAAB6 has been designed for paperless data collection and RAAB7 uses a cloud-based server for data storage. With these modifications, a survey coordinator/principal investigator can monitor/check data collection procedures and clean up data instantly. The most recent RAAB surveys also include assessing the prevalence of diabetes and diabetic retinopathy and related information.

In practice, classical surveys and rapid assessments play complementary roles. In ideal situations, classical epidemiological studies provide the initial baseline, set up priority areas, and help develop realistic, time-bound interventions. The outcome of the interventions is monitored and evaluated using rapid assessment methods. *This is striking a balance between methodologically appropriate and logistically feasible surveys* [7]. Conventional survey methods and rapid assessment methods are compared in Table 8.1.

8.3 History and Evaluation of Rapid Assessment Methods in Eye Care

The RACSS is one of the earliest rapid assessment methods developed in eye care. Venkataswamy et al. reported the use of this method for rapid assessment of cataract blindness for the first time in 1989 [8]. This method was refined further with software development for data entry and analysis by Limburg et al. in 1997.

The RAAB methodology is a modified version of the RACSS [6]. RAAB provides information on the prevalence of visual impairment due to avoidable (and correctable) causes of vision loss like cataract, refractive errors, trachoma, onchocerciasis, corneal scarring, and other anterior segment diseases, in addition to the information provided by RACSS. RAAB software is used for data entry and generation of results. Like its predecessor, RACSS, RAAB overestimates

Table 8.1 Relative differences between conventional versus rapid assessment survey methods

Parameters	Classical epidemiological study designs	Rapid assessment study design
Objective/ outcome	Multiple objectives that include prevalence, risk factors, and associations	One or two inter-related objectives, mainly a prevalence, and service outcome
Application	Where there is no previous data available	Where data are needed immediately so that intervention can be planned; for example, assessing trends in the prevalence of vision impairment
Emphasis	Scientific inquiry for policy formulation, advocacy, and long-term planning	Immediate planning, monitoring, and evaluation of services
Sample size	The sample size is calculated based on the disease with the least prevalence and, hence the sample size would be large	The sample size is calculated based on the most common outcome/objective and in the high-risk age group, hence the sample is relatively smaller
Protocol	Comprehensive examination protocol	Simple examination protocol in most cases
Human resources	Highly technical and cross-functional teams are required, including statisticians, epidemiologists, and other technical personnel other than eye health personnel; in most cases, all participants undergo a similar examination protocol	As the protocol is simple, locally available personnel, general ophthalmologists, and allied ophthalmic personnel (AOP) can perform all data collection, entry, and analysis of data after a short period of training
Technology/ infrastructure	High-end technology required; hence, this is usually an expensive undertaking	Appropriate and simple technology required; hence, easy to undertake in most cases
Setting/ location	Standardized testing conditions required; exclusively developed stations/clinics are set up; subjects are often transported to the study site for examination; for example, visual acuity is measured at constant illumination in all patients	Study teams usually visit the houses of subjects for examination, which is conducted at the subjects' doorsteps; testing conditions are not standardized, though reliability assessments are done for key procedures such as visual acuity assessment, and media and fundus examination
Finances	Expensive	Inexpensive
Duration of data collection	Long; may typically take 2–4 years to complete, depending on the objectives	Short; most rapid assessments can be completed with 8–12 weeks
Data analysis	Exhaustive and needs an expert in biostatistics/public health to decipher results	Relatively simple and straightforward; can be done by a non-expert with some training
Repeatability	Difficult to repeat	Can be repeated at regular intervals
Examples	Andhra Pradesh Eye Disease Study (APEDS)	Rapid Assessment of Cataract Surgical Services (RACSS) Rapid Assessment of Avoidable Blindness (RAAB) Rapid Assessment of Visual Impairment (RAVI)

the prevalence of cataract; however, the examination protocol for RAAB is longer than for RACSS.

The RAAB is now used extensively in different parts of the world and has emerged as the standard method for assessing the prevalence and causes of vision impairment in a given region [9]. The RAAB methodology has evolved over the years to include diabetic retinopathy (DR) and has also incorporated several technological advancements in data collection and analytics [9]. The RAAB repository offers safe storage for data from many rapid assessment studies conducted in different parts of the world (http://raabdata.info/; accessed 31st August 2020). The repository includes data from 137 RAABs, 11 RAABs + DR, and 36 RACSSs, conducted in 70 countries. This repository has been created with a grand vision—to bring as many RAAB study findings as possible into the public domain, so that researchers can have easy access to these data. The upcoming version of RAAB7 includes integration with PEEK (Portable Eye Examination Kit), which is a smart phone-based application [9].

Like RACSS, the RAAB system is also focused on individuals aged 50 years and older, and hence, misses out on collecting data for younger age groups; however, in several places, the data on the population aged ≥50 years may closely reflect the patterns of prevalence in all age groups. The Rapid Assessment of Refractive Errors (RARE) methodology was developed to assess the prevalence of uncorrected refractive errors, presbyopia, spectacle coverage, and barriers to uptake of services for refractive errors and presbyopia [10]. In contrast to RACSS and RAAB, younger age groups of 15–49 years are selected for the RARE survey, as refractive errors are a common cause of visual impairment in this age group.

The Rapid Assessment of Visual Impairment (RAVI) is a more recent rapid assessment method that evolved from other rapid assessment methods [11–13]. RAVI estimates the prevalence and common causes of visual impairment such as presbyopia, spectacle coverage, cataract surgical coverage, visual outcomes after cataract surgery, and barriers to uptake of eye care services. In RAVI, individuals aged ≥40 years are enrolled, which leads to a slightly larger sample size than those of other rapid assessment systems. RAVI protocols include assessment of near vision, which is now included in the World Health Organization (WHO) categories of vision impairment [14]. Although an increase in sample size may impact the use of resources, in RAVI, this increase is unlikely to be too expensive. More recently, RAVI methodology includes a non-mydriatic fundus camera to assess patients for posterior segment disease [15, 16]. To evaluate disabilities beyond impaired vision, a recent version of RAVI methodology also includes assessing disabilities using the Washington Disability Questionnaire. An overview of all rapid methods of population-based study used in eye care is shown in Table 8.2.

Table 8.2 Overview of rapid assessment methods in eye care

A. Rapid Assessment of Cataract Surgical Services (RACSS)	
Objective	Cataract
Outcomes	Prevalence of blindness; cataract surgical coverage (CSC); barriers specific to the uptake of services for cataract surgery; visual outcomes after cataract surgery
Sampling method	Extended Program of Immunization (EPI) random walk method
Age group	≥50 years
Human resources (HR)	Only paramedical personnel
Examination protocol	Vision acuity assessment using a modified Snellen chart (6/18 & 6/60 optotypes); torchlight examination; direct ophthalmoscopy through undilated pupils, if pinhole visual acuity is worse than 6/18
Strengths	Simple protocol; trained paramedical ophthalmic personnel can be used; low cost
Weakness	Diagnosis of posterior segment disease is based on exclusion and marked if the anterior segment is normal
B. Rapid Assessment of Avoidable Blindness (RAAB)	
Objective	Avoidable blindness
Outcomes	Prevalence of the main causes of visual impairment and blindness; cataract surgical coverage (CSC); barriers specific to the uptake of services for cataract surgery; visual outcomes after cataract surgery
Sampling method	Compact segment sampling
Age group	≥50 years
Human resources (HR)	Paramedical ophthalmic personnel/optometrist and an ophthalmologist
Examination protocol	Vision acuity assessment using a modified Snellen chart (6/12, 6/18 & 6/60 optotypes); handheld slit-lamp examination; pupillary dilatation; and direct ophthalmoscopy by an ophthalmologist, if pinhole visual acuity is worse than 6/12
Strengths	Provides information on all avoidable causes of blindness

(continued)

Table 8.2 (continued)

Weakness	Does not provide detailed information on posterior segment eye diseases such as age-related macular degeneration, diabetic retinopathy, or glaucoma; difficult protocol, especially the slit-lamp examination and retinal examination; examinations need to be done by ophthalmologists, hence the cost of the survey is higher
C. Rapid Assessment of Avoidable Blindness (RAAB) + DR	
Objective	Avoidable blindness; diabetic retinopathy
Outcomes	Prevalence of the main causes of visual impairment and blindness; cataract surgical coverage (CSC); effective cataract surgical coverage (eCSC); barriers specific to the uptake of services for cataract surgery; visual outcomes after cataract surgery; prevalence of diabetes and diabetic retinopathy
Sampling method	Compact segment sampling
Age group	≥50 years
Human resources (HR)	Paramedical personnel/optometrists and an ophthalmologist
Examination protocol	Vision acuity assessment using a modified Snellen chart (6/12, 6/18, and 6/60 optotypes); handheld slit-lamp examination; pupillary dilatation, and direct ophthalmoscopy by an ophthalmologist, if pinhole visual acuity is worse than 6/18; also includes fasting blood sugar or oral glucose tolerance test
Strengths	Provides information on all avoidable causes of blindness, including the prevalence of diabetic retinopathy
Weakness	Similar to RAAB, in addition to issues related to blood collection; this is recommended over RAAB only where adequate resources are available
D. Rapid Assessment of Refractive Errors (RARE)	
Objective	Uncorrected refractive errors and presbyopia
Outcomes	Prevalence of refractive error; spectacle coverage (SC); barriers for the uptake of services for uncorrected refractive errors and presbyopia; prevalence of spectacle use
Sampling method	EPI random walk method/compact segment sampling
Age group	15–49 years
Human resources (HR)	Only paramedical personnel/optometrists
Examination protocol	Visual acuity assessment—unaided, aided, and with pinhole if visual acuity worse than 6/12; torchlight examination
Strengths	Simple protocol; HR easily available
Weakness	Limited age group; provides information only on uncorrected refractive errors and presbyopia
E. Rapid Assessment of Visual Impairment (RAVI)	
Objective	Cataract; presbyopia; spectacle coverage
Outcomes	Prevalence of blindness; cataract surgical coverage (CSC); spectacle coverage (SC); barriers for uptake of both avoidable and correctable causes of visual impairment; visual outcomes after cataract surgery; prevalence of spectacle use; near vision impairment/functional presbyopia
Sampling method	Compact segment sampling
Age group	≥40 years
Human resources (HR)	Only paramedical personnel/optometrists
Examination protocol	Visual acuity assessment and torchlight/slit-lamp examination with a portable slit lamp; near vision assessment; direct ophthalmoscopy through undilated pupils if pinhole visual acuity is worse than 6/18; more recently, non-mydriatic retinal imaging and the Washington disability questionnaire have been included
Strengths	Simple protocol; HR easily available; low cost compared to conventional studies; provides information on spectacle coverage
Weakness	Posterior segment disease diagnosis is based on exclusion and marked if the anterior segment is normal; this limitation is minimized by using a non-mydriatic retinal camera

8.4 Application of Results from Rapid Assessment Studies

Vision loss is a considerable burden; however, many vision loss issues have relatively straightforward remedies. Therefore, it is imperative to make adequate plans to address these problems, especially with respect to existing service delivery models. To assess the impact of the current models of service delivery and develop better models, robust data are required to initiate useful service delivery patterns and set realistic time-bound targets. These evaluation methods should provide information on critical success indicators using minimum resources and time. The population-based studies are intended to provide scientifically sound epidemiological data and help in the above process. When repeated at regular intervals, rapid assessment methods can provide trends and an overview of the impacts of services provided in a given area. The WHO Global Action Plan 2014–2019 highlights the need for compiling regional prevalence data that can be used for planning eye care services to address regional priorities. It also recommends repeat surveys in regions where surveys were conducted previously to assess trends in the prevalence of visual impairment over time [17].

There are a few examples where population-based surveys have been repeatedly conducted in specific regions. One such example is our study in south India [15, 16]. We conducted two rapid assessment studies using identical protocols in the same geographical area in 5 years. Our studies have shown a 2.5% decline in vision impairment in 5 years in the region where eye care services were initiated, while the burden of vision impairment remained unchanged in areas where new interventions were not planned [15, 16].

8.5 Population-Based Blindness Studies in South-East Asia

Population-based blindness surveys have been conducted in all ten countries listed in this chapter, and these surveys have also been repeated in a few of these countries. In most situations, a representative sample of people aged ≥50 years proportionate to the size of the population were recruited. In some countries, the age for the sample population is taken as ≥40 years. In all situations, these surveys were door-to-door with basic examination protocols that included: (1) measuring distance vision using a Snellen chart placed at a 6-m distance, which was progressively brought closer for those who could not read the chart; (2) flashlight examination of the eye and adnexa; (3) direct ophthalmoscopy to assess media clarity; and (4) dilated eye examination (in some countries) when the visual acuity was less than 6/18 or 6/12 (unless there were obvious causes such as corneal opacity or cataract). All studies were led by ophthalmologists assisted by optometrists and allied ophthalmic personnel (AOP).

The definitions of diseases were in line with the RAAB instruction manuals. The surgical details were obtained from people who had undergone cataract surgery in the past. Barriers to uptake of cataract surgery were collected from people who had not undergone cataract surgery despite impaired vision due to cataract. The WHO/Prevention of Blindness proforma and its classification system for identifying the main cause of low vision and blindness for each examined subject was used [18].

8.5.1 Bangladesh

The Bangladesh national blindness survey was carried out in 2003 [19]. In this survey, 12,782 adults of age ≥30 years were selected based on multistage cluster random sampling with probability proportional to size procedures. The breakdown of the cluster sites was proportional to the rural/urban distribution of the national population. In this study, the age-standardized prevalence of blindness was 1.53%, and 13.8% of the sampled population had vision <6/12. The main causes of visual impairment were cataract (74.2%), refractive errors (18.7%), and macular degeneration (1.9%). Cataract was the predominant cause (79.6%) of bilateral blindness, followed by uncorrected aphakia (6.2%), and macular degeneration (3.1%).

In 2003, Bangladesh also reported data on the outcomes of cataract surgery [20]. This survey reported that in 88% of the surgeries, intracapsular cataract extraction (ICCE) was carried out, and that 10% of operated eyes had received extracapsular surgery with intraocular lens implantation (ECCE + IOL). Post-surgery, 30.1% of the eyes presented ≥6/12 or better vision, which improved to 50.4% after refraction. However, in 24.8% of the eyes, the presenting visual acuity (PVA) was <3/60, which reduced to 11.1% after refraction. This study also showed that ICCE was more likely to result in a moderate (vision < 6/18) vision gain (Odds Ratio (OR): 4.26) than ECCE + IOL, and that eye camp surgery was more likely to result in poor (vision < 6/60) vision gain (OR: 1.98). However, over the years, the ratio of ECCE + IOL procedures to ICCE procedures has increased in Bangladesh.

In 2010, four RAAB surveys were conducted in Bangladesh [21]. The major findings of these RAABs are shown in Table 8.3. In every survey, cataract was the leading cause of blindness.

8.5.2 Bhutan

Bhutan conducted a national representative blindness survey using the RAAB survey methodology in 2009, and repeated it in 2018 [22, 23]. These two surveys showed that the prevalence of blindness reduced from 1.5% (95% confidence interval, CI: 1.09–1.89) in 2009 to 1.0% (95% CI: 0.5–1.4) in 2018. Incidence of cataract as the major cause of blindness reduced from 67.1 to 48.4% over this time period, and the CSC increased from 72.7 to 86.1%.

In the 2018 RAAB, the prevalence of moderate to severe visual impairment (MSVI) was 5.6% [23]. Extrapolating these data, it was estimated that 16,335 people aged ≥50 years were living with some degree of bilateral visual impairment (PVA < 6/12), and that 1151 people were bilaterally blind. The prevalence of blindness was higher in the rural population (OR: 1.5, $p < 0.13$) and in women (OR: 1.6, $p < 0.06$), though these were not statistically significant.

8.5.3 India

The nation-wide blindness surveys were conducted in India in 2007 and 2015–2019 [24, 25]. These two surveys showed a reduction in the prevalence of blindness (vision < 3/60) from 3.6% in 2007 to 1.9% in 2015–2019 in people ≥50 years of age. The Indian definition of blindness has been changed from 6/60 to 3/60 [26]; this change in the definition of blindness and visual impairment is now at par with the WHO definition. The major differences between these two surveys are shown in Table 8.4.

Table 8.3 Major outcomes of the 2010 RAAB surveys in Bangladesh

Location, District	Sample size	Prevalence of blindness (%)	Principal cause of blindness	CSC (%)	Good visual outcome after cataract surgery (%)
Khulna, Narail	2450	2.7	Cataract, 73.8%	65	73
Jamalpur, Dhaka	3050	1.9	Cataract, 52.6%	75	66
Gajipur, Dhaka	2400	1.9	Cataract, 68.2%	71	74
Cox's Bazar	2500	3.1	Cataract, 76.6%	55	74

CSC cataract surgical coverage

Table 8.4 Major outcomes of the 2007 and 2015–2019 RAAB surveys (for people ≥50 years of age) in India

Year	Area	Sample size	Prevalence of blindness (%)	Principal cause of blindness	CSC	Good visual outcome after cataract surgery
2007	16 districts, 15 states	40,447	3.6	Cataract, 72.2%	NA	NA
2015–2019	31 districts, 22 states	85,135	1.9	Cataract, 66.2%	93.2%	57.8% (PVA) 73.4% (BCVA)

BCVA best corrected visual acuity, *NA* not available, *PVA* presenting visual acuity

In the 0–49 years age group, uncorrected refractive error was the leading cause of visual impairment (29.6%). The proportion of cataract surgeries that included IOL implantation was 94.2%.

The recent survey showed that compared to the 2010 estimation, both visual impairment and blindness have halved (visual impairment has reduced from 5.3 to 2.5%; blindness from 0.68 to 0.36%) [25].

8.5.4 Indonesia

Indonesia carried out a RAAB survey in 15 provinces (of its 34 provinces) between 2014 and 2017 [27]. This study showed that the prevalence of blindness in East Java was highest at 4.4% (95% CI: 3.1–5.6%), followed by Nusa Tenggara Barat (Lesser Sunda Island) at 4.0% (95% CI: 3.0–5.1%). Cataract was the most common cause of blindness in all provinces (range: 71.7–95.5%). Cataract surgical coverage for people with PVA < 3/60 in Bali was the highest at 81.3% and lowest in East Java at 29.6%.

8.5.5 Maldives

The Maldives conducted its first nation-wide population-based blindness survey in 2016 [28]. In this study, the age and gender-adjusted prevalence of blindness was 2.0% (95% CI: 1.5–2.6) and it was higher in women (2.3%; 95% CI, 1.6–3.0) than in men (1.8%; 95% CI 1.0–2.7). The overall prevalence of severe visual impairment (PVA 6/60 < 3/60) was 1.9% (95% CI: 1.4–2.4), and visual impairment (PVA 6/18 < 6/60) was 11.4% (95% CI: 10.0–12.8). The leading cause of blindness was cataract (51.4%), followed by posterior segment anomalies (27.8%). The leading cause of moderate visual impairment was refractive error (50.9%). The in-person cataract surgical coverage at a PVA cut off of <3/60 was 93.5%, and at a PVA cut off <6/18 was 69.1%. After cataract surgery, a good visual outcome was obtained in 67.9% of eyes with PVA (>6/18) and in 76.6% of eyes with BCVA (>6/18). The survey also showed that almost half (48.1%) of the cataract surgeries were performed outside the country.

8.5.6 Myanmar

Myanmar conducted a national blindness survey in 1998, and the overall blindness (for all ages) in the population was 0.58% [29]. Cataract was the leading cause of blindness (63%). Other major causes of blindness were glaucoma (16%), posterior segment disorders (7%), and trachoma (4%).

The RAAB survey was conducted in three districts of Myanmar, namely, Meiktila, Sagaing, and Schwebo [30], from 2001 to 2005 (Table 8.5). The prevalence of blindness, severe visual impairment, and moderate visual impairment in these three districts were as follows: Meiktila—3.4%, 5.9%, and 36.21%; Sagaing—4.25%, 5.91%, and 15.3%, and Shwebo—8.08%, 6.52%, and 21.15%, respectively (Table 8.5).

In 2017, 11 RAABs were conducted to obtain national and regional representative data on blindness and visual impairment (unpublished). These studies showed that the overall age- the sex-adjusted prevalence of blindness in Myanmar was 2.7% (95% CI: 2.2–3.2) in the population aged ≥50 years. Based on this finding, the prevalence of blindness for all ages is extrapolated to be 0.58% for the entire Myanmar population,

Table 8.5 Results of the RAAB survey conducted from 2001 to 2005 in Myanmar

Area	Year	Sample size	Prevalence of blindness, %	Principal cause of blindness, %	CSC, %	Good visual outcome after cataract surgery
Sagaing	2001	3000	8.6	Cataract (71.4)	21.0	28%
Schwebo	2001	3000	4.0.7	Cataract (72.3)	44.0	23%
Meiktila	2005	2076	3.4	Cataract (53.0)	22.3	NA

CSC cataract surgical coverage, *NA* not available

which is the same as it was in 1998. The age-sex adjusted prevalence for severe visual impairment was 3.4% (95% CI: 3.0–3.8%) and moderate visual impairment was 12.8% (95% CI: 10.3–15.3). The prevalence of cataract blindness in this survey was 1.6%, and the prevalence of operable cataracts (pinhole visual acuity <6/60) was 3.5%.

8.5.7 Nepal

The first nation-wide population-based survey on blindness and visual impairment was conducted in 1980–1981 with a total sample of 39,887 people of all ages [31]. This study reported a blindness prevalence of 0.84%. Cataract was the leading cause of avoidable blindness (>80%) and trachoma (6.5%) was the second leading cause of blindness. Results from this survey helped to mobilize support and build an elaborate eye care infrastructure in the country.

Between 2006 and 2010, another population-based survey on blindness and visual impairment was conducted in Nepal's 14 zones. This consisted of customized blindness surveys in 3 zones and RAAB surveys in 11 zones [32–34]. In these surveys, the weighted average sample prevalence of blindness was 2.5% (95% CI: 2.3–2.6%) in people aged ≥50 years. The prevalence of severe visual impairment was 3.0% (95% CI: 2.8–3.2%), and moderate visual impairment was 11.6% (95% CI: 11.3–11.9%). The age and gender-adjusted prevalence of blindness was 2.0% (95% CI: 1.9–2.2%). Cataract was the main cause of bilateral blindness with a weighted average of 62.2%. Other causes of blindness were posterior segment disease (16.5%), glaucoma (5.9%), corneal scar other than trachoma (5.2%), and uncorrected aphakia (3.4%). The CSC was 85% for visual acuity <3/60, 70% for visual acuity <6/60, and 54% for visual acuity <6/18. In 1981, ICCE with aphakic spectacles was the standard of care. Over the years, this has changed to the current ECCE (90% of cataract surgeries) with Small Incision Cataract Surgery (SICS) or phaco and implantation of an IOL.

Nepal, which became a federal state in 2015, is now divided into seven administrative provinces. Health administration was placed under the jurisdiction of the central provincial government. In order to help in program planning for eye health, new province-specific blindness and visual impairment surveys were planned. As of now, data collection has been completed in six provinces, and the preliminary results (unpublished) of these surveys are given in Table 8.6.

8.5.8 Sri Lanka

In 2007, the Kandy Eye Study [35], a randomized cluster sample, examined 1375 people aged ≥40 years in the Kandy district. The prevalence of blindness was 1.1% (95% CI: 0.002–0.020). The prevalence of visual impairment was 5.9% (95% CI, 0.043–0.075). Cataract and age-related macular degeneration were the main causes of visual impairment.

The nation-wide RAAB survey was conducted in 2015 in Sri Lanka [36]. This survey estimated the prevalence of blindness and visual impairment among those aged ≥40 years. The preva-

Table 8.6 Preliminary findings of the RAAB 2020 in Nepal for people aged ≥50 years

Location	Blindness	MSVI	CSC	eCSC	Visual Outcome	DM	DR
Province 1	0.8%	6.3%	84.7%	84.0%	85.9%	NA	Na
Province 2	1.3%	14.0%	76.9%	81.6%	81.0%	5.6%	15.0%
Bagmati Province	0.7%	7.9%	88.2%	84.0%	79.4%	9.4%	16.9%
Gandaki Province	0.9%	6.8%	80.3%	75.7%	76.5%	NA	NA
Lumbini Province	1.7%	13.8%	74.4%	73.4%	77.5%	NA	NA
Karnali Province	0.9%	9.4%	84.9%	77.6%	69.1%	1.9%	5.2%
Sudur Paschim Province	NA	NA	NA	NA	NA	NA	NA

CSC cataract surgical coverage, *DM* diabetes mellitus, *DR* diabetic retinopathy, *eCSC* effective cataract surgical coverage, *MSVI* moderate to severe visual impairment, *NA* not available yet

lence of blindness, severe visual impairment, and moderate visual impairment were 1.7% (95% CI: 1.3–1.99), 1.6%, and 15.4%, respectively. Cataract was the most common cause of blindness (66.7%); among those operated for cataract, 93.8% had received an IOL. The outcome of cataract surgery was good, with a PVA > 6/18 in 59.7% of eyes, which further improved to 75.1% with the BCVA. Cataract surgical coverage was 85.4% at the visual acuity >3/60 cut off level. In this study, 13.8% of the sample population were known diabetic and 20% were known hypertensive. The all age prevalence of disability (as per the Washington Group Disability Questionnaire, short version) was 3.17% [95% CI: 2.87–3.50], which was significantly higher in women, older people, people with lower socioeconomic status, and rural residents [37].

8.5.9 Thailand

The first RAAB survey in Thailand was conducted in 2014 [38]. This survey showed that the age and sex-adjusted prevalence of blindness, severe visual impairment, and moderate visual impairment were 0.6% (95% CI: 0.5–0.8), 1.3% (95% CI: 1.0–1.6), and 12.6% (95% CI: 10.8–14.5), respectively. There were no significant differences in these results between the four regions of Thailand. Cataract was the main cause of vision loss accounting for 69.7% of blindness. CSC in people with cutoff PVA <3/60 was 95.1%. Refractive errors, diabetic retinopathy, glaucoma, and corneal opacities were responsible for 6.0%, 5.1%, 4.0%, and 2.0% of blindness, respectively.

8.5.10 Timor-Leste

The first countrywide RAAB using a national representative sample of people aged ≥50 years was conducted in 2016 [39]. This survey showed that the age and gender-adjusted prevalence of blindness was 2.8% (2.4% for men and 3.1% for women), prevalence of severe visual impairment was 4.5% (4% for men and 4.9% for women), and prevalence of moderate visual impairment was 12.5% (12% for men and 12.5% for women). Cataract was the leading cause of blindness (79.4%). Age and gender-adjusted CSC was 41.5% (52.6% for men and 30.6% for women) among those with PVA < 3/60; CSC was 30.9% (40.3% for men and 22.0% for women) among those with PVA < 6/60; and CSC was 16.8% (23.5% for men and 11.3% for women) for those with PVA < 6/18. Overall, good visual outcome was obtained in 62% of all eyes operated on for cataract.

8.6 Conclusion

Population-based studies provide a unique perspective of vision loss and eye diseases. Analyzing and disseminating such information is needed to assess the health status of the community/country that could subsequently be used in program planning and resource allocation. These studies are the most valid, and often the only, way to determine the prevalence and incidence of a disease. A representative sample that involves the entire population of the community or country is always useful; however, the cost in terms of time and resources is high. A fairly effective alternative methodology is a rapid study that recruits people of certain age groups since many ophthalmic disorders occur in adults and the elderly. In the South-East Asia region, many population studies, including those sampling all age groups and those sampling only the adult/elderly population, have been conducted (Table 8.7). Such studies have helped in eye health program planning by generating evidence, improving the quality and efficacy of eye care programs, and formulating targeted age or disease or geographic location-specific eye care initiatives.

Therefore, new studies are necessary in every region of the world to monitor progress in the ongoing efforts to attain universal eye health and the 2030 sustainable development goals. In this context, the formation and initiatives of the Global Burden of Disease (GBD) are very important. The GBD measures disability and death due to a multitude of causes worldwide. It has grown over the past two decades into an international

Table 8.7 Summary of the results of the most recent status of blindness and visual impairment in the South-East Asia region

				Results Prevalence % (95% CI)		Most common cause of VI Prevalence % (95% CI)	
Country	Year	Study type (Age)	Sample size	Blind	MSVI	Blind	MSVI
Bangladesh [21]	2003	30+	12,782	1.53	13.8	Cataract 79.6	URE 18.7
Bhutan [23]	2018	50+	5050	1.0 (0.5–1.4)	5.6	Cataract 48.4	URE 46.7
India [25]	2019	50+	93,108	1.99	11.8	Cataract 66.2	URE 15.8
Indonesia [27]	2015	50+	45,822	3.0 (2.1–3.9)	10.2	Cataract 81.2	NA
Maldives [28]	2016	50+	3100	1.8 (1.0–2.7)	14.9	Cataract 51.4	URE 43.3
Myanmar [30]	2017	50+	37,369	2.7 (2.2–3.2)	16.2	Cataract 72.0	NA
Nepal [34]	2012	50+	43,307	2.5 (2.3–2.6)	14.6	Cataract 62.2	NA
Sri Lanka [37]	2015	40+	6713	1.7 (1.3–2.0)	17.0	Cataract 66.7	URE 62.4
Thailand [38]	2014	50+	21,000	0.6 (0.5–0.8)	13.9	Cataract 69.7	URE 25.2
Timor-Leste [39]	2016	50+	3350	2.8 (1.8–3.8)	17.0	Cataract 79.4	URE 26.9

CI confidence interval, *MSVI* moderate to severe visual impairment, *NA* not available, *URE* uncorrected refractive error, *VI* visual impairment

consortium of nearly 5500 researchers, and its estimates are being updated annually since 1990 [40]. The Vision Loss Expert Group (VLEG) [41], formed by an international consortium of ophthalmologists and optometrists, has been providing global vision data to the GBD since 2010. These data have been used by the WHO to design the Global Action Plan and International Agency for the Prevention of Blindness Vision Atlas. Therefore, periodic surveys of eye care services and disease burden must continue, as this helps in national planning and/or redesigning eye care strategies.

References

1. Bourne RRA, Flaxman SR, Braithwaite T, et al. Magnitude, temporal trends, and projections of the global prevalence of blindness and distance and near vision impairment: a systematic review and meta-analysis. Lancet Glob Health. 2017;5:e888–e97.
2. Marmamula S, Keeffe JE, Rao GN. Rapid assessment methods in eye care: an overview. Indian J Ophthalmol. 2012;60:416–22.
3. Dandona R, Dandona L, Naduvilath TJ, et al. Design of a population-based study of visual impairment in India: the Andhra Pradesh Eye Disease Study. Indian J Ophthalmol. 1997;45:251–7.
4. Dandona L, Dandona R, Srinivas M, et al. Blindness in the Indian state of Andhra Pradesh. Invest Ophthalmol Vis Sci. 2001;42:908–16.
5. Limburg H, Kumar R, Indrayan A, et al. Rapid assessment of prevalence of cataract blindness at district level. Int J Epidemiol. 1997;26:1049–54.
6. Kuper H, Polack S, Limburg H. Rapid assessment of avoidable blindness. Community Eye Health. 2006;19:68–9.
7. Guha-Sapir D. Rapid assessment of health needs in mass emergencies: review of current concepts and methods. World Health Stat Q. 1991;44:171–81.
8. Venkataswamy G, Lepkowski JM, Ravilla T, et al. Rapid epidemiologic assessment of cataract blindness. The Aravind Rapid Epidemiologic Assessment Staff. Int J Epidemiol. 1989;18:S60–7.
9. Mactaggart I, Limburg H, Bastawrous A, et al. Rapid Assessment of Avoidable Blindness: looking back, looking forward. Br J Ophthalmol. 2019;103:1549–52.
10. Marmamula S, Keeffe JE, Rao GN. Uncorrected refractive errors, presbyopia and spectacle coverage: results from a rapid assessment of refractive error survey. Ophthalmic Epidemiol. 2009;16:269–74.
11. Marmamula S, Narsaiah S, Shekhar K, et al. Visual impairment in the South Indian state of Andhra Pradesh: Andhra Pradesh—rapid assessment of visual impairment (AP-RAVI) Project. PLoS One. 2013;8:e70120.

12. Marmamula S, Madala SR, Rao GN. Rapid assessment of visual impairment (RAVI) in marine fishing communities in South India—study protocol and main findings. BMC Ophthalmol. 2011;11:26.
13. Marmamula S, Khanna RC, Shekhar K, et al. Outcomes of cataract surgery in urban and rural Population in the South Indian state of Andhra Pradesh: rapid assessment of visual impairment (RAVI) project. PLoS One. 2016;11:e0167708.
14. Flaxman SR, Bourne RRA, Resnikoff S, et al. Global causes of blindness and distance vision impairment 1990–2020: a systematic review and meta-analysis. Lancet Glob Health. 2017;5:e1221–34.
15. Marmamula S, Khanna RC, Yellapragada S, et al. Temporal trends in the prevalence and causes of visual impairment in the South Indian state of Telangana: a population-based cross-sectional study. BMJ Open. 2019;9:e029114.
16. Marmamula S, Challa R, Yellapragada S, et al. Temporal trends in the prevalence of spectacle use and spectacle coverage in India. Clin Exp Optom. 2020;103:693–8. https://doi.org/10.1111/cxo.13025.
17. WHO. Universal eye health: a global action plan 2014–2019. www.who.int/blindness. Accessed 25 Sept 2020.
18. https://www.who.int/news-room/fact-sheets/detail/blindness-and-visual-impairment
19. Dinen BP, Bourne RRA, Ali SM, et al. Prevalence and causes of blindness and visual impairment in Bangladesh adults: results of the National Blindness and Low Vision Survey of Bangladesh. Br J Ophthalmol. 2003;87:820–8.
20. Bourne RRA, Dinen BP, Ali SM, et al. Outcome of cataract surgery. Br J Ophthalmol. 2003;87:813–9.
21. http://raabdata.info/repository/. Accessed 6 Oct 2020.
22. Lepcha NR, Chhetri CK, Getshen K, et al. Rapid assessment of avoidable blindness in Bhutan. Ophthalmic Epidemiol. 2013;20:212–9.
23. Lepcha NT, Sharma IP, Sapkota YD, et al. Changing trends of blindness, visual impairment and cataract surgery in Bhutan: 2009–2018. PLoS One. 2019;14:e0216398. https://doi.org/10.1371/journalpone.0216398.
24. Neena J, Rachel J, Praveen V, et al. Rapid assessment of avoidable blindness in India. PLoS One. 2008;3:e2867. https://doi.org/10.1371/journal.pone.0002867.
25. https://npcbvi.gov.in. Accessed 21 Oct 2020.
26. Vashist P, Senjam SS, Gupta V, et al. Definition of blindness under National Programme for Control of Blindness: do we need to revise it? Indian J Ophthalmol. 2017;65:92–6.
27. Rifati L, Halim A, Lestari YD, et al. Blindness and visual impairment situation in Indonesia based on Rapid Assessment of Avoidable Blindness surveys in 15 provinces. Ophthalmic Epidemiol. https://doi.org/10.1080/09286586.2020.1853178.
28. Thoufeeq U, Das T, Limburg H, et al. First rapid assessment of avoidable blindness survey in the Maldives: prevalence and causes of blindness and cataract surgery. Asia Pac J Ophthalmol. 2017;7:1–5.
29. Ocular Morbidity Survey, Myanmar 1997–98. WHO Newsletter July–September 2015. http://origin.searo.who.int/myanmar. Accessed 21 Oct 2020.
30. Casson RJ, Newland HS, Muecke J, et al. Prevalence and causes of visual impairment in rural Myanmar. The Meiktila Eye Study. Ophthalmology. 2007;114:2302–8.
31. Brilliant LB, Pokharel RP, Grasset NC, et al. Epidemilogy of blindness in Nepal. Bull World Health Organ. 1985;63:375–86.
32. Sapkota YD, Pokharel GP, Nirmalan PK, et al. Prevalence of blindness and cataract surgery in Gandaki Zone, Nepal. Br J Ophthalmol. 2006;90:411–6.
33. Sapkota YD, Sunuwar M, Naito T, et al. The prevalence of blindness and cataract surgery in Rautahat district, Nepal. Ophthalmic Epidemiol. 2010;17:82–9.
34. Sapkota YD, Limburg H. Epidemiology of blindness in Nepal 2012. Nepal Netra Jyoti Sangh. https://www.iapb.org/resources/epidemiology-of-blindness-in-nepal. Accessed on 6 Oct 2020.
35. Edussuriya K, Sennanayake S, Senaratne S, et al. The prevalence and causes of visual impairment in Central Sri Lanka, the Kandy Eye study. Ophthalmology. 2009;116:52–6.
36. Rabiu M. National estimates of the magnitude, causes and determinants of blindness and visual impairment in Sri Lanka. Ceylon Med J. 2018;63(S2):s1–2. https://doi.org/10.4038/cmj.v63i5.8734.
37. Bangala C, Gilbert C, Murthy GVS, et al. Prevalence, causes, magnitude and risk factors of visual impairment and blindness in Sri Lanka. Ceylon Med J. 2018;63(S2):s10–7. https://doi.org/10.4038/cmj.v63i5.8735.
38. Isipradit S, Sirimaharaj M, Charukamnoetkanok P, et al. The first rapid assessment of avoidable blindness (RAAB) in Thailand. PLoS One. 2014;9:e114245. https://doi.org/10.1371/journal.pone.0114245.
39. Correia M, Das T, Magno J, et al. Prevalence and causes of blindness, visual impairment, and cataract surgery in Timor-Leste. Clin Ophthalmol. 2017;11:2125–31.
40. www.healthdata.org > gbd. Accessed 23 Oct 2020.
41. www.globalvisiondata.org. Accessed 23 Oct 2020.

Part III

Common Disorders

Cataract in South-East Asia

9

Reeta Gurung, Parikshit Gogate,
Radhika Upreti Oli, A. H. M. Enayet Hussain,
Asela Abeydeera, Indra P. Sharma,
Nor Tshering Lepcha, Phanindra B. Nukella,
and Syumarti

Key Points

- Cataract is the leading cause of blindness in each of the South-East Asian countries.
- Cataract surgical rates and coverage have increased in the past two decades in each country, but there is a considerable variation between countries.
- There is a backlog in each country of the region, and the number of cataract surgeries performed annually must increase.
- Manual small incision cataract surgery has been the mainstay of most blindness control programs, though phacoemulsification is getting more popular.
- Residency training should focus on teaching quality cataract surgery techniques to improve outcomes and, ultimately, coverage.
- Each country must develop a monitoring mechanism for continuous quality improvement.
- Midlevel human resources training is important to improve the quality of care.
- Outreach programs are currently necessary for many countries of the region, but efforts must be made to provide surgical care to people closer to their homes.
- The intraocular lenses constitute the most to cataract surgery costs; currently, the cost is high in some countries.

The International Agency for the Prevention of Blindness (IAPB) South-East Asia Region (SEAR) consists of 11 countries; 6 from the Indian subcontinent (Bangladesh, Bhutan, India, the Maldives, Nepal, and Sri Lanka) and 4 from geographic South-East Asia (Myanmar, Indonesia, Thailand, Timor-Leste, and the

R. Gurung · R. U. Oli
Tilganga Institute of Ophthalmology,
Kathmandu, Nepal
e-mail: reeta.gurung@tilganga.org;
radhika.upreti@tilganga.org

P. Gogate (✉)
Community Eye Care Foundation, Dr. Gogate's Eye
Clinic, Pune, Maharashtra, India

A. H. M. E. Hussain
Directorate General of Medical Education, Ministry
of Health and Family Welfare, Dhaka, Bangladesh

A. Abeydeera
Association of Community Ophthalmologists
of Sri Lanka, Colombo, Sri Lanka

I. P. Sharma · N. T. Lepcha
Department of Ophthalmology, JDW National
Referral Hospital, Thimphu, Bhutan

Faculty of Postgraduate Medicine, Khesar Gyalpo
University of Medical Science of Bhutan,
Thimphu, Bhutan
e-mail: ipsharma@jdwnrh.gov.bt;
nort@jdwnrh.gov.bt

P. B. Nukella
VISION 2020, India, New Delhi, Delhi, India
e-mail: phanindra@vision2020.org

Syumarti
Section of Cataract Blindness Elimination of
Indonesian Ophthalmologist Association West Java,
Bandung, West Java, Indonesia

T. Das, P. D. Nayar (eds.), *South-East Asia Eye Health*,
https://doi.org/10.1007/978-981-16-3787-2_9

Democratic People's Republic of (DPR) Korea). The region is home to nearly 26% of the world population [1]. Cataract is the most common cause of blindness and visual impairment globally and in the region (Fig. 9.1) [2, 3]. Cataract accounts for nearly half to three-fourths of all cases of blindness and severe visual impairment (SVI) [2]. The region has witnessed enormous economic development in the past three decades, which has reduced blindness and SVI. Cataract surgical programs have been the mainstays by which this region has reduced avoidable blindness; many countries in the region now have modern cataract surgery facilities using the latest techniques and technologies [3].

In this region, 12 million people are blind, and 78.5 million people are visually impaired. This amounts to ~30% of global blindness and ~32% of global visual impairment. Cataract is the principal cause of blindness and severe visual impairment in all seven countries (Bangladesh, Bhutan, India, Indonesia, Maldives, Sri Lanka, Thailand, and Timor-Leste) where the RAAB (Rapid Assessment of Avoidable Blindness) survey was conducted recently. In addition, cataract continues to be the principal cause of moderate visual impairment in four countries (Bhutan, Indonesia, Thailand, and Timor-Leste). The outcomes of cataract surgery were suboptimal in the Maldives and Timor-Leste [2, 4–9].

9.1 Definitions

Traditionally, cataract prevalence has been considered a surrogate measure of the quantity and quality of eye care globally. Several nomenclatures have been coined to measure these, and we will repeatedly use these definitions throughout this chapter. These terminologies are: (1) cataract

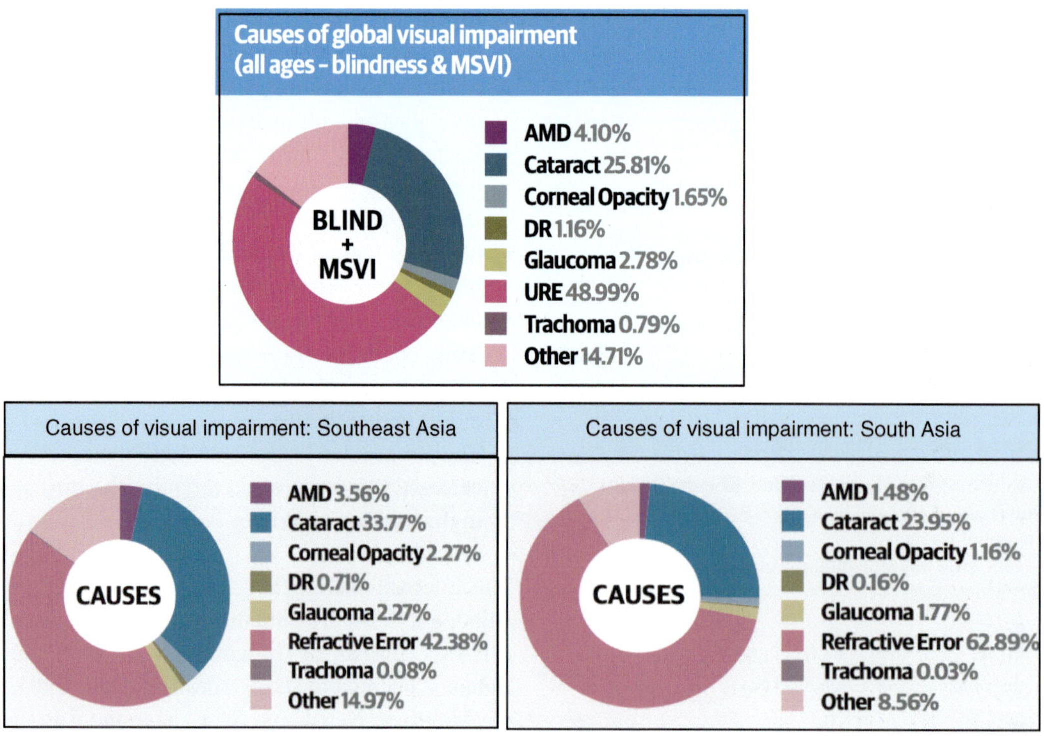

Fig. 9.1 Distribution of causes of visual impairment in the Global Burden of Disease (GBD) regions—global (upper panel), South-East Asia (bottom left) and South Asia (bottom right). (Source: International Agency for the Prevention of Blindness (IAPB) Vision Atlas, 2017). *AMD* age-related macular degeneration, *DR* diabetic retinopathy, *MSVI* moderate to severe visual impairment, *URE* uncorrected refractive error

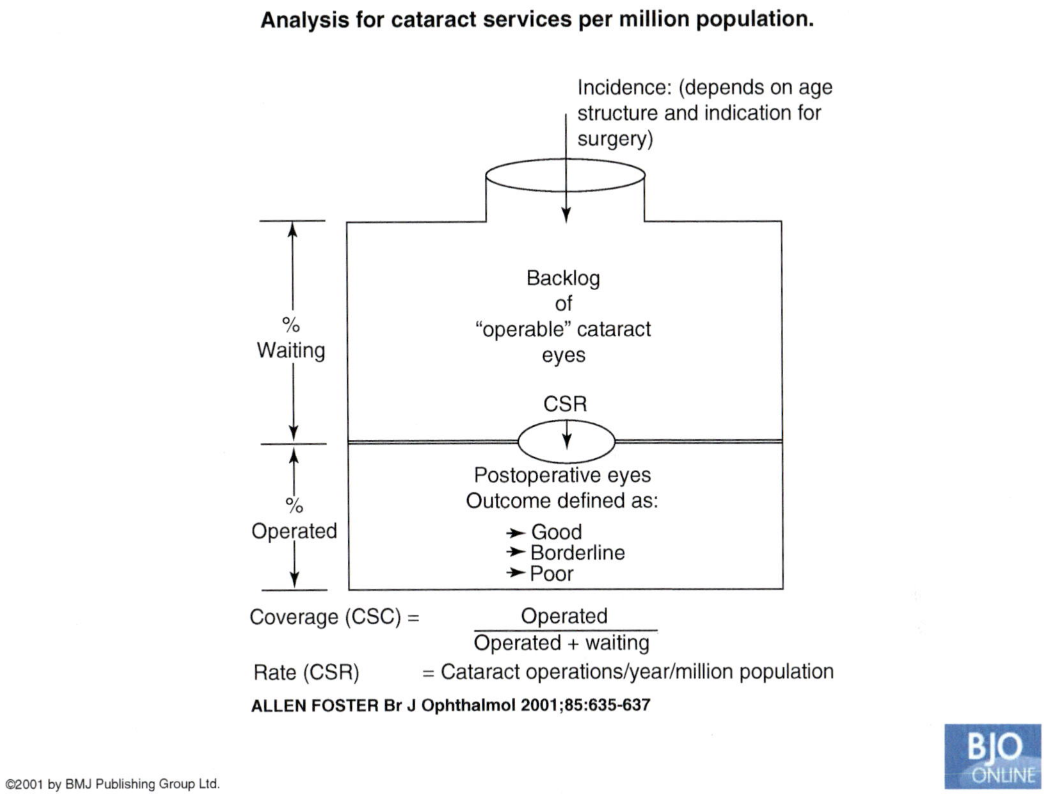

Fig. 9.2 Definition of cataract surgical rate (CSR) and cataract surgical coverage (CSC). (Reprinted with permission from the BMJ publishing group limited, Copy Right 2020) [10]

surgical rate (CSR), (2) cataract surgical coverage (CSC), and (3) effective cataract surgical coverage (eCSC) (Fig. 9.2) [10, 11].

- *Cataract surgical rate (CSR)* is defined as the number of cataract operations performed per million population in one year.
- *Cataract surgical coverage (CSC)* is defined as the proportion of people in a defined population with operated cataract as a proportion of those having operable plus operated cataract.
- *Effective cataract surgical coverage (eCSC)* is defined as the number of people in a defined population with operated cataract and a good outcome (i.e., presenting vision 6/18 or better) as a proportion of those having operable plus operated cataract.

CSR is strongly influenced by resource availability in healthcare delivery. The CSC measures the uptake of services transcending both economic and social barriers. The eCSC measures the quality of care. Two deterrents to an increase in CSC are unaffordable cost and suboptimal quality of care.

The World Health Organization (WHO) classifies vision outcomes after cataract surgery as "good," "moderate," or "poor" based on the presenting visual acuity (PVA) and best-corrected visual acuity (BCVA) of treated patients (Table 9.1).

In the following sections, we will describe country-specific situations vis-à-vis cataract surgery. These are discussed under three broad headings: (1) Facilitators, (2) Barriers, and (3) Strategic planning/recommendations.

Table 9.1 World Health Organization classification of vision after cataract surgery

	Good outcome		Moderate outcome		Poor outcome	
	PVA	BCVA	PVA	BCVA	PVA	BCVA
WHO criteria	>80%	>90%	<15%	<5%	<5%	<5%

BCVA best-corrected visual acuity, *PVA* presenting visual acuity

9.2 Bangladesh

A. H. M. Enayet Hussain

Bangladesh is a densely populated country (population: 165 million; density: 1265 people/km^2—July 2020) [12]. There is also a rich–poor regional divide and the prevalence of blindness in the poorer regions is twice that of the richer regions [13, 14]. In 2005, the National Eye Care (NEC) plan was set in motion along with the Health Nutrition and Population Sector Program (HNPSP), which was subsequently consolidated into the new Health, Population, and Nutrition Sector Development Program (HPNSDP). The objectives of these national plans were to build secondary care and strengthen primary healthcare infrastructure to consolidate preventive care and build a robust referral pathway.

9.2.1 Facilitators

Currently, 344 eye care facilities provide services in Bangladesh and include 78 government, 75 non-government organization (NGO), and 191 private facilities. In Bangladesh, seven international NGOs (INGOs) support local NGOs and the government for health system strengthening and reduction of avoidable blindness. The NEC coordinates and monitors eye care services in Bangladesh [15].

9.2.2 Barriers

1. Inadequate treatment provision: The main source of cataract treatment is the government district hospital for rural populations. Although the cost of treatment in government hospitals is low, cataract surgery is performed in no more than half of the government district hospitals due to an inadequate health workforce.
2. Poor community awareness and service provision: Many people do not know about the causes of blindness and treatment possibilities. A RAAB in 2013 conducted in 14 districts found that about 25% of the survey population with cataract did not feel they needed treatment, and those who knew did not know where to seek treatment [13].
3. Poverty: The national blindness survey found that almost half of the population (48.6%) who had cataract did not seek treatment because they were poor. In Bangladesh, 35.1% of people live below the poverty line of USD1.90 per day [16]. Many do not have the means to bear the transport and ancillary costs related to cataract surgery, even though the surgery itself is free at government facilities.
4. Inadequate training of community health workers: Bangladesh has an extensive networks of community health workers at the rural level. But, these health workers are not adequately trained to identify people with eye problems during regular house visits.
5. Inadequate primary care and referral system: Bangladesh has three tiers of community-based healthcare facilities. The lowest tier is the community health clinics, the mid-tier is union sub-centers, and the upper tier is upazila (sub-district) health complex. Unfortunately, most of these do not address primary eye care; therefore, the opportunity to identify and treat primary eye problems like refractive error and refer people who may need surgery is lost at these levels.
6. Out-of-pocket spending: NGOs and private entrepreneurs provide eye care for a fee in the districts where government eye care services are not available. But without financial assistance, many economically underprivileged people find treatment in these facilities less affordable.

7. Lack of quality surveillance: Currently, Bangladesh does not have any effective system to monitor and maintain the standard of quality of services in eye care.

9.2.3 Strategic Planning/ Recommendations

Despite these constraints, the CSR in Bangladesh had increased from 1100/million people in 2008 to 2594/million people in 2019. Table 9.2 lists the factors that have contributed to this development.

Table 9.2 Measures to improve Cataract Surgical Rate in Bangladesh

Facilitation	Activities
Service	Community outreach camps organized in rural and remote areas Community-level vision centers run by the government, NGOs, and private sector Dedicated eye operation theaters in government district hospitals Trained ophthalmologists and nurses at government district hospitals Equipment provided to government district hospitals Establishment of 344 secondary non-government eye hospitals
Advocacy	Training of government health workers, community volunteers, and "Shastho Sebikas" (women health volunteers) Print and electronic media for information dissemination Linkages with community clinics for the referrals
Treatment	Fee eye care services from the government, international organizations, and corporate philanthropy Financial assistance for transport and daily wages for people undergoing cataract surgery
Strengthening primary care	Community-level vision centers run by the government, NGOs, and private sectors Linkages with community clinics for referrals Using upazila health complexes as eye centers Functional eye departments at government district hospitals Additional private facilities
Financial assistance	Government and international organizations providing free eye care services
Quality surveillance	Development and implementation of National Cataract Surgery Protocol Introduction of patient feedback system Monitoring of visits by NEC and DGHS

NEC National Eye Care, *NGO* non-government organization, *DGHS* Directorate General of Health Services

9.3 Bhutan

Nor Tshering Lepcha and Indra P. Sharma

This small mountainous country had its first population-based survey for blindness and visual impairment in 2009 [5]. Untreated cataract accounted for most cases of blindness (53.8%), severe vision impairment (57.1%), and moderate visual impairment (65.3%). Uncorrected refractive error was the main cause of early visual impairment (46.7%) in a repeat RAAB survey in 2018 [4]. The CSC was 86.1% with relatively better coverage in men (76.7% in men; 73.1% in women) and urban populations (79.2% in urban; 70.2% in rural populations). Good cataract surgical outcomes were achieved in 67.3%, and a leading cause of poor outcomes were ocular co-morbidities (43.6%). The prevalence of blindness and severe visual impairment has been reduced by a one-third in the past decade [17, 18].

9.3.1 Facilitators

Article 9.21 of the Constitution of the Kingdom of Bhutan mandates that the state provides free access to basic public health services to its citizens. All ophthalmic services, including cataract services, are provided free of cost to its citizens by the state. The eye care service in Bhutan is completely integrated with the primary healthcare system. In 1987, the Primary Eye Care Program (PECP) and training for ophthalmic assistants were launched. Ophthalmic services are catered to a population of 773,553 (NSB 2017) through three tiers of the eye health delivery system [18]. Gyalyum Kesang Choeden Wangchuck National Eye Center at the JDW National Referral Hospital serves as the tertiary eye care and referral center. Cataract surgical services and holistic specialized eye care services are provided through community outreach programs to remote locations and unreached populations. Manual small incision cataract surgery (MSICS) is performed more often than phacoemulsification. Age–sex standardized CSCs for blindness (vision < 3/60), severe visual impairment (vision < 6/60), and moderate visual impairment (vision < 6/18) are 88.7%, 86.4%, and 62.6%, respectively. The eCSC has improved between 2009 and 2018 (Table 9.3).

Table 9.3 Visual outcomes after cataract surgery in Bhutan vis-à-vis the WHO criteria

	Good outcome		Moderate outcome		Poor outcome	
	PVA (%)	BCVA (%)	PVA (%)	BCVA (%)	PVA (%)	BCVA (%)
WHO criteria	>80	>90	<15	<5	<5	<5
2009 outcome [6]	56.8	70.0	19.5	15.0	23.6	15.0
2018 outcome [5]	66.2	72.7	19.7	15.8	14.0	11.5

9.3.2 Barriers

The extrapolated magnitude of blindness was 1.0% (95% CI: 0.5–1.4). The adjusted prevalence of severe-, moderate-, and early visual impairment were 0.6% (95% CI: 0.4–0.9), 5.0% (95% CI: 4.2–5.8), and 7.6 (95% CI: 6.6–8.5), respectively [4]. Extrapolating the RAAB 2018 estimates for the country's population, the prevalence of blindness due to cataract was at 0.4% in 2018. This translates to an estimated 466 people blind (vision < 3/60) and 10,460 with impaired vision (vision < 6/18) due to unoperated cataracts. This is Bhutan's cataract backlog. The current average CSR is 984 annually (2016–2019 data), and this has to increase to 1200 to clear the backlog and reduce the waiting time for cataract surgery. Changes in cataract-related numbers between the 2009 and 2018 RAAB are shown in Fig. 9.3. The leading causes of poor outcomes after cataract surgery were comorbidities (43.6%), surgical complications (40.5%), and long-term sequelae (22.2%). Barriers to uptake of cataract surgery were: (1) lack of accompanying person (41.7%), (2) lack of awareness (22.2%), and (3) "no felt need" [mostly for men (35.0%)]. The cost of cataract surgery was not a barrier to uptake of cataract surgery [4].

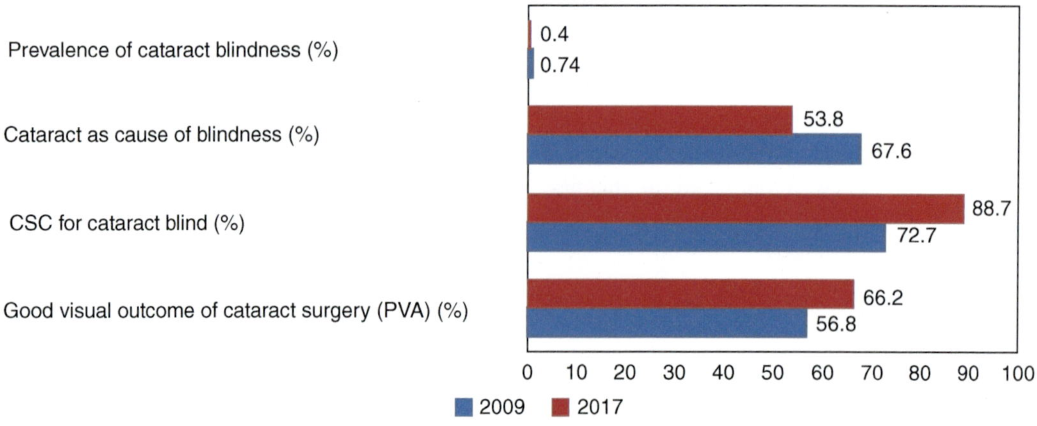

Fig. 9.3 Cataract service indicators to measure progress in reducing blindness due to cataract from 2009 to 2017 [4]

9.3.3 Strategic Planning/ Recommendations

The success of cataract surgeries in reducing blindness prevalence and the documented reduction of blindness and visual impairment between 2009 and 2018 is due to three important factors: (1) the integration of the eye care program with the healthcare program to provide free basic healthcare to all citizens through a three-tier healthcare delivery system with a strong political commitment; (2) a well-established PECP to coordinate, implement, and monitor eye care services; and (3) continued financial and technical support provided by the international agencies and donors.

Despite this progress in Bhutan, other categories of visual impairment are on the rise; the avoidable causes (cataract and refractive error) of low vision/blindness remain high, and gender disparity persists in eye care services. This calls for a need to develop and deploy more human resources, accelerate cataract surgical services, augment refraction services, and strengthen retinal services. The other areas for improvement are advocacy and accessibility, especially for women. The PECP needs further strengthening to make the eye care program effective and sustainable. Some suggestions to achieve these are:

1. Establish a national-level core team for planning, implementing, and monitoring cataract surgical camps, screening programs, mobile clinics, and advocacy.
2. Reduce gender inequity by targeting women and create support mechanisms for elderly women to take up cataract surgery.
3. Strengthen rural cataract services by conducting surgical camps up to Grade I Basic Health Unit level.
4. Increase the numbers and duration of surgical eye camps (up to 10 days) so that more surgeries can be performed in a camp.
5. Increase the numbers of operating days in the apex and regional hospitals.
6. Train and engage village health workers and local leaders for awareness creation.
7. Consider BCVA cut-off at 6/24 for cataract surgery.
8. Monitor cataract surgical outcome and improve the quality of postoperative care.
9. Provide further hands-on training to eye care professionals involved in cataract surgery and care.
10. Include YAG (Yttrium-Aluminum-Garnet) laser capsulotomy services during operative eye camps for people with long-term sequelae of cataract surgery.

9.4 India

India is the most populous country in the WHO SEAR with a large workforce, teaching and training facilities, and well spread-out infrastructure for comprehensive management of all ophthalmic disorders. India has a robust national plan and large, systematically collected data. The country has shown tremendous improvement in CSR, intraocular lens coverage, and improved cataract surgical outcomes in the past two decades.

9.4.1 Facilitators

India is the first country to launch the National Program for Control of Blindness (NPCB) in 1976, as a 100% centrally sponsored program. Over a period, the NPCB (now, NPCB VI) has enlarged its focus beyond cataract to many other eye diseases. Five national-level eye care surveys (1971–1974, 1986–1989, 1999–2001, 2006–2007, and 2015–2019) have been conducted in India over the past five decades. As per the last survey, unoperated cataracts are the principal cause of blindness (66.2%) in the elderly population. Unoperated cataracts account for 71.2% of visual impairment in India in the population aged >50 years [19]. The CSC in the population aged ≥50 years for those who are blind due to cataracts (VA < 3/60 in the better eye) is 93.2% (94.8% in men and 91.9% in women). The CSC among those who are visually impaired due to cataracts (VA < 6/18 in the better eye) is 74.0%. The most important reasons for poor visual outcomes after cataract surgery were ocular co-morbidities (41.4%) and operative complications (31.2%); borderline visual outcome after cataract surgery were operative complications (33.9%) and refractive error (25.9%). The national program, NPCB VI provides financial assistance to many registered non-government organizations for cataract surgery to economically underprivileged sections of the society. Currently, the grant-in-aid is extended to few other emerging causes of blindness, such as glaucoma, diabetic retinopathy, and retinopathy of pre-maturity. The national program also supports short-term skill enhancement training of ophthalmologists in modern techniques of cataract surgery.

9.4.2 Barriers

In 2020, the estimated number of people aged >50 years, blind due to untreated cataract is 3,527,189 [19]. In 2018, India's CSR was 5300. India has to increase its annual CSR to 12,000 and maintain it for the next 6 years to clear its backlog in cataract and maintain a backlog-free status. The gap between current and target CSR is huge. It requires a strong policy commitment by the government and a well-coordinated approach under private and public partnerships.

9.4.3 Strategic Planning/ Recommendations

1. Develop strategies to achieve cataract backlog-free India.
2. Reduce Goods and Service Tax (GST) on intraocular lenses (IOLs).
3. Increase the budget allocated to the cataract treatment program.
4. Ensure seamless grant-in-aid.
5. Use strategic information (human resources and infrastructure mapping) for program and policy planning.
6. Develop sustainable approaches for scale-up of low-cost yet high-volume models.

9.5 The World Bank-Assisted Cataract Program in India

Phanindra B. Nukella

9.5.1 Origin/Context

Five national-level eye care surveys have been conducted in India over the past five decades. The results of the first survey (1971–1974) led to the inception of the National Program for Control of Blindness (NPCB) in 1976 [20]. The second survey, 1986–1989, evaluated the impact of this program [21]. This survey reported a cataract backlog of over 22 million blind eyes (or 12 million blind people) [22]. This resulted in India seeking a loan of USD117.8 million (INR 5772 million) from the World Bank in 1994 [22]. The national objectives for the World Bank-assisted project were: upgrade the quality of cataract surgery, expand the coverage of the NPCB to underprivileged areas with particular attention to women, tribal, and isolated, and assist in reducing cataract blindness prevalence by >50% and bilateral blindness incidence by >30% in the participating states.

Seven states which accounted for over 70% of cataract blindness in India were selected for the project. These were Andhra Pradesh (includes current Telangana), Madhya Pradesh (includes current Chhattisgarh), Maharashtra, Orissa (now called Odisha), Rajasthan, Tamil Nadu, and Uttar Pradesh (includes current Uttarakhand). The 7-year project sought to eliminate the backlog of cataract cases by conducting more than 11 million cataract surgeries.

An important project goal was to shift from intracapsular cataract extraction (ICCE) and aphakic correction to technologically advanced extracapsular cataract extraction (ECCE) with intraocular lens (IOL) implantation. A mid-term review in 1997–1998, while recording good program implementation, also extended the project by 1 year to end in June 2002, instead of June 2001.

The project provided 747 operating microscopes, 600 slit lamps, 821 A-scans, 681 keratometers, 178 YAG lasers, and 393 indirect ophthalmoscopes. Under the project, 943 ophthalmologists were trained in modem cataract surgery including 100 trainers, 301 new operating rooms, and 5089 beds for ophthalmic patients were added.

9.5.2 Benefits

1. A cumulative 15.35 million cataract surgeries were performed under the project, against the stated target of 11 million cataract surgeries.
2. There was an increase in ECCE/IOL surgeries up to 91% in 2001, compared to <3% at the start of the project.
3. Technical skill enhancement for ophthalmic surgeons in performing IOL surgeries.
4. Strengthening of infrastructure, including the procurement of appropriate equipment for conducting high-quality cataract surgeries.
5. There was a decline in camp eye surgeries.
6. Increased access for women, tribal, and marginalized people.
7. Strengthened involvement of the private/NGO sector in service delivery and outreach programs.
8. The prevalence of cataract blindness reduced from 1.49% at baseline to 1.1% at the end of the project (a reduction of 26%).

A dramatic, albeit unforeseen outcome, has been the expansion of manufacturing capacity for high-quality ophthalmic materials such as IOLs and suture materials at an affordable cost for surgery; India currently exports these ophthalmic materials to other counties.

9.5.3 Ancillary Benefits

During the program, standards for eye care manuals were developed and distributed; there was a shift to microsurgery and use of IOLs, and provisions were made for non-recurring and recurring grants to participating NGOs. Additionally, there were capacity building, increased advocacy, collaborations with NGOs, and private eye care providers, putting in place a feedback mechanism with the formation of the National Program Management Cell (NPMC).

9.5.4 Constraints

Major impediments to project implementation were human resources management (frequent staff turnover), procurement management (delay and non-standardization), building of facilities (civil work delays), and finance (ease of allocated fund disbursement).

9.5.5 Lessons Learned

The 8-year experience of implementing the project has yielded lessons useful for other health sector projects in India. The project strengthened the national program, NPCB VI, created greater public–private trust and partnership, promoted effective reach to the rural community, and demonstrated the importance of support staff, including paramedics, for the healthcare community.

9.6 Indonesia

Syumarti

Indonesia is a large archipelago with 18,000 islands and 5 time zones. Cataract is the leading cause of blindness in Indonesia (RAAB survey, 2014–2016 conducted in 15 of 34 provinces); the prevalence of blindness in people >50 years of age was 2.8% (1.4–4.4%), the prevalence of severe visual impairment was 2.3%, and the prevalence of moderate visual impairment was 8.9%.

9.6.1 Facilitators

Untreated cataract was the leading cause (77.7%) of avoidable blindness (71.7–95.5%). Cataract was also the leading cause of MSVI. CSC for people with VA < 3/60 in the better eye was

52.7% (29.6–81.3%) [23]. The government health system plays a major role in access to cataract surgery, accounting for around 80% of all cataract surgeries.

The Indonesian Ophthalmologists Association, Perhimpunan Dokter Spesialis Mata Indonesia (PERDAMI) regularly conducts charity programs for cataract surgery with collaborations with Indonesian and/or INGOs. Indonesia has 12 ophthalmologist training centers under the Ministry of Education.

9.6.2 Barriers

The CSR in Indonesia was 2000 in 2018. There is only one report of outcome analysis from the RAAB 2014–2016 (15 provinces). This study reported that the postoperative VA > 6/18 with available correction was in a range of 50.9–68.7% [23]. The government insurance system has included cataract surgery since 2014. However, this has not yielded the desired results because of high indirect cost (mostly related to travel in this large archipelago) and the nearly non-existent referral system from primary to secondary and/or tertiary levels.

9.6.3 Strategic Planning/ Recommendations

The Ministry of Health established the "National Eye Committee" along with the Indonesian Ophthalmology Association (IOA), NGOs, professional organizations, and the International Agency for the Prevention of Blindness (IAPB). The main goal of the National Eye Committee is to create the required support system for prevention of blindness, reduce cataract-related blindness, and establish monitoring and evaluation systems. The committee has charted a roadmap of the visual impairment control program 2017–2030. The IAPB recommends this roadmap as a reference for short- and long-term planning at the regional and national levels. This planning is aligned with the six pillars of the WHO-recommended healthcare system building blocks [24].

9.7 The Maldives

This island country spends the maximum on healthcare in the region. But reaching out to a small population spread over a cluster of islands and atolls has its challenges.

9.7.1 Facilitators

A RAAB survey in 2016 showed that the age–sex standardized prevalence of blindness at 2.0% (95% CI: 1.5–2.6) was relatively higher than the rest of the SEAR countries. Cataract was the leading cause of blindness (51.4%), and uncorrected refractive error was the leading cause of visual impairment (50.9%) [6]. Blindness was more prevalent in older age groups and women. The CSC was 86% in cataract blind eyes and 93.5% in cataract blind persons.

9.7.2 Barriers

Good visual outcome in cataract operated eyes was 67.9% (presenting) and 76.6% (best corrected). Nearly half of the patients operated for cataract (48.1%) had undergone surgery in neighboring countries. Significant barriers for not using eye care services were "not felt need" (29.7%) and "treatment deferred" (33.3%) [6].

9.8 Myanmar

In the RAAB 2018, the prevalence of blindness was 0.58% among people >50 years of age. Cataract was the major cause of blindness accounting for 72.9% of overall blindness; it was also responsible for 9.5% of visual impairment. Other major causes of blindness were glaucoma (11.7%), corneal opacity other than trachoma (2.9%), surgical complications (2.3%), trachoma (1.6%), and diabetic retinopathy (0.9%) [25]. This survey also reported that 70.9% of all cataract surgeries had good outcomes by presenting vision and 82% by best-corrected vision. These numbers varied in different states from 59% (Nay Pyi Taw state) to 90% (Keyn state).

9.8.1 Facilitators

Eye care service is provided by the Ministry of Health and Sports (MoHS) through a tiered system in both rural and urban areas. Five tertiary eye care institutions provide regular cataract services with some sub-specialties. Likewise, secondary eye care services comprising of ambulatory eye care and cataract surgical services are provided by ophthalmologists based in 83 general hospitals. Though integrated into primary healthcare in rural health centers, primary eye care services are limited to some parts of the country. Besides, the MoHS, local NGOs, local charity associations, religious chief monks, and INGOs also provide primary and secondary eye care services.

9.8.2 Barriers

The major barriers for cataract surgery among cataract blind people were: "not felt need" (25.8%), fear of surgery (24.2%), economic reasons (16.2%), unaware of treatment (16.1%), difficulties in accessing the service (9.7%), and longer waiting for surgery in hospital (8.0%). In the mountain region (Chin state), accessibility to service was the major barrier (58.6%) [25].

The overall CSCs among cataract eyes were 61.9%, 49.1%, and 31.5% for visual acuity of 3/60, 6/60, and 6/18, respectively. The highest surgical coverage was in Yangon (87.5%) and lowest in Ayeyarwaddy (43.4%) [25]. The CSR was 2038 surgeries per million population in 2015 [26].

There are 309 ophthalmologists, 32 optometrists, 3 orthoptists, and 150 nurses (73 specially trained) in eye care. But there is an unequal distribution of ophthalmologists; 150 are in Yangon (six million population) and 32 are in Mandalay (three million people). Of the 309 ophthalmologists in Myanmar, 81 are in private practice [27].

The overall prevalence of blindness estimated in 1998 and in 2018 showed that it has remained unchanged at 0.58% [25, 26]. There is a large backlog of cataract causing bilateral blindness and visual impairment. Other emerging or persistent eye care problems are glaucoma, diabetic retinopathy, and corneal lesions.

9.8.3 Strategic Planning/ Recommendations [27]

1. Expansion of cataract surgical services to rural areas.
2. Improvement in cataract surgical outcomes that will result in improved health-seeking behavior of people.
3. Building human resources in cataract surgery and equitable distribution to rural and remote areas.
4. Make mid-level ophthalmic personnel responsible for refraction services and primary eye care.
5. Expansion of refraction and optical dispensing services.
6. Greater awareness and advocacy.
7. Surveillance and quality assurance.
8. Consolidated and unified effort of NGOs, monasteries, and the government towards eye health service delivery.
9. Strengthening of the National Blindness Committee and Task Force.

9.9 Nepal

Blindness and vision impairment are major public health problem in Nepal. In the early 1980s, the prevalence of bilateral blindness was 0.84% among people of all age groups [28]. The burden of blindness reduced by more than half by 2010, with an extrapolated blindness prevalence of 0.35% and low vision of 1.3% in all age groups [29]. In both of these surveys, there was a higher prevalence of blindness in women. Despite a decrease in the prevalence of cataract, it has remained a major cause of blindness and vision impairment in Nepal. However, cataract-induced bilateral blindness has reduced from 72.1% in 1980 to a weighted average of 62.2% in 2010 [29]. In 2010, the prevalence of bilateral cataract blindness with BCVA < 6/60 in people aged >50 years was 3.2% (95% CI: 3.0–3.4%; men: 2.8%; women: 3.5%) It was estimated that around 35,900 people aged >50 years were blind due to cataract (against 87,500 in 1981 survey) [28, 29].

9.9.1 Facilitators

After the first national blindness survey in 1981, two-pronged strategies were developed to control and prevent blindness in Nepal: (1) development of training programs for eye care professionals; and (2) establishment of primary, secondary, and tertiary eye care centers in areas where services were most needed. Substantial support came from international organizations for both these programs.

Multi-disciplined, highly specialized, and trained physicians, nurses, and administrators provide eye care in Nepal using a standardized system engineered for high-volume cataract surgery that enables a large reduction in unit cost. A cross-subsidy for cataract surgery is offered to patients who cannot afford to pay. The surplus gained from patients who can afford to pay is used to provide subsidized costs for those living in remote areas and/or for those who cannot pay for the service.

There are two kinds of eye care services in Nepal, the fixed facilities and the outreach programs. The outreach programs include a team approach with one or two ophthalmologists, a cadre of ophthalmic technicians, and local volunteers, including local NGOs. The surgery is provided at subsidized and affordable cost to people in the community. In these outreach clinics, high-volume cataract surgery is performed by the MSICS technique with highest acceptable quality and outcome [30, 31].

A recent RAAB of Bagmati province (a centrally located province with the capital city, Kathmandu, and other big towns and with a relatively better Human Development Index than other areas in Nepal) showed that cataract accounted for 61.4% of blindness and 67.6% of severe vision impairment. The estimated prevalence of blindness due to cataract among people aged >50 years was estimated to be 0.3% (0.1% in men and 0.4% in women) [32]. The quality of cataract surgery has improved since the 1980s. The two major population-based studies in Nepal reported good outcomes (PVA > 6/18) ranging from 61.4 to 72.4% [33, 34]. The 2019 RAAB study in Bagmati province showed a further improvement in cataract surgery outcome with 79.4% for PVA > 6/18 [32].

In Nepal, IOLs are manufactured with support from the Fred Hollows Foundation. This has significantly reduced the unit cost of IOLs from USD200 to less than USD4. The IOLs manufactured by the Fred Hollows Foundation at the Tilganga Institute of Ophthalmology are low-cost alternatives with similar visual outcomes to the premium lens in the western markets [35]. There has also been a sharp rise in IOL use from 25% in 1994 to 99.5% in 2008 (Fig. 9.4).

Eye hospitals in Nepal have a strong network of community eye centers in the districts and pri-

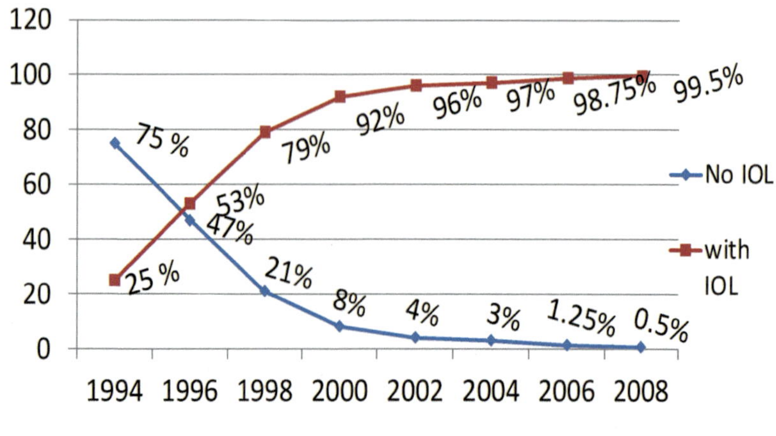

Fig. 9.4 Trends in the use of intraocular lenses (IOLs) in Nepal (Source: Program Department, Tilganga Institute of Ophthalmology)

mary care in more rural areas. These community eye centers serve people in areas who were previously dependent solely on outreach campaigns. In 2018, approximately 150,000 cataract surgeries were performed in Nepal, excluding the surgeries provided to people from neighboring countries; 15% of cataract surgeries were performed in an outreach setting [36].

There has been significant growth of human resources in eye health, from 7 ophthalmologists in the 1980s to more than 308 ophthalmologists in 2017, 470 optometrists in 2018, and 970 allied ophthalmic personnel in 2018 [37]. The Second Long-term Health Plan (1997–2017) and Health Sector Strategy III have stressed the public–private partnerships in the health sector [36]. Eye health service provision has been included in National Health Insurance Schemes.

Consequent to all these measures, the CSC has also increased over the years. In the 2019 Bagmati Province RAAB, the CSC in people aged >50 years was 95.9%, and eCSC was 84% [32]. The CSR of Nepal has seen a manifold increase over the last three decades, to the current estimated 4364 per million population [38].

9.9.2 Barriers

A survey conducted in some select eye hospitals in Nepal found that, on average, a patient had to pay around NPR 2030 (USD1 = NPR 100) for a cataract surgery. The cost range is from NPR 20 for a patient who receives a full subsidy to around NPR 12,000 for a patient who pays in full for the service. Around three quarters (73%) of patients are required to pay out of pocket [39]. Health insurance is not available to all in 77 districts. Eye care NGOs provide most of Nepal's eye care services; these organizations subsidize the treatment cost or provide treatment at no cost to patients who cannot pay for the service.

Eye care in Nepal is considered a model that can be replicated in less developed countries. However, eye care in Nepal is mostly operated by NGOs with minimal governmental participation. The concept of integrating basic eye care at the primary level has just been approved at the national policy level but is not yet implemented.

There is an unequal distribution of the eye health workforce that adversely impacts the eye care services. More ophthalmologists work in provinces # 3 and #1—35.4% of all ophthalmologists work in province # 3, serving 20.8% of the total population, and 20.8% of all ophthalmologists work in province # 1, serving 17.1% of the total population. Only 0.65% of all ophthalmologists are currently working in province # 6, serving 5.9% of the total population. The situation is similar for ophthalmic assistants and optometrists [36].

9.9.3 Strategic Planning/Recommendations

1. Integration of primary eye care centers with the existing primary healthcare system.
2. Use of the latest technologies in eye care.
3. Good coordination at every level to prevent duplication among eye care service providers.
4. Multi-sectoral collaboration of good eye care with education, women and social welfare, drinking water, and sanitation.
5. Information flow in healthcare through scientific research and publications.
6. Low vision and rehabilitation programs in all eye hospitals.
7. Teleophthalmology to connect to remote areas.
8. Surveillance and quality monitoring.

9.10 Sri Lanka

Asela Abeydeera

In Sri Lanka, the eye care services are mostly conducted by the National Eye Hospital and eye units attached to government health institutions. Private sector and charity hospitals play a minor role in eye care service delivery. There are around 50 eye units established within government hospitals. The Colombo National Eye Hospital is the largest eye care institution in the country and has one of the region's busiest out-patient departments. Eighty clinical ophthalmologists serve within the government health system, but one-fourth of them belong to other sub-specialties and are restricted to perform cataract surgeries.

9.10.1 Facilitators

Sri Lanka had conducted a scientific blindness survey in 2014–2015. The prevalence of blindness and low vision was 1.7% and 17%, respectively [40]. The most common cause of blindness was unoperated cataract (66%). Wide variations were observed in different provinces; Uva province (mid-Eastern Sri Lanka) had the highest prevalence of blindness (2.65%).

9.10.2 Barriers

The CSR in Sri Lanka was above 4000 in 2016, and after that, there was a decline. The backlog of unoperated cataracts increased from 1.2 million to a much higher number. Factors contributing to the backlog of cataract are lack of human resources (ophthalmologists, nurses, and optometrists), infrastructure deficiencies including dedicated eye operation theaters, competency of operating eye surgeons, non-operating eye surgeons, unavailability of free IOLs, and restrictions on obtaining IOLs from different sources.

9.10.3 Strategic Planning/Recommendations

1. Re-establishment of a National Eye Care Program within the Ministry of Health for the central coordination of all eye health-related activities.
2. Formation of a donor forum (international and local) to support the eye care activities.
3. Stronger advocacy for eye care.
4. Short-term plans: Provision of free IOLs and consumables to needy patients attending government eye units for cataract operations.
5. Mid-term plans: Improvement of current infrastructure and skill of eye health personnel.
6. Long-term plans: Capacity building for infrastructure and human workforce. Sri Lanka needs 200 ophthalmologists, 400 optometrists, and matching numbers of eye nurses per the 2020 requirement.

9.11 Thailand

Vision impairment was designated as a national health priority, and a primary eye care program was initiated in 1981. A comparison of five national eye surveys conducted in Thailand from 1983 to 2013 (Table 9.4) [41]. Cataract remains as the major cause of blindness in all these surveys. However, the surgical backlog for blinding cataract has continuously decreased from 270,000 in 1983 to 70,071 in 2013 [41].

In RAAB 2013, the age–sex adjusted prevalence of blindness was 0.6% (95% CI: 0.5–0.8), severe visual impairment was 1.3% (95% CI: 1.0–1.6), and moderate visual impairment was 12.6% (95% CI: 10.8–14.5) among people >50 years of age. The prevalence of vision impairment and blindness increased with age. Women had a higher burden of MSVI than men, but there were no gender differences in the burden of blindness [41]. Cataract remained a major cause of overall and avoidable blindness (69.7%)

Table 9.4 Comparisons between five national eye surveys in Thailand [41]

National eye survey	Year	Blindness prevalence %	% Cataract blindness	Cataract surgical backlog
First	1983	1.14	47.3	270,000
Second	1987	0.56	731	220,000
Third	1994	0.31	74.7	134,000
Fourth	2006	0.59	51.6	99,336
Fifth	2013	0.60	69.7	70,071

and vision impairment. Other causes of blindness were refractive errors, including uncorrected aphakia (6.0%), diabetic retinopathy (5.1%), glaucoma (4.0%), corneal opacities (2.0%), and complications after cataract surgery (1%) [41].

9.11.1 Facilitators

The CSC in the study population was 95.1% for the blind, 85.3% for those with severe visual impairment, and 46.6% for those with moderate visual impairment; there was higher coverage in women in each category. The higher coverage across all Thailand regions can be attributed to strong primary eye care. Basic eye care is integrated into the primary healthcare delivery system and the existing national programs. The backlog of blinding cataract (VA < 3/60) was 70,071, but as per the Universal Coverage Scheme (UCS), the cut-off for cataract surgery is 6/36 in Thailand. Hence, the absolute numbers of people needing cataract surgery may be a lot higher [41].

In 2002, the UCS was introduced in Thailand, but cataract surgery was included in the scheme by the National Health Security Office only in 2006. This included an exclusive mobile service for case finding and treatment in remote areas and a grant-in-aid for hospitalized surgery. In 2015, cataract surgical facilities were available in 365 hospitals, and nearly 200,000 cataract surgeries were performed. This figure was twice the number of surgeries in 2005 before the inclusion of cataract surgery in the UCS. A major proportion (76.7%) of the surgeries were conducted at public healthcare facilities.

In 2015, the CSR of the country was 7653 per million population [42]. The higher CSC and CSR indicate that Thailand is on track to achieve the targets set for VISION 2020. To accomplish this and reduce the backlog in cataract surgery, eye care is planned to be integrated into the "Service Plan" wherein the need for referral is minimized by using local expertise and public health volunteers.

9.11.2 Barriers

The triple burden of eye diseases, including the global trend of increased chronic eye diseases, glaucoma, diabetic retinopathy, and age-related macular degeneration, are new challenges to Thailand. It requires political will, commitment, cooperation between various professional bodies, and the use of new technology and techniques to overcome these challenges.

9.12 Timor-Leste

Timor-Leste is the youngest country in the region (it became independent in 1999) and was war-torn and impoverished at its independence.

9.12.1 Facilitators

In June 2000, the Royal Australian College of Surgeons (RACS) set up the East Timor Eye Program (ETEP) to address the substantial burden of ophthalmic trauma and the backlog of cataract blindness. In 2005, the Fred Hollows Foundation, New Zealand, assisted in establishing eye care services in Timor-Leste by training allied ophthalmic personnel and local medical graduates in ophthalmology. (The Fred Hollows Foundation, New Zealand discontinued its activities in Timor-Leste in 2015). In 2012, a dedicated building, the National Eye Centre, was opened at the Hospital Nacional Guido Valadares (HNGV) grounds in Díli, the capital city. Currently, the HNGV is the only place for post-graduate ophthalmology training in Timor-Leste. It offers a Postgraduate Diploma of Ophthalmology (PGDO)—an 18-month program that trains medical graduates to be cataract surgeons. Additional masters-level training, coordinated by the Department in conjunction with the RACS and the ETEP, is offered to successful PGDO graduates in either Nepal or Fiji.

9.12.2 Barriers

The 2016 RAAB, an overall age and gender-adjusted prevalence of blindness in Timor-Leste was 2.8% (in people) and 4.6% (in the eyes). The prevalence of blindness was higher in women (3.1%) than in men (2.4%) [43]. The main cause of blindness was cataract (79.4%), followed by posterior segment disease (6.2%), and glaucoma (5.2%). Most cataract surgeries (91%) were performed in hospital and the remaining in eye camps. The major barriers to uptake of cataract surgery were related to access barrier (45.5%) and lack of attendants (24.8%). CSR was low at 775 per million persons (crude rate) and CSC low at 48.6% for blinding cataracts.

The CSC among blind people (due to cataract) was higher in men (65.8%) than in women (31.3%) [43]. The 2016 RAAB also reported that postoperative vision did not meet the WHO standards [43]. Overall, good visual outcomes of cataract surgery was 62.0% (against the WHO standard of >80%), and good BCVA was achieved in only 75% of the cases (against the WHO standard of >90%). Causes for poor cataract surgery outcomes were long-term complications (52.4%) and complications related to cataract surgery (33.3%) [43]. Although the Ministry of Health in Timor-Leste regularly supplies consumables and drugs, in general, eye care is mostly dependent on INGOs.

9.12.3 Strategic Planning/ Recommendations

1. Cataract must be considered as the number one priority disease in the National Ophthalmic Strategy 2020–2050 (Draft Version 3.2, January 2018) [44]
2. The actions required to improve the CSR must involve training and incentives to ophthalmologists (PGDO graduates) to complete Masters training; build cadres of eye health workers and nurses; train traditional healers to recognize cataracts and refer for surgery.
3. Improve mobile surgery outreach at less accessible areas of the country.
4. Improved advocacy.
5. Build mid-level ophthalmic human resources.

The actions required to improve the quality of cataract surgery are: (1) training of technicians, eye care nurses, and eye care workers in biometry, (2) availability of B-scan at the district level; and (3) better surgical training in newer techniques such as phacoemulsification for ophthalmologists.

Timor-Leste has recently formulated a robust public eye health policy [45]. This is based on the 2016 RAAB survey results.

1. The Ministry of Health has approved the long-term Eye Care Strategy Plan (ECSP). Its main target is to: (a) eliminate avoidable blindness caused by cataract, (b) establish an eye care network in the entire country over the next 30 years, (c) promote academics and research through the Timor-Leste Institute of Ophthalmology, (d) develop sub-specialty services, and (e) introduce the latest technologies in eye care.
2. Continue to conduct outreach; currently, at least one outreach (eye camp) per month per district using the RAAB data to identify dense cataract cluster zones.
3. Training all general practitioners in primary eye care by the National Eye Center team throughout the country, focusing on those blind due to cataract and refractive errors, and refer them for further care.
4. Establish permanent surgery centers in four main referral hospitals in the country starting from 2021. Infrastructure development and human resource training for the expansion of services.

9.13 Current Evidence-Based Treatment Strategy

ICCE was the mainstay of all cataract surgery programs in public health domains till the 1990s in South-East Asia, after which ECCE surgery with posterior chamber intraocular lens implantation (ECCE-PCIOL) became popular [46]. Phacoemulsification, in which an ultrasound

Table 9.5 Costs of various techniques of cataract surgery in some countries in South-East Asia [48, 49, 61, 62]

Country	Author	Year of Publication	ECCE, IOL used	Phaco, IOL used	MSICS, IOL used
India	Gogate et al. [61]	2003	15.82	–	15.68
India	Muralikrishnan et al. [62]	2004	16.25	25.55	17.03
India	Gogate et al. [48]	2007	–	42.10	15.34
Nepal	Ruit et al. [49]	2007	–	70.00	15.00

ECCE extracapsular cataract extraction, *IOL* intraocular lens, *MSICS* manual small incision cataract surgery, *Phaco* phacoemulsification

probe pulverizes the cataract through a 3 mm incision, became the mainstay in the developed world by early 2000 [47]. MSICS, in which the nucleus is removed through a 6 mm scleral tunnel, became popular in the Indian subcontinent. It was proven to be as effective and safe as phacoemulsification [48–50]. Today, phacoemulsification is also performed under injection-free anesthesia for early and predictable visual rehabilitation [51]. In the past few years, femtosecond laser assisted cataract surgery (FLACS) in which the corneal tunnel and capsulorhexis steps of phacoemulsification are performed using a femtosecond laser is in vogue. While many studies did not demonstrate a clear superiority of FLACS over phacoemulsification, it is a significant technological improvement for steps that require experience and skill, like tunnel construction and capsulorhexis [52]. As of now, MSICS forms the mainstay of the most public- and NGO-funded hospitals and in residency training programs in India [53, 54].

Cataract surgery accounts for the majority of all spending in most blindness control programs. This is because cataract surgery is one of the most cost-effective surgical interventions for restoring quality of life [55, 56]. A study from India has estimated that cataract causes a loss of USD4.4 billion annually to the country, and that the cumulative loss over an entire life could be USD22.2 billion. However, the cost of tackling cataract blindness is not more than USD0.15 billion [57]. The World Bank-assisted cataract project provided a significant qualitative and quantitative boost to cataract surgery in India [22].

The cost of surgery includes the direct and indirect cost to the service provider and the patient [58]. Due to high volumes of surgery, reduced overheads, and shared costs, cataract surgery costs are less in eye camps or NGO hospitals [59]. Higher volumes divide the cost of infrastructure, maintenance, and equipment amongst more recipients, and human resources are also more efficiently utilized [60]. Table 9.5 shows the cost calculation for various types of cataract surgeries published over the years in India and Nepal. Surgical techniques that depend on capital-intensive equipment, its maintenance, and numerous disposable consumables are less inexpensive.

Two countries in South-East Asia, India, and Nepal, are known for performing high-volume cataract surgeries. Sometimes this practice is shunned and considered a possible compromise on the quality of care and outcome. However, studies from India have shown that high-volume cataract surgeons show improved visual acuity outcomes, both after phacoemulsification and MSICS procedures [63]. This is important in many developing South-East Asia countries where there is a large backlog of untreated cataracts and there is a need for high-volume cataract surgeons.

Globally, cataract blindness accounts for a substantial proportion of blindness, including all countries in South-East Asia. Apparently, there is a strong correlation between national-level socio-economic development and cataract surgery. An analysis of 266 RAABs across 73 countries that looked for a relationship between the human development index (HDI), gross domestic product (GDP) per capita, CSC, eCSC, and visual outcome of cataract surgeries performed between 2010 and 2015 showed strong associations between HDI with the prevalence of cataract blindness, the proportion of IOL implantations, and the proportion of cases with good postoperative vision [64]. These socioeconomic indicators should be considered as important factors for developing strategies aimed at improving cataract surgery service delivery worldwide.

References

1. The International Agency for the Prevention of Blindness—South East Asia. www.iapb.org/connect/regions/south-east-asia/. Accessed 24 Nov 2020.
2. Das T. Blindness and visual impairment profile and rapid assessment of avoidable blindness in South East Asia: Analysis of new data. 2017 APAO holmes lecture. Asia-Pacific J Ophthalmol. 2018;7:312–5. https://doi.org/10.22608/APO.2017425.
3. Flaxman SR, Bourne RRA, Resnikoff S, et al. Global causes of blindness and distance vision impairment 1990–2020: a systematic review and meta-analysis. Lancet Glob Health. 2017;5:e1221–34. https://doi.org/10.1016/S2214-109X(17)30393-5.
4. Lepcha NT, Sharma IP, Sapkota YD, et al. Changing trends of blindness, visual impairment and cataract surgery in Bhutan: 2009–2018. PLoS One. 2019;14(5):1–13. https://doi.org/10.1371/journal.pone.0216398.
5. Lepcha NT, Chettri CK, Getshen K, Rai BB, Bindiganavale Ramaswamy S, Saibaba S, et al. Rapid assessment of avoidable blindness in Bhutan. Ophthalmic Epidemiol. 2013;20(4):212–9. https://doi.org/10.3109/09286586.2013.794902.
6. Thoufeeq U, Das T, Limburg H, et al. First rapid assessment of avoidable blindness survey in the Maldives: prevalence and causes of blindness and cataract surgery. Asia-Pacific J Ophthalmol. 2017;7(5):316–20. https://doi.org/10.22608/APO.2017332.
7. Wing K, Low G, Sharma M, et al. Building a national eye-care service in post-conflict Timor-Leste. Bull World Health Organ. 2018;96:716–22. https://doi.org/10.2471/BLT.18.212506.
8. Ramke J, Brian G, Naduvilath T, et al. Prevalence and causes of blindness and low vision revisited after 5 years of eye care in timor-leste. Ophthalmic Epidemiol. 2012;19(2):52–7. https://doi.org/10.3109/09286586.2011.645108.
9. Ramke J, Palagyi A, Naduvilath T, et al. Prevalence and causes of blindness and low vision in Timor-Leste. Br J Ophthalmol. 2007;91(9):1117–21. https://doi.org/10.1136/bjo.2006.106559.
10. Foster A. Cataract and "Vision 2020- the right to sight" initiative. Br J Ophthalmol. 2001;85:635–9. https://doi.org/10.1136/bjo.85.6.635.
11. Ramke J, Gilbert CE, Lee AC, et al. Effective cataract surgical coverage: an indicator for measuring quality-of-care in the context of universal health coverage. PLoS One. 2017; https://doi.org/10.1371/journal.pone.0172342.
12. Worldometer. Bangladesh population. 2020. www.worldometers.info/world-population/bangladesh-population/. Accessed 15 Sept 2020.
13. Muhit M, Wadud Z, Islam J, et al. Generating evidence for program planning: rapid assessment of avoidable blindness in Bangladesh. Ophthalmic Epidemiol. 2016;23:176–84. https://doi.org/10.3109/09286586.2016.1155716.
14. Wadud Z, Kuper H, Polack S, et al. Rapid assessment of avoidable blindness and needs assessment of cataract surgical services in Satkhira District, Bangladesh. Br J Ophthalmol. 2006;90:1225–9. https://doi.org/10.1136/bjo.2006.101287.
15. Cambridge Economic Policy Associates Ltd. Strategic evaluation of the vision Bangladesh project. 2014. https://www.sightsavers.org/wp-content/uploads/2017/11/Vision-Bangladesh-Evaluation.pdf. Accessed 30 Nov 2020.
16. United Nations. The millennium development goals report 2012. New York; 2012. https://www.un.org/millenniumgoals/pdf/MDG%20Report%202012.pdf. Accessed 16 Nov 2020.
17. National Statistical Bureau of Bhutan. Population Projections of Bhutan 2005–2030 www.nsb.gov.bt/publication/publications.php?id=2. Accessed 1 Sept 2020.
18. Ministry of Health Royal Government of Bhutan. Annual health bulletin 2020. HMIS and research section, Policy and Planning Division (PPD). 2020. http://www.moh.gov.bt/wp-content/uploads/ict-files/2017/06/health-bulletin-Website_Final.pdf. Accessed 30 Nov 2020.
19. Directorate General of Health Services Government of India. National blindness and visual impairment survey, India, 2015–2020—a summary report. www.dghs.gov.in/content/NationalProgrammeforControlofBlindnessVisual.aspx. Accessed 24 Nov 2020.
20. Mohan M. Collaborative study on blindness (1971–1974): a report. Delhi. 1987.
21. Mohan M. National survey of blindness-India. NPCB-WHO Report. New Delhi. 1989.
22. Jose R, Bachani D. World bank-assisted cataract blindness control project. Indian J Ophthalmol 1995;43:35–43. https://www.ijo.in/text.asp?1995/43/1/35/25277. Accessed 29 Nov 2020.
23. Rini M, Ratnanina N, Halim A, et al. Prevalence and causes of blindness in people age 50 years and above, the intervention category and action required reducing blindness in West Java province. Indonesia. J Ophthalmol Clin Res. 2017;1:1–4. https://doi.org/10.33140/JOCR/01/01/00005.
24. IAPB. Roadmap of visual impairment control program in Indonesia 2017–2030. 2017. https://www.iapb.org/learn/resources/roadmap-of-visual-impairmentcontrol-program-in-indonesia2017-2030/. Accessed 17 Nov 2020.

25. Ministry of Health and Sports, The Republic of Myanmar. Report of rapid assessment of avoidable blindness survey. 2018.
26. Department of Public Health, Ministry of Health and Sports, The Republic of Myanmar. Trachoma control and prevention of blindness program. 2016.
27. Pokharel GP, Khanna R. Prevention of blindness in Myanmar: situation analysis and strategy for change. 2013. https://www.iapb.org/learn/resources/situational-analysis-and-strategy-for-change-in-myanmar/. Accessed 30 Nov 2020.
28. Brilliant LB, Pokhrel RP, Grasset NC, Lepkowski JM, Kolstad A, Hawks W, et al. Epidemiology of blindness in Nepal. Bull World Health Organ 1985;63(2):375–386. https://www.ncbi.nlm.nih.gov/pmc/articles/PMC2536402/. Accessed 25 May 2020.
29. Sapkota YD. Epidemiology of blindness in Nepal. Kathmandu; 2012.
30. Nowak R, Grzybowski A. Outcome of an outreach microsurgical project in rural Nepal. Saudi J Ophthalmol. 2013;27(1):3–9. https://doi.org/10.1016/j.sjopt.2012.09.002.
31. Ruit S, Tabin G, Nissaman S, Paudyal G, Gurung R. Low-cost high-volume extracapsular cataract extraction with posterior chamber intraocular lens implantation in Nepal (abstract). Ophthamology. 1999;106(10):1887–92. https://doi.org/10.1016/S0161-6420(99)90397-4.
32. Gurung R, Thapa SS, Rai N, et al. Rapid assessment of avoidable blindness (RAAB) survey in Bagmati Province of Nepal. Kathmandu; 2020.
33. Kandel RP, Sapkota YD, Sherchan A, Sharma MK, Aghajanian J, Bassett KL. Cataract surgical outcome and predictors of outcome in Lumbini zone and Chitwan district of Nepal. Ophthalmic Epidemiol. 2010;17(5):276–81. https://doi.org/10.3109/09286586.2010.508355.
34. Thapa SS, Berg RVD, Khanal S, Paudyal I, Pandey P, Maharjan N, et al. Prevalence of visual impairment, cataract surgery and awareness of cataract and glaucoma in Bhaktapur district of Nepal: The Bhaktapur Glaucoma Study. BMC Ophthalmol. 2011;11(1) https://doi.org/10.1186/1471-2415-11-2.
35. Constantinou M, Jhanji V, Jing X, Lamoureux EL, Boffa U, Taylor HR, et al. A randomized, single-center study of equivalence of 2 intraocular lenses used in cataract surgery. Ophthalmology. 2013;120(3):482–8.
36. Department of Health Services, Ministry of Health and Population, Government of Nepal. Annual report. 2018.
37. International Agency for the Prevention of Blindness. Vision atlas. Available from: http://atlas.iapb.org/global-action-plan/gap-implementation/. Accessed 9 Nov 2020.
38. Vision 2020 Australia. Universal eye health: a global action plan 2014–2019. Available from: https://www.vision2020australia.org.au/resources/universal-eye-health-a-global-action-plan-2014-2019/. Accessed 30 Nov 2020.
39. Tilganga Institute of Ophthalmology. Baseline study report: effectiveness of eye health care package to increase access to eye health care for women: A pragmatic trial in selected districts of Nepal. 2018.
40. Banagala C, Gilbert C, Murthy GVS, et al. Prevalecnce, causes, magnitude and risk factors of visual impairment and blindness in Sri Lanka. Ceylone Med J. 2018;63(S2):s10–7. https://doi.org/10.4038/cmj.v63i5.8735.
41. Isipradit S, Sirimaharaj M, Charukamnoetkanok P, et al. The first rapid assessment of avoidable blindness (RAAB) in Thailand. PLoS One. 2014;9(12):1–12. https://doi.org/10.1371/journal.pone.0114245.
42. Limwattananon C, Limwattananon S, Tungthong J, et al. Association between a centrally reimbursed fee schedule policy and access to cataract surgery in the universal coverage scheme in Thailand. JAMA Ophthalmol. 2018;136:796–802. https://doi.org/10.1001/jamaophthalmol.2018.1843.
43. Correia M, Das T, Magno J, et al. Prevalence and causes of blindness, visual impairment, and cataract surgery in Timor-Leste. Clin Ophthalmol. 2017;11:2125–31. https://doi.org/10.2147/OPTH.S146901.
44. National Directorate for Diseases Control Ministry of Health Timor-Leste. National ophthalmic strategy 2020 to 2050 draft version 3.2. 2018.
45. Ministry of Health. Action plan arising from the RAAB survey Timor-Leste. 2017.
46. Prajna V, Chandrakanth KS, Kim R, et al. The Madurai intraocular lens study II: clinical outcomes. Am J Ophthalmol. 1998;125:14–25. https://doi.org/10.1016/s0002-9394(99)80230-x.
47. Minassian DC, Rosen P, Dart JKG, et al. Extracapsular cataract extraction compared with small incision surgery by phacoemulsification: a randomized trial. Br J Ophthalmol. 2001;85:822–9. https://doi.org/10.1136/bjo.85.7.822.
48. Gogate P, Deshpande M, Nirmalan PK. Why do phacoemulsification? Manual small-incision cataract surgery is almost as effective, but less expensive. Ophthalmology. 2007;114:965–8. https://doi.org/10.1016/j.ophtha.2006.08.057.
49. Ruit S, Tabin G, Chang D, et al. A prospective randomized clinical trial of phacoemulsification vs manual sutureless small-incision extracapsular cataract surgery in Nepal. Am J Ophthalmol. 2007;143(1):32–8. https://doi.org/10.1016/j.ajo.2006.07.023.
50. Gogate PM, Kulkarni SR, Krishnaiah S, et al. Safety and efficacy of phacoemulsification compared with manual small-incision cataract surgery by a randomized controlled clinical trial: six-week results. Ophthalmology. 2005;112:869–74. https://doi.org/10.1016/j.ophtha.2004.11.055.
51. Fichman RA. Use of topical anesthesia alone in cataract surgery (abstract). J Cataract Refract Surg. 1996;22(5):612–4. https://doi.org/10.1016/s0886-3350(96)80019-8.
52. Day AC, Gore DM, Bunce C, Evans JR. Laser-assisted cataract surgery versus standard ultrasound phaco-

emulsification cataract surgery. Cochrane Database Syst Rev. 2016; https://doi.org/10.1002/14651858.CD010735.pub2.
53. Gogate P, Biswas P, Nataranjan S, et al. Residency evaluation and adherence design study: young ophthalmologists' perception of their residency programs—clinical and surgical skills. Indian J Ophthalmol 2017;65:452–460. https://www.ijo.in/text.asp?2017/65/6/452/208891. Accessed 29 Nov 2020.
54. Biswas P, Gogate PM, Maskati QB, et al. Residency evaluation and adherence design study III: ophthalmology residency training in India: then and now–improving with time? Indian J Ophthalmol 2018; 66:785–792. https://www.ijo.in/text.asp?2018/66/6/785/232822. Accessed 29 Nov 2020.
55. Marseille E. Cost-effectiveness of cataract surgery in a public health eye care programme in Nepal. Bull World Health Organ 1996;74(3):319–324. https://apps.who.int/iris/handle/10665/53988. Accessed 17 Nov 2020.
56. Porter RB. Global initiative: the economic case. Community Eye Heal 1998;11(27):44–45. https://www.ncbi.nlm.nih.gov/pmc/articles/PMC1706060/. Accessed 17 Nov 2020.
57. Shamanna BR, Dandona L, Rao GN. Economic burden of blindness in India. Indian J Ophthalmol 1998; 46:169–172. https://www.ijo.in/text.asp?1998/46/3/169/14954. Accessed 29 Nov 2020.
58. Johnson GJ, Minassian DC, Weale R. The epidemiology of eye disease. Community Eye Health 1999;12(29):10. https://www.ncbi.nlm.nih.gov/pmc/articles/PMC1705990/. Accessed 17 Nov 2020.
59. Singh AJ, Garner P, Floyd K. Cost-effectiveness of public-funded options for cataract surgery in Mysore, India. Lancet. 2000;355(9199):180–4. https://doi.org/10.1016/S0140-6736(99)07430-9.
60. Thulasiraj RD, Sivakumar AK. Cost containment in eye care. Community Eye Heal 2001;14(37):4–6. https://www.cehjournal.org/article/cost-containment-in-eye-care/ Accessed 17 Nov 2020.
61. Gogate PM, Deshpande M, Wormald RP. Is manual small incision cataract surgery affordable in the developing countries? A cost comparison with extracapsular cataract extraction. Br J Ophthalmol. 2003;87:843–6. https://doi.org/10.1136/bjo.87.7.843.
62. Muralikrishnan R, Venkatesh R, Venkatesh Prajna N, et al. Economic cost of cataract surgery procedures in an established eye care centre in Southern India. Ophthalmic Epidemiol. 2005;11:369–80. https://doi.org/10.1080/09286580490888762.
63. Cox JT, Ganesh-Babu BS, Munoz B, et al. Visual acuity outcomes after cataract surgery: high-volume versus low-volume surgeons. Ophthalmology. 2019;126:1480–9. https://doi.org/10.1016/j.ophtha.2019.03.033.
64. Wang W, Yan W, Müller A, He M. A global view on output and outcomes of cataract surgery with national indices of socioeconomic development. Invest Ophthalmol Vis Sci. 2017;58:3669–76. https://doi.org/10.1167/iovs.17-21489.

Refractive Error and School Eye Health

10

Krupa Philip, Prakash Paudel, Jerry Vincent,
Srinivas Marmamula, Timothy Fricke,
and Padmaja Sankaridurg

Key Points

- The prevalence of refractive errors across the South-East Asia Region and the associated burden is substantial. The prevalence of presbyopia is high, with an estimated 20% of the population affected in 2015, and is continuing to rise. There is also evidence of a rising prevalence of myopia that will continue to grow significantly in the coming years.
- The prevalence of uncorrected and under-corrected refractive error across the region is high. Data indicate inequalities in spectacle coverage rate across countries in the region; additionally, the spectacle coverage rate is lesser for near vision impairment, for the rural population, and in older age groups.
- Primary barriers to refractive care in the region are poverty, lack of public awareness of eye health, lack of "felt need," and limited availability of adequate eye care services.
- In addition to directing efforts to increase affordability and availability of eye care and related human resources, strategies should include greater advocacy, systematic school eye health programs, self-screening, or e-tools.
- Newer myopia control strategies are required to reduce the burden of myopia.

Uncorrected refractive error is the largest cause of global vision loss in 2020; 161 million people have distance vision impairment or blindness and 570 million people suffer from near vision impairment. Cataract (100 million people), age-related macular degeneration (8.1 million people), glaucoma (7.8 million people), and diabetic retinopathy (4.4 million people) are other leading causes of vision loss (Fig. 10.1). Uncorrected refractive error in South-East Asia (adjusted from the relevant Global Burden of Disease-defined regions to the World Health Organization (WHO)-defined South-East Asia Region, SEAR)

K. Philip
Brien Holden Vision Institute,
Sydney, NSW, Australia
e-mail: k.philip@bhvi.org

P. Paudel · T. Fricke
Brien Holden Foundation, Sydney, NSW, Australia
e-mail: p.paudel@brienholdenfoundation.org; t.fricke@bhvi.org

J. Vincent
Department of Optometry, Rangsit University,
Bangkok, Thailand

S. Marmamula
Allen Foster Community Eye Health Research Centre, Gullapalli Pratibha Rao International Centre for Advancement of Rural Eye Care, L V Prasad Eye Institute, Hyderabad, Telangana, India
e-mail: sri.marmamula@lvpei.org

P. Sankaridurg (✉)
Brien Holden Vision Institute,
Sydney, NSW, Australia

Department of Optometry and Vision Sciences,
University of New South Wales,
Sydney, NSW, Australia
e-mail: p.sankaridurg@bhvi.org

T. Das, P. D. Nayar (eds.), *South-East Asia Eye Health*,
https://doi.org/10.1007/978-981-16-3787-2_10

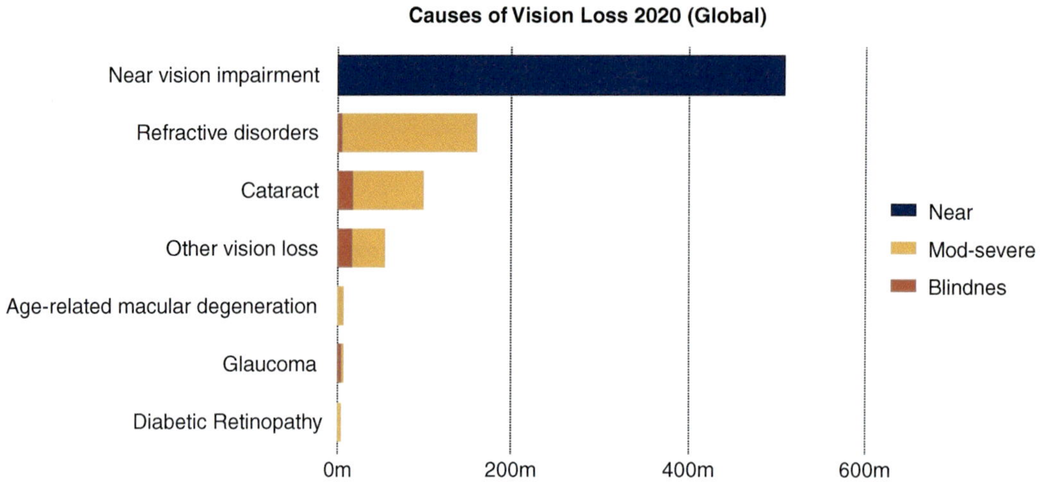

Fig. 10.1 Causes of vision loss (Source: Vision Atlas, 2020)

accounted for 46.1% (95% CI: 42.19–49.51) of moderate to severe vision impairment (MSVI) and 12.6% (95% CI: 10.79–14.33%) of blindness [1]. Given that these data are for adults aged 50 years and above, the relative burden of vision impairment due to uncorrected refractive error is likely to be higher when data on younger adults and children are added.

10.1 Prevalence of Refractive Errors

Refractive errors are common, may result in reduced vision either for distance, near, or both, and are a significant public health issue resulting in substantial health and economic burden. Two important factors in the global burden of refractive error are: (1) the rising prevalence of myopia [2, 3] and (2) vision impairment from uncorrected and under-corrected refractive error.

In the following section, we discuss the prevalence and burden of refractive errors in South-East Asia countries.

10.1.1 Myopia

Myopia is the most frequent refractive error and a leading cause of avoidable blindness and vision impairment. Commonly, the condition is characterized by an excessive increase in axial length of the eye resulting in light rays falling in front of the retinal plane and causing blurred vision for distance. Myopia generally begins in childhood, is progressive, and is associated with an increased risk of potentially sight-threatening complications such as glaucoma, lattice degeneration, retinal detachment, cataract, and myopic macular degeneration in later life. Although both genetic and environmental factors play a role in the development of myopia, both increased near-based activities and lack of outdoor activities have also been identified as significant factors [4].

Evidence indicates that the prevalence of myopia is steadily rising worldwide, and it is estimated that 50% of the world's population could have some degree of myopia by 2050 [2]. Currently, the prevalence and incidence of myopia varies across countries and is already high in many East Asian countries. For example, 80–90 % of young adults in Taiwan are affected [5]. Data on myopia prevalence are limited to a few countries in the South-East Asia region; however, given that the WHO SEAR is home to more than a quarter of the world's population (>2 billion), even at moderate to low prevalence, the impact of vision impairment due to uncorrected/under-corrected myopia and myopia-related complications would be substantial. Furthermore, the economic burden is considerable as a greater proportion of health expenditure in South-East Asia relies on out-of-pocket spending by individuals rather than government-implemented health measures [6].

A recent meta-analysis reported an overall low prevalence of myopia (4.9%, 95% CI: 1.6–8.1, among 5–15 years old) in South-East Asia [7], but there is a marked variation in myopia prevalence in children across countries in the region (Table 10.1) [8–26]. Evidence indicates that the rising prevalence of myopia in South-East Asia is mainly due to increasing urbanization and technology, which focus on near-based activities. For example, in urban North India, myopia prevalence in children increased from 7.4 to 13.1% from 2001 to 2015 and increased further to 21.1% in 2018 [7, 14, 18]. In Nepal, myopia prevalence varied markedly between Tibetan and Sherpa children at 21.7% and 2.9%, respectively, despite a common ancestry and it was attributed to more rigorous schooling in Tibetan children [8]. The prevalence of myopia was low in children at 1.2 % in rural Nepal in the late 1990s, but increased to 3.9% (non-cycloplegic) in 2011 and 6.9% in 2013 [9, 11, 12]. One study from Bangladesh reported a low prevalence of myopia in children. There are no reports from other countries of WHO SEAR.

Myopia prevalence in adults is generally higher than in children (Table 10.2) [27–44]. However, it is acknowledged that the presence of nuclear opacities may confound these figures [40]. A meta-analysis in 2018 reported the pooled prevalence of myopia at 32.9% [95% CI: 25.1–40.7] in adults from urban and rural areas in the South-East Asian region [7].

The limited available data on the myopia prevalence from the SEAR preclude exploration of the underlying risk factors except for the fact that there is a rural–urban difference (higher prevalence in urban areas) and association with years spent in education [45].

The prevalence of high myopia is low (Tables 10.1 and 10.2). In a population-based cross-sectional study from rural central India, high myopia (> −6 D) was present in 0.5% of eyes and myopic retinopathy in 0.17% of 4711 participants [46]. Prevalence of high myopia was also associated with an increased risk of nuclear cataract [47].

10.1.2 Hypermetropia

In hypermetropia, light rays from a distance are focused behind the retinal plane with accommodation at rest; however, clear vision can often be achieved with an accommodative effort. Although a shorter axial length of the eye characterizes the condition, the relation between corneal curvature, lenticular power, and axial length plays an important role in hyperopia [48]. In infants, hyperopia is normal, with up to +3.50 D. There is a significant relation between the decreasing prevalence of hyperopia with increasing age. A meta-analysis of 40 cross-sectional studies and cut-off criteria of children with ≥+2.00 D reported a prevalence of 5% at age 7, 2–3% between ages 9 and 14, and approximately 1% at age 15 [49]. Emmetropization is considered failed if a significant amount of hyperopia continues at the age of 6 years [48].

Low hyperopia does not produce any vision impairment. Past infancy, high hyperopia (>+3.00 D) is associated with a greater risk of visual deficit and/or may lead to strabismus, amblyopia, anisometropia, and astigmatism [50]. In the absence of consensus on the management guidelines, it is agreed that higher hyperopia with vision impairment requires treatment.

The prevalence of hyperopia in children and young adults across the SEAR countries (Tables 10.1 and 10.2) is lower than myopia. Indeed, using cut-off criteria of spherical equivalent ≥+2.00 D, hyperopia prevalence in children aged 5–15 years was reported at 2.2% (95% CI: 1.2–3.3) [7], and may vary across the region, from 0.17% to 7.7%. In the South-East Asia region, Nepal, India, Thailand, Indonesia, and Bangladesh have reported data on hyperopia prevalence; there are no reports or limited information from other countries. In one study, the prevalence of hyperopia (≥+1.00 D) among urban preschool children from Bangladesh, aged

Table 10.1 Prevalence of refractive errors among children

Country	Year	Sample size	Location	Age range (years)	Prevalence %						Authors
							Hyperopia		Astigmatism		
					Myopia	High myopia	≥+0.50	≥+2.00 D	≤−0.50 D	≤−0.75 D	
Nepal [8]	1999	825	Tibet, Sherpa	–	Sherpa: 2.9%, Tibetan: 21.7%	–	–	–	–		Garner et al. (1999)
Nepal [9]	1999	5067	Mechi zone	5–15	1.2%	–	–	1.4%	–	3.50%	Pokharel et al. (2000)
Nepal [10]	2010	440	Sunsari district	7–15	Urban: 15.5%, Rural: 8.2%, Overall: 11.8%	–	Urban: 6.4%, Rural: 5.9%, Overall: 6.1%	–	–	Urban: 1.8%, Rural: 1.8%, Overall: 1.8%	Pokharel et al. (2010)
Nepal [11]	2003	2000	Kathmandu	5–16	6.85%	–	1.40%	0.5%	–	0.65%	Adhikari et al. (2013)
Nepal [12]	2009	1150	Jhapa, Mechi zone	5–16	3.9%	0.6%	-	1.70%	–	3%	Shrestha et al. (2011)
India [13]	1997	4029	Hyderabad	3–18	8.6%	–	22.6%	–	–	10.3%	Kalikivayi et al. (1997)
India [14]	2001	6447	New Delhi	5–15	7.4%	–	–	7.70%	–	10.19%	Murthy et al. (2002)
India [15]	2000	2859	Hyderabad	≤15	3.19%	–	62.62%	–	–		Dandona et al. (2002)
India [16]	~2008	3214	Hyderabad	7–15	Urban: 51.4%, Rural: 16.7%	–	–	Urban: 3.3%, Rural: 3.1%	–		Uzma et al. (2009)
India [17]	2004–2005	12,422	Maharashtra	5–15	Urban: 3.16%, Rural: 1.45%	–	–	Urban: 1.06%, Rural: 0.39%	–	Urban: 0.16%, Rural: 0.21%	Padhye et al. (2009)
India [18]	2014	9884	Delhi	5–15	13.1%	1.5%	–	–	–		Saxena et al. (2015)
India [19]	2012	1378	Bangalore	7–15	4.40%	–	–	1.03%	–	1.60%	Pavithra et al. (2013)
India [20]	2016	5990	Odisha	5–15	4.9%	–	–	0.2%	–	5.4%	Panda et al. (2020)
India [21]	2000–2001	4074	Mahabubnagar	7–15	5.60%	0.27%	–	0.68%	–	6.30%	Dandona et al. (2002)

Indonesia [22]	2015	410	Yogyakarta	10–12	Urban: 53.16%, Rural: 20.41%, Overall: 32.7%	–	0.73%	0.24%	–		Mahayana (2017)
Indonesia [23]	2015	435	Java	11–15	34.71%	None	None	None	–	1.3%	Nikmah et al. (2016)
Thailand [24]	2006	1202	Entire country	<10	27.54%	–	≥+1.00D: 6.41%	>+3.00D: 0.17%	–		Jenchitr and Raiyawa (2012)
Thailand [24]	2006	2097	Entire country	10–20	37.96%	–	≥+1.00D: 3.20%	>+3.00D: 0.29%	–		Jenchitr and Raiyawa (2012)
Thailand [25]	2008–2009	2340	Bangkok, Nakhonpathom	6–12	11.1%	–	–	1.40%	–	0.30%	Yingyong (2010)
Bangladesh [26]	2015	900	Chittagong	4–6	4.00%	–	>+1.00 D: 2.80%	–	–	0.70%	Uddin et al. (2016)

Table 10.2 Prevalence of refractive errors among adults

					Prevalence (%)							
							Hyperopia		Astigmatism			
Country	Year	Sample	Location	Age range (years)	Myopia	High myopia	≥+0.50 D	≥+2.00 D	≤−0.50 D	≤−0.75 D	Presbyopia	Authors
India [27]	–	1414	Tamil Nadu	>40	19.40%	–	39.70%	–	–		–	Rani (2010)
India [28]	2001–2004	7774	Chennai	>39	Urban—16.8%, Rural—27%	Urban—1.6%, Rural—3.7%	Urban—52.3%, Rural—18.7%	–	Urban—53.0%, Rural—54.8%	–	–	Prema et al. (2008)
India [29]	1996–2000	3642	Andhra Pradesh	40–92	36.50%	4.80%	18.40%	–	–	38.20%	–	Krishnaiah et al. (2009)
India [30]	–	2472	Maharashtra	> 30	17.00%	0.40%	18.00%		–		–	Nangia et al. (2010)
India [31]	2001–2003	2508	Chennai	>39	26.99%	3.71%	18.70%	–	–		–	Raju et al. (2004)
India [32]	–	1722	–	>15	<−0.75 D 19.39%	–	>+1.00 D 9.83%	–	–	12.94%	–	Dandona et al. (1999)
Bangladesh [33]	–	11624	–	>30	22.10%	1.80%	20.60%	–	–	32.40%	–	Bourne et al. (2004)
Bangladesh [34]	2010–2012	3050	Sirajganj	15–49	39%	–	55%	–	–	6.8%	62%	Muhit et al. (2018)
Myanmar [35]	–	2076	Meiktila district	≥40	42.70%	6.50%	15%	–	–	30.60%	–	Gupta et al. (2008)
Indonesia [36]	–	1043	Sumatra	≥ 21	26.10%	–	9.20%	–	–	18.50%	–	Saw et al. (2002)
India [37]	1996–2000	5587	Andhra Pradesh	>30	–	–	–	–	–		69.9%	Nirmalan et al. (2006)
India [38]	–	Meta-analysis	South India	>30	27.7%	–	22.9%	–	–		33%	Sheeladevi et al. (2019)
India [39]	–	2848	Andhra Pradesh	≥40	–	–	–	–	–		35.1%	Marmamula et al. (2013)

India [40]	–	3267	Pondicherry, Tamil Nadu	≥40	39.6%	–	30.3%	SE ≥ +1 D −17.0%	–	32.6%	–	Joseph et al. (2018)
Indonesia [41]	2009–2010	858	Jakarta	≥35	25.1%	–	16.6%	–	–	30.3%	66.4%	Ehrlich et al. (2013)
Nepal [42]		2165	Kaski district	>35	–	–	–	–	–		66.1%	Sapkota et al. (2012)
Timor-Leste [43]	2005	1414	–	≥40	–	–	–	–	–		43.7 %	Ramke et al. (2007)
Nepal [44]	2016	101	Hospital based Nepal	Mean age: 34.4 ± 15.1	55.4%	–	20.8%	–	–		27.7%	Kandel et al. (2018)

4–6 years, was 2.8% [26]; in another study on children <15 years of age, the prevalence was 3.24% [51]. In SEAR, the estimated pooled prevalence of hyperopia (≥+0.50 D) by meta-analysis is 28% (23.4–32.7%) [7]. A study in rural India has reported a higher prevalence of hyperopia in adult females, hypothesized to relate to a shorter axial length of female eyes in India. Some studies have associated diabetes with hyperopia [31, 40].

Unlike myopia, there is no urban–rural divide or life-style related factors associated with the occurrence of hypermetropia.

10.1.3 Astigmatism

Astigmatism results from unequal curvatures of the two principal meridians of either the anterior/posterior corneal surfaces or lenticular surface and/or as a result of tilt or decentration of the crystalline lens. In most cases, the condition occurs mainly due to cornea. It is established that infants generally have a high prevalence of "against-the-rule" astigmatism that gradually reduces and changes to "with-the-rule astigmatism" by approximately 4–5 years of age [52]; after that, the condition usually remains relatively stable until late adulthood, when there may be a change toward "against-the-rule" astigmatism again. Evaluation of both magnitude and type of astigmatism are necessary to estimate the prevalence of astigmatism that may impair vision. Only a few studies have systematically addressed the prevalence of astigmatism in the South-East Asian region.

A cut-off criterion for astigmatism at ≤−0.50 D is commonly used to define astigmatism. Using this criterion, the reported global prevalence was 9.8% (95% CI: 6.3–13.2) in children and 44.8% (95% CI: 36.6–53.1) in adults [7, 14]. It was 3.5% in children in Nepal [9], 0.3% in children in Thailand [25], 0.7% in children in Bangladesh [26], and ranged from 0.2 to 10.2% in children in India [14, 17, 32]. There are no data from other SEAR countries.

10.1.4 Presbyopia

Presbyopia, an age-related refractive condition, occurs due to a gradual loss of the crystalline lens's ability to change its optical power, thereby rendering the human eye unable to focus clearly on near vision targets. The inability to see N6 or N8 (*N* = Times New Roman font and the number denotes the point size in print) at either 40 cm or preferred distance is considered the threshold for near vision impairment [3]. It has been estimated that globally, in 2015, there were approximately 1.8 billion (95% CI, 1.7–2.0 billion) people living with functional presbyopia, and 826 million (95% CI: 686–960 million people) of them with near visual impairment because of inadequate or no vision correction (Fig. 10.2) [3]. Prevalence of presbyopia in the South-East Asian region was estimated at 20% (~125 million people) in 2015, of which 60% (~75 million people) are either under-corrected or uncorrected (Table 10.2) [3]. The prevalence of presbyopia in the region ranges from 27.7 to 70.0%.

One study reported the prevalence of uncorrected presbyopia in south India at 33% (95% CR: 19.1–51.0) [38]. Yet, another study from rural south India reported an unwillingness to wear presbyopia correction despite facing difficulties in near work [53]. There is evidence of increased productivity and economic gain by correcting presbyopia among Indian tea plantation workers [54]. There are no data on the prevalence of presbyopia from many countries in SEAR—Bhutan, DPR Korea, Indonesia, Myanmar, Sri Lanka, Thailand, and Timor-Leste.

10.2 Barriers to Managing the Burden

10.2.1 Spectacle Coverage

The "spectacle coverage rate" indicates the number of people with corrected vision using spectacles for either distance and/or near vision impairment (met need) compared to the total need for spectacles in a specific population.

Limited data are available on the spectacle coverage for most countries worldwide, and where available, the reported data are not directly comparable due to varying definitions used to categorize refractive error and related vision impairment [55]. There is no internationally

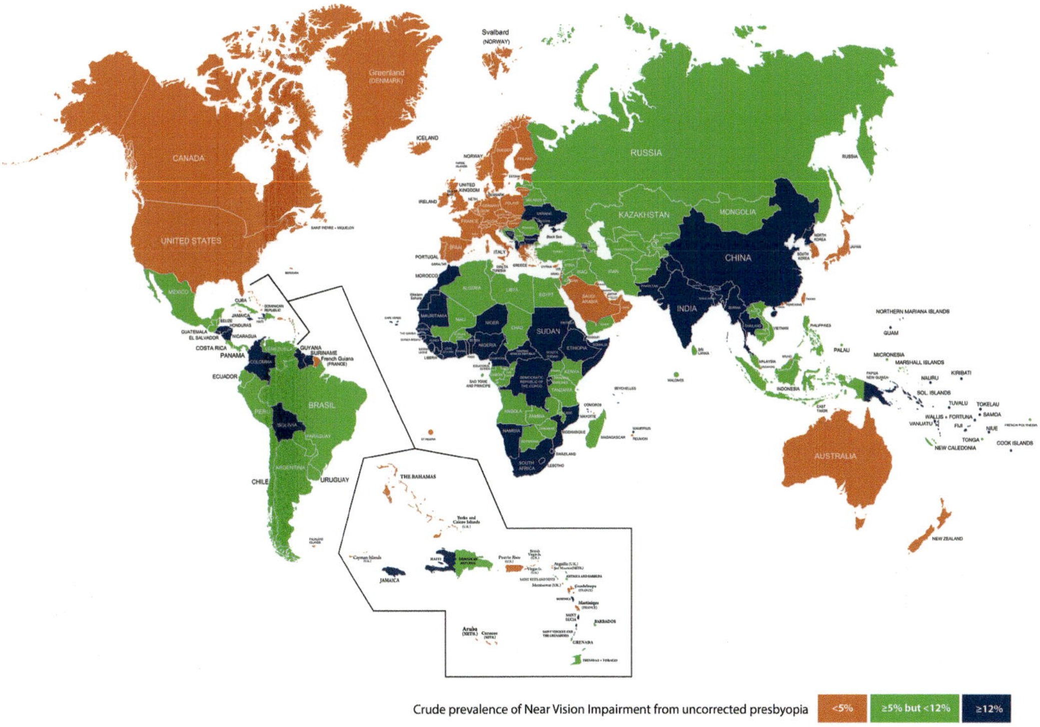

Fig. 10.2 The global prevalence of vision impairment from uncorrected presbyopia [3]

accepted definition/threshold/cut-off criteria for distance and near vision that meets the criteria for spectacle need. The proposed cut-off at 6/12 applies only to distance vision impairment; it is defined as follows [56]:

$$\frac{\text{Met Need}}{\text{Met need} + \text{Under-met need} + \text{Unmet need}}$$

where in a person's better eye has:

1. *Met need* = Presenting/habitual visual acuity (VA) of 6/12 or better, but with uncorrected VA worse than 6/12.
2. *Under-met need* = Presenting/habitual VA better than uncorrected VA, but worse than 6/12, improving to 6/12 or better with pinhole (pinhole VA) or new refraction (best-corrected VA).
3. *Unmet need* = Presenting/habitual VA is the same as uncorrected VA and is worse than 6/12 but can improve to 6/12 or to that of the better eye with pinhole [57].

A systematic review and meta-analysis of 37 studies from 36 countries (combined sample size, 174,736 participants) found that older people in the rural areas of the least developed countries carry the greatest burden of visual impairment from uncorrected refractive error [57]. The potential productivity loss from vision impairment associated with uncorrected myopia, globally, is estimated at USD244 billion, and productivity loss from blindness associated with myopic macular degeneration is estimated at USD6 billion. Productivity loss significantly affects individuals in the age group of 25–29 years. The productivity loss due to myopia in South-East Asia is estimated at USD35 billion [56]. In LMICs (low- and middle-income countries), the rate of presbyopia could be as low as 10% [58].

These data indicate a suboptimal spectacle coverage despite a greater need for spectacles. It is also anticipated that a significant portion of the population does not wear spectacles for mild vision impairment. The discrepancy may relate to service availability, affordability, and compliance. One study from India has shown increased usage of spectacles when services are available in the community [59].

In 2017, the International Agency for the Prevention of Blindness (IAPB) investigated (from RAAB (rapid assessment of avoidable blindness) repository data for the population (>50 years) spectacle coverage for distance vision correction from 27 countries (about 4.4% of the world's population) and near vision correction from 17 countries [55]. These data included two countries from the South-East Asia region—the Maldives and Nepal. In these countries, the usage of spectacles corrections for distance and near vision were 77.6% and 63.6%, respectively, in the Maldives, and 51.8% and 45%, respectively, in Nepal. In the past 10 years, RAAB studies have been completed in 8 of the 11 South-East Asian countries (Bangladesh, Bhutan, India, Indonesia, the Maldives, Sri Lanka, Thailand, and Timor-Leste); the results of these studies have shown that refractive error was the principal cause of moderate vision impairment in 4 countries (Bangladesh, India, the Maldives, and Sri Lanka) [60], but these studies did not report spectacle coverage.

Since published data on spectacle coverage are scarce and limited for the SEAR countries, we calculated the prevalence of myopia (distance vision) and presbyopia (near vision) using the Brien Holden Vision Institute (BHVI) data sets that underpin the global estimates of these conditions [2, 3, 61]. The coverage was calculated for three age ranges (<15 years, 15–49 years, and >50 years). According to the BHVI model, spectacle coverage was: (1) lower for near vision compared to distance vision impairment; (2) lower in rural than in urban areas; (3) lower in older age groups than in younger age groups for distance visual impairment; and (4) lower in Bangladesh, Myanmar, Nepal, and Timor-Leste (Table 10.3).

Similar to BHVI data, earlier studies from the South-East Asian region had reported low spectacle coverage and high unmet needs for refractive error correction. For example, there was only 25–35% spectacle coverage among the population of >40 years in India [59, 62, 63]; 33.3% (95% CI: 30.0–36.7) coverage in rural North India [34]; 52.9% coverage in urban Tamil Nadu, and 17.6% in rural Tamil Nadu [28]. Among school children in North India, spectacle coverage improved from 29.3 to 58.8% after subsidizing the cost of spectacles [64]. Spectacle coverage was only 17.7% in Sri Lanka (BHVI model reported a higher coverage though) for distance vision impairment among individuals aged >40 years [65]. In Bangladesh, the RARE (rapid assessment of refractive errors) study reported spectacle coverage for refractive errors and presbyopia in 15–49 years age group at 13.3% and 3.2%, respectively [34, 42]. In early 2000, the spectacle coverage in the Bangladeshi population of age >30 years was 25.2% (cut-off vision 6/12) [66]. In Timor-Leste, refractive error and presbyopia correction coverage were 15.7% and 26.2%, respectively, among people >40 years [43]. In the Kaski district, Nepal, over 90% of the population >35 years of age with near visual impairment did not have a pair of spectacles [42].

10.2.2 Spectacle Compliance

Spectacle compliance is defined as the regular use of spectacles prescribed for refractive errors and assessed either by interviewing (children or parents) or observing children in schools at an unannounced visit. Both wearing spectacles or having it in the bag during interviews are both considered compliant to spectacle wear. Spectacle compliance identifies the factors that hinder the wearing of spectacles as required. For example, a child prescribed with and wearing spectacles following a school screening may have discontinued wear due to progression of refractive error. The reported reasons for non-compliance, identified in three systematic reviews, were: broken/lost spectacles, forgetfulness, parental disapproval, headaches, teasing by peers, dislike for spectacles, use only when required, unclear vision, unattractive frames/poor appearance, fear of injuries, unaffordability, uncomfortable spectacles, and negative attitude of society to spectacles usage [67–69]. Overall, the spectacle compliance collated from 20 studies (mostly from Asia) was low at 40.14%

Table 10.3 Spectacle coverage (weightage rates) for distance vision and near vision based on BHVI (Brien Holden Vision Institute) myopia and presbyopia model

	5–14 years		15–49 years		35–49 years		50+ years			
	Distance		Distance		Near		Distance		Near vision[a]	
Country	Urban (%)	Rural (%)	Urban (%)	Rural (%)	Urban (%)	Rural (%)	Urban (%)	Rural (%)	Urban (%)	Rural (%)
Bangladesh	51.1	29.5	51.1	29.5	32.0	20.4	39.7	22.9	33.1	25.5
Bhutan	59.0	37.7	59.0	37.7	33.6	21.7	45.4	29.0	35.6	27.4
India	59.8	38.6	59.8	38.6	35.9	23.6	46.0	29.7	38.5	29.6
Nepal	53.8	29.0	53.8	29.0	28.9	18.2	28.0	15.0	29.8	22.9
Sri Lanka	93.8	86.7	93.8	86.7	46.1	52.7	72.3	65.7	52.0	52.0
Thailand	86.0	76.0	86.0	76.0	46.5	53.2	66.6	57.8	52.5	52.5
Timor-Leste	56.6	35.1	56.6	35.1	33.8	23.9	43.8	26.7	38.7	29.8
Maldives	81.7	68.7	81.7	68.7	51.8	66.1	64.7	53.5	65.3	65.3
Myanmar	50.6	26.3	50.6	26.3	22.5	14.3	29.4	14.6	22.7	17.5
Indonesia	76.7	60.8	76.7	60.8	39.8	30.7	61.1	47.7	48.8	37.5
DRP Korea	86.4	76.6	86.4	76.6	46.0	51.8	68.3	59.6	51.2	51.2

[a]In personal communication with the IAPB country chair in Thailand, people of older age usually purchase ready-made reading glasses for near activities. Therefore, the spectacle coverage for near vision should be higher in the 50+ population. However, when they are asked about whether they have spectacles for near vision, most answers were "no" as they are relating to prescribed spectacles

(95% CI: 32.78–47.50) and varied from 9.84% (95% CI: 2.36–17.31) to 78.57% (95% CI: 68.96–88.18) [67]. The common causes for non-compliance were personal factors (25.8%) and breakage/loss/forgetfulness (23.3%).

Table 10.4 [19, 70–77] summarizes spectacle compliance rates from countries in the South-East Asian region; most of these studies are from children in India and show low to moderate compliance. These studies have also identified the barriers to spectacle usage and their remedies. While loss and breakage of devices and affordability can be managed with better investment in resources, factors such as peer influence and negative attitudes require education on vision impairment and eye health.

10.2.3 Barriers to Refraction Care and Services

Access to refractive correction and eye care at the individual or community level may be impeded due to various factors. These specific barriers may vary between places and communities, and even across individuals within a community. These include lack of awareness, local geographic factors, perceived need or lack of it, quality of care, perceptions of care, fear (of the care process, or that glasses could weaken eyes), cosmesis/perceived cosmesis of glasses, economics (including the cost of care, cost of time off work to access care, transport to care), social acceptance, and fatalism (accepting vision loss as unavoidable) [78].

There are limited data on barriers to refractive services in SEAR. Studies from rural Andhra Pradesh, India, and north India, examining individuals aged 15–49 years, reported two main barriers to the uptake of refractive correction services—poverty and/or a lack of "felt need" [79, 80].

10.3 Provision of Care for Refractive Errors

Managing the extensive scale of vision impairment resulting from uncorrected refractive error and refractive error-related complications requires expansion, improvement, and/or innovations in all aspects of refractive care—prevention, improved awareness, human resource development, infrastructure, service delivery, and supply chain management. Traditionally, emphasis and attention has mainly been focused on refractive services and service delivery; however, improvements are not sustainable without the other components of the health system, such as governance and leadership; human resource; finance; health information systems; technology and goods; and health service delivery [81]. The following section reviews some of these components.

10.3.1 Governance and Leadership

Governance includes licensure and regulation of personnel to conduct refraction and/or dispense prescription spectacles, contact lenses, and other optical devices. Professional optometry and ophthalmology societies may also play a part in licensure and will often provide leadership and input on shaping laws and policies related to eye care. Additionally, professional societies, academic institutes, and non-governmental organizations often work in partnership with the government to help shape and develop national eye plans.

In South-East Asia, national eye health plans have been made in all countries except Bhutan and Nepal (at the time of writing, Nepal is developing a national eye health plan) (Table 10.5) [82–90]. The burden of refractive error is acknowledged in all of these national plans, but the urgency of prioritization and the inclusion of specific targets or indicators for refractive error vary significantly between these plans.

10.3.2 Human Resource

Simple refractive error management falls under the primary eye care domain with the key deliverables of addressing the burden, including refraction and dispensing of optical devices, mainly spectacles. In the South-East Asian region,

Table 10.4 Spectacle compliance from South-East Asia

Authors	Country	Age (years)	Year	Study design	Compliance measure	Type of prescription	Duration of follow-up (months)	Sample size	Compliant (%)
Narayanan et al. [70]	India	13–17	2017	Cross-sectional (Qualitative)	Questionnaire/Interview based	No specific type	–	32	–
Bhatt NK et al. [71]	India	6–15	2017	Cross-sectional	Wearing spectacles on a surprise visit	No specific type	3	200	78 (39.0)
Kumar et al. [72]	India	6–17	2017	Cross-sectional	Wearing spectacles on a surprise visit	Children with visual acuity <6/9	6	82	52 (63.4)
Bhandari et al. [73]	Nepal	5–16	2016	Cross-sectional	Wearing spectacles on surprise visit or in bag	No specific type	No follow-up	170	48 (28.2)
Sumana et al. [74]	India	9–16	2015	Cross-sectional	Wearing spectacles on a surprise visit	No specific type	6	362	139 (38.4)
Pavithra et al. [19]	India	7–15	2014	Cross-sectional	Wearing spectacles on a surprise visit	Myopia SE ≥−0.5 D, hypermetropia SE ≥+1.00 D, and astigmatism ≥1.00 D	3	83	48 (57.8)
Gogate et al. [75]	India	8–16	2014	Cross-sectional	Wearing spectacles on surprise visit followed by an interview	Myopia ≥−0.50D or hyperopia ≥+1.00D	6–12	1018	300 (29.4)
Khandekar et al. [76]	India	School going	2008	Cross-sectional	Questionnaire/Interview based	Myopia (>−0.75 D spherical, unilateral, or bilateral)	3–4	70	55 (78.5)
Morjaria et al. [77]	India	11–15	2017	Cross-sectional	Wearing spectacles or had them at school Unannounced observation	Children's vision screening at the 6/9 level in each eye	3–4	Ready-made arm: 232 Custom-made arm: 228	Ready-made arm: 75.5% Custom-made arm: 73.6%

Table 10.5 Selected indicators for eye and refractive services in South-East Asia by country

Country (population)	GDP per capita	Per capita government health spending	Eye service budget[a]	National eye plan (NEP)	Refractive error (RE) in NEP[b]	Vision screening in NEP[b]	Human resources for handling refractive errors in NEP[b]
Bangladesh (161,356,000)	$1855	$36.28	$2,000,000	2014–2020	2	1	2
Bhutan (754,000)	$3243	$96.80	$200,000	–	–	2	–
India (1,353,000,000)	$2104	$69.29	$58,000,000	Yes	Yes	–	–
Indonesia (267,663,000)	$4135	$114.97	$5,000,000	2017–2030	1	2	No
Maldives (516,000)	$10,790	$1006.94	–	2010–2020	2	1	No
Myanmar (53,708,000)	$1407	$58.04	$8,409,000	2018–2030	1	–	–
Nepal (28,088,000)	$1071	$47.92	$1,000,000	–	–	–	–
North Korea (25,550,000)	–	–	–	2010–2015	1	–	–
Sri Lanka (21,670,000)	$3853	$159.48	$9,132,000	2013–2017	1	2	–
Thailand (69,429,000)	$7868	$247.04	–	Yes	1	1	1

Population data (2018), GDP: Gross Domestic Product (2017), and health spending data (2017) from World Bank
[a]2010 data in US Dollars [91, 92] except for Bangladesh (2017) [27, 92] Bhutan (2018) [57, 84] and Timor-Leste (2017) [55, 82]
[b]1 = included in plan without targets or indicators; 2 = included in plan with specific targets or indicators

refraction services are provided at the primary eye care level staffed typically by allied ophthalmic personnel (AOP). The AOP cadre includes eye care personnel such as ophthalmic assistants, ophthalmic technicians, and ophthalmic nurses. Optometrists are considered independent eye care personnel and provide primary eye care predominantly in the private sector in this region. Complications related to refractive errors, such as myopic retinopathy, are managed by ophthalmologists and are delivered mostly at tertiary eye care facilities.

Well-trained human resources for refraction services in adequate numbers with equitable geographical distribution are prerequisites to providing high-quality primary eye care. Globally, in 2007, there were 167,000 full-time clinical refractionists dealing with vision impairments caused by uncorrected refractive error [93]. According to BHVI's current data sets, eye care practitioners are inadequate in most countries in Africa, Latin America, and South-East Asia (Fig. 10.3). This is a challenge for refraction services, particularly in rural and far-flung areas in the SEAR. It is estimated that by 2030, the South-East Asian region would need an eye care infrastructure of a minimum of 429,802 community, 43,374 primary, 4334 secondary, and 434 tertiary care facilities (with the most numbers needed in India); and a minimum workforce of 429,802 community workers, 164,784 AOPs, and 14,744 ophthalmologists (70.5% comprehensive ophthalmologists) [94].

In the public health system, refraction services are provided by AOPs in primary health centers, but these numbers are often inadequate. Independent optometrists and non-governmental organizations also support primary eye care, including refraction service, but this support is still inadequate to meet the growing need in this

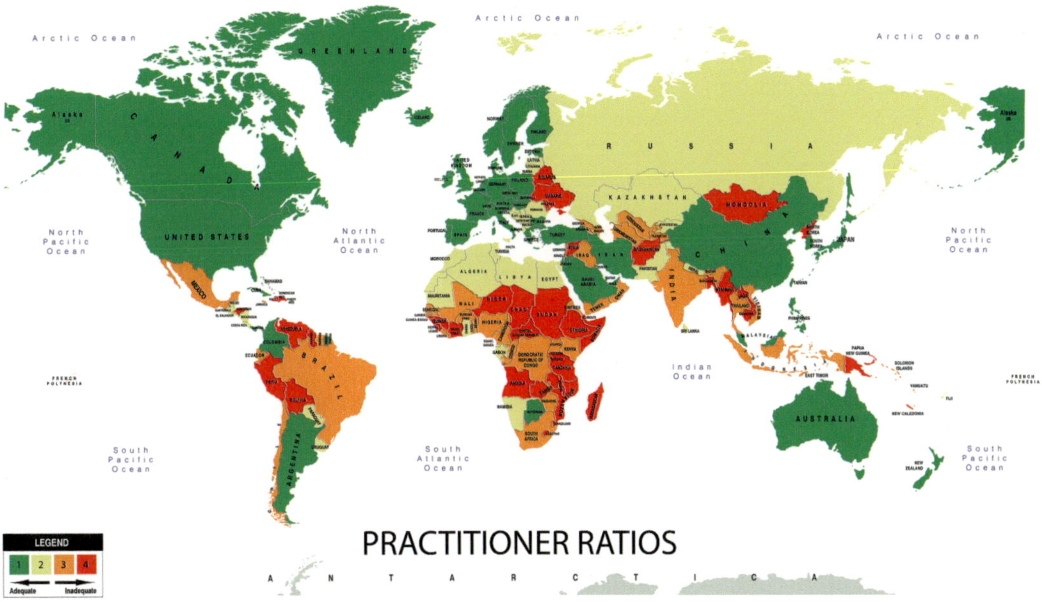

Fig. 10.3 Global eyecare practitioner ratios [94]

region [95]. The governments of India, Bangladesh, Nepal, and Sri Lanka recognize AOPs and optometrists as essential eye care providers, though the nomenclature for these workers varies, adding to the complexity of the system. Nepal has more structured primary eye care and ophthalmic assistants provide most of the refraction services [95].

In addition to the specifically trained workforce in eye health, the grassroots-level personnel involved in primary healthcare at the community level in the South-East Asian region can be trained to conduct preliminary eye screenings and referrals for refraction or other services [96]. For example, the basic eye screening test (BEST) has been implemented very effectively in the south Indian state of Telangana, using the ASHA (accredited social health activist) workforce and a simple test protocol. BEST is one of the largest universal eye health initiatives with a focus on cataracts, uncorrected refractive errors, and presbyopia with 15 million people screened, and 0.5 million spectacles dispensed in 6–8 months; this model is now being replicated in the state of Andhra Pradesh, India (Table 10.6).

10.3.3 Finance

The per capita spending on health in South-East Asia varies from USD36 in Bangladesh to over USD1000 in the Maldives (Table 10.5). National eye care budgets vary greatly and are not always available. International non-government organizations (INGOs) make significant contributions to eye care in some countries. In 2000, there was no indigenous eye care system in Timor-Leste, and eye services were entirely dependent upon INGO funding and personnel. As the national capacity was built, the Ministry of Health has assumed increasing responsibility for funding and providing eye services [97]. In Bangladesh, the combined budget of the INGOs in 2014 was about 10 times higher than the government's eye health budget [86]. Government eye care services are provided at no cost to patients in Bhutan, Myanmar, Sri Lanka, and Timor-Leste; these services are highly subsidized in Thailand and are available with government-provided insurance in the Maldives [83]. However, free government eye services do not always include refraction correction or spectacles. Private sector optical shops

Table 10.6 Human resources for eye health in South-East Asia[a]

S. No.	Country	Population	HR Cadre	Number	Ratio per million	Comments
1	Bangladesh	260,000,000	Ophthalmologist	1100	4	–
			Optometrist	200	0.7	–
			AOP	1000	4	–
2	Bhutan	750,000	Ophthalmologist	8	10	–
			Optometrist	4	5	–
			AOP	54	72	–
3	India	1,200,000,000	Ophthalmologist	20,000	16	–
			Optometrist	9000	7	–
			AOP	40,000	33	–
4	Nepal	30,000,000	Ophthalmologist	308	10	–
			Optometrist	470	15	–
			AOP	950	31	–
5	Pakistan	200,000,000	Ophthalmologist	2590	13	–
			Optometrist	1605	8	–
			AOP	2156	11	–
6	Maldives	350,000	Ophthalmologist	10	28	(8 are expatriates)
			Optometrist	10	28	(All are expatriates)
7	Sri Lanka	21,000,000	Ophthalmologist	195	9	–

[a]Adapted from Sapkota YD. Human Resources for eye health in South Asia. Community Eye Health. 2018; 31 (102): S1–S2

currently bridge this gap, but at a cost that could be a barrier to many people.

10.3.4 Provision of Eye Care for Refractive Errors

10.3.4.1 Eye Care Service Delivery Models

The government is the main provider of eye care in Bhutan, DPR Korea, and the Maldives; the governments provide nearly 95% of all required eye care in Sri Lanka and Timor-Leste [82]. There is a strong INGO presence in Bangladesh, India, Indonesia, Nepal, Myanmar, and Sri Lanka [83]. Besides, national-level NGOs, civil society organizations and social enterprise entities also provide eye care services.

Standard government eye care systems using three or more tiers of service remain a mainstay for government eye services in most SEAR countries. Historically, these services had placed emphasis on hospital-based eye care but are increasingly adopting variations of the eye health pyramid model (developed in India by the LV Prasad Eye Institute [98]) and placing more emphasis on primary eye care (PEC) through vision centers. The eye health pyramid model has been replicated across the South-East Asian region with relevant modifications to suit local needs [99].

Even when there are eye services available for free, correction of refractive error and provision of spectacles are not always included or integrated into these services. Throughout the region, there is a vibrant and thriving presence of private sector optical outlets, and in some countries, these are in large numbers. Optometrists are few in Thailand, and ophthalmologists do not routinely offer refraction correction services; thus, private optical shops are the main providers of eyeglasses.

10.3.4.2 Eye Care Delivery Through School Eye Health

Children's eye health services are typically accessed through one of two systems: (1) health settings such as community health centers, eye clinics, and hospitals; or (2) school-based health interventions, where teachers or other personnel screen children's vision and visiting health practitioners provide eye care on site to the extent possible [69]. School interventions are a unique opportunity to provide comprehensive eye health services to >700 million children throughout the world. This service can potentially address issues such as vitamin A deficiency or trachoma and provides a cost-effective solution to detecting and treating uncorrected refractive errors [100–102]. These activities are potentially more cost-effective than other primary eye care models [103].

However, to be successful, school eye health services should interface directly with the broader health system [98]. The essential parameters are proper referral and examination of all screening failures and the provision of affordable and accessible care for refractive errors. The guiding principles for school eye health programs are: (1) engagement of school leadership and teachers, (2) active collaboration between ministries of health and education, (3) integration of inclusive education and school eye health into the ministries, (4) an education component for teachers and parents on eye health and treatment, (5) referral systems to connect children to advanced care [104, 105].

Most countries in the South-East Asian region have national school health programs (Table 10.7). Primary vision screening person differs. School eye nurses perform vision screening (schoolteachers are not permitted) in the Maldives and Myanmar. Although teachers conduct vision screenings in Timor-Leste schools, the National Education Strategic Plan 2011–2030, which includes school health, does not have a vision screening component [106].

In Sri Lanka, the "School Medical Inspection" (SMI) program began in 1918 (considered one of the earliest eye care programs in the country) and included periodic examination for general health including vision problems [107]. Later, the VISION 2020 Program of the Ministry of Health of Sri Lanka initiated an action plan to correct refractive errors in children, including the provision of spectacles. The National Eye Health Plan 2012–2017 included medical inspections for children enrolled in grades 4, 7, and 11. Children with vision problems were referred to the government hospitals where eye examinations are free, but spectacles are not dispensed for free [107].

Nepal has a holistic approach to eye health that includes eye screening, health education, and promoting inclusive education in schools [108]. Nepal's National School Health policy includes eye health; however, NGOs and private institutes mostly conduct vision screenings and eye examinations at schools. In Bangladesh, school-based vision testing is an established National Eye Care plan priority and is currently being implemented on a small scale [109].

India launched the National Child Health Program in 2018, which included vision screening, eye examination, and provision of spectacles [110]. In India, many schoolteachers are trained to conduct preliminary-level vision screening for children in schools [111]. Typically, children studying in 5th to 10th grades are included in the

Table 10.7 School health policy and eye care program coverage at schools [75–79]

Country	National school health policy	Vision screening	Eye exam	Spectacles provision	Free spectacles
Bhutan	Yes	Yes	Yes	Yes	NA
Maldives	Yes	Yes	NA	NA	Yes
Myanmar	NA	NA	NA	NA	NA
Timor-Leste	NA	NA	NA	NA	NA
Sri Lanka	Yes	Yes	Yes	Yes	NA
India	Yes	Yes	Yes	Yes	NA
Bangladesh	Yes	Yes	Yes	Yes	NA
Nepal	Yes	Yes	Yes	Yes	NA
DPR Korea	–	–	–	–	–
Indonesia	Yes	Yes	Yes	Yes	NA
Thailand	Yes	Yes	Yes	Yes	NA

NA Not available

screening programs though there is a recent emphasis on including primary school children as well. All children who fail the initial screening are referred to AOPs for refraction. Spectacles are provided free of cost to these children. Despite a large variation among teachers in how they conduct preliminary screening, this system appears to be the most cost-effective modality for screening for vision impairment in school children [112, 113]. Two well-designed and executed school eye health programs in India are the REACH (Refractive Error Among Children) and I-SCREEN (Initiative for Screening Children for Refractive Errors and other Eye Health Needs) programs [114, 115].

10.3.4.3 Optical Supply Chains

Spectacles are the mainstay of refractive correction. Although contact lenses and refractive surgery each have their place in refractive correction, we will center our discussion on spectacles in this chapter.

Spectacles come in four broad forms, with all forms in use across SEAR countries:

1. *Custom-made spectacles* are the most adaptable/customizable (to provide for the broadest range of refractive errors and inter-pupillary distances) and of the highest quality, but are expensive.
2. *Ready-to-assemble spectacles* are reasonably adaptable/customizable (a broad range of refractive errors can be accommodated, not astigmatism; partially customizable for inter-pupillary distance), can be assembled on-site from stock materials, provide reasonable quality, and are reasonably priced.
3. *Ready-made spectacles* are the cheapest, can be delivered on-site, but are of lower quality and not appropriate for higher powers, astigmatism, anisometropia, or non-standard inter-pupillary distances.
4. *Recycled spectacles* were popular in the past, but sorting, cleaning, stock management, and transport make them more expensive and less friendly than ready-made or ready-to-assemble options. Besides, variability in quality makes such spectacles difficult to deliver.

Published evidence suggests that spectacle coverage varies with Human Development Index (healthier, wealthier, and more educated countries generally have higher spectacle coverage), equality (greater financial equality generally allows higher spectacle coverage), health expenditure (more health expenditure improves spectacle coverage), and urbanization (urban areas typically appear to have the best spectacle coverage) [3, 56]. While the specific barriers related to individuals and communities exist, it is reasonable to suggest that spectacle accessibility decreases with resource limitations. This coverage pattern should be considered when analyzing the current state of and in planning future optical supply chains in South-East Asian countries.

Two eye care distribution strategies have been pioneered in South-East Asian countries with the specific aim of improving care for refractive errors in low resource areas, the free-standing optical outlets, and vision centers. Both sell low-cost spectacles and promote some degree of cross-subsidization to improve eye care access to the very poor. Vision centers provide an additional focus on eye health with referral networks as needed. Cost-recovery and cross-subsidy mechanisms enable vision centers and optical outlet staff to provide outreach services in schools and even more remote communities. Both have been measurably successful at improving refraction correction services in the areas where they have been established. Of late, e-commerce provides another potential optical supply chain mechanism as wireless data technology spreads faster than healthcare improvements in some places.

10.4 What Next for Refractive Error Care in the South-East Asia Region?

10.4.1 Looking Ahead

The current evidence on refractive errors from the South-East Asian region indicates a steadily growing public health challenge particularly associated with myopia and presbyopia. The health impact of uncorrected distance and near vision impairment, complications related to myopia, and the economic costs related to the burden (such as health expenditure and loss of productivity) are significant. Besides, data indicate that even for those with access to corrective glasses, compliance is less than desirable [116]. Irrespective of the reasons, poor visual health consequences are substantial and include loss of income and productivity, impaired or reduced functional capacity, increased risk of injury and accident, and increased future health expenditure at both the individual and societal level. In younger individuals, there is an additional risk of impaired education that may impact their future productivity.

The strategies to address these issues include strengthening the service model, increasing human resources at all levels of eye care, and reducing the cost of care. A few of these factors are discussed below.

10.4.1.1 School-Based Eye Health

The school eye health intervention is a promising strategy and alleviates some of the burdens associated with uncorrected refractive error. School-based health promotion activities also improve the student's awareness of health. The involvement of teachers, educators, and the entire school is valuable to children. There are growing bodies of evidence that outdoor time reduces the risk of myopia [117]. The protective benefits of outdoor time extended to all children, both myopic and non-myopic, through school-based intervention is long-lasting. A study in Taiwan had shown that the schoolchildren who spent at least 11 h per week outdoors (approximately 2 h per day of school-oriented outdoor activities) with exposure to a light intensity of at least 1000 lux had significantly less myopic shift in refractive error [118]. Such interventions also provide an opportunity for early detection and management of other eye conditions.

The success of this simple model depends on several factors. These are: (1) availability of resources, including tools and training; (2) appropriate referral pathways; (3) economic and physical accessibility for specialist and treatment pathways; and (4) the socio-economic setting of the school with parental and cultural attitudes. Though the school may be successful in adopting and improving awareness of good eye health in children, these changes may not translate entirely to correction and management of refractive errors, particularly in rural or more impoverished socio-economic settings with suboptimal parental attitudes, social behavior, and limited access to healthcare. This would be all the more important for conditions such as myopia, where the progressive nature of the condition demands a regular and frequent evaluation of the child's refractive error.

10.4.1.2 Self-screening or eHealth Tools

The improved access to digital and on-line media via smartphones provides a unique opportunity. It has enormous potential to empower individuals and their families to better manage the risks of poor eye health, including refractive errors using self-screening strategies that involve eHealth tools. Importantly, they can be universally applied across all ages, as compared to strategies such as school eye health that serve only a particular demographic. Such on-line tools or health apps include visual acuity checks [119], evaluation of refraction [91], methods to monitor screen time, and outdoor time. The tools also enable the provision of valuable information to fill in gaps in knowledge and intervention strategies. The wide virtual network allows access in poorly resourced communities. However, it must be remembered that economically underprivileged people and those with significant vision impairment or language barriers may have difficulty accessing these electronic tools. Besides, the application of many of these resources are not yet validated and may be used with caution in certain circumstances.

10.4.1.3 Availability and Affordability

Spectacle coverage is less in underdeveloped and rural communities due to access barrier and poverty. It calls for increased investment in eye health to reduce out-of-pocket spending and consequent financial hardship. Providing appropriate mechanisms that include higher governmental health expenditure and support from various community and public health organizations, as well as NGOs, are critical for reducing both distance and/or near vision impairment in children and adults in many countries in the South-East Asian region.

10.4.1.4 Newer Myopia Control Treatments

Several optical and pharmacological interventions are currently practiced to slow myopia progression. Utilizing one or more of these treatments reduces the risk of progression and vision impairment and complications associated with high myopia. These measures reduce the burden of poor vision on individuals, their families, and the community. Presently, optical interventions for myopia control include peripheral defocus correcting spectacle lenses, bifocal spectacles, progressive addition spectacles, multifocal soft contact lenses, and orthokeratology [92]. Atropine (0.01%) is the most widely used pharmacological intervention to reduce myopia progression. Though some of these interventions may be more expensive than traditional approaches, the broader benefits in reduced risk of vision impairment or further complications and reduced health expenditure in future years suggest that they are useful considerations.

10.5 Conclusion

Evidence shows a growing prevalence of myopia and presbyopia in the South-East Asia region. There is also a high prevalence of uncorrected and under-corrected refractive errors across the region. With barriers to eye health services such as lack of resources for refractive correction and lack of awareness of eye health services, there is a clear and urgent need to strengthen the human resource at all levels of eye care, from primary to advanced eye care. There is a need for greater advocacy for school eye health programs, so also, self-screening and e-tools. Reduced out-of-pocket health expenditure, higher governmental health expenditure and support from various NGOs, community and public health organizations are of critical importance for improving eye health services in this region.

References

1. Flaxman SR, Bourne RRA, Resnikoff S, Ackland P, Braithwaite T, Cicinelli MV, et al. Global causes of blindness and distance vision impairment 1990–2020: a systematic review and meta-analysis. Lancet Glob Health. 2017;5:e1221–e34.
2. Holden BA, Fricke TR, Wilson DA, et al. Global prevalence of myopia and high myopia and temporal trends from 2000 through 2050. Ophthalmology. 2016;1(23):1036–42.
3. Fricke TR, Tahhan N, Resnikoff S, et al. Global prevalence of presbyopia and vision Impairment from uncorrected presbyopia: systematic review, meta-analysis, and modelling. Ophthalmology. 2018;125:1492–9.
4. Morgan IG, Rose KA. Myopia: is the nature-nurture debate finally over? Clin Exp Optom. 2019;102:3–17.
5. Lin LL, Shih YF, Hsiao CK, et al. Prevalence of myopia in Taiwanese schoolchildren: 1983 to 2000. Ann Acad Med Singap. 2004;33:27–33.
6. Majumder M. Economics of healthcare financing in WHO South East Asia. South East Asia J Public Health. 2012;2:3–4. https://doi.org/10.3329/seajph.v2i2.15936.
7. Hashemi H, Fotouhi A, Yekta A, et al. Global and regional estimates of prevalence of refractive errors: systematic review and meta-analysis. J Curr Ophthalmol. 2018;30:3–22.
8. Garner LF, Owens H, Kinnear RF, et al. Prevalence of myopia in Sherpa and Tibetan children in Nepal. Optom Vis Sci. 1999;76:282–5.
9. Pokharel GP, Negrel AD, Munoz SR, et al. Refractive Error Study in Children: results from Mechi Zone, Nepal. Am J Ophthalmol. 2000;129:436–44.
10. Pokharel A, Pokharel PK, Das H, et al. The patterns of refractive errors among the school children of rural and urban settings in Nepal. Nepal J Ophthalmol. 2010;2:114–20. https://doi.org/10.3126/nepjoph.v2i2.3717.
11. Adhikari S, Nepal BP, Shrestha JK, et al. Magnitude and determinants of refractive error among school children of two districts of Kathmandu, Nepal. Oman J Ophthalmol. 2013;6:175–8.
12. Shrestha GS, Sujakhu D, Joshi P. Refractive error among school children in Jhapa, Nepal. J Optom. 2011;4:49–55.
13. Kalikivayi V, Naduvilath TJ, Bansal AK, et al. Visual impairment in school children in southern India. Indian J Ophthalmol. 1997;45:129–34.
14. Murthy GV, Gupta SK, Ellwein LB, et al. Refractive error in children in an urban population in New Delhi. Invest Ophthalmol Vis Sci. 2002;43:623–31.

15. Dandona R, Dandona L, Srinivas M, et al. Population-based assessment of refractive error in India: the Andhra Pradesh eye disease study. Clin Exp Ophthalmol. 2002;30:84–93. https://doi.org/10.1046/j.1442-6404.2002.00492.x.
16. Uzma N, Kumar BS, Khaja Mohinuddin Salar BM, et al. A comparative clinical survey of the prevalence of refractive errors and eye diseases in urban and rural school children. Can J Ophthalmol. 2009;44:328–33.
17. Padhye AS, Khandekar R, Dharmadhikari S, et al. Prevalence of uncorrected refractive error and other eye problems among urban and rural school children. Middle East Afr J Ophthalmol. 2009;16:69–74.
18. Saxena R, Vashist P, Tandon R, et al. Prevalence of myopia and its risk factors in urban school children in Delhi: the North India Myopia Study (NIM Study). PLoS One. 2015;10(2):e0117349. https://doi.org/10.1371/journal.pone.0117349.
19. Pavithra MB, Maheshwaran R, Sujatha R. A study on the prevalence of refractive errors among school children of 7–15 years age group in the field practice areas of a medical college in Bangalore. Int J Med Sci Public Health. 2013;2 https://doi.org/10.5455/ijmsph.2013.220420131.
20. Panda L, Nayak S, Khanna RC, et al. Tribal Odisha Eye Disease Study (TOES) # 7. Prevalence of refractive error in children in tribal Odisha (India) school screening. Indian J Ophthalmol. 2020;68:1596–9.
21. Dandona R, Dandona L, Srinivas M, et al. Refractive error in children in a rural population in India. Invest Ophthalmol Vis Sci. 2002;43:615–22.
22. Mahayana IT, Indrawati SG, Pawiroranu S. The prevalence of uncorrected refractive error in urban, suburban, exurban and rural primary school children in Indonesian population. Int J Ophthalmol. 2017;10:1771–6.
23. Nikmah ST, Rifada RM, Santoso PTR. Refractive errors in state junior high school students in Bandung. Althea Med J. 2016;3:545–8. https://doi.org/10.15850/amj.v3n4.936.
24. Jenchitr W, Raiyawa S. Refractive errors: the major visual impairment in Thailand. Rangsit J Arts Sci. 2012;2:133–41. https://doi.org/10.14456/rjas.2012.13.
25. Yingyong P. Refractive errors survey in primary school children (6-12-year-old) in 2 provinces: Bangkok and Nakhonpathom (one-year result). J Med Assoc Thail. 2010;93:1205–10.
26. Uddin M, Omar R, Feizal V, et al. Ocular morbidity among preschool children in urban area of Chittagong in Bangladesh. Int Eye Sci. 2017;17:16–20.
27. Rani PK, Raman R, Rachapalli SR, Kulothungan V, Kumaramanickavel G, Sharma T. Prevalence of refractive errors and associated risk factors in subjects with type 2 diabetes mellitus SN-DREAMS, report 18. Ophthalmology. 2010;117(6):1155–62. https://doi.org/10.1016/j.ophtha.2009.10.025.
28. Prema R, George R, Sathyamangalam Ve R, et al. Comparison of refractive errors and factors associated with spectacle use in a rural and urban South Indian population. Indian J Ophthalmol. 2008;56:139–44.
29. Krishnaiah S, Srinivas M, Khanna RC, et al. Prevalence and risk factors for refractive errors in the South Indian adult population: the Andhra Pradesh Eye disease study. Clin Ophthalmol. 2009;3:17–27.
30. Nangia V, Jonas JB, Sinha A, et al. Refractive error in central India: the Central India Eye and Medical Study. Ophthalmology. 2010;117:693–9.
31. Raju P, Ramesh SV, Arvind H, et al. Prevalence of refractive errors in a rural South Indian population. Invest Ophthalmol Vis Sci. 2004;45:4268–72.
32. Dandona R, Dandona L, Naduvilath TJ, et al. Refractive errors in an urban population in Southern India: the Andhra Pradesh Eye Disease Study. Invest Ophthalmol Vis Sci. 1999;40:2810–8.
33. Bourne RR, Dineen BP, Ali SM, et al. Prevalence of refractive error in Bangladeshi adults: results of the National Blindness and Low Vision Survey of Bangladesh. Ophthalmology. 2004;111:1150–60.
34. Muhit M, Minto H, Parvin A, et al. Prevalence of refractive error, presbyopia, and unmet need of spectacle coverage in a northern district of Bangladesh: Rapid Assessment of Refractive Error study. Ophthalmic Epidemiol. 2018;25:126–32.
35. Gupta A, Casson RJ, Newland HS, et al. Prevalence of refractive error in rural Myanmar: the Meiktila Eye Study. Ophthalmology. 2008;115:26–32.
36. Saw SM, Gazzard G, Koh D, et al. Prevalence rates of refractive errors in Sumatra, Indonesia. Invest Ophthalmol Vis Sci. 2002;43:3174–80.
37. Nirmalan PK, Krishnaiah S, Shamanna BR, et al. A population-based assessment of presbyopia in the state of Andhra Pradesh, south India: the Andhra Pradesh Eye Disease Study. Invest Ophthalmol Vis Sci. 2006;47:2324–8.
38. Sheeladevi S, Seelam B, Nukella PB, et al. Prevalence of refractive errors, uncorrected refractive error, and presbyopia in adults in India: a systematic review. Indian J Ophthalmol. 2019;67:583–92.
39. Marmamula S, Narsaiah S, Shekhar K, et al. Presbyopia, spectacles use and spectacle correction coverage for near vision among cloth weaving communities in Prakasam district in South India. Ophthalmic Physiol Opt. 2013;33:597–603.
40. Joseph S, Krishnan T, Ravindran RD, et al. Prevalence and risk factors for myopia and other refractive errors in an adult population in southern India. Ophthalmic Physiol Opt. 2018;38:346–58.
41. Ehrlich JR, Laoh A, Kourgialis N, et al. Uncorrected refractive error and presbyopia among junior high school teachers in Jakarta, Indonesia. Ophthalmic Epidemiol. 2013;20:369–74.
42. Sapkota YD, Dulal S, Pokharel GP, et al. Prevalence and correction of near vision impairment at Kaski, Nepal. Nepal J Ophthalmol. 2012;4:17–22. https://doi.org/10.3126/nepjoph.v4i1.5845.

43. Ramke J, du Toit R, Palagyi A, et al. Correction of refractive error and presbyopia in Timor-Leste. Br J Ophthalmol. 2007;91:860–6.
44. Kandel H, Khadka J, Shrestha MK, et al. Uncorrected and corrected refractive error experiences of Nepalese adults: a qualitative study. Ophthalmic Epidemiol. 2018;25:147–61.
45. Tay MT, Au Eong KG, Ng CY, et al. Myopia and educational attainment in 421,116 young Singaporean males. Ann Acad Med Singap. 1992;21:785–91.
46. Jonas JB, Nangia V, Gupta R, et al. Prevalence of myopic retinopathy in rural Central India. Acta Ophthalmol. 2017;95:e399–404. https://doi.org/10.1111/aos.13301.
47. Praveen MR, Vasavada AR, Jani UD, et al. Prevalence of cataract type in relation to axial length in subjects with high myopia and emmetropia in an Indian population. Am J Ophthalmol. 2008;145:176–81.
48. Flitcroft DI. Emmetropisation and the aetiology of refractive errors. Eye (Lond). 2014;28:169–79.
49. Castagno VD, Fassa AG, Carret ML, et al. Hyperopia: a meta-analysis of prevalence and a review of associated factors among school-aged children. BMC Ophthalmol. 2014;14:163. https://doi.org/10.1186/1471-2415-14-163.
50. Kulp MT, Ying G, Huang J, et al. Associations between hyperopia and other vision and refractive error characteristics. Optom Vis Sci. 2014;91:383–9.
51. Hussain A, Roy T, Ferdausi N, et al. Prevalence of childhood ocular morbidity in a peri-urban setting in Bangladesh: a community-based study. Public Health. 2019;170:103–12.
52. Read SA, Collins MJ, Carney LG. A review of astigmatism and its possible genesis. Clin Exp Optom. 2007;90(1):5–19.
53. Gajapati CV, Pradeep AV, Kakhandaki A, et al. Awareness of presbyopia among rural female population in North Karnataka. J Clin Diagn Res. 2017;11:NC01–NC5. https://doi.org/10.7860/JCDR/2017/26125.10608.
54. Reddy PA, Congdon N, MacKenzie G, et al. Effect of providing near glasses on productivity among rural Indian tea workers with presbyopia (PROSPER): a randomised trial. Lancet Glob Health. 2018;6:e1019–e27. https://doi.org/10.1016/S2214-109X(18)30329-2.
55. Adler D, Millodot M. The possible effect of under correction on myopic progression in children. Clin Exp Optom. 2006;89:315–21.
56. Naidoo KS, Fricke TR, Frick KD, et al. Potential lost productivity resulting from the global burden of myopia: systematic review, Meta-analysis, and Modeling. Ophthalmology. 2019;126:338–46.
57. McCormick I, Mactaggart I, Bastawrous A, et al. Effective refractive error coverage: an eye health indicator to measure progress towards universal health coverage. Ophthalmic Physiol Opt. 2020;40:1–5.
58. Chan VF, MacKenzie GE, Kassalow J, et al. Impact of presbyopia and Its correction in Low- and Middle-Income countries. Asia Pac J Ophthalmol (Phila). 2018;7:370–4.
59. Marmamula S, Challa R, Yellapragada S, et al. Temporal trends in the prevalence of spectacle use and spectacle coverage in India. Clin Exp Optom. 2020;103:693–8.
60. Das T. Blindness and visual impairment profile and Rapid Assessment of Avoidable Blindness in South East Asia: Analysis of new data. 2017 APAO Holmes Lecture. Asia Pac J Ophthalmol (Phila). 2018;7:312–5.
61. Holden BA, Fricke TR, Ho SM, et al. Global vision impairment due to uncorrected presbyopia. Arch Ophthalmol. 2008;126:1731–9.
62. Marmamula S, Khanna RC, Kunuku E, et al. Near visual impairment and spectacle coverage in Telangana, India. Clin Exp Ophthalmol. 2017;45:568–74.
63. Marmamula S, Khanna RC, Kunuku E, et al. Spectacles use in a rural population in the state of Telangana in South India. Indian J Ophthalmol. 2017;65:509–15.
64. Gupta V, Saxena R, Vashist P, et al. Spectacle coverage among urban schoolchildren with refractive error provided subsidized spectacles in North India. Optom Vis Sci. 2019;96:301–8.
65. Gilbert C, Murthy GV, Schmidt E, et al. Prevalence and types of refractive errors, and spectacle coverage in Sri Lankan adults: the Sri Lanka National Survey of Blindness and Visual Impairment. Ceylon Med J. 2018;63(S2):s33–9.
66. Bourne RR, Dineen BP, Huq DM, et al. Correction of refractive error in the adult population of Bangladesh: meeting the unmet need. Invest Ophthalmol Vis Sci. 2004;45:410–7.
67. Dhirar N, Dudeja S, Duggal M, et al. Compliance to spectacle use in children with refractive errors—a systematic review and meta-analysis. BMC Ophthalmol. 2020;20:71. https://doi.org/10.1186/s12886-020-01345-9.
68. Morjaria P, McCormick I, Gilbert C. Compliance and predictors of spectacle wear in schoolchildren and reasons for non-wear: a review of the literature. Ophthalmic Epidemiol. 2019;26:367–77.
69. Burnett AM, Yashadhana A, Lee L, et al. Interventions to improve school-based eye-care services in low- and middle-income countries: a systematic review. Bull World Health Organ. 2018;96:682–94. https://doi.org/10.2471/BLT.18.212332.
70. Narayanan A, Kumar S, Ramani KK. Spectacle compliance among adolescents: a qualitative study from Southern India. Optom Vis Sci. 2017;94:582–7.
71. Bhatt N, Rathi M, Dhull CS, et al. Spectacle compliance amongst school children of Rohtak, Haryana, India. Int J Com Med Public Health. 2017;4(3) https://doi.org/10.18203/2394-6040.ijcmph20170749.
72. Kumar MR, Mallika OU. Study of refractive errors, amblyopia and compliance of spectacles in school children. J Med Sci Clin Res. 2017;5:1–8. https://doi.org/10.18535/jmscr/v5i4.67.

73. Bhandari G, Pradhan S, Shrestha MK. Eye glasses compliance among children undergoing school visual acuity screening in Nepal. Adv Ophthalmol Vis Syst. 2016;5:286–90. https://doi.org/10.15406/aovs.2016.05.00162.
74. Sumana M, Sreelatha CY, Sagar K, et al. Prevalence of refractive error and other ocular morbidities and follow-up study on compliance to spectacles use among school going children aged 9–16 years in selected village of Hassan. J Evolution Med and Dental Sci. 2015;4:16163–7. https://doi.org/10.14260/jemds/2015/2372.
75. Gogate P, Mukhopadhyaya D, Mahadik A, et al. Spectacle compliance amongst rural secondary school children in Pune district, India. Indian J Ophthalmol. 2013;61:8–12.
76. Khandekar R, Sudhan A, Jain BK, et al. Compliance with spectacle wear and its determinants in school students in central India. Asian J Ophthalmol. 2008;10:174–7.
77. Morjaria P, Evans J, Murali K, et al. Spectacle wear among children in a school-based program for ready-made vs custom-made spectacles in India: A randomized clinical trial. JAMA Ophthalmol. 2017;135:527–33.
78. Holden B, Fricke TR, Naidoo K, et al. IAPB Refractive Error Program Committee Strategy for the elimination of vision impairment from uncorrected refractive error. International Agency for the Prevention of Blindness (IAPB). 2008. www.iapb.org. Accessed 30 Nov 2020.
79. Marmamula S, Keeffe JE, et al. Population-based cross-sectional study of barriers to utilisation of refraction services in South India: Rapid Assessment of Refractive Errors (RARE) Study. BMJ Open. 2011;1:e000172. https://doi.org/10.1136/bmjopen-2011-000172.
80. Malhotra S, Kalaivani M, Rath R, et al. Use of spectacles for distance vision: coverage, unmet needs and barriers in a rural area of North India. BMC Ophthalmol. 2019;19:252. https://doi.org/10.1186/s12886-019-1262-3.
81. Blanchet K, Patel D. Applying principles of health system strengthening to eye care. Indian J Ophthalmol. 2012;60:470–4.
82. The International Agency for the Prevention of Blindness. National eye health strategy 2014–2019. Ministry of Health, Government of Timor-Leste. 2017. www.iapb.org. Accessed 30 Nov 2020.
83. Das T, Ackland P, Correia M, et al. Is the 2015 eye care service delivery profile in Southeast Asia closer to universal eye health need! Int Ophthalmol. 2018;38:469–80.
84. WHO Regional office for South-East Asia. Situation analysis of vision 2020 in the WHO South-East Asia Region. World Health Organization. 2012. www.who.int. Accessed 30 Nov 2020.
85. Sightsavers. Bangladesh quadruples its eye care budget. 2017.www.sightsavers.org. Accessed 30 Nov 2020.
86. Zakir Hussain AM. Strategy for national eye care for vision 2020 in Bangladesh. 2014. www.ssmf-bd.org. Accessed 30 Nov 2020.
87. The International Agency for the Prevention of Blindness (IAPB). Roadmap of visual impairment control program in Indonesia 2017–2030. 2018. www.iapb.org. Accessed 30 Nov 2020
88. Ministry of Health, Male, Republic of Maldives. Planning and international health division Maldives health profile. 2016. Available from: http://www.health.gov.mv. Accessed 30 Nov 2020.
89. Ministry of Health and Sports, Republic of the Union of Myanmar. National eye health plan 2017–2021. 2017. www.iapb.org. Accessed 30 Nov 2020.
90. The International Agency for the Prevention of Blindness. Vision 2020 Sri Lanka: right to sight. National Program for Prevention of Blindness, Sri Lanka. Comprehensive eye care plan (2013–2017 five years). 2017. www.iapb.org. Accessed 30 Nov 2020.
91. Wisse RPL, Muijzer MB, Cassano F, et al. Validation of an independent web-based tool for measuring visual acuity and refractive error (the Manifest versus Online Refractive Evaluation Trial): Prospective open-label noninferiority clinical trial. J Med Internet Res. 2019;21:e14808. https://doi.org/10.2196/14808.
92. Wildsoet CF, Chia A, Cho P, et al. IMI—Interventions Myopia Institute: Interventions for controlling myopia onset and progression report. Invest Ophthalmol Vis Sci. 2019;60:M106–M31. https://doi.org/10.1167/iovs.18-25958.
93. Fricke TR, Holden BA, Wilson DA, et al. Global cost of correcting vision impairment from uncorrected refractive error. Bull World Health Organ. 2012;90:728–38.
94. Das T, Keeffe J, Sivaprasad S, et al. Capacity building for universal eye health coverage in South East Asia beyond 2020. Eye (Lond). 2020;34(7):1262–70.
95. Sapkota YD. Human Resources for eye health in South Asia. Community Eye Health. 2018;31(102):S1–2.
96. Shukla P, Vashist P, Senjam SS, et al. Evaluation of a training program on primary eye care for an Accredited Social Health Activist (ASHA) in an urban district. Indian J Ophthalmol. 2020;68:356–60.
97. Wing K, Low G, Sharma M, et al. Building a national eye-care service in post-conflict Timor-Leste. Bull World Health Organ. 2018;96:716–22.
98. Mehta MC, Narayanan R, Thomas AH, et al. The L V Prasad Eye Institute: a comprehensive case study of excellent and equitable eye care. Healthcare (Amst). 2020;8:100408. https://doi.org/10.1016/j.hjdsi.2019.100408.
99. Misra V, Vashist P, Malhotra S, et al. Models for primary eye care services in India. Indian J Community Med. 2015;40:79–84.
100. Gilbert C, Minto H, Morjaria P, et al. Standard guidelines for comprehensive school eye health programs. Sight Savers International, London: London

School of Hygiene and Tropical Medicine, Brien Holden Vision Institute. 2016. www.iceh.ishtm.ac.uk. Accessed 30 Nov 2020.
101. Minto H, Ho M. What is comprehensive school eye health? Community Eye Health. 2017;30(98):21–5.
102. Frick KD, Riva-Clement L, Shankar MB. Screening for refractive error and fitting with spectacles in rural and urban India: cost-effectiveness. Ophthalmic Epidemiol. 2009;16:378–87.
103. Lester BA. Comparing the cost-effectiveness of school eye screening versus a primary eye care model to provide refractive error services for children in India. Community Eye Health. 2007;20(61):15.
104. Wodon Q, Male C, Nayihouba A, et al. The price of exclusion: disability and education looking ahead: visual impairment and school eye health programs. World Bank Group, EYElliance, DECDG, USAID. 2019. www.pubdocs.worldbank.org. Accessed 30 Nov 2020.]
105. Smith E, Chen W, Congdon N, et al. Eyeglasses for global development: Bridging the visual divide. World Economic Forum, Schwab Foundation for Social Entrepreneurship, Eyelliance. www.weforum.org. Accessed 30 Nov 2020.
106. The World Bank and Brien Holden Vision Institute Foundation report 2018. Situational analysis of child eye health—individual country profiles (2016 survey result). www.visionimpactinstitue.org. Accessed 30 Nov 2020.
107. Abeydeera A. School eye health services in Sri Lanka: an innovative way of approaching eye health in children. Comm Eye Health. 2017;30(98):S21–3.
108. Singh SK, Thakur S, Anwar A. School eye health in Nepal: a holistic model. Community Eye Health. 2017;30(98):S18–20.
109. Sightsavers. Paediatric eye care services in Bangladesh. 2018. www.sightsavers.org/wp-content/uploads/2019/03/Paediatric-eye-care-services-in-Bangladesh-evaluation-report-1.pdf. Accessed 29 Nov 2020.
110. Government of India. Operational guidelines on school health programme under Ayushman Bharat. Available from www.nhm.gov.in/guidelines/Operational_guidelines_on_School_Health_Programme_under_Ayushman_Bharat.pdf. Accessed 29 Nov 2020.
111. Jose R, Sachdeva S. School eye screening and the National Program for Control of Blindness. Indian Pediatr. 2009;46:205–8.
112. Marmamula S, Khanna RC, Mettla AL, et al. Agreement and diagnostic accuracy of vision screening in children by teachers, community eye-health workers and vision technicians. Clin Exp Optom. 2018;101:553–9.
113. Saxena R, Vashist P, Tandon R, et al. Accuracy of visual assessment by school teachers in school eye screening program in Delhi. Indian J Community Med. 2015;40:38–42.
114. Jan CL, Timbo CS, Congdon N. Children's myopia: prevention and the role of school programmes. Community Eye Health. 2017;30(98):37–8.
115. Panda L, Khanna RC. Metla AL, et al Causes of vision impairment and blindness among children in schools for the blind in South Indian States of Andhra Pradesh and Telangana. Indian J Ophthalmol. 2020;68:345–50.
116. Ramke J, Brian G, Naduvilath T. Refractive error and presbyopia in Timor-Leste: the impact of 5 years of a national spectacle program. Invest Ophthalmol Vis Sci. 2012;53:434–9.
117. Xiong S, Sankaridurg P, Naduvilath T, et al. Time spent in outdoor activities in relation to myopia prevention and control: a meta-analysis and systematic review. Acta Ophthalmol. 2017;95:551–66.
118. Wu PC, Chen CT, Lin KK, et al. Myopia prevention and outdoor light intensity in a school-based cluster randomized trial. Ophthalmology. 2018;125:1239–50.
119. Yeung WK, Dawes P, Pye A, et al. Erratum: Author Correction: eHealth tools for the self-testing of visual acuity: a scoping review. NPJ Digit Med. 2019;2:117. https://doi.org/10.1038/s41746-019-0195-9.

Childhood Blindness and Visual Impairment

11

Clare Gilbert, P. Vijayalakshmi, Sahithya Bhaskaran, Tavisha Udupihille, Habibah S. Muhiddin, Dyah Ayu Windy, Idayani Panggalo, Sanduk Ruit, Srijana Adhikari, A. H. M. Enayet Hussain, and Khaleda Islam

Key Points

- The number of blind children in a given population is determined by the prevalence of blindness and the proportion of the population who are children. Both reflect socio-economic development and access to public healthcare and healthcare services, including eye care.
- In Asian countries, between 50 and 250 children are blind per 10 million total population.
- The main causes of blindness in this region are congenital anomalies of the whole globe (such as microphthalmos and anophthalmos), corneal disease (principally corneal scarring), cataract, and retinal conditions (including dystrophies and retinopathy of prematurity). Cerebral visual impairment is an emerging cause of blindness.
- The main avoidable causes of blindness are corneal scarring, cataract, and retinopathy of prematurity.
- A comprehensive, integrated approach is required for control; prevention, and health promotion in the community through to specialist tertiary care provided by highly competent, well-equipped teams, with rehabilitation for children with irreversible vision impairment.
- Greater emphasis is needed for comprehensive eye care services, which are integrated into child health policies, programs, and services, as illustrated by some of the case studies in the region.
- Further research is needed in the region on the prevalence and causes of blindness, and studies which assess the effectiveness and challenges of integrating eye care for children into the health system.

C. Gilbert (✉)
International Centre for Eye Health, Department of Clinical Research, London School of Hygiene & Tropical Medicine, London, UK
e-mail: clare.gilbert@lshtm.ac.uk

P. Vijayalakshmi · S. Bhaskaran
Aravind Eye Care System, Madurai, India
e-mail: p.vijayalakshmi@aravind.org

T. Udupihille
Sirimavo Bandaranaike Specialized Children's Hospital, Peradeniya, Central Province, Sri Lanka

H. S. Muhiddin · D. A. Windy · I. Panggalo
South Sulawesi Indonesian Ophthalmologists Association, Makassar, South Sulawesi, Indonesia

S. Ruit · S. Adhikari
Tilganga Institute of Ophthalmology, Kathmandu, Nepal
e-mail: srijana.adhikari@tio.org

A. H. M. Enayet Hussain
Directorate General of Medical Education, Ministry of Health and Family Welfare, Dhaka, Bangladesh

K. Islam
Directorate General of Health Services, Ministry of Health and Family Welfare, Dhaka, Bangladesh

T. Das, P. D. Nayar (eds.), *South-East Asia Eye Health*,
https://doi.org/10.1007/978-981-16-3787-2_11

11.1 Epidemiology

11.1.1 Prevalence and Magnitude of Blindness in South-East Asian Children

Epidemiology is defined as the study of the frequency, distribution, determinants, and control of health conditions in the population. In other words, it addresses how common a condition is, who is most affected, what is causing the condition, and what can be done to control it.

Studying the epidemiology of blindness and visual impairment in children is challenging, as they are relatively rare at the population level. Most population-based surveys have focused on adults, and there are only a limited number of surveys of children, for the following reasons: (1) a very large sample is required due to the low prevalence and clustering of conditions within households, such as congenital cataract and vitamin A deficiency; (2) reliably measuring visual acuity in a field setting is challenging, particularly for children under the age of 5 years; (3) there are multiple causes of blindness in children and field teams need more expertise to identify the causes accurately; (4) children aged 7–15 years are likely to be in school; and lastly, (5) children who are blind may be away from home in residential schools or staying with relatives. Faced with these challenges, other sources of data or methods have been used, which include the key informant method, active surveillance, data from registers, or house-to-house surveys using questionnaires administered to the caregivers.

Using the available data, it appears that the prevalence of blindness in children is associated with under-5 mortality rates; countries with higher under-5 mortality rates have a higher prevalence of blindness [1]. This is expected, as many of the causes of child mortality are also causes of blindness, such as vitamin A deficiency, measles infection, meningitis, malaria, birth hypoxia, retinoblastoma, and congenital rubella syndrome. Indeed, under-5 mortality rates are now used to assess whether vitamin A deficiency is likely to be a public health problem, as it can predispose young children to succumbing to infections [2]. Besides this, children with congenital eye anomalies, such as microphthalmos or coloboma, may have syndromes with anomalies affecting other organs. Children with cerebral visual impairment (CVI) and cerebral palsy also have high mortality rates. In the absence of population-based data, under-5 mortality rates can be used as a proxy for the prevalence of blindness, as outlined in Table 11.1.

Table 11.1 Prevalence estimates for blindness and severe visual impairment in children using under-5 mortality rates as a proxy [1]

Under-5 mortality/1000 live births[a]	Prevalence estimate/10,000 children
0–19	3
20–39	4
40–59	5
60–79	6
80–99	7
100–119	8
120–139	9
140–159	10
160–179	11
180–199	12
200–219	13
220–239	14
240+	15

[a]The under-5 mortality rates for the year 7–8 years before the required time period should be used, as this is the midpoint of the 16 years of childhood

Applying this approach to the 11 countries in South-East Asia, there are an estimated 283,151 blind children in 2020, the vast majority of whom live in India (72.9%) and Bangladesh (10%) (Table 11.2, Fig. 11.1).

The number of blind children per million total population allows comparisons between countries regarding the burden of blindness (Fig. 11.2). As can be seen, Myanmar has the highest rate, and the Democratic Republic of Korea has the lowest. These values reflect the proportion of the population who are children and the prevalence of blindness, both of which are indicators of development.

It is important to bear in mind that prevalence data only refer to the situation at a particular point in time—children who became blind and died or who have had their sight restored before the study would not have been counted, which-

Table 11.2 Estimates of the numbers of blind and severely visually impaired children aged 0–15 years in South-East Asian countries in 2020

Country	Population aged 0–15 years in 2020	U5MR in 2013	Prevalence estimate of blindness/10,000	Estimate of number of blind children	% of all blindness
Bangladesh	47,326,339	41	6	28,396	10.0%
Bhutan	283,340	36	4	113	0.0%
DPR Korea	7,346,774	4	3	2204	0.8%
India	413,046,276	53	5	206,523	72.9%
Indonesia	70,744,920	29	4	28,298	10.0%
Maldives	111,266	10	3	33	0.0%
Myanmar	14,753,235	51	5	7377	2.6%
Nepal	9,795,291	40	5	4898	1.7%
Sri Lanka	5,310,983	10	3	1593	0.6%
Thailand	11,485,102	13	3	3446	1.2%
Timor-Leste	539,848	55	5	270	0.1%
Total	580,743,374	–	4.9	283,151	100%

U5MR under-5 mortality rate, *DPR Korea* Democratic Republic of Korea

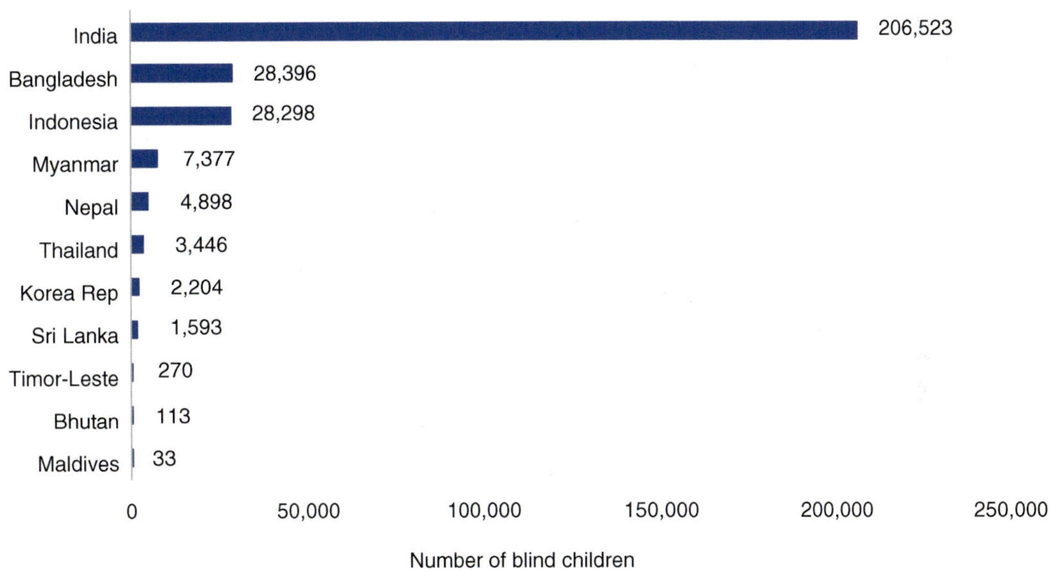

Fig. 11.1 Estimated number of blind children aged 0–15 years in South-East Asian countries in 2020

ever methodology was used. Indeed, there is some evidence that blind children have a higher mortality than their sighted counterparts; but data for this are scant. Hence, for these reasons, prevalence data and estimates for numbers of blind children are likely to underestimate the magnitude of the actual problem as they do not take into account those children who have died.

Data on the number of new cases of blindness and visual impairment that occur over time (i.e., the incidence) are even more challenging to obtain because longitudinal studies are required. The only data available come from a few studies of registers of children with visual impairment in Scandinavian countries and active surveillance studies in the United Kingdom.

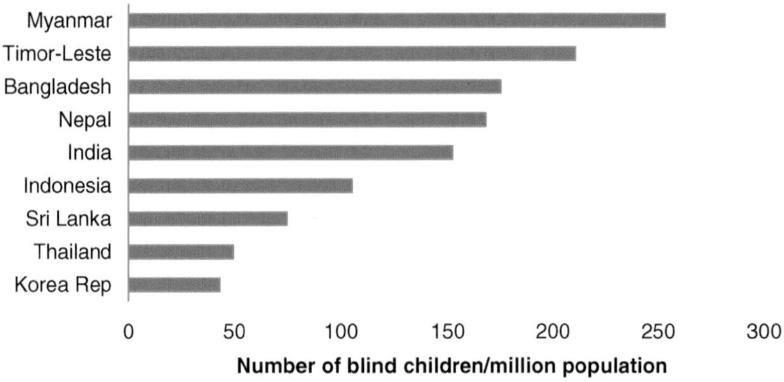

Fig. 11.2 Number of blind children per million population in the nine South-East Asian countries with a total population of over 1 million

11.1.2 Causes of Blindness in Children

In 1993, the World Health Organization (WHO) developed a system for classifying the causes of blindness and severe visual impairment (SVI) in children [3]. This classification uses two different approaches: (1) to describe the main cause of blindness according to which part of the eye or higher visual pathways are affected (anatomical site); and (2) to describe the time of onset of the condition leading to blindness (etiology). For example, for genetic conditions and intrauterine infections, this would be prenatal even if the visual impairment is not apparent until many years later; ophthalmia neonatorum and retinopathy of prematurity (ROP) would be classified as perinatal conditions. Unfortunately, although these data are much more useful for identifying strategies and planning for control, these are far more challenging to obtain. Most studies report data on the anatomical site of abnormality after clinical examination.

Data on the causes of blindness in children are more plentiful than prevalence data. These data come from examining children in schools for the blind, hospital eye care services, key informant, or house-to-house studies. The last two sources are likely to be more reliable, as the first two are likely to suffer from selection bias. For example, if an eye hospital is known for its excellent pediatric surgery, this will attract more children with conditions such as cataract, glaucoma, or ROP.

Data on the major causes of blindness in children in South-East Asian countries come from 23 studies of 7401 blind/SVI children published from 2000 to 2020 from India (11 studies), Bangladesh (6), Nepal (2), Indonesia (2), Sri Lanka (1), and Myanmar (1) (Table 11.3). The four major sites of abnormality are the whole globe (mainly microphthalmos and anophthalmos), lens (unoperated cataract or complications following cataract surgery), and retinal conditions (predominantly retinal dystrophies with some ROP) (Fig. 11.3).

From these figures, the numbers of blind children in the region can be estimated (classified according to cause of blindness), but this assumes that the causes are very similar across countries, which is unlikely (Table 11.4).

For example, in the South-East Asian region, over 77,000 children are blind due to lesions of the whole eye (i.e., microphthalmos, anophthalmos, or disorganized eyes); over 60,000 have corneal conditions (i.e., scarring from a range of conditions, keratoconus, dystrophies) and over 48,000 are blind due to lesions of the lens (cataract or poor outcomes following cataract surgery). Usually, CVI and other lesions of the central nervous system are uncommon.

From a public health and clinical perspective, it is also useful to segregate causes of blindness as avoidable and unavoidable, bearing in mind that vision rehabilitation can reduce or prevent developmental delay and disability in children with irreversible causes of vision loss. Avoidable causes of blindness are those which can be prevented, such as most cases of corneal scarring and ROP, as well as those which can be managed clinically to improve visual function or prevent

Table 11.3 Studies on the causes of blindness and severe visual impairment in children aged 0–15 years in the WHO South-East Asia Region between 2000 and 2020 [4–24]

Country/location	Author	N	Whole globe	Cornea	Lens	Uvea	Retina	Glaucoma	Optic nerve	CVI	Other
India South	Gogate et al. 2009 [4]	891	39%	14%	14%	0%	20%	2%	4%	0%	7%
India North East	Bhattacharjee et al. 2008 [5]	258	32%	36%	11%	2%	6%	4%	5%	1%	3%
India Maharashtra	Gogate et al. 2007 [6]	1778	46%	22%	6%	1%	11%	0%	5%	0%	9%
India Andhra Pradesh	Hornby et al. 2000 [7]	267	20%	24%	8%	3%	31%	7%	5%	0%	2%
India South	Krishnaiah et al. 2012 [8]	113	41%	8%	10%	5%	19%	8%	5%	0%	4%
India North & South	Magdula 2009 [9]	103	32%	13%	13%	2%	22%	4%	11%	0%	3%
India North	Pal et al. 2006 [10]	133	6%	7%	31%	17%	16%	0%	17%	0%	6%
India North	Titiyal et al. 2003 [11]	650	27%	22%	11%	9%	15%	5%	11%	0%	0%
India	Bhalerao et al. 2015 [12]	90	51%	25%	10%	1%	3%	3%	7%	0%	0%
India	Kemmanu et al. 2018 [13]	8	25%	13%	13%	25%	13%	0%	0%	13%	0%
India	Prakash et al. 2017 [14]	302	2%	17%	13%	4%	19%	7%	25%	0%	14%
Bangladesh	Hussain et al. 2019 [15]	25	28%	4%	16%	0%	12%	4%	8%	20%	8%
Bangladesh (a)	Muhit et al. 2007 [16]	394	18%	31%	23%	1%	17%	4%	6%	0%	0%
Bangladesh (b)	Muhit et al. 2007 [16]	1245	11%	25%	36%	2%	12%	4%	9%	0%	1%
Bangladesh (c)	Muhit et al. 2007 [16]	296	15%	28%	29%	2%	11%	5%	9%	0%	1%
Bangladesh (d)	Muhit 2010 [17]	45	13%	13%	38%	0%	9%	0%	11%	0%	16%
Bangladesh	Mactaggart 2013 [18]	184	9%	8%	27%	3%	5%	3%	18%	0%	27%
Nepal	Adhikari et al. 2015 [19]	7	14%	0%	29%	0%	14%	0%	0%	0%	43%
Nepal	Byanju et al. 2019 [20]	23	22%	0%	13%	4%	0%	0%	9%	4%	48%
Indonesia, Java	Sitorus et al. 2007 [21]	82	40%	6%	15%	7%	21%	0%	11%	0%	0%
Indonesia	Muhit et al. 2018 [22]	113	7%	8%	31%	2%	12%	1%	4%	0%	36%
Myanmar	Muecke et al. 2009 [23]	202	19%	44%	14%	2%	7%	7%	4%	1%	2%
Sri Lanka	Gao et al. 2011 [24]	192	18%	8%	11%	3%	36%	4%	11%	3%	6%
Total		7401	27%	21%	17%	3%	15%	3%	8%	0%	6%

CVI cerebral visual impairment; (a–d) How children were identified: (a) special education, (b) key informants, (c) community-based rehabilitation, or (d) house-to-house survey

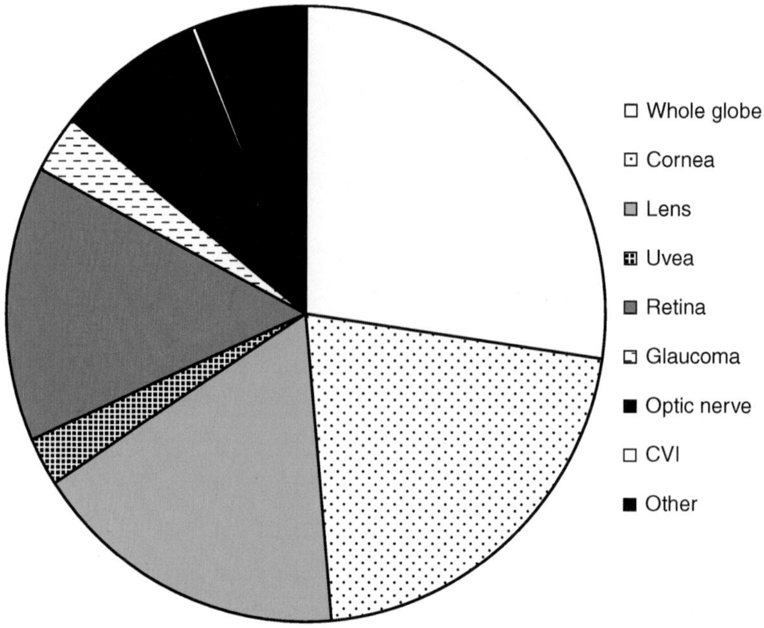

Fig. 11.3 Causes of blindness and severe visual impairment (classified according to anatomical site of abnormality) in children aged 0–15 years in countries in the WHO South-East Asia Region in 2020

Table 11.4 Proportion of blindness in the WHO South-East Asia Region by anatomical site, and most frequent eye conditions

Anatomical site	%	N	Principle conditions
Whole globe	27.3	77,244	Microphthalmos, disorganized, anophthalmos
Cornea	21.3	60,372	Scarring, staphyloma, phthisis from ulceration
Lens	17.1	48,397	Cataract, complications of surgery
Uvea	2.6	7384	Uveitis
Retina	14.5	41,090	Dystrophies, ROP
Glaucoma	3.0	8608	Buphthalmos or other glaucoma
Optic nerve	8.0	22,611	Optic atrophy, hypoplasia
CVI	0.2	689	Cortical blindness
Other	5.9	16,757	High myopia, cannot be determined
Total	100	283,151	

ROP retinopathy of prematurity, *CVI* cerebral visual impairment

visual impairment, such as cataract, glaucoma, ROP, and some cases of retinoblastoma. Irreversible causes are structural abnormalities of the eye, such as microphthalmos, anophthalmos, and coloboma, and other conditions such as genetic retinal dystrophies and lesions of the central nervous system.

11.1.3 Changes in the Major Causes of Blindness over Time

Corneal scarring has declined dramatically over the last 20–39 years in all regions of the world [25]. This is attributable to increasing measles immunization coverage, declining incidence of vitamin A deficiency due to a combination of improving socio-economic development, vitamin A supplementation of preschool-age children, and other control measures such as better water supply and sanitation, less overcrowding, and nutritional interventions.

Over the same period of time, governments in the South-East Asian region have also been paying closer attention to neonatal mortality rates (which comprise around 40% of all deaths before the age of 1 year) by expanding neonatal intensive care provision. This has and continues to lead to better survival of preterm infants. Indeed, in 2010, there were an estimated 15 million preterm births globally [26], almost 5 million of which occurred in South-East Asia. It was also estimated that nearly 80,000 of these 5 million preterm infants survived neonatal care, and 5300 of them developed severe ROP warranting treatment [27]. This number is likely to have increased over the last decade as services for sick and preterm neonates continue to expand in many countries in the region. In addition to visual loss from ROP, very or extremely preterm infants can also develop CVI, with visual field defects, optic atrophy, and disruption of higher visual processing, including poor visual-motor integration (perceptual visual impairment) [28, 29]. Consequently, blindness due to ROP is increasing in countries such as India, Bangladesh, and Indonesia, and an increase in CVI is also likely. Assessing these children is complex and challenging (Box 1).

Box 1. Assessing Children with Cerebral Visual Impairment

P. Vijayalakshmi; Sahithya Bhaskaran
Aravind Eye Care System, Madurai, India

Cerebral visual impairment (CVI) refers to visual and perceptual abnormalities from perinatal damage to or dysfunction of retrogeniculate visual pathways [30], i.e., to and within the visual cortex, and/or from the visual cortex in the ventral or dorsal streams to centers involved in higher-order visual processing and attention (Fig. 11.4). Lesions can lead to vision loss, visual field defect (often inferior), impaired saccades and pursuits, unstable and eccentric fixation, and perceptual difficulties in the absence of clinical signs in the eyes. Affected children often also have ocular morbidities such as refractive errors (20–50%), anomalies of accommodation (mostly hypo-accommodation; 12%), strabismus and amblyopia, nystagmus, cataract, optic nerve hypoplasia, and optic atrophy [31, 32].

Children with CVI may have cerebral palsy, developmental delays, seizures, and be cognitively impaired. Children with or suspected to have CVI should have a comprehensive assessment, although this can be challenging to perform.

Assessment

A good history includes asking about motor problems associated with cerebral palsy, developmental milestones, and difficulties the child experiences. The following difficulties which do not correlate with visual acuity suggest CVI: (1) difficulty going down steps; (2) inability to fixate an object at a distance; (3) frequently bumping into objects; (4) inability to locate an object in a crowded environment (simultagnosia); and (5) difficulty seeing moving objects, recognizing faces, or being able to find way along a route which should be familiar. Birth history and events during the neonatal period may indicate the cause, which includes hypoxic-ischemic encephalopathy (particularly in children born preterm), seizures, hydrocephalus, trauma, and infections.

One should observe the child for abnormal head posture, eccentric viewing, and abnormal head or eye movements. This should be followed by an assessment of ocular movements (smooth pursuit, saccades), fixation, and alignment, noting associated head and body movements. Anterior segment examination (preferably with a handheld slit lamp) should include pupil light reflexes. Other assessments include dynamic retinoscopy to assess accommodation, cycloplegic refraction, and a detailed fundus evaluation.

In CVI, visual acuity can range from normal to no light perception. Children cooperate better with binocular acuity testing (start with an age-appropriate method). If this is not possible, one uses forced preferential looking tests (Lea gratings, Cardiff or Teller cards). Children with simultagnosia should be tested with single optotypes. Near vision must also be assessed as this affects functional vision for most tasks. It is also necessary to determine the child's ability to fix, follow, and hold fixation on a target.

Contrast sensitivity can be assessed using a Hiding Heidi (for non-verbal children) or a Pelli Robson chart (for verbal children); color vision can be tested with Ishihara plates; and visual fields can be tested by confrontation. If an inferior field defect is suspected, use the leg raising test or their ability to negotiate around objects on the floor without help.

Recognition of size and shape can be assessed using Lea's rectangle game or puzzle; orientation can be assessed using Lea's mailbox. A clinical protocol has been developed in south India to assess simultagnosia, recognition of emotions (emojis of happy, sad, angry faces), motion perception, and visual closure using simple in-house techniques/games. This protocol increases the proportion of children who can be assessed [33].

To simplify these tests and make them quicker for children with CVI, a tertiary vision rehabilitation center in collaboration with a software company in south India has developed VIKAS (Visual Intervention Kit with Analytics for children with Special needs), which tests 10 major visual skills using 34 simple games. Apart from assessment, VIKAS can also be used as an intervention kit. Repeated training improves visual cerebral abilities in children with special needs and aids in overall development [34].

Investigations

Although MRI (magnetic resonance imaging) is better than CT (computed tomography) in detecting CVI, a "normal" scan does not exclude CVI, and the extent of the changes in the brain does not always correlate with the severity of CVI. Functional MRI may be more valuable than other imaging techniques [32, 35]; VEP (visual evoked potential) may also be of value as a prognostic tool.

Interventions

Correcting refractive errors and poor accommodation is important, but the benefits of visual stimulation remain controversial [32]. A 52 item questionnaire (Insight Inventory) can be used to identify specific areas of functional difficulty [36]. The Inventory has corresponding vision support strategies for caregivers to improve their child's functioning, such as decluttering the environment, removing low furniture, telling the child to look down at their feet when going downstairs [37]. The realization that their child has a clinical problem rather than being stupid, awkward, or disobedient can also benefit parents.

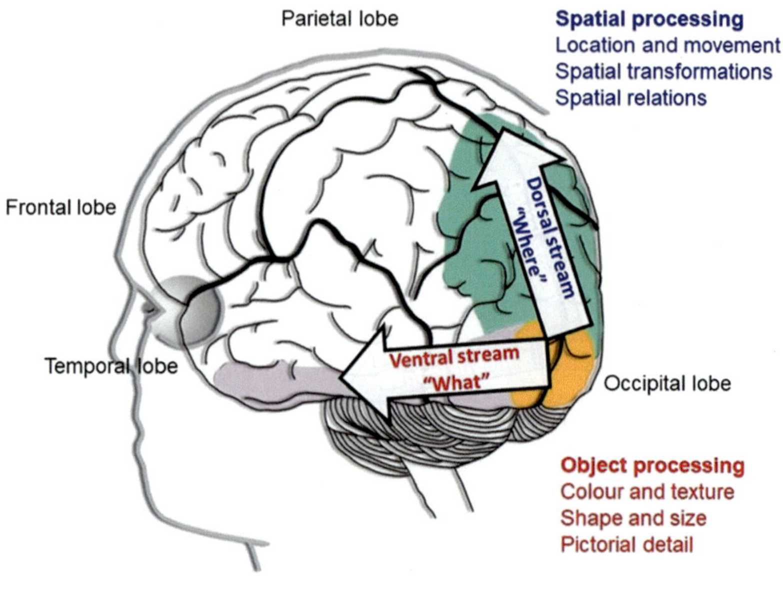

Fig. 11.4 Dorsal and ventral streams which transmit visual information to higher visual centers

11.1.4 Myopia in Children

In addition to the causes outlined above, refractive errors, particularly myopia, are an important and increasing cause of visual impairment and blindness in children [38]. Indeed, in 2004, there were an estimated 12.81 million children with visual impairment (<6/18 in the better eye) due to uncorrected refractive errors, principally myopia; roughly 1.6 million of these children lived in India [39]. Many more children will have milder degrees of impairment and require optical correction. The current epidemic of myopia is particularly acute in children and adolescents in South-East and East Asia. Myopia has an earlier age of onset in these regions, starting around the age of 6–10 years, and progresses to high myopia (more than −5.0 dioptres) in an increasing number of adolescents [38, 40]. Myopia has a genetic component but the current rapid increase is also likely to be due to environmental factors, such as reduced time spent outdoors in daylight [41], more intensive close work, increasing academic pressure, and the use of electronic devices from a very young age [42, 43].

11.1.5 Strategies for Control of Visual Impairment in Children

The strategies from a public health perspective are outlined below.

11.1.5.1 Primordial Prevention

Reduction in exposure to the risk factors for diseases causing blindness could benefit. Examples include preventing multiple births and teenage pregnancies to reduce the number of preterm births, and improving water supplies, sanitation, and young children's dietary intake to reduce the risk of vitamin A deficiency. Many of these interventions extend beyond eye care or even healthcare and will not be considered further.

11.1.5.2 Primary Prevention

These are specific interventions to prevent conditions causing blindness. Examples include measles immunization, vitamin A supplementation, ocular prophylaxis to prevent ophthalmic neonatorum, high-quality neonatal care from immediately after birth to reduce the incidence of sight-threatening ROP (ST-ROP) (i.e., Type 1), and reducing the intensity of close work and increasing the amount of time children spend outdoors to prevent myopia.

11.1.5.3 Secondary Prevention

This entails managing a potentially blinding eye condition to reduce the risk that it progresses to blindness. This includes diagnosing and treating corneal ulcers, screening for and treating ROP, as well as early detection and management of pediatric glaucoma.

11.1.5.4 Tertiary Prevention

Tertiary prevention has two components: (1) interventions that restore visual function in visually impaired children such as cataract surgery and spectacle correction for refractive errors; and (2) vision rehabilitation for irreversibly blind children to reduce disability by improving functioning, activities, and participation [44].

Ideally, all these different control strategies should be in place in any given catchment population to provide comprehensive eye care. Interventions and services are required at all service delivery levels, such as in the community, primary healthcare level, and in district and tertiary level facilities. Many interventions should be integrated into other services for children, such as newborn eye screening as part of the general examination of all newborns; eye care needs to be integrated into general primary child healthcare programs, and ROP services in all neonatal units caring for sick and preterm infants (Box 2). General ophthalmologists at the secondary level ideally should know more about eye care in children and have the required resources to manage less complex conditions, and refer children requiring more specialized management to tertiary level facilities, when required. Vision rehabilitation must also be available for children, with referral to special education or other support services.

Box 2. The National ROP Program in Sri Lanka

Tavisha Udupihille

Sirimavo Bandaranaike Specialized Children's Hospital, Peradeniya, Central Province

In Sri Lanka ROP screening and treatment are fully integrated into the health system. Healthcare in Sri Lanka is mainly publicly funded, with a parallel private sector that provides services for a small proportion of the population's healthcare needs.

Public healthcare is delivered by a series of regional hospitals, along with several referral centers. There are 2 national hospitals, 9 teaching hospitals, 6 specialized teaching hospitals, 10 other specialized hospitals, 2 provincial general hospitals, 20 district general hospitals, 28 base hospitals (type A), and 53 base hospitals (type B) to provide specialized care. Most of these hospitals have neonatal units, which vary in size and care level. Most are run by consultant pediatricians, and a few have consultant neonatologists.

Most of the type A base hospitals and above have consultant general ophthalmologists who perform ROP screening in 46 units. Hospitals without a consultant ophthalmologist, particularly type B base hospitals, refer babies needing ROP screening to the nearest hospital with a general ophthalmologist. Babies needing treatment for ROP are referred and transported by ambulance, if needed, to the nearest center that can provide laser treatment. There are six such units distributed across the country (Fig. 11.5), and all but one provide treatment at no cost to the parents. Occasionally, babies needing treatment, are too unstable to be transferred; these babies are initially treated with anti-VEGF (vascular endothelial growth factor) therapy at the screening unit and are then referred to a treatment center once stable.

The College of Ophthalmologists, Sri Lanka is the professional body responsible for formulating the ROP national guidelines. These were first developed in 2010, and the last revision was made in 2019 after a series of discussions involving pediatric ophthalmologists and vitreoretinal surgeons involved in ROP treatment. The College recommends ROP screening for babies who meet the following criteria: (1) gestational age <32 weeks; (2) birth weight <1500 g; or (3) any of the following sickness criteria in more mature babies—septicemia, hypothermia, respiratory distress syndrome, cyanotic congenital heart disease, oxygen therapy, or blood transfusion. It is recommended that the first screening takes place between 3 and 4 weeks of age.

This system has resulted in a high rate of prevention of ROP blindness. For example, one treatment unit in central Sri Lanka, which is the referral center for 20 of the 46 ROP screening units in Sri Lanka, screened/examined 286 babies in 2019. This included babies directly screened in the neonatal unit and other babies referred from other screening units for specialist opinion and/or treatment. Thirty babies were treated with laser and/or anti-VEGF therapy. Only one of these babies progressed to stage 4 ROP, and this baby became blind despite retinal surgery.

While the rate of ROP-related blindness is low, several challenges remain. The major challenges are: (1) reducing the incidence of ROP by improving the quality of neonatal care; (2) improving the detection of sight-threatening ROP by general ophthalmologists with timely referral to treatment units, and (3) reducing dropouts from the screening program by better educating parents and the general population. A national ROP data monitoring system would be of value but challenging to implement.

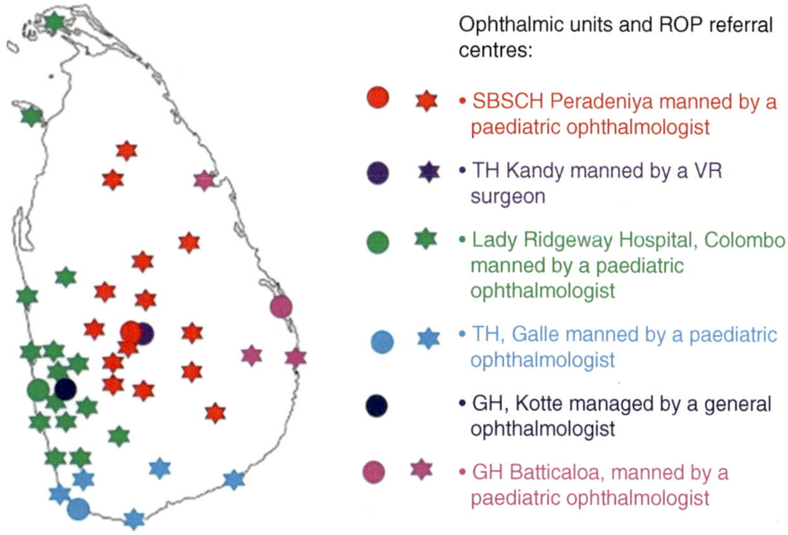

Fig. 11.5 Map of Sri Lanka showing ROP regions with screening sites (stars) and treatment centers (circles). *SBSCH* Sirimavo Bandaranayake specialized children hospital, *TH* tertiary hospital, *GH* general hospital

11.1.6 Control of Major Blinding Eye Diseases of Children in South-East Asia

1. **Primary prevention**

Primary prevention includes vitamin A supplementation, measles and rubella immunization, ocular prophylaxis of the newborn, and high-quality care to reduce the risk of sight-threatening (ST-ROP), Type 1 ROP.

Vitamin A deficiency

Despite global efforts to control vitamin A deficiency in preschool-age children through a range of interventions, it remains a public health problem in several South-East Asian countries; serum retinol levels remain low in many children in this area (Fig. 11.6) [45].

Vitamin A supplementation, delivered at the primary level or during community outreach, is one of the strategies adopted at the primary level for prevention of visual impairment in children. But the coverage with 6-monthly doses of retinyl palmitate to children aged 9–59 months remains low in several Asian countries (Fig. 11.7) [46]. In 2018, only 59% of preschool-age children in these countries had received two or more vitamin A doses. This situation must improve because vitamin A deficiency also increases the risk of mortality in preschool-age children. It is acknowledged that other interventions are possibly more sustainable, such as nutrition education, biofortification (e.g., red maize) [47], fortification of commonly consumed foods with vitamin A precursors, such as cooking oil, sugar, and flour [48], and adding micronutrient powders to young children's food [49]. The use of genetically modified "golden rice" remains controversial for many reasons, including loss of biodiversity [50]. However, focusing on just one micronutrient will not address the under-nutrition that affects a relatively high proportion of young children in some South-East Asian countries. Improving the nutritional status of children will require concerted, broad-based approaches such as those outlined in "Scaling up Nutrition" [51].

Measles infection and congenital rubella syndrome

Measles immunization is also an important strategy, as children with measles can develop corneal blindness due to several reasons, including vitamin A deficiency. Measles infection can cause acute vitamin A deficiency through several mechanisms: (1) lower dietary intake due to anorexia, herpes stomatitis, or customs about what to feed sick children; (2) increased demand for vitamin A due to fever and to repair epithelial damage (which requires vitamin A); and (3) loss of serum

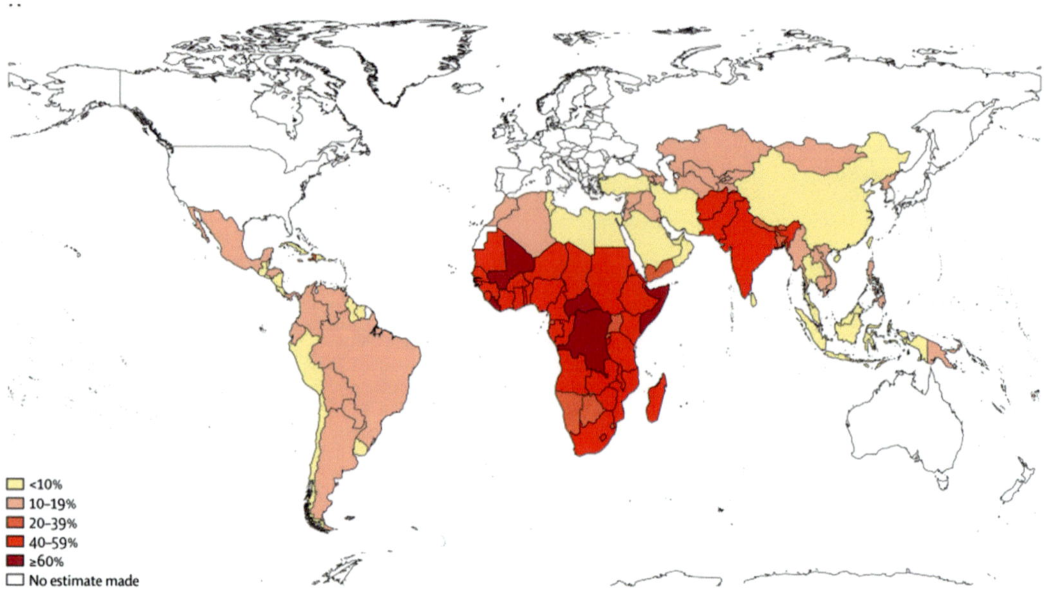

Fig. 11.6 Prevalence of vitamin A deficiency (serum retinol levels) in preschool children between 1991 and 2013 [45]

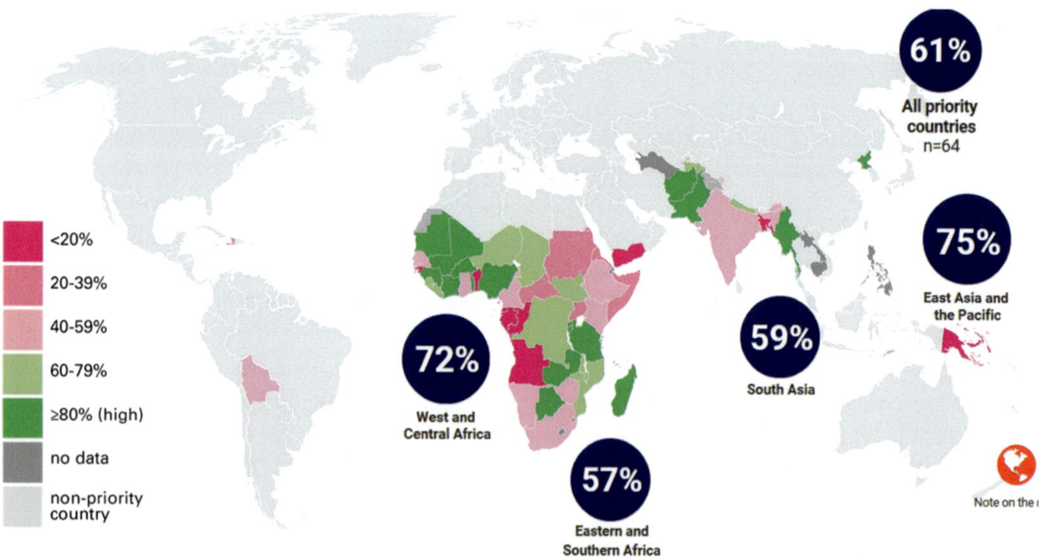

Fig. 11.7 Vitamin A supplementation coverage with two doses in 2018 [United Nations Children's Fund (UNICEF)] [46]

retinol in feces and urine from infection of the mucosa in the gut and bladder. Other causes of corneal ulceration include herpetic and bacterial corneal ulceration, and in some regions of the world, the use of harmful traditional remedies [52]. The measles immunization coverage is not as high as it should be (>95% coverage is required to prevent epidemics) (Fig. 11.8) [54], and this is falling in many regions, including Europe, partly as a result of ill-founded fears that vaccination may lead to autism. Coverage is likely to fall further because of the COVID-19 pandemic. India has the largest number of children unvaccinated for measles in the region (Table 11.5).

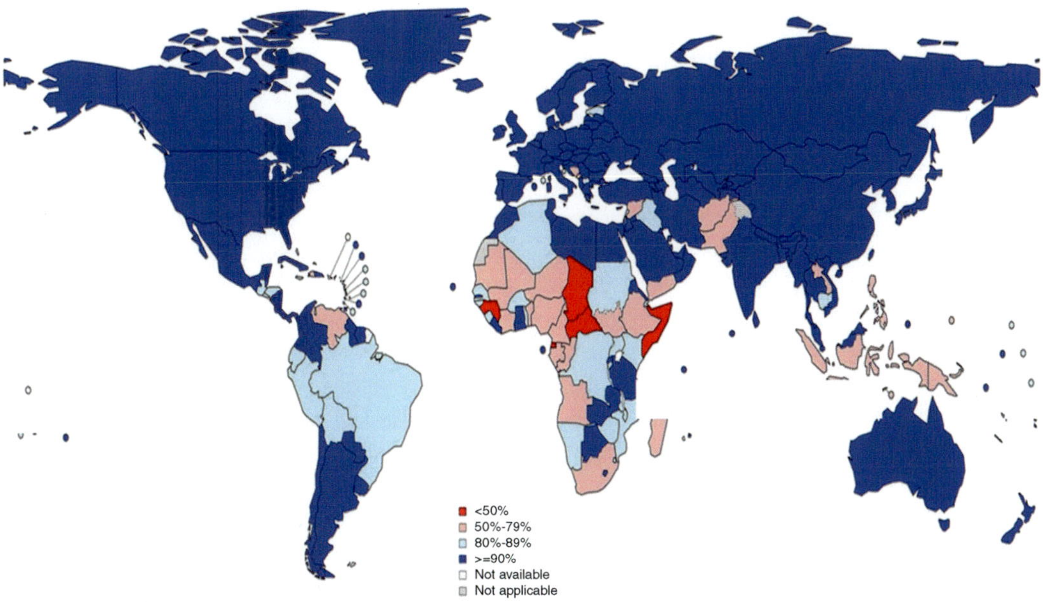

Fig. 11.8 Measles immunization coverage with the first dose in 2018 [53]

Table 11.5 Number of children not receiving their first dose of measles vaccine in the WHO South-East Asia Region [54]

Country	Number unvaccinated against measles	As a % of unvaccinated children in SEAR
India	1,169,000	57
Bangladesh	85,000	4
Nepal	44,000	2
Indonesia	556,000	28
Myanmar	145,000	7
Thailand	28,000	1
Korea	7,000	<1
Total	2,034,000	100

No data from Bhutan, Maldives, Sri Lanka, and Timor-Leste

Many countries in this region also immunize against rubella to prevent congenital rubella syndrome. It is also important to maintain high coverage to prevent unvaccinated girls from becoming infected during epidemics when they reach childbearing age [55].

Ophthalmia neonatorum
Conjunctivitis of the newborn, which manifests within 28 days of birth, is caused by an infection acquired during delivery. It can be due to a wide range of organisms; of all others, gonococcal infection is the most virulent, and without treatment, up to 3% of newborns developing this condition can go blind [56]. Primary prevention entails detecting and treating sexually transmitted diseases during pregnancy. Many countries have policies in place to conduct ocular prophylaxis, i.e., cleaning the eyelids at birth and instilling an antibiotic or antiseptic agent in the eyes. However, in the absence of robust evidence from clinical trials, there is no consensus regarding the optimal prophylactic agent [57]. The extent to which *Gonococcus neisseria* is resistant to penicillin or other antibiotics also needs to be considered. Many countries recommend the use of topical erythromycin (tetracycline cannot be used due to side effects in neonates).

Retinopathy of prematurity (ROP)
The WHO recommends a course of antenatal steroids to women with threatened preterm delivery as an important primary preventive strategy for ROP [58]. This is usually a good strategy as steroids also mature the lungs, and reduces the need for respiratory support. Other primary preventive

measures include high-quality neonatal care from immediately after birth. Evidence-based interventions during the "first golden hour" after birth include not clamping the umbilical cord until 60–90 s after birth to prevent hypovolemia, keeping the newborn warm by using an occlusive wrap, or putting the baby's body in a plastic bag; avoiding all forms of respiratory support, including ventilation and supplemental oxygen, unless absolutely necessary [59], and administration of caffeine soon after birth to improve systemic blood flow and blood pressure [60].

High-quality care is needed to reduce exposure to modifiable risk factors during the neonatal stay, including careful delivery of supplemental oxygen with monitoring of oxygen saturation to prevent hyperoxia and fluctuating hypoxia/hyperoxia. A report from India has shown extensive damage to the retinal circulation and very aggressive ROP secondary to unmonitored 100% supplemental oxygen use. This confirms that oxygen is highly toxic to retinal blood vessels (and other tissues) [61]. To safely deliver oxygen, one requires blenders to mix 100% oxygen with air to the lowest concentration needed to maintain oxygen saturation within the target of 89–94% [62]; use of humidifiers so that the air/oxygen mix is not too dry; appropriate devices to deliver the oxygen to the baby (nasal prongs and systems for continuous positive airway pressure, CPAP, that keep the lungs expanded); and pulse oximeters with monitors to continuously measure oxygen saturation. The monitors have alarms set to go off if the oxygen saturation levels fluctuate beyond the set limits which is 88–94%, based on evidence from clinical trials [63]. Besides, the neonatal staff must possess skills to use and maintain the equipment, respond if an alarm goes off, and very importantly, be taught that high oxygen saturation levels are damaging to the developing retinal blood vessels, and that this condition is a precursor for ROP.

Another modifiable risk factor is sepsis; this can be reduced by acceptable infection control practices, including handwashing and reducing unnecessary handling and venepuncture. Ensuring that preterm infants have adequate nutrition so that they gain weight is equally important [64], and human milk [65], including colostrum, is vital for a healthy gut microbiome [66], which also reduces infection. Human milk can be given in very small amounts from within days of birth; enteral feeding may be required to ensure an adequate calorie and nutrient intake. Other risk factors include blood transfusions and, more recently, thrombocytopenia, which was first recognized as a risk factor in India [67, 68]. Developmental supportive care is also important as it promotes neurodevelopment, keeps preterm infants stable, and improves bonding with caregivers. Supportive care includes kangaroo mother care, keeping the temperature stable and reducing noise and pain, allowing babies time to sleep, and nursing the infant in a "nest" that can be made from a towel or foam roll under the bedsheet. Supportive care requires few additional resources and can be successfully implemented in Asia [69].

There is conclusive evidence that high-quality care can almost eliminate the risk of ST-ROP and aggressive posterior ROP in infants with a birth weight above 1250 g; however, extremely preterm infants (less than 1000 g) are still at risk. As indicated above, providing this level of care is challenging in low resource settings, where functioning equipment and adequately trained neonatal and nursing staff can be in short supply. In many countries in Asia, the provision of neonatal care does not yet meet the demand, and units can be overcrowded, which increases the risk of infection, and babies are sometimes discharged home early. There is a great need to train members of the neonatal team to be aware of the factors which increase the risk of ROP and the means to minimize them.

Myopia

Control of myopia by modifying the amount of time children spend outdoors and reducing prolonged close work is an intense area of research, and there is some evidence that increasing the amount of time children spend outdoors reduces the incidence (i.e., the development of myopia) but has little impact on the progression of preexisting myopia [70]. Also, there are a range of other potentially beneficial pharmacological and optical interventions [71].

2. **Secondary prevention**

Secondary prevention entails managing eye conditions to prevent the consequences of visual impairment.

Measles and vitamin A deficiency
All children with measles infection must be given two doses of vitamin A on day 1 and day 2, either orally, and parenterally, if they are too sick to swallow. The dose is: children aged >12 months—200,000 IU retinyl palmitate; infants aged 6–11 months—100,000 IU retinyl palmitate; and infants <6 months 50,000 IU retinyl palmitate. Restoring the vitamin A levels of children with measles reduces the risk of keratomalacia and increases their chance of survival [72]. The same applies to all children with signs of vitamin A deficiency (xerophthalmia). The required dose depends on the child's age (as above), given on day 1, day 2, and 2 weeks later. This simple, low-cost intervention saves both sight and life.

ROP screening and treatment
Screening and treatment of ROP require a good understanding of the International Classification of ROP (ICROP) [73], which describes the degree of maturity of the retinal blood vessels, five stages and three zones of ROP, and the presence of plus or pre-plus disease depending on the degree of dilation and tortuosity of retinal blood vessels. The indications for treatment use a combination of these signs, which is largely driven by the presence of plus disease. The ICROP is currently being revised.

Timely screening of preterm infants at risk, followed by urgent treatment of ST-ROP prevents ROP-related blindness. In each setting, evidence of the birth weight (BW) and gestational age (GA) of preterm infants who develop ST-ROP should be used to define screening criteria, which can be modified over time as better evidence becomes available. One set of screening criteria is not suitable for all settings, [74] as larger, more mature infants also develop ST-ROP in settings where neonatal care is suboptimal compared with settings where the quality of care is high [75]. Most countries use a combination of BW and GA criteria, and some add a "sickness" criteria for more mature infants who were exposed to other risk factors, such as prolonged exposure to oxygen.

Timing of the first screening is also important; too early before the ROP features have developed, or too late after the disease has advanced, does not help. Some countries use post-menstrual age (chronological age plus gestational age) to determine when screening should start [76], but in settings where GA is unreliable, chronological age is used, such as by 30 days of life, as in India [77]. The latter is easy for providers and parents to remember.

Ophthalmologists who visit the neonatal unit usually undertake screening by examining infants using a binocular indirect ophthalmoscope, with the assistance of a trained ROP nurse [78]. Wide-field imaging systems can also be used, either with bedside interpretation of the image or remote reading by ROP experts [79, 80]; in India, a pilot study of image analysis using artificial intelligence has recently been undertaken [81]. In either situation, it is the responsibility of the neonatal team to identify and list infants eligible for screening. At each screening, the findings and management decisions must be documented in the medical records. If further screening or treatment is required, this must also be communicated to the neonatal team and caregivers. There is evidence in India and elsewhere that not all infants who should be screened are screened; in addition, many do not complete the follow-up screenings [82, 83]. Systems must be put in place to ensure that no eligible infants miss screening; one way to increase screening coverage is for the first screening to be done before the baby is discharged from the neonatal care center, even if this is a bit early [84]. A package of different interventions, including parental counseling, can increase uptake of screening services [84]. Operational guidelines, such as those drawn up for India, and protocols are useful for all aspects of screening [85, 86].

The gold standard treatment for ST-ROP is confluent laser photocoagulation to the peripheral, avascular retina. A high degree of skill is required to administer the treatment, given either under analgesia with or without sedation or general anesthesia. Intravitreal injection of agents which block vascular endothelial growth factors (anti-VEGF agents) is sometimes used instead of or in addition to the laser treatment. These agents have some advantages over lasers, as the treatment is quicker and can lead to complete resolution of ROP, and there is some evidence that high degrees of myopia are less likely than after laser treatment [87]. However, in a significant proportion of cases, the ROP recurs at an unpredictable time after treatment with intravitreal anti-VEGF, which means that regular long-term follow-up is essential. As the anti-VEGF agents can pass into the systematic circulation and block endogenous VEGF when the brain, lungs, and other organs are developing, there are concerns about negative neurodevelopmental and other long-term consequences of this treatment [87–89]. For these reasons, many countries recommend that anti-VEGF agents only be used as "rescue" therapy after careful explanation to parents; this usually happens when laser treatment is not possible for clinical reasons or where the risk of progression to stages 4 and 5 is very high, such as in aggressive posterior ROP. Extensive research is currently underway to investigate the most effective anti-VEGF agent, the minimum required dose which in the case of bevacizumab was a fraction of the dose used in the BEAT-ROP trial, and whether lower doses are associated with better ocular outcomes [90–92].

Regardless of the type of treatment, infants must be followed up in the short term to ensure complete regression of ROP, with repeated treatments if required. Regular and long-time follow-up is also needed, particularly for treated infants to detect and manage complications, including early-onset (i.e., during the first year of life) refractive errors, strabismus, and cataract [93].

Correction of refractive errors

The correction of refractive errors in school children is covered in another chapter. The International Agency for the Prevention of Blindness (IAPB) has produced guidelines for school eye health programs for low and middle-income countries, which could be adapted for countries in the South-East Asian region [94].

Children with congenital eye anomalies such as microphthalmos and coloboma can also have refractive errors, which need to be corrected at an early age to prevent amblyopia.

3. **Tertiary prevention**

Surgery

High-quality surgery is required for children with congenital and developmental cataract, but surgery with or without an intraocular lens is only the first step in their vision rehabilitation. Regular follow-up is required to detect and manage short- and long-term complications and ensure optical correction of the eyes as the child grows and the visual demands change. The outcomes of surgery for developmental cataract are better than those for congenital cataracts, as surgery for cataract surgery is often delayed due to late presentation. There is also some evidence that girls with cataracts in Asia are less likely to access surgery than boys, an issue of gender bias which must be addressed [95].

Complex vitreoretinal surgery for stage 4 ROP is often indicated, and the structural and functional outcomes of such a surgery can be useful. However, the visual outcomes following surgery for stage 5 ROP are usually inferior even if the retina can be reattached, and this is why surgery for stage 5 ROP is generally not performed in high-income settings.

Vision rehabilitation

Vision rehabilitation is required for children with a wide range of eye conditions. This is best delivered by teams who understand visual and child development, and other professionals such as physiotherapists, speech therapists, and educationalists. Early intervention is recommended for infants with profound visual impairment, as lack of vision at this age can be associated with developmental delays in many areas. There are three potential outcomes of rehabilitation—improvement in vision function (i.e., visual acuity, visual fields), improvement of visual functioning (i.e., activities and behavior using vision), and coping with visual disabilities [96].

There are different schools of thought about which interventions are the most beneficial, which can broadly be described as vision stimulation (such as moving or flashing lights or shapes) or visual training/vision promotion where carers use other senses, such as touch, sound, and speech to aid the child interpret and interact with their surroundings. The latter has been described as interventions to improve "seeing" (i.e., paying attention and responding to what is seen or experienced rather than "looking" which is more passive [97]. Although limited, the available evidence supports vision promotion rather than visual stimulation using interventions which maximize use of the available vision for the child's general development [96]. There is some evidence that the more frequent the input that parents can provide after training and support, the more the child will benefit compared with other forms of intervention [98]. However, more research is needed in this area but rehabilitation is a challenging area to study because of heterogeneity in the characteristics of the children affected, the wide range of interventions possible, and the variety of possible outcomes.

Counseling

Counseling parents or guardians is of critical importance, using language and/or materials appropriate to their education level. Repeated counseling is often required, and in large tertiary units, a trained, dedicated counselor is recommended.

11.1.7 Bringing the Strategies Together

The main causes of avoidable blindness and visual impairment in children must be known so that relevant strategies can be identified to control visual impairment. Some of the strategies may be implemented in the community, while others are implemented at the primary, secondary, and/or tertiary levels of the health system (Fig. 11.9) (Box 3). In addition to providing high-quality clinical and rehabilitation services in the hospital, the staff working in tertiary level facilities should ideally take the lead to improve comprehensive eye care services in the catchment population of

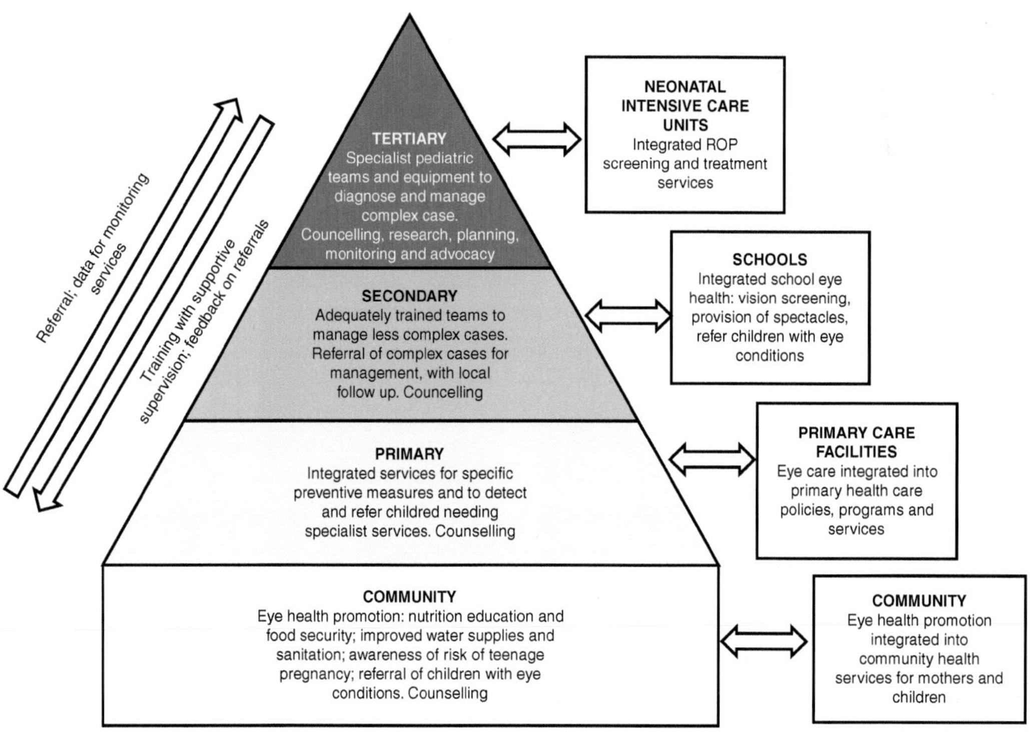

Fig. 11.9 Comprehensive, integrated eye care services for children

Box 3. Childhood Blindness Prevention Program in South Sulawesi, Indonesia

Habibah S. Muhiddin, Dyah Ayu Windy, Idayani Panggalo

South Sulawesi Indonesian Ophthalmologists Association

In 2014, a program to prevent blindness in children was established by the South Sulawesi Regional Government in collaboration with the South Sulawesi Health Department, South Sulawesi Indonesian Ophthalmologists Association (IOA), the Ophthalmology Department Faculty of Medicine Hasanuddin University, and Hasanuddin University Hospital. The program includes early detection of refractive errors, white pupil screening in primary healthcare (PHC) facilities, and an ROP network in South Sulawesi Province. The program collaborated with Helen Keller International, ORBIS International, and CBM, and was supported by Standard Chartered Bank's "Seeing is Believing" program (2015–2020).

Early detection of refractive error

This program component was initially carried out as a pilot program in the schools of six districts in South Sulawesi between 2016 and 2018. By 2020, it had expanded to 24 districts. Teams were built at the provincial, city, and district levels. Agreements were drawn between Hasanuddin University Hospital, South Sulawesi Educational Department, South Sulawesi Health Department, South Sulawesi IOA, and South Sulawesi IROPIN organization of refractionists and opticians in Indonesia.

Initially IOA and IROPIN conducted a training of trainers at the provincial level, with 3–5 delegates from each district. Those trained then trained district-level school health teachers, primary health care (PHC) staff, and community volunteers attached to PHC clinics. In this program, 1096 PHC staff, 521 teachers, and 6859 volunteers were trained. By 2020, 173,858 children had been screened, 3129 of whom received glasses, and 5068 were referred to eye care services.

Screening for white pupils

In collaboration with the Indonesian Pediatricians Association, 10,000 general practitioners, midwives, and other staff in 4594 PHC clinics and maternal and child health posts in 24 districts were trained to detect leucocoria using a penlight/torch or direct ophthalmoscope, when available. White pupil screening is now a standard operating procedure during immunization and monthly monitoring of child development for children under 5. During this program, 85,452 babies and young children were screened, and 3801 were referred to eye care providers.

ROP network

In a study in 2012, 15.5% of preterm infants screened for ROP developed ROP. In another study, 6.5% of 682 infants screened between 2013 and 2019 at the Wahidin Sudirohusodo Hospital and Hasanuddin University Hospital, Makassar developed ROP. Nine babies with ST-ROP were treated with laser therapy and/or anti-VEGF injection, of which four infants developed Stage 5 ROP because of late intervention. To expand the scope of screening and treatment services, an ROP network was created. Training was a key component in which capacity building was carried out with fellowships and training of ophthalmologists and ophthalmic nurses in India and Scotland, which was also supported by VISION 2020 UK. Ophthalmic nurses were trained to screen children using a RetCam that was provided by the program.

In December 2019, the South Sulawesi IOA signed a tripartite agreement with Hasanuddin University Hospital, South Sulawesi Provincial Health Department, other hospitals involved in the project, South Sulawesi IDAI (Ikatan Dokter Anak Indonesia), Indonesian Anesthesiologist Association, and Indonesian Midwives Association for an ROP Program. A call center was established to contact parents and to respond to their concerns or questions. A team of ROP professionals was established, comprising of three pediatric ophthalmologists, four vitreo-retina experts, two screening nurses, and two administration staff. We now have agreements with ten hospitals that have joined the network, and services are expanding, with screening being undertaken using a portable RetCam.

Sustainability of all of these initiatives after the "Seeing is Believing" funded ended is assured because of the widespread collaboration and agreements between services providers, professional groups, provincial Education and Health Departments, and the Regional Eye Committees. School eye health is now routine in elementary and junior high schools, and white pupil screening for young children has become a standard procedure. Funding for ROP screening and treatment will continue as the costs are covered by national health insurance or private insurance, even in private hospitals.

their hospital. This may include identifying all the neonatal intensive care units in the area and advocating for and providing ROP services, if these are not already in place. The tertiary level team's function is also to provide training, mentoring, and supportive supervision for ophthalmologists working at the district and secondary level eye care facilities (Box 4).

School eye health programs can also be planned at the tertiary level, working closely with the Departments of Education so that the services are integrated into school health policies and activities. Implementation of school eye health programs can also be carried out by secondary level teams, with referral of children with serious eye conditions to the tertiary level if required. Primary eye care (PEC) for children (and adults) has been a neglected area. The best way to achieve high coverage of services is to advocate with the Ministries of Health to ensure that eye care is included in the training curriculum for primary level child healthcare workers, as has been done in Tanzania [99] and Bangladesh (Box 5).

Box 4. Tertiary Level Pediatric Eye Care Team: The Tilganga Story

Sanduk Ruit, Srijana Adhikari

Tilganga Institute of Ophthalmology, Kathmandu, Nepal

The Tilganga Institute of Ophthalmology (TIO) is a tertiary referral hospital with six main wings—hospital services; outreach; academic and training department; research; and the Fred Hollows intraocular lab and eye bank. The Department of Pediatric Ophthalmology and Strabismus is one of the ten subspecialties at TIO. The work is primarily focused on four areas—hospital services; research; academics and training; and outreach. The Department has its own director and a manager and the following eye care professionals: consultant pediatric ophthalmologists, ophthalmology fellows, optometrists, ophthalmic assistants, orthoptists, and eye health workers trained in eye diseases in children and their management. There are also pediatrician, pediatric anesthesiologist, and geneticist.

Mid-level eye health personnel, including eye health workers, ophthalmic assistants, and optometrists, are the backbone of eye care service delivery in Nepal. They work as a team and assist in pediatric refraction, orthoptics, counseling, investigations, and anesthetic assistants. At TIO there is a strong workforce and infrastructure to undertake ~3000 pediatric surgeries throughout the year. Cataract surgery is the most common procedure, followed by surgery for strabismus, trauma, pediatric retina, glaucoma, and oculoplastics.

Creating future leaders in pediatric ophthalmology is one of our goals. Short- and long-term fellowship programs, modular training, and continuous medical education are conducted throughout the year. Trainees from within and outside the country undertake training; TIO pediatric department has trained ophthalmologists and paramedics from Africa (Ethiopia, Ghana, Tanzania), and Asia (Indonesia, Bangladesh, Cambodia, Myanmar, and Bhutan). The TIO faculty members are also involved in hospital-based training programs in many countries.

Box 5. Incorporating Eye Care in Integrated Management of Childhood Illness (IMCI) in Bangladesh

AHM Enayet Hossain and Khaleda Islam
Bangladesh

In Bangladesh, primary health care in the public sector is delivered in community clinics, union sub-centers, and Upazila (sub-district) Health Complexes. District hospitals provide secondary care, and medical college hospitals and specialized institutes deliver tertiary care.

A study in 2003 showed that there were approximately 40,000 blind children in Bangladesh, 68% from avoidable causes, mainly vitamin A deficiency, cataracts, and corneal scarring. About 85% of blind children were either born blind or became blind before 6 years [100]. Another study estimated the prevalence of blindness to be 6.3/10,000 children, and 84% of the causes were congenital [15]. Over the last two decades, several initiatives have been made to address childhood blindness, including strengthening tertiary eye care across the country, but it continues to remain a public health problem.

Aligned with the WHO's Global Action Plan [101] to ensure primary eye care in primary level facilities, the Ministry of Health and Family Welfare in its 4th Health Population Nutrition Sector Program [102] has prioritized eye care and developed the National Eye Care Operational Plan (NEC OP). As a result, 70 community vision centers were established in 24 districts, staffed by trained ophthalmic nurses who are connected via telemedicine to the district or medical college hospitals. By June 2022, 200 vision centers are planned [103]. But, primary eye care for children was not adequately represented in the Government's essential service package; it is sporadically supported by non-government organizations (NGOs). Eye care is not included in the WHO's Integrated Management of Childhood Illness (IMCI) program at primary level; routine eye screening and eye care for children aged 0–5 years is therefore inadequate.

To address this, in 2016, with support from WHO, a pilot package of interventions to identify and refer children with eye conditions by PHC workers was developed and delivered in one sub-district [104]. Given the success of this initiative, it was decided to include eye care in the IMCI program, which has been operational across Bangladesh since 1998 [105]. IMCI is now included in the curriculum of medical, nursing, and paramedical students for effective implementation.

Several consultation meetings were held in 2017 involving a wide range of stakeholders in newborn care, child health, and eye care from the government, United Nations agencies, NGOs, professional associations, and district program managers. Delegates decided that including eye care and screening in IMCI would benefit around 7.5 million children every year, using the same resources and workforce with some additional training. In May 2018, government policymakers, WHO, UNICEF, and technical experts agreed to include eye care in IMCI, and Sightsavers supported a pilot project in one district [106].

A technical group developed the curriculum and training materials, which included screening using a torch [107]. Guidelines for identifying eye problems were produced, and strong referral mechanisms to the district hospital eye department were developed. IMCI recording forms for children <2 months and 2–59 months of age were updated to include eye conditions, and referral slips and reporting forms were designed. The eye conditions screened for in children aged 0–59 months were a white pupillary reflex, watering, red or discharging eye(s), and structural abnormalities. Eye injuries, squints, and concerns about vision were added for older children.

The project started in July 2018. The IMCI staff started screening children, and cases requiring further eye care interventions were referred to the sub-district medical officer for treatment or were referred to the district hospital ophthalmologist. Working group members conducted regular monitoring and supportive supervision to ensure the quality of care and reporting. The IMCI national database, District Health Information Software 2 (DHIS2), of the DGHS was modified to include eye conditions, and facilities used this system for monthly reporting. This project mostly focused on health system strengthening.

Based on the lessons learned from the pilot project, the Government included the eye care component of the IMCI protocol in the National New-Born Health Program (NNHP) and scaled it up nationwide. A budget was allocated in the HHNP operation plan to train IMCI staff. National data are being recorded in the updated DHIS2 platform, and NNHP monitors and provides supportive supervision. All these initiatives showed an increasing number of children benefitting from eye care services.

Lessons Learned

- IMCI staff could screen and refer cases confidently after basic training. Additional in-service training increased performance.
- The eye care component of the IMCI was included in monthly facility coordination meetings, which increased awareness among all stakeholders.
- The orientation of community health workers on eye care in IMCI clinics increased awareness and referrals from the community to PHC clinics.
- Good follow-up, coordination, and strong referral mechanisms improved the quality of eye care.

Conclusions and Recommendations

Integrating eye care into the IMCI program was a feasible, efficient, effective, and sustainable way to address primary eye care for children in Bangladesh. Success depends on the facility readiness in terms of logistics, equipment, and trained health workforce. Basic training and refresher training (as trained staff may be transferred) are essential. Incorporating eye care into IMCI is an excellent example of using available resources to address avoidable blindness in children by strengthening the health system to ensure universal eye care in Bangladesh.

These examples and some of the other case studies from the region demonstrate the importance of engaging the Ministries of Health and other key stakeholders from the beginning. This approach leads to affordable, scalable, and sustainable services.

Primary eye care services should include newborn eye screening, which is included in the Government of India's child eye care policy and program, Rashtriya Bal Swasthya Karyakram (RBSK). The program ensures the detection and referral of children with white pupils or other serious eye conditions, ensuring high coverage of measles immunization, vitamin A supplementation and ocular prophylaxis, health education, and counseling. The most effective way to ensure health promotion in the community is to collaborate with organizations and agencies who work in

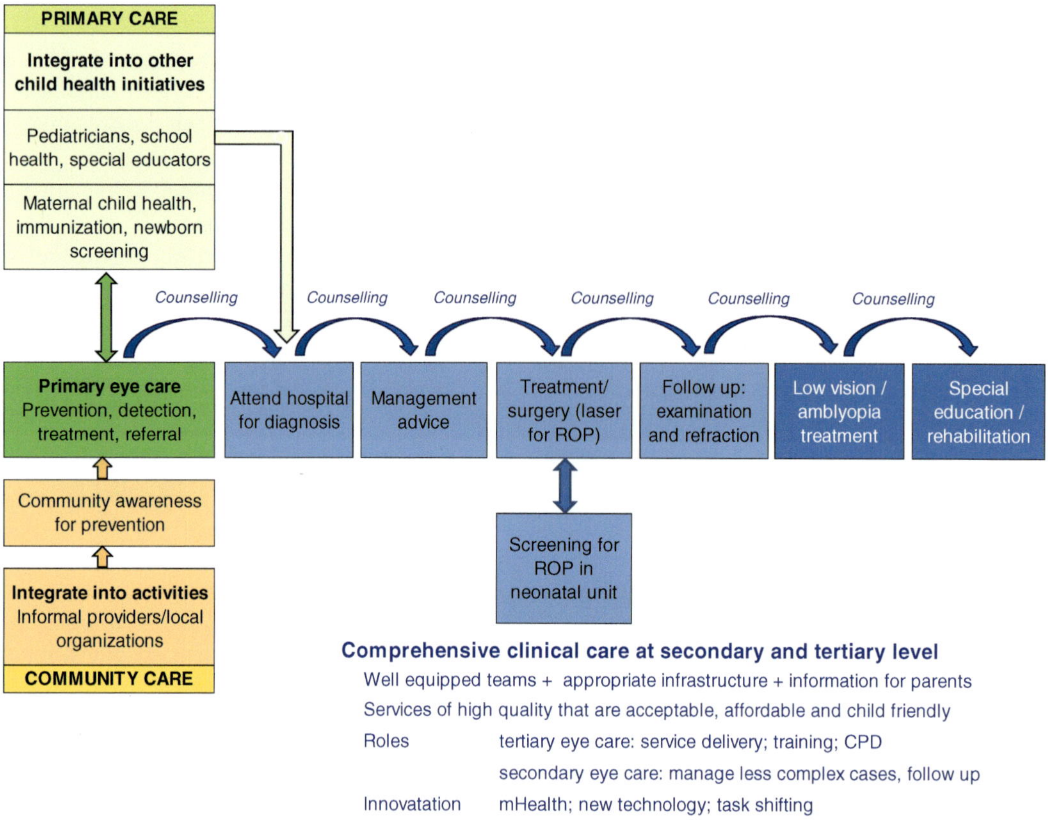

Fig. 11.10 The continuum of care (Adapted from Dr. P. Vijayalakshmi, Aravind Eye Care System). *CPD* continuing professional development

the community on maternal and child health (Fig. 11.9). Health information management systems to track follow-up and referrals at and between levels would also be highly desirable to ensure a continuum of care (Fig. 11.10).

VISON 2020—the "Right to Sight" initiative of the WHO and IAPB, which prioritized the control of blindness in children, closed at the end of 2020. Many countries in the WHO South-East Asia region have achieved a great deal thanks to the leadership, commitment, dedication, hard work, and support of many. However, children are still becoming blind and are remaining blind despite effective strategies for control due to lack of adequately trained and equipped eye care personnel and teams, and lack of accessible primary eye care for children. The WHO's approach to equitable, affordable, and sustainable healthcare through universal health coverage [108] offers a unique opportunity to address some of these challenges. The WHO's World Report on Vision [109] recommends Integrated People-Centered Eye Care. To address this, the WHO is developing evidence-based packages of eye care interventions, supported by a planning and financing tool (OneHealth). The packages are principally for the Ministries of Health so that eye care can be included in their national strategic development and health plans, for health workforce planning, for example. The WHO package of eye care interventions specifically includes congenital cataract and glaucoma, ROP, strabismus, and amblyopia [110].

Another key recommendation of the World Report on Vision is to integrate eye care into the health system at all levels, which is particularly important for child eye health; interventions need to be integrated into the care of healthy and sick newborns, into primary level child health programs [99], and into school and adolescent health. Eye care be an integral part of rehabilitation care, and more importantly, must be integrated into child health policies [111]. Many eye care interventions are complex or entail packages of interventions; a systematic evaluation is required to assess the effectiveness of integration [111, 112]. Universal health coverage provides a mechanism for integrating sustainable, affordable eye care services for all ages, including children, even in the poorest countries, with appropriate health workforce planning, financing, and monitoring indicators.

References

1. Preventing blindness in children. Geneva: World Health Organization; 2000. WHO/PBL/00.77.
2. Sommer A, Davidson FR. Assessment and control of vitamin A deficiency: the Annecy Accords. J Nutr. 2002;132(9 Suppl):2845S–50S.
3. Gilbert C, Foster A, Negrel AD, et al. Childhood blindness: a new form for recording causes of visual loss in children. Bull World Health Organ. 1993;71:485–9.
4. Gogate P, Kishore H, Dole K, et al. The pattern of childhood blindness in Karnataka, South India. Ophthalmic Epidemiol. 2009;16:212–7.
5. Bhattacharjee H, Das K, Borah RR, et al. Causes of childhood blindness in the northeastern states of India. Indian J Ophthalmol. 2008;56:495–9.
6. Gogate P, Deshpande M, Sudrik S, et al. Changing pattern of childhood blindness in Maharashtra, India. Br J Ophthalmol. 2007;91:8–12.
7. Hornby SJ, Adolph S, Gothwal VK, et al. Evaluation of children in six blind schools of Andhra Pradesh. Indian J Ophthalmol. 2000;48:195–200.
8. Krishnaiah S, Subba Rao B, Lakshmi Narasamma K, et al. A survey of severe visual impairment in children attending schools for the blind in a coastal district of Andhra Pradesh in South India. Eye (Lond). 2012;26:1065–70.
9. Magdula I. Childhood blindness in India – regional variations. J Clin Diagn Res. 2009;3:1255–60.
10. Pal N, Titiyal JS, Tandon R, et al. Need for optical and low vision services for children in schools for the blind in North India. Indian J Ophthalmol. 2006;54:189–93.
11. Titiyal JS, Pal N, Murthy GV, et al. Causes and temporal trends of blindness and severe visual impairment in children in schools for the blind in North India. Br J Ophthalmol. 2003;87:941–5.
12. Bhalerao SA, Tandon M, Singh S, et al. Visual impairment and blindness among the students of blind schools in Allahabad and its vicinity: a causal assessment. Indian J Ophthalmol. 2015;63:254–8.
13. Kemmanu V, Giliyar SK, Shetty BK, et al. Emerging trends in childhood blindness and ocular morbidity in India: the Pavagada Pediatric Eye Disease Study 2. Eye (Lond). 2018;32:1590–8.
14. Prakash MV, Sivakumar S, Dayal A, et al. Ocular morbidity patterns among children in schools for the blind in Chennai. Indian J Ophthalmol. 2017;65:733–7.
15. Hussain A, Ferdoush J, Mashreky SR, et al. Epidemiology of childhood blindness: a community-based study in Bangladesh. PLoS One. 2019;14:e0211991. https://doi.org/10.1371/journal.pone.0211991.
16. Muhit MA, Shah SP, Gilbert CE, et al. Causes of severe visual impairment and blindness in Bangladesh: a study of 1935 children. Br J Ophthalmol. 2007;91:1000–4.
17. Muhit MA. Developing a comprehensive approach to blindness and disability in children: epidemiological and qualitative studies in Bangladesh. PhD Thesis. International Centre for Eye Health, London School of Hygiene & Tropical Medicine; 2010.
18. Mactaggart I, Murthy G. The key informant child disability project in Bangladesh and Pakistan. London School of Hygiene & Tropical Medicine; 2013. https://www.lshtm.ac.uk/media/23736. Accessed 6 Nov 2020.
19. Adhikari S, Shrestha MK, Adhikari K, et al. Causes of visual impairment and blindness in children in three ecological regions of Nepal: Nepal Pediatric Ocular Diseases Study. Clin Ophthalmol. 2015;9:1543–7.
20. Byanju RN, Kandel RP, Sharma P, et al. Childhood blindness and visual impairment in the Narayani Zone of Nepal: a population-based survey. Ophthalmic Epidemiol. 2019;26:257–63.
21. Sitorus RS, Abidin MS, Prihartono J. Causes and temporal trends of childhood blindness in Indonesia: study at schools for the blind in Java. Br J Ophthalmol. 2007;91:1109–13.
22. Muhit M, Karim T, Islam J, et al. The epidemiology of childhood blindness and severe visual impairment in Indonesia. Br J Ophthalmol. 2018;102:1543–9.
23. Muecke J, Hammerton M, Aung YY, et al. A survey of visual impairment and blindness in children attending seven schools for the blind in Myanmar. Ophthalmic Epidemiol. 2009;16:370–7.
24. Gao Z, Muecke J, Edussuriya K, et al. A survey of severe visual impairment and blindness in children attending thirteen schools for the blind in Sri Lanka. Ophthalmic Epidemiol. 2011;18:36–43.
25. Gilbert C, Bowman R, Malik AN. The epidemiology of blindness in children: changing priorities. Community Eye Health. 2017;30:74–7.
26. Blencowe H, Lawn JE, Vazquez T, et al. Preterm-associated visual impairment and estimates of retinopathy of prematurity at regional and global levels for 2010. Pediatr Res. 2013;74(Suppl 1):35–49.
27. Blencowe H, Moxon S, Gilbert C. Update on blindness due to retinopathy of prematurity globally and in India. Indian Pediatr. 2016;53(Suppl 2):S89–92.

28. Geldof CJA, Van Wassenaer AG, de Kieviet JT, et al. Chapter 2. Visual perception and visual-motor integration in very preterm and/or very low birth weight children: a meta-analysis. Res Developmental Disabil. 2012;33:726–36.
29. Pehere N, Chougule P, Dutton GN. Cerebral visual impairment in children: causes and associated ophthalmological problems. Indian J Ophthalmol. 2018;66:812–5.
30. Dutton GN. Cognitive vision, its disorders and differential diagnosis in adults and children: knowing where and what things are. Eye (Lond). 2003;17:289–304.
31. Geetha VKP. Cerebral visual impairment in children. Kerela J Ophthamol. 2020;32:27–35.
32. Chang MY, Borchert MS. Advances in the evaluation and management of cortical/cerebral visual impairment in children. Surv Ophthalmol. 2020;65:708–24.
33. Bhaskaran S, Lawrence L, Flora J, et al. Functional and cognitive vision assessment in children with autism spectrum disorder. J AAPOS. 2018;22:304–8.
34. VIKAS: Visual Intervention Kit with Analytics for Special children. https://play.google.com/store/apps/details?id=com.mindtree.vikas. Accessed 6 Nov 2020.
35. Good WV, Jan JE, Burden SK, et al. Recent advances in cortical visual impairment. Dev Med Child Neurol. 2001;43:56–60.
36. Tsirka A, Liasis A, Kuczynski A, et al. Clinical use of the Insight Inventory in cerebral visual impairment and the effectiveness of tailored habilitational strategies. Dev Med Child Neurol. 2020;62:1324–30.
37. Duke R, Eyong K, Burton K, et al. The effect of visual support strategies on the quality of life of children with cerebral palsy and cerebral visual impairment/perceptual visual dysfunction in Nigeria: study protocol for a randomized controlled trial. Trials. 2019;20:417. https://doi.org/10.1186/s13063-019-3527-9.
38. Holden BA, Fricke TR, Wilson DA, et al. Global prevalence of myopia and high myopia and temporal trends from 2000 through 2050. Ophthalmology. 2016;123:1036–42.
39. Resnikoff S, Pascolini D, Mariotti SP, et al. Global magnitude of visual impairment caused by uncorrected refractive errors in 2004. Bull World Health Organ. 2008;86:63–70.
40. Rudnicka AR, Kapetanakis VV, Wathern AK, et al. Global variations and time trends in the prevalence of childhood myopia, a systematic review and quantitative meta-analysis: implications for aetiology and early prevention. Br J Ophthalmol. 2016;100:882–90.
41. Ho CL, Wu WF, Liou YM. Dose-response relationship of outdoor exposure and myopia indicators: a systematic review and meta-analysis of various research methods. Int J Environ Res Public Health. 2019;16. https://doi.org/10.3390/ijerph16142595.
42. Sherwin JC, Reacher MH, Keogh RH, et al. The association between time spent outdoors and myopia in children and adolescents: a systematic review and meta-analysis. Ophthalmology. 2012;119:2141–51.
43. Fan Q, Verhoeven VJ, Wojciechowski R, et al. Meta-analysis of gene-environment-wide association scans accounting for education level identifies additional loci for refractive error. Nat Commun. 2016;7:11008. https://doi.org/10.1038/ncomms11008.
44. World Health Organization. International classification of functioning, disability and health: ICF. 2001. https://apps.who.int/iris/handle/10665/42407. Accessed 6 Nov 2020.
45. Stevens GA, Bennett JE, Hennocq Q, et al. Trends and mortality effects of vitamin A deficiency in children in 138 low-income and middle-income countries between 1991 and 2013: a pooled analysis of population-based surveys. Lancet Glob Health. 2015;3:e528–36. https://doi.org/10.1016/S2214-109X(15)00039-X. Accessed 6 Nov 2020.
46. UNICEF. Percentage of children aged 6–59 months that received two high-dose vitamin A supplements in 2018. 2018. https://data.unicef.org/topic/nutrition/vitamin-a-deficiency/. Accessed 6 Nov 2020.
47. Talsma EF, Melse-Boonstra A, Brouwer ID. Acceptance and adoption of biofortified crops in low- and middle-income countries: a systematic review. Nutr Rev. 2017;75:798–829.
48. World Health Organization. Guideline: Fortification of maize flour and corneal meal with vitamins and minerals. Geneva: World Health Organization; 2016.
49. World Health Organization. Guideline on use of multiple micronutrient powders for point-of-use fortification of foods consumed by infants and young children aged 6–23 months and children aged 2–12 years. Geveva: World Health Organization; 2016. https://www.who.int/publications/i/item/9789241549943. Accessed 6 Nov 2020.
50. Then C. The campaign for genetically modified rice is at the crossroads. A critical look at Golden Rice after nearly 10 years of development. www.scouting--biotechnology.net, January 2009, Commissioned by Foodwatch, Germany. https://www.gmwatch.org/files/golden-rice-10yrs-on.pdf. Accessed 6 Nov 2020.
51. Scaling up nutrition: a framework for action. 2011. https://scalingupnutrition.org/wp-content/uploads/2013/05/SUN_Framework.pdf. Accessed 6 Nov 2020.
52. Semba RD, Bloem MW. Measles blindness. Surv Ophthalmol. 2004;49:243–55.
53. World Health Organization. Immunization coverage with 1st dose of measles continaing vaccines, 1980–2018. https://www.who.int/immunization/monitoring_surveillance/burden/vpd/surveillance_type/active/mcv1_1980_2018.gif?ua=1. Accessed 6 Nov 2020.
54. UNICEF. Immunization coverage estimates data visualization. https://data.unicef.org/resources/immunization-coverage-estimates-data-visualization/. Accessed 6 Nov 2020.

55. World Health Organization, Regional Office for South-East Asia. Strategic plan for measles elimination and rubella and congenital rubella syndrome control in the South-East Asia Region, 2014–2020. 2015. https://apps.who.int/iris/handle/10665/205923. Accessed 6 Nov 2020.
56. Schaller UC, Klauss V. Is Crede's prophylaxis for ophthalmia neonatorum still valid? Bull World Health Organ. 2001;79:262–3.
57. Kapoor VS, Evans JR, Vedula SS. Interventions for preventing ophthalmia neonatorum. Cochrane Database Syst Rev. 2020;9:CD001862. https://doi.org/10.1002/14651858.CD001862.pub3.
58. Travers CP, Clark RH, Spitzer AR, et al. Exposure to any antenatal corticosteroids and outcomes in preterm infants by gestational age: prospective cohort study. BMJ. 2017;356:j1039. https://doi.org/10.1136/bmj.j1039.
59. Deorari A, Darlow BA. Preventing sight-threatening ROP: a neonatologist's perspective. Community Eye Health. 2017;30:50–2.
60. Katheria A, Rich W, Finer N. Optimizing Care of the preterm infant starting in the delivery room. Am J Perinatol. 2016;33:297–304.
61. Shah PK, Narendran V, Kalpana N. Aggressive posterior retinopathy of prematurity in large preterm babies in South India. Arch Dis Child Fetal Neonatal Ed. 2012;97:F371–5.
62. Askie LM, Darlow BA, Davis PG, et al. Effects of targeting lower versus higher arterial oxygen saturations on death or disability in preterm infants. Cochrane Database Syst Rev. 2017;4:CD011190. https://doi.org/10.1002/14651858.CD011190.pub2.
63. Darlow BA, Husain S. Primary prevention of ROP and the oxygen saturation targeting trials. Semin Perinatol. 2019;43:333–40.
64. Lin L, Binenbaum G. Postnatal weight gain and retinopathy of prematurity. Semin Perinatol. 2019;43:352–9.
65. Zhou J, Shukla VV, John D, et al. Human milk feeding as a protective factor for retinopathy of prematurity: a meta-analysis. Pediatrics. 2015;136:e1576–86.
66. Skondra D, Rodriguez SH, Sharma A, et al. The early gut microbiome could protect against severe retinopathy of prematurity. J AAPOS. 2020; https://doi.org/10.1016/j.jaapos.2020.03.010.
67. Cakir B, Liegl R, Hellgren G, et al. Thrombocytopenia is associated with severe retinopathy of prematurity. JCI Insight. 2018;3(19):e99448. https://doi.org/10.1172/jci.insight.99448.
68. Vinekar A, Hegde K, Gilbert C, et al. Do platelets have a role in the pathogenesis of aggressive posterior retinopathy of prematurity? Retina. 2010;30(4 Suppl):S20–3.
69. Sathish Y, Lewis LE, Noronha JA, et al. Promoting developmental supportive care in preterm infants and families in a level III neonatal intensive care unit (NICU) setting in India. Nurse Educ Pract. 2019;40:102612. https://doi.org/10.1016/j.nepr.2019.08.006.
70. Xiong S, Sankaridurg P, Naduvilath T, et al. Time spent in outdoor activities in relation to myopia prevention and control: a meta-analysis and systematic review. Acta Ophthalmol. 2017;95:551–66.
71. Wildsoet CF, Chia A, Cho P, et al. IMI – Interventions Myopia Institute: Interventions for controlling myopia onset and progression report. Invest Ophthalmol Vis Sci. 2019;60(3):M106–M31. https://doi.org/10.1167/iovs.18-25958.
72. Moss WJ. Measles. Lancet. 2017;390(10111):2490–502.
73. International Committee for the Classification of Retinopathy of P. The International Classification of Retinopathy of prematurity revisited. Arch Ophthalmol. 2005;123:991.
74. Gilbert CE. Screening for retinopathy of prematurity: does one size fit all? Arch Dis Child Fetal Neonatal Ed. 2016;101:F280–1. https://doi.org/10.1136/archdischild-2015-310129.
75. Gilbert C, Fielder A, Gordillo L, et al. Characteristics of infants with severe retinopathy of prematurity in countries with low, moderate, and high levels of development: implications for screening programs. Pediatrics. 2005;115:e518–25. https://doi.org/10.1542/peds.2004-1180.
76. Fierson WM. Screening examination of premature infants for retinopathy of prematurity. Pediatrics. 2018;142(6). https://doi.org/10.1542/peds.2018-3061.
77. Singh A. Guidelines for universal eye screening in newborns including retinopathy of prematurity. Rashtriya Bal Swasth ya Karyakram, Ministry of Health & Family Welfare, Government of India. 2016. https://nhm.gov.in/images/pdf/programmes/RBSK/Resource_Documents/Revised_ROP_Guidelines-Web_Optimized.pdf. Accessed 6 Nov 2020.
78. Gilbert C, Shukla R, Murthy GVS, et al. Retinopathy of prematurity: overview and highlights of an initiative to integrate prevention, screening, and management into the public health system in India. Indian J Ophthalmol. 2020;68(Suppl 1):S103–S7.
79. Quinn GE, Vinekar A. The role of retinal photography and telemedicine in ROP screening. Semin Perinatol. 2019;43:367–74.
80. Shah PK, Narendran V, Kalpana N. Evolution of ROP screening at Aravind Eye Hospital, Coimbatore – Lessons learnt and the way ahead. Community Eye Health. 2018;31:S23–S4.
81. Campbell JP, Redd TK, Brown JM, et al. Applications of artificial intelligence for retinopathy of prematurity screening. Pediatrics. 2020; in press.
82. Zepeda-Romero LC, Meza-Anguiano A, Barrera-de Leon JC, et al. Case series of infants presenting with end stage retinopathy of prematurity to two tertiary eye care facilities in Mexico: underlying reasons for late presentation. Matern Child Health J. 2015;19:1417–25.
83. Kulkarni S, Gilbert C, Zuurmond M, et al. Blinding retinopathy of prematurity in Western India:

characteristics of children, reasons for late presentation and impact on families. Indian Pediatr. 2018;55:665–70.
84. Vinekar A, Jayadev C, Mangalesh S, et al. Initiating retinopathy of prematurity screening before discharge from the Neonatal Care Unit: effect on enrolment in rural India. Indian Pediatr. 2016;53(Suppl 2):S107–S11.
85. Prevention of Blindness from Retinopathy of Prematurity in Neonatal Care Units. Project Operational Guidelines, India. https://drropindia.org/retinopathy-of-prematurity/policy-makers-rop/#operationalguidelines. Accessed 6 Nov 2020.
86. Shukla R, Murthy GVS, Gilbert C, et al. Operational guidelines for ROP in India: a summary. Indian J Ophthalmol. 2020;68(Suppl 1):S108–S14.
87. Klufas MA, Chan RV. Intravitreal anti-VEGF therapy as a treatment for retinopathy of prematurity: what we know after 7 years. J Pediatr Ophthalmol Strabismus. 2015;52:77–84.
88. Natarajan G, Shankaran S, Nolen TL, et al. Neurodevelopmental outcomes of preterm infants with retinopathy of prematurity by treatment. Pediatrics. 2019;144(2):e20183537. https://doi.org/10.1542/peds.2018-3537.
89. Morin J, Luu TM, Superstein R, et al. Neurodevelopmental outcomes following Bevacizumab injections for retinopathy of prematurity. Pediatrics. 2016;137(4). https://doi.org/10.1542/peds.2015-3218.
90. Mintz-Hittner HA, Kennedy KA, Chuang AZ, et al. Efficacy of intravitreal bevacizumab for stage 3+ retinopathy of prematurity. N Engl J Med. 2011;364:603–15.
91. Wallace DK, Dean TW, Hartnett ME, et al. A dosing study of bevacizumab for retinopathy of prematurity: late recurrences and additional treatments. Ophthalmology. 2018;125:1961–6.
92. Crouch ER, Kraker RT, Wallace DK, et al. Secondary 12-month ocular outcomes of a Phase 1 dosing study of bevacizumab for retinopathy of prematurity. JAMA Ophthalmol. 2020;138:14–20.
93. Vijayalakshmi P, Gilbert C. Following up children born preterm. Community Eye Health. 2017;30:62–4.
94. Standard school eye health guidelines for low and middle-income countries. IAPB School Eye HealthWork Group, International Agency for the Prevention of Blindness, February 2018. https://www.iapb.org/wp-content/uploads/Guidelines-School-Eye-Health-Programmes-English-Final.pdf. Accessed 6 Nov 2020.
95. Gilbert CE, Lepvrier-Chomette N. Gender inequalities in surgery for bilateral cataract among children in low-income countries: a systematic review. Ophthalmology. 2016;123:1245–51.
96. Vervloed MP, Janssen N, Knoors H. Visual rehabilitation of children with visual impairments. J Dev Behav Pediatr. 2006;27:493–506.
97. Sonksen PM, Petrie A, Drew KJ. Promotion of visual development of severely visually impaired babies: evaluation of a developmentally based programme. Dev Med Child Neurol. 1991;33:320–35.
98. Dale NJ, Sakkalou E, O'Reilly MA, et al. Home-based early intervention in infants and young children with visual impairment using the Developmental Journal: longitudinal cohort study. Dev Med Child Neurol. 2019;61:697–709.
99. Mafwiri MM, Kisenge R, Gilbert CE. A pilot study to evaluate incorporating eye care for children into reproductive and child health services in Dar-es-Salaam, Tanzania: a historical comparison study. BMC Nurs. 2014;13:15. https://doi.org/10.1186/1472-6955-13-15.
100. Gilbert C, Muhit M. Twenty years of childhood blindness: what have we learnt? Community Eye Health. 2008;21:46–7.
101. World Health Organization. Universal eye health: a Global Action Plan 2014-2019. Geneva, 2013. http://www.who.int/blindness/actionplan/en/. Accessed 6 Nov 2020.
102. Ministry of Health and Family Welfare, Government of People's Republic of Bangladesh. The 4th Health, Nutrition and Population Sector Program (HNPSP) (January 2017–June 22), Program Implementation Plan (PIP), Vol. 1, January 2017.
103. Ministry of Health and Family Welfare, Government of People's Republic of Bangladesh. 4th Health Population Nutrition Sector program (HNPSP), National Eye Care (NEC) Operation Plan (OP).
104. Preventing avoidable childhood blindness in Bangladesh: a pilot intervention. 2016. https://www.who.int/bangladesh/news/detail/24-04-2017-preventing-avoidable-childhood-blindness-in-bangladesh-a-pilot-intervention. Accessed 20 Sep 2020.
105. Directorate General of Health Services (DGHS) and UNICEF. IMCI Newsletter, Issue 4, March 2013. https://dghs.gov.bd/bn/licts_file/images/IMCI/IMCI4.pdf. Accessed 6 Nov 2020.
106. Sightsavers Bangladesh. Paediatric eye care services in Bangladesh. https://www.sightsavers.org/reports/2019/03/paediatric-eye-care-services-in-bangladesh/. Accessed 6 Nov 2020.
107. World Health Organization, Country office of Bangladesh. No more avoidable childhood blindness. A training manual for the community health workers. 2016. https://www.who.int/docs/default-source/searo/bangladesh/pdf-reports/year-2016-2018/no-more-avoidable-childhood-blindness%2D%2Da-training-manual-for-the-community-health-workers.pdf?sfvrsn=f4a12170_2. Accessed 20 Sept 20 2020.

108. World Health Organization. Universal health coverage. https://www.who.int/news-room/fact-sheets/detail/universal-health-coverage-(uhc).
109. World Health Organization. World report on vision. Geneva: World Health Organization; 2019.
110. Keel S, Evans JR, Block S, et al. Strengthening the integration of eye care into the health system: methodology for the development of the WHO package of eye care interventions. BMJ Open Ophthalmol. 2020;5(1):e000533. https://doi.org/10.1136/bmjophth-2020-000533.
111. Malik ANJ, Mafwiri M, Gilbert C. Integrating primary eye care into global child health policies. Arch Dis Child. 2018;103:176–80.
112. World Health Organization and UNICEF. SURVIVE and THRIVE- Transforming care for every small and sick newborn. Geneva: WHO; 2019. http://apps.who.int.

The Burden of Non-communicable Diseases and Diabetic Retinopathy

12

Ramachandran Rajalakshmi, Vijayaraghavan Prathiba, Rajiv Raman, Paisan Ruamviboonsuk, Rajendra Pradeepa, and Viswanathan Mohan

Key Points

- Non-communicable diseases (NCDs) are a major public health problem in South-East Asia.
- Four NCDs, cardiovascular diseases (coronary heart disease and stroke), diabetes mellitus (DM), cancer, and chronic respiratory diseases account for the majority of morbidity and mortality caused by NCDs.
- Mortality attributable to NCDs accounts for ~70% of all deaths and >50% of the global burden of disease.
- DM is a global epidemic/pandemic, and three quarters of those with DM live in low- and middle-income countries.
- Four modifiable behavioral risk factors, tobacco use, unhealthy diet, physical inactivity, and harmful use of alcohol are largely responsible for the majority of NCDs.
- The global increase in DM has resulted in an increased prevalence of diabetic retinopathy (DR).
- It has been estimated that one-third of those with DM have DR, and 1 out of 10 people with DM have sight-threatening DR.
- It is estimated that globally, by 2040, 642 million adults will be living with DM, 224 million people will have some form of retinopathy, and 70 million people will have sight-threatening retinopathy.
- The prevalence of DR in South-East Asia countries is likely to increase from 11.3% in 2019 to 12.2% in 2030.
- Lifelong repetitive screening for DR is essential for early detection and timely management to avoid visual impairment due to sight-threatening diabetic retinopathy.

Non-communicable diseases (NCDs) are a global health and developmental crisis. They cause premature mortality, aggravate poverty, and threaten global economies [2]. Four NCDs, cardiovascular diseases (CVDs), diabetes mellitus (DM), cancer, and chronic respiratory diseases, are the major causes of morbidity and mortality in the South-East Asia Region (SEAR), accounting for 55% of all deaths each year (~7.9 million) [3, 4].

R. Rajalakshmi (✉) · V. Prathiba
Department of Ophthalmology, Dr. Mohan's Diabetes Specialties Centre and Madras Diabetes Research Foundation, Chennai, India
e-mail: drraj@drmohans.com; drprathiba@drmohans.com

R. Raman
Shri Bhagwan Mahavir Vitreoretinal Services, Sankara Nethralaya, Chennai, India
e-mail: drrrn@snmail.org

P. Ruamviboonsuk
Department of Ophthalmology, Rajavithi Hospital, Bangkok, Thailand

R. Pradeepa · V. Mohan
Dr. Mohan's Diabetes Specialties Centre and Madras Diabetes Research Foundation, Chennai, India
e-mail: pradeepa@drmohans.com; drmohans@diabetes.ind.in

T. Das, P. D. Nayar (eds.), *South-East Asia Eye Health*,
https://doi.org/10.1007/978-981-16-3787-2_12

In 2011, the World Health Organization (WHO) estimated a 21% increase in deaths due to NCDs over the next decade [5]. Furthermore, NCDs claim lives at a younger age in South-East Asia than in other WHO regions [6].

DM is a global epidemic/pandemic, where three quarters of those with DM reside in low- and middle-income countries (LMICs). With rapid industrialization and urbanization in the last five decades, many traditionally classified LMICs like India have faced an alarming increase in the incidence of DM in a relatively short time. Diabetic retinopathy (DR) consequent to DM is the leading cause of visual impairment in working-age adults. It has been estimated that 1 in 3 people with DM have DR, and 1 in 10 people with DM have sight-threatening diabetic retinopathy (STDR).

12.1 Non-communicable Diseases

12.1.1 Disease Burden

12.1.1.1 Global Burden of Diabetes Mellitus

Diabetes mellitus is a constellation of metabolic diseases characterized by hyperglycemia resulting from defects in insulin secretion, insulin action, or both [7]. The two main types of DM are: (1) type 1 DM (T1DM), caused by autoimmune destruction of beta cells in the pancreas resulting in absolute insulin deficiency; and (2) type 2 DM (T2DM), caused due to a progressive loss of adequate beta-cell insulin secretion and insulin resistance. T2DM accounts for 90–95% of all diagnosed cases of DM. The increasing number of people with T2DM in LMICs is of greater concern [8, 9]. DM increases the risk of both macrovascular diseases (coronary artery disease, cerebrovascular disease, and peripheral vascular disease) and microvascular diseases (retinopathy, nephropathy, and neuropathy) [10].

The International Diabetes Federation (IDF) has estimated that in 2019, 463 million people worldwide had DM (9.3% of the world's population). The DM population could rise to 578 million (10.2% of the world population) by 2030 and 700 million (10.9% of the world population) by 2045 [1]. Among the IDF regions, the Western Pacific region has the largest number of people with DM (133 million), followed by the South-East Asia Region (SEAR) (88 million) (Fig. 12.1) [1]. The prevalence of DM is higher in urban than rural populations in developing countries

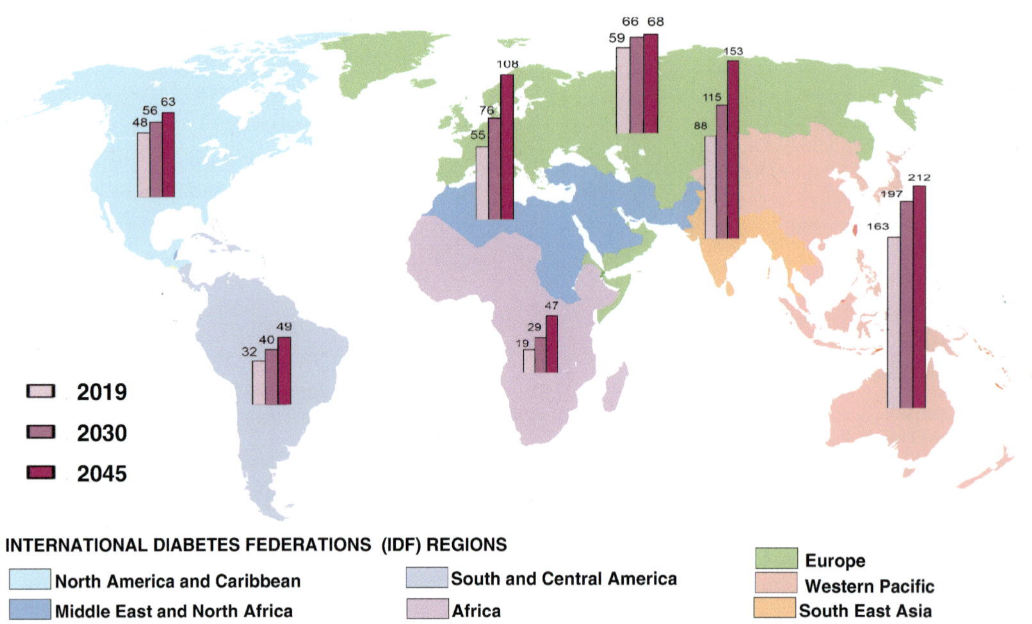

Fig. 12.1 Global burden of diabetes mellitus in 2019 and its projection in 2030 and 2045 in the International Diabetes Federation (IDF) regions (in millions) (Source: IDF [1])

[11]. But this trend is also quickly changing due to rapid urbanization.

A systematic review of 109 population-based studies reported that globally the prevalence of DM in rural areas has increased from 5.7% during 1985–1989 to 8.7% during 2005–2011 [12]. The incidence of DM is rising equally in affluent and impoverished sections of society [13]. The two main concerns regarding T2DM in LMICs are: onset of T2DM at a younger age; and frequent occurrence of T2DM in younger and productive (35–64 years) of life [14, 15]. The incidence of T1DM is also increasing worldwide though there is considerable regional variation [16]. In 2019, over 1.1 million children and adolescents had T1DM [1]. DM accounted for 11.3% of global all-cause mortality among adults aged 20–79 years in 2019 (nearly 4.0 million). This equates to one death every 8 s. Almost 46% of deaths associated with DM are in the working-age group (<60 years of age) [1].

12.1.2 South-East Asia Burden of DM

The IDF SEAR (seven countries: Bangladesh, Bhutan, India, the Maldives, Mauritius, Nepal, and Sri Lanka) is home to nearly 88 million adults with DM as of 2019 and this number is expected to exceed 115 and 153 million in 2030 and 2045, respectively [1]. In 2019, India was home to the 2nd largest number of adults with DM (77 million); Indonesia and Bangladesh were 7th and 10th (with 10.7 million and 8.4 million, respectively, in the age groups of 20–79 years) [1, 11]. People with undiagnosed DM accounts for 57% of adults in the IDF SEAR. Over 1 million people in this region die due to DM; this is the second highest number of deaths in all the IDF regions [1].

The WHO SEAR, consisting of 11 countries, is home to over a quarter of the world's population and has an estimated 96 million people with DM [17]. There has been a dramatic increase in DM in these countries (inadequate information from the Democratic People's Republic of (DPR) Korea). Figure 12.2 presents the trends in regional DM prevalence in 10 SEAR countries between 2000 and 2019 [1, 18–25]. In 2019, the highest prevalence of DM was in India (8.9%), and the lowest was in Myanmar (3.7%).

There are significant differences in DM occurrence between and within SEAR countries because of the geographical diversity, socioeco-

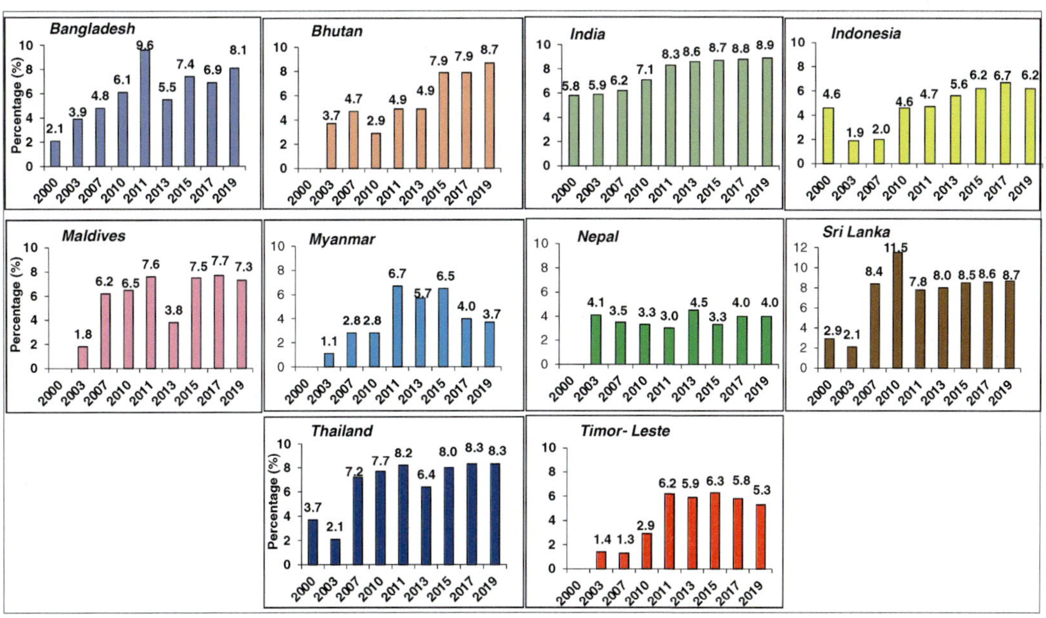

Fig. 12.2 Trends in regional diabetes mellitus prevalence in 10 South-East Asia Region countries between 2000 and 2019 [1, 18–25]

nomic factors, demographic alterations, lifestyle changes, and perhaps ethnic susceptibility to DM [26–30]. For example, the prevalence of DM in Nepal is 8.1% in urban and 1.0% in rural populations [26]; in the neighboring country, India, the prevalence of DM is 11.2% and 5.2% in the urban and rural areas, respectively [11].

The IDF has estimated that 184,100 children and adolescents aged <20 years have T1DM in the SEAR. In the year 2019 alone, ~21,300 children and adolescents had developed T1DM in this region. Globally, there are 171,300 children and adolescents with T1DM, and India is home to the second largest number of such children and adolescents [1].

12.1.3 Global Burden of Other NCDs

Other than DM, CVDs, cancer, and respiratory diseases constitute the world's biggest NCD challenges. The total number of disability-adjusted life years (DALYs) due to DM, CVDs, and cancer is significantly higher than other NCDs. Between 1990 and 2010, the DALYs due to DM, CVDs, and cancer have increased by 69%, 22.6%, and 27.3%, respectively [31].

CVDs consist of ischemic heart disease, stroke, heart failure, peripheral arterial disease, and several other cardiac and vascular conditions; these remain a major cause of health loss and are the leading cause of global mortality and reduced quality of life [32]. The Global Burden of Disease (GBD) study estimated that there were nearly 423 million cases of CVD and 18 million CVD deaths in 2015; ischemic heart disease was the leading cause of CVD health loss, followed by stroke [33].

In 2018, the WHO reported that cancer was the second leading cause of death globally and was responsible for an estimated 9.6 million deaths, and that ~70% of deaths due to cancer occurred in LMICs [34]. Globally, it is the single most important barrier to increasing life expectancy in the twenty-first century [35]. Lung, prostate, colorectal, stomach, and liver cancers are the more common types of cancer in men; breast, cervical, colorectal, lung, and thyroid cancers are most common in women [34]. In 2018, 36 cancers in 185 countries were responsible for 18.1 million new cancer cases and 9.6 million deaths [35]. Lung cancer (in both genders) was the most commonly diagnosed cancer and the leading cause of death due to cancer (11.6% of the total cases and 18.4% of the total deaths due to cancer) [36].

Chronic obstructive pulmonary disease (COPD), asthma, acute lower respiratory tract infections, tuberculosis, and lung cancer are the most common causes of severe illness and death due to respiratory diseases worldwide [36]. In 2017, the GBD reported that globally, nearly 545 million people suffered from chronic respiratory diseases [37].

12.1.4 The Burden of Other NCDs in South-East Asia

Cardiovascular disease, cancer, DM, chronic respiratory diseases are the leading causes of morbidity and mortality in the SEAR [38]. The WHO Global Health Observatory reported that the estimated number of deaths due to NCDs exceeds 50% of all deaths in 10 SEAR Member States [39]; mid-80s in the Maldives and Sri Lanka, mid-70s in Thailand and Indonesia; mid to high 60s in Myanmar, Bangladesh, Bhutan, Nepal, and India, and mid-40s in Timor-Leste. In absolute numbers, India and Indonesia together account for 80% of NCD deaths in the SEAR. Figure 12.3 shows the estimated percentage of mortalities in 2016, by cause, in 10 of the SEAR countries (WHO Global Health Observatory) [39].

CVDs alone accounted for nearly 25% of all deaths in the SEAR. CVDs caused the highest number of deaths in the Maldives and lowest number of deaths in Timor-Leste. In India, the age-standardized CVD mortality rate of 272/100,000 population is higher than the global average of 235/100,000 population [40]. The burden of CVD, mortality, and morbidity is also on the rise in Bangladesh [41].

There is high incidence of breast cancer in South-East Asians [35]. In Bangladesh, about 141,000 patients are newly diagnosed with cancer each year [42]. In India, 8.3% of the total deaths and 5.0% of the total DALYs were due to

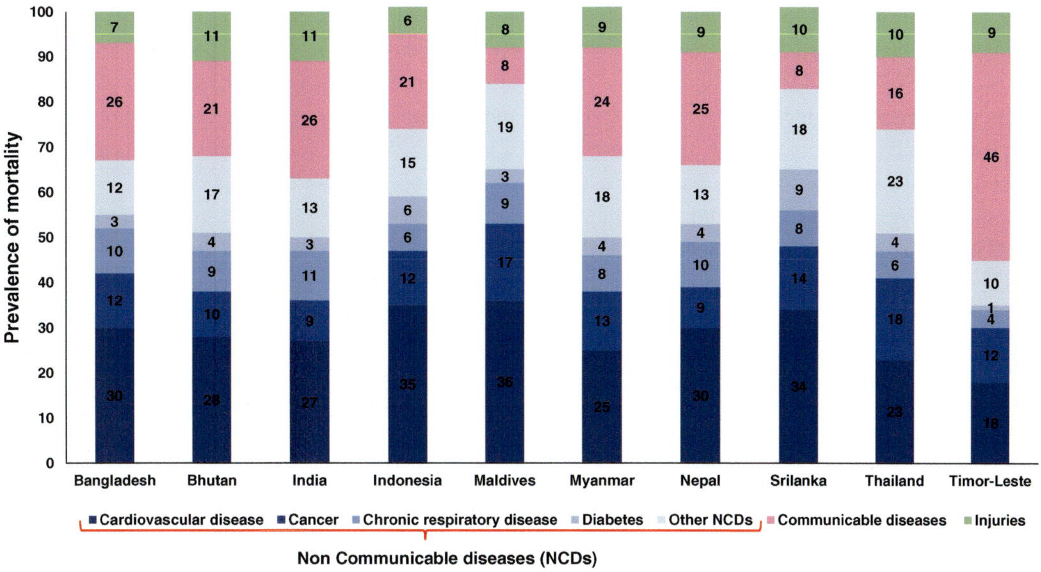

Fig. 12.3 Estimated percentage mortality, by cause, in 10 of the South-East Asia Region countries in 2016 [36]

Fig. 12.4 Prevalence of new cancer cases in India in 2018 (all ages) [37]

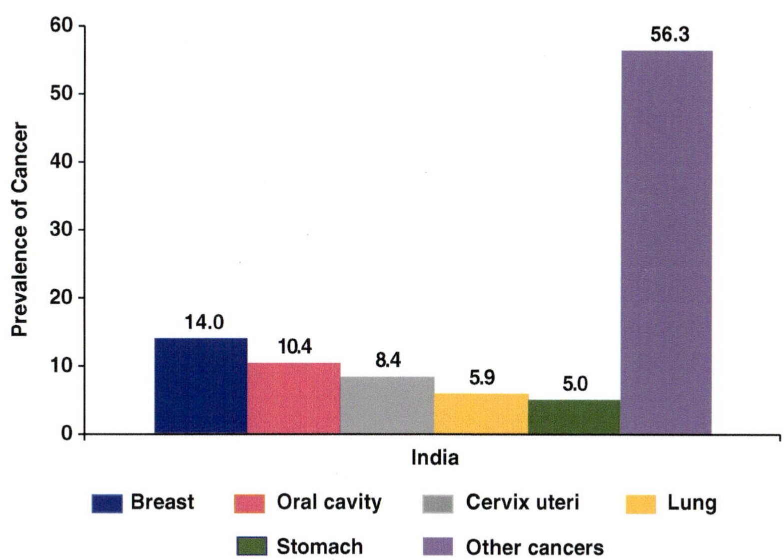

cancer in 2016; this number has doubled since 1990. In 2016, the top 10 cancers accountable for a high proportion of cancer DALYs in India were stomach (9.0%), breast (8.2%), lung (7.5%), lip and oral cavity (7.2%), pharynx other than nasopharynx (6.8%), colon and rectum (5.8%), leukemia (5.2%), cervical (5.2%), esophageal (4.3%), and brain and nervous system (3.5%) cancers. Figure 12.4 presents the prevalence of new cancer cases in India in 2018 (all ages); breast cancer had the highest prevalence [43]. An increasing trend in cancer incidence has also been reported in Nepal and Thailand [44–46].

In 2016, 32% of the total global DALYs due to chronic respiratory diseases occurred in India. COPD and asthma were responsible for 75.6% and 20% of the chronic respiratory disease DALYs, respectively [46]. Asthma (23.7%) and COPD (8%) were two frequently diagnosed chronic respiratory diseases in Thailand (Asia-Pacific Burden of Respiratory Diseases, APBORD study) [47].

12.1.5 Risk Factors for NCDs in South-East Asia

NCDs share many common preventable antecedents. Most NCDs result from four modifiable risk factors: (1) use of tobacco, (2) harmful use of alcohol, (3) physical inactivity, and (4) unhealthy diet. These risk factors, in turn, lead to four key metabolic changes: (1) being overweight/obese, (2) high blood pressure, (3) higher blood sugar, and (4) higher blood cholesterol levels.

Rapid socio-cultural and epidemiological transitions have led to drastic changes in the diet and physical activity of many populations. Some of these diet changes include increased consumption of packaged and processed foods, mainly refined carbohydrates, added sugars, refined edible oils, and fats, along with decreased consumption of whole grains, nuts, fruits, and vegetables [48–50], so also consumption of cheaper and more readily available energy-dense foods by many people in the LMICs [51]. Consumption of adequate servings of vegetables reduces the risk of CVDs, T2DM, and some cancers. On the other hand, foods with high fat and sugar promote obesity, the main risk factors for CVDs, DM, and many cancers [52].

The Global School-Based Health Survey (GSHS) conducted on school-going adolescents (aged 13–15 years) of five South-East Asian countries (India, Indonesia, Myanmar, Sri Lanka, and Thailand) reported that 76.3% of students had <5 servings/day of fruits and vegetables, 28% consumed <1 serving/day of fruits, and 13.8% consumed <1 serving/day of vegetables [53]. The high cost of fruits and vegetables could be a major barrier to shifting to a healthier diet.

There is also evidence of high salt consumption in many SEAR countries, an important risk factor for hypertension and other NCDs. Against the WHO recommendation of <5 g/day, salt intake is 10.8 g/day in Thailand, 8.3 g/day in Sri Lanka, 13.3 g/day in Nepal, 8.5 g/day in south India, and 17 g/day in Bangladesh [54–58].

Other areas of concern are high fat intake, high intake of saturated fatty acids (SFAs), and low intake of both polyunsaturated and monounsaturated fatty acids (PUFAs and MUFAs, respectively). Consumption of SFA contributes to an increased risk of T2DM.

Evidence shows good physical activity could reduce the incidence of major NCDs such as CVD, T2DM, and breast and colon cancers by 6–10% and increase life expectancy [59]. A systemic review on physical activity patterns among South-Asian adults reported that 19–88% of Indians and 11–32% of Sri Lankans were physically inactive [60]. The Indian Council or Medical Research (ICMR)–INDIAB (India DIABetes) study has reported physical inactivity in ~55% Indians [61]. The WHO STEPS (STEP wise approach to Surveillance) reported a prevalence of 25% inactivity in 11% people in Sri Lanka, 45.9% people in the Maldives, and 3.5% people in Nepal [62–65].

Bangladesh, India, Indonesia, and Thailand are among the top 20 tobacco-producing countries in the world, and its use (smoking and smokeless) is a serious public health problem in the SEAR [66]. Three quarters of world tobacco users live in this region, and 2.3 million tobacco-related premature deaths occur annually in this region [67]. Globally, tobacco use is the second major cause of all deaths due to NCDs and the fourth most common risk factor for NCDs [68]. The WHO SEAR accounts for 81% of smokeless tobacco users and is home to more than 22% of the global adult smoker population (aged >15 years) [69]. India (24.3% in men) and Indonesia (63.1% in men) are the highest tobacco consuming countries in the world [69, 70]. The prevalence of smokeless tobacco use is from 1.3% (Thailand) to 31.8% (Myanmar) in men, and 4.6% (Nepal) to 27.9% (Bangladesh) in women [66].

The WHO estimates that >10% of NCD burden is due to harmful use of alcohol consumption globally and is responsible for more than 1 in 20 deaths [71–73].

12.1.6 Challenges and Strategies in Tackling NCDs in South-East Asia

12.1.6.1 Challenges

The specific challenges in NCD prevention and control are:

1. Lack of strong national partnerships for multi-sectoral actions.
2. Lack of robust surveillance and research data on NCDs.
3. Lack of access to basic prevention/management of NCDs in primary health care, including access to affordable medicines.
4. Disproportionate fund allocation for NCD programs.
5. Difficulties in engaging the industry and private sector.
6. Limited human resources for NCDs.
7. Inadequate community mobilization and weak coordination among civil societies and between the civil societies and government agencies for NCDs.

12.1.6.2 Strategies

Tackling NCDs calls for a fundamental change—from addressing each NCD separately to collectively addressing a cluster of disorders in an integrated manner, a shift from a biomedical to a public health approach [2]. The key strategies for the prevention/control of NCDs should include:

1. *Prevention*: reduced exposure to risk factors through health promotion and primary care
2. *Treatment*: early diagnosis and management
3. *Surveillance*: monitoring the risk factors

12.1.7 Health Policy

Some of the policy issues to reverse the growing burden of NCDs in the SEAR are [3]:

1. *National food policy*: Improve production and distribution of wholesome food; improve availability, affordability, and food safety standards.
2. *Health policy*: Reduce harmful behaviors such as smoking, harmful use of alcohol, consumption of trans fat foods; create amenities in public places (walking, cycling) to encourage physical activities.
3. *Health information*: Improve public awareness of NCDs
4. *Essential medicines*: Reduce the cost of essential drugs and ensure easy availability

All these efforts need collaboration between health, information, education, and agriculture ministries to facilitate a healthy lifestyle.

Recommendations related to non-communicable diseases

1. Improved surveillance of chronic NCDs and risk factors
2. Strengthening of existing primary healthcare systems.
3. Creating an integrated approach to four major NCDs
4. Multisectoral actions and adoption of "Health in All Policies" (HiAP).
5. Promotion of healthy behavior.
6. Early diagnosis and management
7. Easy access and affordable healthcare.
8. Partnership: public, private, philanthropic, and civil society
9. Health system strengthening.

12.2 Diabetic Retinopathy

The global burden of DM has increased the prevalence of diabetic retinopathy (DR). It is a microvascular complication and all people with DM will potentially develop it if they live long enough. It is one of the most important causes of preventable blindness. Lifelong repetitive screening is essential for early detection and timely management to prevent visual impairment due to DR.

12.2.1 Global Burden

In 2012, a meta-analysis of an estimated 285 million people worldwide with T1DM and T2DM showed that over one-third of them had DR, and a third of these were afflicted with STDR, defined as the presence of proliferative DR (PDR) and/or the presence of diabetic macular edema (DME) [74]. Despite the differences in the prevalence of DR across populations, the risk factors for DR are similar. It is increased with the duration of DM and results from uncontrolled hyperglycemia and hypertension. The estimated lifetime risk of developing DR is 90% and 60% in people with T1DM and T2DM, respectively [74]. The meta-analysis showed that the prevalence of DR was highest in African Americans (49.6%) and lowest in Asians (19.6%) [74].

In 1990–2010 estimation, DR was ranked as the fifth most common cause of preventable blindness and moderate to severe visual impairment (MSVI) [75, 76]. A systematic review of eight DR studies conducted after 2000 (five from Asia, and one each from North America, the Caribbean, and Africa) indicated that the annual incidence of DR is from 2.2% to 12.7% and yearly progression to STDR is from 3.4% to 12.3% [77]. The prevalence of various stages of DR is declining since 1980 in populations with improved diabetes control [74, 77]. But the crude prevalence of visual impairment and blindness caused by DR worldwide has increased, largely because of the increasing prevalence of T2DM in LMICs [75]. It is predicted that globally, by 2040, 642 million adults will be living with DM, 224 million will have some form of DR, and 70 million will have STDR [78]. The incidence of DR is decreasing in high-income countries (such as the UK, the USA) due to a combination of public health effort, increased awareness, national-level DR screening, and improved therapies [79–81]. However, with the rising prevalence of DM and a growing population of aged people worldwide, the absolute number of people with DR is expected to increase.

12.2.2 Prevalence of DR in the SEAR

India, Indonesia, Bangladesh, and China account for 45% of people with DR worldwide [1]. The age-adjusted prevalence of DR in the SEAR countries is likely to increase from 11.3% in 2019 to 12.2% in 2030 [1]. Several studies from individual countries in the region give an approximate estimate of the disease burden. Table 12.1 lists the prevalence of DR, DME, and STDR based on various published studies conducted in the SEAR countries [1, 27, 82–119]. The WHO DR report on "Strengthening the diagnosis and treatment of DR in South-East Asia 2020" provides an update on various aspects of DR services in the SEAR [120]. Table 12.2 provides the country profiles and details of DM, DR screening, and management services in the SEAR countries [120].

Several countries have conducted country-wide surveys [121–125]. In the International Agency for the Prevention of Blindness (IAPB) South-East Asia region 12 million people are blind and 78.5 million are visually impaired; the main causes are cataract, refractive errors, glaucoma, and DR [122]. Rapid Assessment of Avoidable Blindness (RAAB) surveys have been conducted in Bhutan, the Maldives, Sri Lanka, Thailand, and Timor-Leste; two important barriers to uptake of eye care were poor accessibility (Maldives and Timor-Leste) and poor affordability (Sri Lanka) [122–125].

12.2.3 Awareness Regarding DM and DR in the SEAR

Awareness of DM and DR depends on the socioeconomic status, availability and accessibility of health care to the general population, and literacy [81]. Knowledge, attitude, and practice (KAP) patterns of people with regard to DM and DR can help identify barriers to compliance for treatment and follow. Table 12.3 lists the details of KAP studies on DM and DR in the SEAR countries [26, 30, 110, 126–183]. These studies suggest suboptimal patient and physician awareness.

12.2.3.1 Real-World Situation of DR Services in SEAR

The unique challenges in detecting and treating DM and DR are: (1) both conditions could be asymptomatic; (2) there is a shortage of trained professionals for treating these conditions; and (3) once diagnosed, there is life-long health-related expenditure to keep these conditions from progressing.

A brief description of country-specific real-world situation in the region follows.

Table 12.1 Epidemiology of diabetic retinopathy, diabetic macular edema, and sight-threatening diabetic retinopathy in South-East Asia Region countries

Country	DM disease burden (20–79 years)			Author	Year	Number of subjects	Type of study	Prevalence/ incidence of diabetes	Prevalence of DR	Prevalence of DME	Prevalence of STDR
	Estimated in 2019	Projected in 2045	% increase								
Bangladesh	8.4 million	14.9 million	79	Ahmed et al. [82]	2012	977	Retrospective, hospital-based		50.6% (incidence over 15 years)		
				Muqit et al. [83]	2019		Hospital-based population	–	33%	19.2%	7.8%
				Biswas et al. [27]	2016	51,252	Review	7.4% (overall pooled prevalence)	–	–	–
				IDF [1]	2019		–	9.2%	–	–	–
				Akhter et al. [84]	2013		Population-based study		5.4%		
				Billah et al. [85]	2016	94	Hospital-based population	36.2%	6.06%	9.09%	
Bhutan	46,000	88,000	91	IDF [1]	2019			10.3%	–	–	–
				Rai et al. [86]	2020	2913	Hospital-based	12.4%	15.8% (DR with macular edema)		9.7% referable DR
				Chhetri et al. [87]	2020	641 (2014); 1590 (2018)		2.91%	–	–	

(continued)

Table 12.1 (continued)

Country	DM disease burden (20–79 years)			Author	Year	Number of subjects	Type of study	Prevalence/ incidence of diabetes	Prevalence of DR	Prevalence of DME	Prevalence of STDR
	Estimated in 2019	Projected in 2045	% increase								
India	77.0 million	134.2 million	74	Agarwal et al. [88]	2003	4067	Hospital-based		28.9%		
				Rema et al. [89]	2000	448	Hospital based		7.3% (at time of diagnosis of DM)		
				Rema et al. [90]	2005	1382	Population-based (urban)		17.6%	5.0%	
				Raman et al. [91]	2009	5999	Population-based (urban)	28.2%	18.0%		
				Namperumalsamy et al. [92]	2009	25,969	Population-based	10.8%	12.2%		
				Raman et al. [93]	2014	13,079	Population-based (rural)	10.1%	10.3%		3.8%
				Jonas et al. [94]	2013	4711	Population-based (rural)	5.5%	9.6%		
				Ramavat et al. [95]	2013	168	Hospital-based		33.9%	6.5%	
				Gadkari et al. [96]	2016	6218	Nationwide		21.7%		
				Rajalakshmi et al. [97]	2020	11,182	Hospital-based (multi-centric)		32.3%	9.1%	19.1%
Indonesia	10.7 million	16.6 million	56	IDF [1]	2019			6.3%			
				WHO [98]	2016			7% (men: 6.6%, women: 7.3%)	–	–	–
				Sasongko et al. [99]	2017	1184	Population-based		43.1%	17.1%	26.3% PDR:12.1%
Maldives	22,800	48,500	113	IDF [1]	2019			9.2%			
				WHO Steps survey [100]	2012			4.5%			
				Thoufeeq et al. [101]	2018		Population-based		Severe VI due to DR: 3.1%		

Myanmar	1.28 million	2.00 million	56	WHO [100]	2012		Census data	6.6%			
				Patel et al. [102]	2017	97	Hospital-based		34%		23.5% PDR: 13.5%
				IDF [1]	2019			3.9%			
				Latt et al. [103]	2019	8575	Proportional cluster approach	10.8%			
Nepal	0.69 million	1.59 million	129	Thapa et al. [104]	2018	1860	Population-based	9%	23.8%	4.2%	9.5%
				Mishra et al. [105]	2016	5400	Population-based	12%	9.9%	5.5%	PDR: 0.5%
				IDF [1]	2019		Population-based	7.2%			
				Paudyal et al. [106]	2019	8855	Retrospective review		19.4%	6.9%	PDR: 4.6%
				Agrawal et al. [107]	2017	698	Cross-sectional	15.3%	2.1%	1.4% + 2.1%	
Sri Lanka	1.23 million	1.54 million	25	Katulanda et al. [108]	2014	5000	Cross-sectional	12.0%	27.4%	5.3%	5.3%
				IDF [1]	2019		Population-based	10.7%			
				Ranasinghe et al. [109]	2015		Systematic review	10.3%			
				VISION 2020 Srilanka [110]	2013–2017		National program		14.2% in men; 13.5% in women		5% blind

(continued)

Table 12.1 (continued)

Country	DM disease burden (20–79 years)			Author	Year	Number of subjects	Type of study	Prevalence/incidence of diabetes	Prevalence of DR	Prevalence of DME	Prevalence of STDR
	Estimated in 2019	Projected in 2045	% increase								
Thailand	4.28 million	5.07 million	18	Chetthakul et al. [111, 112]	2006	9419	Cross-sectional		T1DM: 21.6%, T2DM: 31.4%		10.7%
				IDF [1]	2019		Population-based	7.0			
				Public Health Regional Service Provider sixth, Thailand [113]	2018	191,776 and 85,786	Population-based	Increased from 2.3% in 1991 to 6.9% in 2009	14.48%		PDR: 2%
				Jongsareejit [114], Phoksunthorn and Thatsnarong [115], Sriwijitkamol et al. [116], Silpa-Archa and Sukhawarn [117]	2007–2013				24–31%		2.3–9.4%
Timor-Leste	32,000	645,000	102	Dawkins et al. [118]	2015	283	Hospital-based	15.2%	19%		
				TImor-Leste DHS [119]	2016		Population-based	2.3% women, 1.8% men			
				IDF [1]	2019		Population-based	16.3% (2010), 32% (2019)	2.7%		

DM diabetes mellitus, *IDF* International Diabetes Federation, *PDR* proliferative diabetic retinopathy, *VI* visual impairment

Table 12.2 Services in South-East Asia Region countries available to treat diabetic retinopathy [120]

Parameters	Bangladesh	Bhutan	India	Indonesia	Maldives	Myanmar	Nepal	Srilanka	Thailand
Prevalence of DR in rural areas	5%	Not known	10.4%	Not known	Not known	Not known	18%	Not known	35%
Prevalence of DR in urban areas	33%	Not known	18%	43.1%	Not known	Not known (minimal data)	30%	27.4%*	8.4%
Awareness about DR/Knowledge Attitude Practices (KAP) for DR	4% aware about DR		37.1% aware				50%		Low awareness
National guidelines on DR	No	No	Yes	Yes	No	No	Yes	Yes	Yes
DR screening at PHC level	No	Limited	No	Yes	No	No	Limited	Yes	No
DR screening at SHC level	Yes	Present	Yes	Yes	No, only at THC level	Present	Yes	Yes	Yes
Funding for DR screening programs	Yes (Hellen Keller International, Fred Hallows Foundation and Orbis International)	Himalayan cataract project may be used	Yes (World Diabetic Foundation, RD TATA trust, Queen Elizabeth Diamond Jubilee trust, Lions Club International Foundation)	Hellen Keller International	Government, World Diabetes Foundation	Yes, Helen Keller International, WHO and Sight for all	Yes (Fred Hallows and World Diabetic Foundation)	Ministry of health	Fundus photography and ophthalmoscopy
Government support for DR screening	Yes, through National Eye Care (NEC)	Yes	Yes—through the All India Ophthalmological Society	Yes	Government will fund if requested by service provider	No	Yes, but limited	Yes	Yes
DR screening as part of national program	Yes	Yes, but lack of human resources is a problem	Yes	Yes	No	No	Yes	No	Yes
Mode of screening	Fundus camera, direct and indirect ophthalmoscopy, and smart phone	Ophthalmoscopy	Fundus camera, direct and indirect ophthalmoscopy and smartphone	Fundus photography	Fundus camera, direct and indirect ophthalmoscopy	Fundus camera and ophthalmoscopy	Targeted/ mass screening/ integration of DR screening	Fundus photography and direct ophthalmoscopy	Fundus photography and ophthalmoscopy

(continued)

Table 12.2 (continued)

Parameters	Bangladesh	Bhutan	India	Indonesia	Maldives	Myanmar	Nepal	Srilanka	Thailand
Screening system for DR	Targeted/ opportunistic	Opportunistic	Targeted/ opportunistic	Targeted	Opportunistic	Targeted	Targeted/ opportunistic	Targeted	Targeted
Fundus photography	Yes	Not done	Yes	Yes	Yes	Yes		Yes	Yes
Data maintenance	Paper	Paper	Electronic and paper-based	Electronic and paper-based	Paper	Electronic and paper-based	Electronic and paper-based	Paper	Electronic and paper-based
Ophthalmologists trained in DR	Yes, medical and surgical	Severe deficiency	Yes, medical and surgical	Yes	Medical retina alone, not surgical	Yes, at THC level	Yes, medical and surgical	Yes (medical and surgical)	Yes
Laser facility	Yes, at THC level	Only at THC level	Yes, at secondary and tertiary levels	Yes	Yes	Yes, at THC level	Yes, at THC level	Yes	Yes
Injection facility	Yes, at THC level	Only at THC level	Yes, at tertiary level	Yes	Yes	Yes, at THC level	Yes, at THC level	Yes	Yes
Country-based registry for DR	No	Available	No	Yes	No	No	No	No	No

DR diabetic retinopathy, *PHC* primary healthcare, *SHC* secondary healthcare, *THC* tertiary healthcare

Table 12.3 Knowledge Attitude and Practice with respect to diabetes mellitus and diabetic retinopathy in South-East Asia Region countries.

Country	Author, year	Diabetes KAP	Author, year	Diabetic retinopathy KAP
Bangladesh	Rahman et al. 2015 (Population-based) [126]	39.7% aware about DM	Ahmed et al. 2017 (Hospital-based) [127]	Only 50% knew that eye screening was essential
	Fottrell et al. 2018 (Rural) [128]	Only 14% had diabetes checkup	Islam et al. 2018 (Rural) [129]	Poor health literacy and reduced confidence on ophthalmic assistants
Bhutan	Zam et al. 2015 (Nation-wide) [130]	40% attrition (4 of 10) in people registered for DM care	–	–
India	Prabhu et al. 2016 (Hospital-based) [131]	Only 11.5% of patients knew about importance of HbA1c	Venugopal et al. 2020 (Hospital-based) [132]	Only 34.9% of the individuals with DM were aware about DR
	Hussain et al. 2016 [133]	40.7% had good knowledge of DM; only 9.6% had undergone DR screening	Shah et al. 2018 (Hospital-based) [134]	Two-thirds of those with T2DM were unaware that the retina can get affected in DM
			Kulkarni et al. 2019 (RAAB survey) [135]	69.3% of patients with DM did not have any previous ophthalmic examination
			Rajalakshmi et al. 2020 (Hospital-based T1DM) [136]	Three-quarters of all participants were compliant with the annual follow-up retinal examination
			Lingam et al. 2018 [137]	Over three-fifths of all patients with DM were aware of DR
			Rani et al. 2005 (Population-based) [138]	50% of urban individuals with DM and STDR had never undergone a fundus evaluation before.
Indonesia	Widyahening et al. 2014 [139]	89% of primary care physicians were aware of the DM guidelines	Sasongko et al. 2020 [140] (Community-based)	In the Jakarta Eye Diabetic Study, 95% of the study population had not had any prior ocular examination
	Arifin et al. 2019 [141]	Participants in primary care had 3.7 times greater diabetic distress than patients in tertiary care	Adriono et al. 2011 [142]	85% had not undergone an ocular examination in the previous year. Less than 50% of DM patients were told of the need for eye examinations by their physicians.
	Rudijanto et al. 2018 [143]	A high proportion of individuals with T1DM and T2DM had impaired hypoglycemic awareness		
Maldives	No KAP studies			
Myanmar	Aung et al. 2019 WHO STEPS [144]	Awareness levels of DM increased from 44.3% in 2004 to 69.4% in 2014	Muecke et al. 2008 [145]	49% of general physicians never assessed the fundus of patients with DM; 86% patients were aware that diabetes affects their vision, but only 57% visited ophthalmologist

(continued)

Table 12.3 (continued)

Country	Author, year	Diabetes KAP	Author, year	Diabetic retinopathy KAP
Nepal	Gyawali et al. 2018 [146]	Awareness level of DM was 65% among T2DM; only 21% of them had their diabetes under control	Thapa et al. 2014 (Hospital-based) [147]	46.6% not aware of DR; 44.4% had first retinal examination only after inpatient admission
	Sapkota et al. 2018 [148]	Poor lifestyle and knowledge/awareness of diabetic control in patients on insulin or those living with DM for a long time	Thapa et al. 2012 (Hospital-based) [149]	Almost half of all diabetic patients in Nepal unaware of DR screening
			Dahal et al. 2017 (Hospital-based) [150]	88.5% were aware of DR; but about two-thirds of patients with DM underwent fundus evaluations for the first time
Sri Lanka	Wijesinghe et al. 2016 (Hospital-based) [151]	70% of patients had a good or very good overall knowledge of DM; poor knowledge regarding hypoglycemia, neuropathy, and foot ulcer prevention	Piyasena et al. 2019 [152] (Population-based)	Uptake of DR services is low due to poor knowledge
	Perera et al. 2013 (at PHC level) [153]	90% of the individuals were unable to recognize hyperglycemic/ hypoglycemic symptoms; 42% not aware of target blood glucose level or annual check-ups	Seneviratne et al. 2016 (Hospital-based [154]	69% had poor knowledge of DR
	Herath et al. 2017 (Population-based) [155]	Majority (77%) had either moderate or above moderate knowledge of DM; >50% of the public never had their blood sugar checked		
Thailand	Porapakkham et al. (NHS Survey), 2008 [156]	Almost half of them unaware of hypertension (56%) and DM (41%) due to old age, low income, and low education	Sriwijitkamol et al. 2011 (Hospital-based) [116]	Only 38% of patients with DM had had a retinal assessment by an ophthalmologist
	Tiptaradol et al. (Population-based) 2012 [157]	>80% were unaware of having DM and hypertension, only 6% achieved target blood sugar and blood pressure control		
Timor-Leste	Dawkins et al. 2015 [118]	Only 68.8% of known diabetic patients received any treatment and mean HbA1c levels of patients was 9.9%	Ramke et al. 2012 [158]	Only 3.6% thought that DM causes eye problems
	Ramke et al. 2012 [159]	Only 6% knew about the symptoms of DM		

KAP Knowledge Attitude Practice, *PHC* primary healthcare, *RAAB* Rapid Assessment of Avoidable Blindness

1. **Bangladesh**

The IDF has estimated that there were 8.4 million people with DM in Bangladesh in 2019, and by 2030, this number is projected to increase to >11 million [1]. The cost of care for DM is high (average annual cost USD864.7/patient). This is significantly higher for women, those who use insulin, those who have had DM for a longer duration, and those with complications [160].

The cumulative incidence of DR over the last 15 years is reported at 50.6% [82]. In one population-based study, the prevalence of DR was 33%, MSVI was 12.2%, and DR-associated blindness was 2.5% [83]. In a hospital-based study of people with T2DM, the proportion of patients with DR, cataract, glaucoma, and diplopia was 55%, 40%, 44%, and 30%, respectively [127].

The Bangladesh DR screening program uses an international-standard grading center with DR software. The grading center reviews fundus photographs, electronically transmitted from three screening centers, and sends recommendations for further management almost immediately. The Bangladesh National Eye Care plan found this modality more cost-effective than screening by ophthalmologists [161]. The National Blindness and Low Vision Survey of Bangladesh recommended screening DR in people with DM by non-medical health workers, and availability of such screening facilities in all hospitals [83, 161].

ORBIS International has supported the Bangladesh Diabetes Somiti (BADAS) in establishing two facilities to treat DR; the World Diabetes Foundation (WDF) has supported BADAS to extend DR care throughout the country.

2. **Bhutan**

Despite being a hilly country where most people undertake daily physical labor, Bhutan's population has a high proportion of overweight and obese people [162]. This number is likely to increase with population ageing, nutrition transitions, and higher rural-to-urban migrations [162]. In 1996, the Ministry of Health of Bhutan started the National Diabetes Control Program, and diabetic clinics were set up in all district hospitals. In a hospital-based study of all new patients examined over 3 years at the National Referral Hospital, Thimphu, 15.8% had DR with DME, and 18.9% had hypertensive retinopathy [86]. The first countrywide review of DM care in Bhutan showed a 40% attrition in people registered for DM care, and only one-third of patients retained in the care had good glycemic control [130].

3. **India**

DM and its associated complications are increasing in India [11, 97]. But, very little has been done at the national level for promoting mass awareness [163]. The main challenge for India is its inability to replicate established National DR screening programs of high-income countries that recommend use of high-end retinal cameras, infrastructure, and trained personnel.

India has used some unique models for DR case finding. These are:

- *Screening camps:* Camps to screen for DM and DR have good turnover, are relatively quick, and offer direct consultation with an ophthalmologist. But such camps require a team of eye health professionals and an accessible location.
- *Telemedicine:* India has used the emerging technology of retinal photography for tele-screening for DR by trained non-ophthalmic technicians. There is good agreement between indirect ophthalmoscopy and tele-screening [165]. It could be well suited for India, given its diverse geography and inadequate number of ophthalmologists.

The Government of India, through its National Program for Control of Blindness and Visual Impairment (NPCBVI), has included support for laser treatment for DR in its 11th five-year plan.

The Public Health Foundation of India (PHFI, published) [166] and Vitreoretinal Society of India (VRSI; doi: 10.4103/ijo) have developed national DR guidelines in India.

4. **Indonesia**

Indonesia is home to the fifth largest adult-onset DM population in the world. This is projected to increase from the current 6.5 million to >20 million population by 2030 [99]. A population-based cross-sectional study on T2DM showed a high prevalence of DR at 43.1% and STDR at 26.3% [99]. Among those with STDR, 1 in 12 was bilaterally blind [99]. The Jakarta Eye Diabetes Study reported that the estimated healthcare cost of DR in Indonesia was nearly 2% of the 2017 national budget and was projected to increase more than threefold in 2025 [140]. The study also reported that 95% of the study population did not have a prior eye examination before screened for DR and that the DR screening was not available to many communities [140]. A guideline for preventing and managing DM has been introduced in Indonesia [168].

5. **Maldives**

National-level reports from the Maldives indicate a low prevalence of DM and pre-diabetes, although approximately two-thirds of the population is overweight (highest in the region) [169]. The prevalence of T2DM is 8.1% (IDF) [1]. The mean annual incidence of T1DM in the age groups <15 and <20 years is increasing—from 3.6 and 2.7/100,000 people in 2009 to 11.0 and 9.1/100,000 in 2018, respectively, an annualized increase of 12% and 13%, respectively [170]. The WDF, with "Project Hope (DM and cancer)" is creating awareness and build resources needed to meet the disease burden in the Maldives [171].

6. **Myanmar**

Myanmar reports a high prevalence of undiagnosed DM and STDR [102, 103]. A major challenge for eye care in Myanmar is the lack of trained personnel.

7. **Nepal**

The WHO estimates that the prevalence of DM in Nepal would rise by more than three times by 2030 [174]. In the Bhaktapur Retina Study, the prevalence of DR was 23.8% in people with known DM and 6.5% in people with newly diagnosed DM [104]. The prevalence of STDR was 9.5%. Cost of care is a major barrier to people seeking healthcare.

8. **Sri Lanka**

The highest recorded prevalence of DM is 18.6% in the Western province of Sri Lanka [176] and 5% of all blindness in Sri Lanka is due to DR [110]. DR service uptake is low, despite the government offers free eye care in Sri Lanka [152].

9. **Thailand**

Thailand has a high prevalence of DM and obesity, as well as an aging population. The age-adjusted prevalence of DM increased from 7.7% in 2004 [30] to 8.3% in 2019 [1]. In recent years, DR care has improved in Thailand. The country has implemented a health care initiative, the "Service Plan," integrating 13 centers of excellence for certain specialties, including ophthalmology. The Ministry of Public Health of Thailand has recognized eye care as a fundamental right. This policy implementation is aimed at reducing preventable blindness and visual impairment from various posterior segment eye diseases [179].

The Ministry of Public Health directly governs the DR screening program in Thailand. The program uses trained health personnel to grade retinal images and detect referable DR at the point of care [179]. The Ministry has set a target of screening at least 60% of people with DM as the performance indicator for the national program. Thailand is also exploring the possibility of using artificial intelligence (AI) for DR screening. An initial retrospective study found the AIs are ~20% more sensitive but 2% less specific than trained personnel in detecting referable DR cases [180]. A prospective study on real-world screening using AI is currently conducted [181]. Thailand is also one of the few countries where bevacizumab is included in the National List of Essential Medications to treat DME [182].

10. **Timor-Leste**

Timor-Leste is the least economically developed country in the SEAR. There is a lack of data on both DM and DR from this country [159]. Dawkins et al. (2015) have reported that only 68.8% of known DM patients received any treatment, and the mean HbA1c among such patients was 9.9% [118]. Over two-thirds of people with DM were undiagnosed. The prevalence of DM at 15.2% in Timor-Leste is similar to those of other countries in the region.

12.2.4 Screening for DR

DR is a prime candidate disorder suitable for universal screening [184]. Traditionally, ophthalmologists screen for DR by dilated eye examination using a direct/indirect ophthalmoscope and slit-lamp biomicroscope.

The WHO has laid four cardinal principles for screening for any medical condition as follows:

1. The condition should be an important health problem with a recognizable pre-symptomatic state.
2. The screening procedure(s) should be acceptable to both, the public and healthcare professionals.
3. Treatment for individuals with recognizable disease should be safe, effective, and universally agreeable.
4. The cost-effectiveness of early diagnosis and treatment should be considered in relation to total healthcare expenditure, including the consequences of leaving the disease untreated.

Numerous studies in high-income countries have demonstrated a reduction in the prevalence of blindness and visual impairment in people with DM where a national program for DM exists [79, 184–187].

Screening for DR can be done either opportunistically or proactively, rolling into the existing health infrastructure with public–private partnerships, where required. Understandably, community participation is critical to its success. In some SEAR countries, DR screening is conducted as part of primary care and many of these programs use a non-mydriatic retinal camera. In SEAR, only Thailand has established systematic DR screening programs [179].

The clinical course of DR has a long asymptomatic phase. Hence, individuals with DM may not regularly visit the ophthalmologist for DR screening unless they are aware of visual loss due to STDR. A universal screening program for DR aims for early identification of people with DR who are at high risk of vision impairment and ensures timely referral to the ophthalmologist/retina specialist to initiate treatment before advanced damage to the eye [184]. Lifelong evaluation for DR by repetitive retinal screening of people with DM is valuable. Color fundus photography is a proven means of effective DR screening [188]. Figure 12.5 shows the stages and varying severities of non-sight threatening and sight-threatening DR. Referral is based on the International Clinical Classification of DR and DME (Table 12.4) [189].

Manual grading of fundus photographs for a large number of people with DM by trained graders incurs substantial costs to the healthcare systems. The advent of artificial intelligence (AI) and deep learning (DL) techniques have raised the possibility of automated detection of retinopathy [190]. Tele ophthalmology that relies on remote screening of DR using digital retinal cameras and retinal image grading can facilitate larger population coverage and timely referrals to ophthalmologists. Tables 12.5 and 12.6 list the

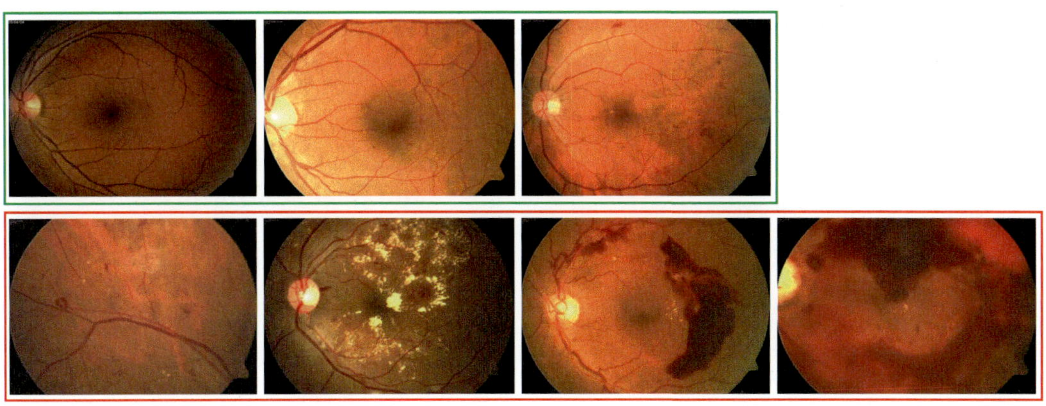

Fig. 12.5 Upper panel—Non-sight threatening DR (green border, left to right: no DR, mild DR, and moderate DR) indicates non-referable DR; these people require observation and good glycemic control. Lower panel—Sight-threatening DR (red border, left to right: severe non-proliferative diabetic retinopathy, diabetic macular edema, proliferative diabetic retinopathy (with preretinal hemorrhage, PDR with vitreous hemorrhage); these people require urgent referral for further management

Table 12.4 (A) Diabetic Retinopathy International Disease Severity Scale [189]. (B) Classification of diabetic macular edema (DME)

(A)	
Severity of DR	**Findings on ophthalmoscopy**
No apparent retinopathy (No DR)	No abnormalities
Mild NPDR (non-proliferative diabetic retinopathy)	Microaneurysms only
Moderate NPDR	More than just microaneurysms but less than severe NPDR
Severe NPDR	Any one of the following: (4:2:1 rule) • More than 20 intraretinal hemorrhages in each of four quadrants • Definite venous beading in 2+ quadrants • Prominent intraretinal microvascular abnormalities (IRMA) in 1+ quadrant *and* no signs of PDR
Proliferative diabetic retinopathy (PDR)	One or more of the following: • Neovascularization • Vitreous/preretinal hemorrhage
(B)	
Diabetic macular edema (DME) classification based on ophthalmoscopy	
No apparent DME	No retinal thickening or hard exudates at macula
Mild DME	Some retinal thickening or hard exudates in posterior pole but distant from the center of the macula
Moderate DME	Retinal thickening or hard exudates approaching the center of the macula, but not involving the center
Severe DME	Retinal thickening or hard exudates involving the center of the macula
DME classification based on Optical Coherence Tomography (OCT)	
Non-center involving DME	Retinal thickening in the macula that does not involve central subfield zone in OCT (1 mm diameter)
Center-involving DME	Retina thickening in the macula that involves the central subfield zone in OCT (1 mm diameter)

DME diabetic macular edema, *DR* diabetic retinopathy, *NPDR* non-proliferative diabetic retinopathy, *PDR* proliferative diabetic retinopathy

Table 12.5 Recommendations for DR screening [191, 192]

American Diabetes Association (ADA) recommendations for timing of eye examination for different types of diabetes mellitus (DM)	
Type 1 DM	Within 5 years after onset of diabetes and annually thereafter
Type 2 DM	At the time of diagnosis and annually thereafter
Women with pre-existing diabetes who plan pregnancy	Before planning pregnancy; at 6 weeks of pregnancy; monitoring every trimester; and for 6 weeks post-partum, as indicated by the degree of retinopathy and advised by ophthalmologist
ADA recommends that patients with DM should have an initial dilated and comprehensive eye examination by an ophthalmologist	
International Council of Ophthalmology (ICO) recommendations for eye examination for people with diabetes	
Visual acuity	Distant vision (with pin hole improvement) and near vision
Retinal assessment/ examination	1. Direct or indirect ophthalmoscopy or slit-lamp biomicroscopy of the retina 2. Retinal photography with any of the following: (a) 30-degree single field or multiple field, (b) wide field, (c) mono or stereo photography, (d) non-mydriatic or mydriatic fundus photography; can be done remotely (telemedicine)

DM diabetes mellitus

screening recommendations for people with DM and the follow-up advice for individuals with and without DR [191, 192].

12.2.5 Artificial Intelligence and Telemedicine in DR Detection

It is expected that automated computer-based analysis of fundus images could partly overcome the problems caused by shortage of health workforce for the enormous burden of screening a large number of people with DM [190, 193, 194]. Such analyses are usually quicker, more accurate,

Table 12.6 Screening and follow-up for people with and without diabetic retinopathy

Status of DR	Referral to ophthalmologist	Follow-up	Recommended intraocular treatment
No diabetic retinopathy (No DR)	Within 1 year	Every 1–2 years	None
Mild NPDR	Within 1 year	Every year	None
Moderate NPDR	Within 3–6 months	Every 6 months	None
Severe NPDR	Immediate	Every 3 months	Can consider PRP under specific circumstances
PDR	Immediate	Every 3 months	PRP and/or intra-vitreal anti-VEGF therapy, especially if high risk characteristics are present
No DME	Within 1 year	Every 1 year	None
Non-center involving DME	Within 3–6 months	Every 3 months	Focal laser photocoagulation, and observe carefully for progression to Center involving DME
Center involving DME	Immediate	Every 1–2 months	Anti-VEGF as first-line therapy. Consider focal macular laser therapy as rescue therapy in eyes with persistent CiDME despite anti-VEGF treatment. Intravitreal steroids can be used as an alternative in pseudophakic eyes or in select cases if anti-VEGF therapy is contraindicated (like a recent episode of MI or CVA)

CVA cerebrovascular accident, *DME* diabetic macular edema, *MI* myocardial infarction, *NPDR* non-proliferative diabetic retinopathy, *PDR* proliferative diabetic retinopathy, *VEGF* vascular endothelial growth factor

consistent, and scalable. Currently, in the absence of legal approvals for the use of AI in DR screening in some countries, it is empirical for ophthalmologists to grade all AI-referable retinal images and reconfirm the diagnosis.

Multiple inexpensive portable imaging devices, validated in terms of sensitivity, specificity of performance, and ease of use even by non-ophthalmological health workers, have been developed in recent years [164]. With the expansion of the information technology and digital imaging fields, image capture, compression, and transmission; data storage; and computational analysis of images has advanced substantially, potentially allowing telemedicine to become more cost-effective. Currently, telemedicine programs for DR are available in three SEAR countries, India, Indonesia, and Thailand. The WDF has provided support to various organizations for the establishment of telemedicine services [164, 165, 195, 196].

Barriers to DR screening are lack of knowledge and awareness about DR in people; and lack of training, skills, screening equipment, and infrastructure for care providers [142, 167].

12.2.6 Support by International Non-Governmental Organizations (INGOs) in DR Care

Many international NGOs (INGOs) support many aspects of DR care in SEAR countries [195–212]. These organizations are the World Diabetes Foundation (WDF), Sight First, Lions Club International Foundation (LCIF), Orbis International, Helen Keller International (HKI), VISION 2020, Sight For All (SFA), and Queen Elizabeth Diamond Jubilee Trust (QEDJT) (Table 12.7). These organizations support advocacy, disease detection, capacity building, infrastructure development, and health system building. At the time of writing, no INGO is working in the Timor-Leste diabetes program.

12.2.6.1 Strategies to Tackle Global Blindness Due To DR

We need broad, population-based strategies to address DM-related vision problems divided into primary, secondary, and tertiary intervention stages (Fig. 12.6).

Table 12.7 Major international non-government organizations supporting diabetic retinopathy care in South-East Asia Region countries [193–210]

Country	NGO	Project/Program
Bangladesh	WDF	Integrated model for comprehensive eye care in people with diabetes
	Orbis	Screening children with T1DM
	HKI	Digital tracking system for tracking blindness from diabetes for government hospitals, increasing awareness among public about DM & DR
Bhutan	WDF	Strengthening DM and NCDs in all districts of the country
India	WDF	Telemedicine DR screening
	LCIF	Screening camps, increasing awareness, capacity building
	QEDJT	Health system building in DR care
Indonesia	WDF	Screening and treatment of vulnerable population
	HKI	DR screening in PHC, increasing awareness among public about DM/DR
Maldives	WDF	Establishment of eye clinics
Myanmar	WDF	Integration of DM/DR care in primary care. WHO-PEN model
	SFA	Setup of secondary eye care centers
Nepal	WDF	Develop national guidelines, capacity building, and integrated eye care
Thailand	WDF	Raising awareness about DM and DR among rural communities.
Timor-Leste	–	–

HKI Helen Keller International, *LCIF* Lions Club International Foundation, *SFA* sight for all, *QEDJT* Queen Elizabeth Diamond Jubilee Trust, *WDF* World Diabetes Foundation

PREVENTION OF BLINDNESS DUE TO DIABETIC RETINOPATHY (DR)

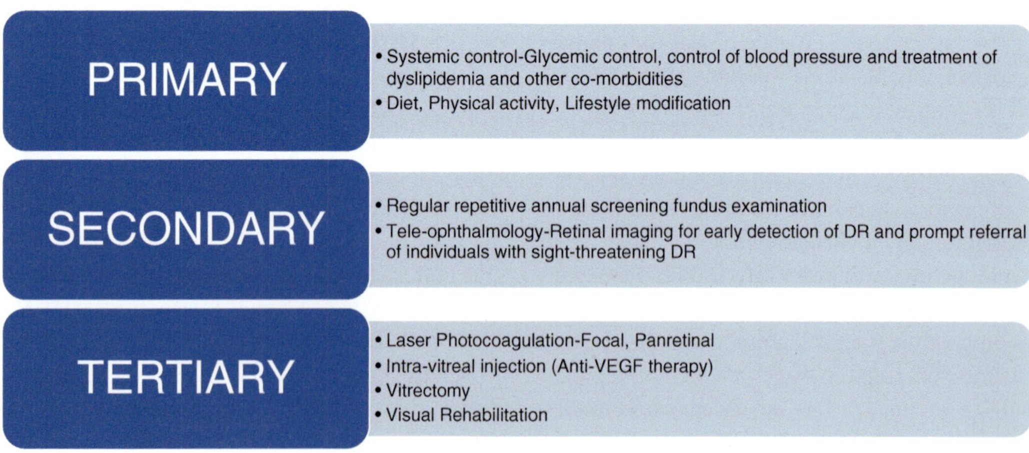

Fig. 12.6 Modes of prevention of blindness at different levels of care

Primary prevention is for individuals with DM without DR that aims to prevent/delay onset of DR; secondary prevention is for those with early stages of DR that aims to prevent DR progression to STDR; and tertiary prevention is for those with STDR that aims to prevent blindness, restore vision, and improve the quality of life of those with visual impairment.

Table 12.8 provides solutions for the various challenges in DR prevention and management in South-East Asia.

Table 12.8 Challenges and solutions for prevention and management of diabetic retinopathy in South-East Asia

Challenge	Solutions
Awareness regarding DR is poor among people with DM	1. Patient education materials to be available at primary, secondary, and tertiary healthcare centers. 2. Structured education for patients with DM to manage their blood sugar levels, to ensure compliance with regular annual eye examinations, and information regarding the risk to their vision due to DM.
Awareness about regular DR screening is not optimal among primary care/general physicians	1. Education (CME) programs for primary healthcare general physicians/ diabetologists. 2. Good inter-referral practice and communication between physicians and ophthalmologists regarding patients' retinal findings and a clear documentation of the care pathway.
Motivate lifestyle modifications in patients with DM	1. Educational and media campaigns to promote healthy food choices; reduce the consumption of unhealthy foods. 2. The primary care physician, in discussion with an endocrinologist/ diabetologist and other specialists can develop individualized plans tailored to each patient. 3. Empower patients with DM to self-manage their health though diet, exercise, and monitoring of blood pressure (BP) and blood glucose levels. 4. Deploy technologies/devices to track activities that promote lifestyle changes such as use of smart phones and mobile apps for monitoring blood sugar and BP, setting reminders for medications
DR management variation across settings/difficulty in implementing guidelines in resource-limited settings	Adoption of DR management based on the type of resource setting (as recommended in the International Council of Ophthalmology (ICO) guidelines)
Limited access to DR screening in poor-resource settings	1. Telemedicine-based DR screening. 2. Engagement of non-governmental organizations (NGOs)/other voluntary organizations to implement DR screening programs and providing free equipment/fundus camera 3. Public–private partnership (PPP). Engage private partners to assist in DR management.
Sustainability of DR screening programs	1. Integrating DR screening into existing NCD programs. 2. Artificial intelligence-assisted DR screening with careful monitoring. 3. Screening based on risk stratification; e.g., extending the screening interval from annually to once in 2 years in people with low risk.
Inadequate capacity of healthcare services to deliver primary and secondary prevention in low- and middle-income countries (LMICs)	Partnering with the World Diabetes Foundation, international NGOs, and private partners, to improve DR care by providing medicines, equipment, training for eye care professionals, screening and treatment of DR, and rehabilitation
Securing policies by commitment of decision-makers in the Health Ministry to promote the prevention of avoidable blindness due to DR	1. Policy changes to encourage lifestyle changes like taxing unhealthy foods, food labels at supermarkets, parks/exercise tracks in the neighborhood, smoking restrictions in public places, etc. 2. Integrating eye care into routine diabetes care/primary care and integrating DR policies, guidelines, and training into all relevant national health policies and guidelines. 3. Development of national action plans for addressing DR in consultation with relevant stakeholders such as those involved in diabetic care and eye care, patients with DM, and the public and private sector, and integrating these plans into national diabetes strategies. 4. Promote surveillance and research for assessing the burden of DR and the needs; evaluate the cost-effectiveness of screening and interventions, especially in LMICs.

DM diabetes mellitus

12.3 Conclusion

South-East Asian countries are ethnically diverse and geographically dispersed. Identification barriers and implementation of country-specific cultural and resource-specific strategies are required to reduce the burden of DM and DR. Studies in the SEAR have shown need for greater awareness and advocacy. This will be possible with participation of all stakeholders—government, INGOs, civil societies, and communities. There is urgent need for capacity building, infrastructure development, increasing funding for primary and secondary prevention, health promotion, and implementation of DM/DR guidelines, along with validation/use of emerging technologies/techniques for DR screening and treatment.

Recommendations for Integrated DM, NCDs, and DM Eye Care

I. Integration of eye care and routine DM care
   - Training of general physicians and diabetologists to educate and raise awareness of DR in people with DM.
   - Regular retinal screening as part of diabetes care by service providers.
   - Robust referral pathways for people detected as having referable DR/STDR.
   - Effective management of available resources for health and wellness including lifestyle management and glycemic control.

II. Integration of DM with comprehensive/primary eye care
   - Capacity building and skill enhancement of health personnel relevant to understanding DM and DR.
   - Patient support with appropriate management to reduce DM-related vision loss.

III. Services and continuum of care
   - Improved referral and recall pathways.
   - Innovative methods to improve compliance and encourage continuum of care.

IV. Integration of DR policies into national health policies and guidelines
   - Integration of DR specific policies in national NCD strategic plans and other public policies.
   - Creation of national action plans for DR.
   - Inclusion of DR in health insurance schemes to ensure sufficient financial coverage for screening and treatment.
   - Standard operating procedures for care at different levels, from primary to tertiary care.

References

1. International Diabetes Federation. IDF Diabetes Atlas. 9th ed. Brussels: International Diabetes Federation; 2019.
2. Narain JP, Garg R, Fric A. Non-communicable diseases in the South-East Asia region: burden, strategies, and opportunities. Natl Med J India. 2011;24:280–7.
3. World Health Organization. Action plan for the prevention and control of noncommunicable diseases in South-East Asia, 2013–2020. New Delhi: WHO Regional Office for South-East Asia; 2013.
4. World Health Organization. Noncommunicable diseases in South-East Asia. https://www.who.int/southeastasia/health-topics/noncommunicable-diseases. Accessed 19 Sept 2020.
5. World Health Organization. Noncommunicable diseases in the South-East Asia Region: Situation and response 2011. New Delhi: WHO Regional Office for South-East Asia; 2011.
6. World Health Organization, South East Asian Region-Noncommunicable Diseases. https://www.who.int/nmh/ncd-tools/who-regions-south-east-asia/en/. Accessed 19 Sept 2020.
7. American Diabetes Association. Classification and diagnosis of diabetes: standards of medical care in diabetes—2020. Diabetes Care. 2020;43(S1):S14–31.
8. Unnikrishnan R, Pradeepa R, Joshi SR, et al. Type 2 Diabetes: demystifying the global epidemic. Diabetes. 2017;66:1432–42.
9. Danaei G, Finucane MM, Lu Y, et al. National, regional, and global trends in fasting plasma glucose and diabetes prevalence since 1980: systematic analysis of health examination surveys and epidemiological studies with 370 country-years and 2.7 million participants. Lancet. 2011;378:31–40.

10. Pradeepa R, Mohan V. Prevalence of type 2 diabetes and its complications in India and economic costs to the nation. Eur J Clin Nutr. 2017;71:816–24.
11. Anjana RM, Deepa M, Pradeepa R, et al., ICMR–INDIAB Collaborative Study Group. Prevalence of diabetes and prediabetes in 15 states of India: results from the ICMR-INDIAB population-based cross-sectional study. Lancet Diabetes Endocrinol. 2017;5:585–96.
12. Zabetian A, Sanchez IM, Narayan KM, et al. Global rural diabetes prevalence: a systematic review and meta-analysis covering 1990–2012. Diabetes Res Clin Pract. 2014;104:206–13.
13. Bird Y, Lemstra M, Rogers M, et al. The relationship between socioeconomic status/income and prevalence of diabetes and associated conditions: a cross-sectional population-based study in Saskatchewan, Canada. Int J Equity Health. 2015;14:93. https://doi.org/10.1186/s12939-015-0237-0.
14. Tabish SA. Is diabetes becoming the biggest epidemic of the twenty-first century? Int J Health Sci (Qassim). 2007;1:V–VIII. PMID: 21475425.
15. Gujral UP, Pradeepa R, Weber MB, et al. Type 2 diabetes in South Asians: similarities and differences with white Caucasian and other populations. Ann N Y Acad Sci. 2013;1281:51–63.
16. Oldroyd J, Banerjee M, Heald A, Cruickshank K. Diabetes and ethnic minorities. Postgrad Med J. 2005;81:486–90.
17. Bulletin of the World Health Organization. 2017;95:550–1. https://www.who.int/bulletin/volumes/95/8/17-020817/en/
18. International Diabetes Federation. IDF Diabetes Atlas. 1st ed. Brussels: International Diabetes Federation; 2000.
19. International Diabetes Federation. IDF Diabetes Atlas. 2nd ed. Brussels: International Diabetes Federation; 2003.
20. International Diabetes Federation. IDF Diabetes Atlas. 3rd ed. Brussels: International Diabetes Federation; 2007.
21. International Diabetes Federation. IDF Diabetes Atlas. 4th ed. Brussels: International Diabetes Federation; 2010.
22. International Diabetes Federation. IDF Diabetes Atlas. 5th ed. Brussels: International Diabetes Federation; 2011.
23. International Diabetes Federation. IDF Diabetes Atlas. 6th ed. Brussels: International Diabetes Federation; 2013.
24. International Diabetes Federation. IDF Diabetes Atlas. 7th ed. Brussels: International Diabetes Federation; 2015.
25. International Diabetes Federation. IDF Diabetes Atlas. 8th ed. Brussels: International Diabetes Federation; 2017.
26. Gyawali B, Sharma R, Neupane D, et al. Prevalence of type 2 diabetes in Nepal: a systematic review and meta-analysis from 2000 to 2014. Glob Health Action. 2015;8:29088. https://doi.org/10.3402/gha.v8.29088.
27. Biswas T, Islam A, Rawal LB, et al. Increasing prevalence of diabetes in Bangladesh: a scoping review. Public Health. 2016;138:4–11.
28. Wangdi K, Jamtsho T. Risk factors for self-reported diabetes among Bhutanese adults: a nationally representative survey data analysis. PLoS One. 2018;15:e0206034. https://doi.org/10.1371/journal.pone.
29. Latt TS, Zaw KK, Ko K, Hlaing MM, et al. Measurement of diabetes, prediabetes and their associated risk factors in Myanmar 2014. Diabetes Metab Syndr Obes. 2019;12:291–8.
30. Aekplakorn W, Chariyalertsak S, Kessomboon P, et al. Prevalence of diabetes and relationship with socioeconomic status in the Thai population: National Health Examination Survey, 2004-2014. J Diabetes Res. 2018;1654530 https://doi.org/10.1155/2018/1654530.
31. Hunter DJ, Reddy KS. Noncommunicable diseases. N Engl J Med. 2013;369:1336–43.
32. Mensah GA, Roth GA, Fuster V. The Global burden of cardiovascular diseases and risk factors: 2020 and beyond. J Am Coll Cardiol. 2019;74:2529–32.
33. Roth GA, Johnson C, Abajobir A, et al. Global, regional, and national burden of cardiovascular diseases for 10 causes, 1990 to 2015. J Am Coll Cardiol. 2017;70:1–25.
34. World Health Organization. Cancer. https://www.who.int/health-topics/cancer#tab=tab_1. Accessed 22 Sept 2020.
35. Bray F, Ferlay J, Soerjomataram I, et al. Global cancer statistics 2018: GLOBOCAN estimates of incidence and mortality worldwide for 36 cancers in 185 countries. CA: A Cancer J Clin. 2018;68:394–424.
36. GBD 2015 Mortality and Causes of Death Collaborators. Global, regional, and national life expectancy, all-cause mortality, and cause-specific mortality for 249 causes of death, 1980–2015: a systematic analysis for the Global Burden of Disease Study 2015. Lancet. 2016;388:1459–544.
37. GBD Chronic Respiratory Disease Collaborators. Prevalence and attributable health burden of chronic respiratory diseases, 1990-2017: a systematic analysis for the Global Burden of Disease Study 2017. Lancet Respir Med. 2020;8:585–96.
38. World Health Organization, Regional Office for South-East Asia. Noncommunicable diseases in the South-East Asia Region, 2011: situation and response. WHO Regional Office for South-East Asia. 2012. https://apps.who.int/iris/handle/10665/205578
39. Global Health Observatory. World Health Organization 2020. http://apps.who.int/ghodata/?region=searo. Accessed 22 Sept 2020.
40. Prabhakaran D, Jeemon P, Roy A. Cardiovascular diseases in India: current epidemiology and future directions. Circulation. 2016;133:1605–20.

41. Al Mamun M, Rumana N, Pervin K, et al. Emerging burden of cardiovascular diseases in Bangladesh. J Atheroscler Thromb. 2016;23:365–75.
42. Noronha V, Tsomo U, Jamshed A, et al. A fresh look at oncology facts on south central Asia and SAARC countries. South Asian J Cancer. 2012;1:1–4.
43. India State-Level Disease Burden Initiative Cancer Collaborators. The burden of cancers and their variations across the states of India: the Global Burden of Disease Study 1990-2016. Lancet Oncol. 2018;19:1289–306.
44. Pun CB, Pradhananga KK, Siwakoti B, et al. Malignant neoplasm burden in Nepal – Data from the seven major cancer service hospitals for 2012. Asian Pac J Cancer Prev. 2015;16:8659–63.
45. Virani S, Bilheem S, Chansaard W, et al. National and subnational population-based incidence of Cancer in Thailand: assessing cancers with the highest burdens. Cancers (Basel). 2017;9:108. https://doi.org/10.3390/cancers9080108.
46. India State-Level Disease Burden Initiative CRD Collaborators. The burden of chronic respiratory diseases and their heterogeneity across the states of India: the Global Burden of Disease Study 1990-2016. Lancet Glob Health. 2018;6:e1363–74. https://doi.org/10.1016/S2214-109X(18)30409-1.
47. Thanaviratananich S, Cho SH, Ghoshal AG, et al. Burden of respiratory disease in Thailand: results from the APBORD observational study. Medicine (Baltimore). 2016;95:e4090. https://doi.org/10.1097/MD.0000000000004090.
48. Radhika G, Van Dam RM, Sudha V, et al. Refined grain consumption and the metabolic syndrome in urban Asian Indians (Chennai Urban Rural Epidemiology Study 57). Metabolism. 2009;58:675–81.
49. Radhika G, Sudha V, Mohan Sathya R, et al. Association of fruit and vegetable intake with cardiovascular risk factors in urban south Indians. Br J Nutr. 2008;99:398–405.
50. Anand SS, Hawkes C, De Souza RJ, et al. Food consumption and its impact on cardiovascular disease: importance of solutions focused on the globalized food system: a report from the Workshop Convened by the World Heart Federation. J Am Coll Cardiol. 2015;66:1590–614.
51. Schmidhuber J, Shetty P. The nutrition transition to 2030. Why developing countries are likely to bear the major burden. Acta Agric Scand C. 2005;2:150–66.
52. World Health Organization. Diet, nutrition and the prevention of chronic diseases. Report of a joint WHO/FAO expert consultation. Geneva: World Health Organization; 2003.
53. Peltzer K, Pengpid S. Fruits and vegetables consumption and associated factors among in-school adolescents in five Southeast Asian countries. Int J Environ Res Public Health. 2012;9:3575–87.
54. World Health Organization 2010. Creating an enabling environment for population-based salt reduction strategies. Report of a joint technical meeting held by WHO and the Food Standards Agency, UK. 2010.
55. Jayatissa R, Yamori Y, De Silva AH, et al. Estimation of salt intake, potassium intake and sodium-to-potassium ratio by 24-hour urinary excretion: an urban rural study in Sri Lanka. https://doi.org/10.1101/2020.04.17.20068833.
56. Neupane D, Rijal A, Henry ME, et al. Mean dietary salt intake in Nepal: a population survey with 24-hour urine collections. J Clin Hypertension. 2020;22:273–9.
57. Radhika G, Sathya RM, Sudha V, et al. Dietary salt intake and hypertension in an Urban South Indian population – [CURES - 53]. J Assoc Physicians India. 2007;55:405–11.
58. Zaman MM, Choudhury SR, et al. Salt intake in an adult population of Bangladesh. Glob Heart. 2017;12:265–6.
59. Lee IM, Shiroma EJ, Lobelo F, et al., Lancet Physical Activity Series Working Group. Effect of physical inactivity on major non-communicable diseases worldwide: an analysis of burden of disease and life expectancy. Lancet. 2012;380:219–29.
60. Ranasinghe CD, Ranasinghe P, Jayawardena R, et al. Physical activity patterns among South-Asian adults: a systematic review. Int J Behav Nutr Phys Act. 2013;10:116. https://doi.org/10.1186/1479-5868-10-116.
61. Anjana RM, Pradeepa R, Das AK, et al., ICMR–INDIAB Collaborative Study Group. Physical activity and inactivity patterns in India-results from the ICMR-INDIAB study (Phase-1) [ICMR-INDIAB-5]. Int J Behav Nutr Phys Act. 2014;11:26. https://doi.org/10.1186/1479-5868-11-26.
62. Ministry of Healthcare and Nutrition Healthcare Sector Development Project/World Bank. National Noncommunicable Disease Risk Factor Survey. Colombo: Directorate of Noncommunicable Disease Ministry of Healthcare and Nutrition Sri Lanka; 2008. https://www.who.int/ncds/surveillance/steps/2006_STEPS_Survey_SriLanka.pdf. Accessed 25 Sept 2020.
63. Katulanda P, Jayawardana R, Ranasinghe P, et al. Physical activity patterns and correlates among adults from a developing country: the Sri Lanka Diabetes and Cardiovascular Study. Public Health Nutr. 2013;16:1684–92.
64. World Health Organization Country Office for the Republic of Maldives. WHO STEPS survey on risk factors for noncommunicable diseases. Maldives, 2011. New Delhi: Regional Office form South-East Asia; 2014. SEA-NCD-91; http://www.searo.who.int/entity/noncommunicable_diseases/data/maldives_2011-steps-survey-report.pdf. Accessed 25 Sept 2020.
65. Aryal KK, Neupane S, Mehata S, et al. Non communicable diseases risk factors: STEPS survey Nepal 2013. Kathmandu: Nepal Health Research Council; 2014. www.who.int/chp/steps/2012-13_Nepal_STEPS_Report.pdf. Accessed 25 Sept 2020.

66. Thakur JS, Garg R, Narain JP, et al. Tobacco use: a major risk factor for non-communicable diseases in South-East Asia region. Indian J Public Health. 2011;55:155–60.
67. Anderson I. Tobacco as a development issue: latest estimates from WHO. 2012. http://devpolicy.org/tobacco-as-a-development-issue-latest-estimates-from-who20120430. Accessed 24 Sept 2020.
68. World Health Organization. Noncommunicable diseases in the Western Pacific Region. Manila: WHO Office of the Western Pacific Region; 2012.
69. World Health Organization. Tobacco control in South East Asia. https://www.who.int/southeastasia/health-topics/tobacco. Accessed 25 Sept 2020.
70. World Health Organization. Health situation in the South-East Asia Region 2001-2007. New Delhi: SEARO; 2008. https://apps.who.int/iris/handle/10665/205256. Accessed 25 Sept 2020.
71. World Health Organization. Non communicable diseases: harmful use of alcohol. http://www.emro.who.int/noncommunicable-diseases/causes/harmful-use-of-alcohol.html. Accessed 25 Sept 2020.
72. World Health Organization. Regional Office for South-East Asia. Making South-East Asia SAFER from alcohol-related harm: current status and way forward. 2019. https://apps.who.int/iris/handle/10665/326535.
73. Jakkaew N, Pinyopornpanish K, Jiraporncharoen W, et al. Risk of harm from alcohol use and heavy alcohol consumption: its association with other NCD risk factors in Thailand. Sci Rep. 2019;9:16343. https://doi.org/10.1038/s41598-019-52754-w.
74. Yau JW, Rogers SL, Kawasaki R, et al. Global prevalence and major risk factors of diabetic retinopathy. Diabetes Care. 2012;35:556–64.
75. Bourne RR, Stevens GA, White RA, et al. Causes of vision loss worldwide, 1990–2010: a systematic analysis. Lancet Glob Health. 2013;1(6):e339–49. https://doi.org/10.1016/S2214-109X(13)70113-X.
76. Leasher JL, Bourne RR, Flaxman SR, et al., Vision Loss Expert Group of the Global Burden of Disease Study. Global estimates on the number of people blind or visually impaired by diabetic retinopathy: a meta-analysis from 1990 to 2010. Diabetes Care. 2016;39:1643–9.
77. Sabanayagam C, Banu R, Chee ML, et al. Incidence and progression of diabetic retinopathy: a systematic review. Lancet Diabetes Endocrinol. 2019:140–9. https://doi.org/10.1016/S2213-8587(18)30128-1.
78. https://www.iapb.org/learn/vision-atlas/. Accessed 22 Sept 2020.
79. Liew G, Michaelides M, Bunce C. A comparison of the causes of blindness certifications in England and Wales in working age adults (16-64 years), 1999-2000 with 2009-2010. BMJ Open. 2014:e004015. https://doi.org/10.1136/bmjopen-2013-004015.1.
80. Claessen H, Kvitkina T, Narres M, et al. Markedly decreasing incidence of blindness in people with and without diabetes in southern Germany. Diabetes Care. 2018;41:478–84.
81. Wong TY, Sabanayagam C. Strategies to tackle the global burden of diabetic retinopathy: from epidemiology to artificial intelligence. Ophthalmologica. 2020;243:9–20.
82. Ahmed KR, Karim MN, Bhowmik B, et al. Incidence of diabetic retinopathy in Bangladesh: a 15-year follow-up study. J diabetes. 2012;4:386–91.
83. Muqit MM, Kourgialis N, Jackson-deGraffenried M, et al. Trends in diabetic retinopathy, visual acuity, and treatment outcomes for patients living with diabetes in a fundus photograph–based diabetic retinopathy screening program in Bangladesh. JAMA Network open. 2019;2:e191628. https://doi.org/10.1001/jamanetworkopen.
84. Akhter A, Fatema K, Ahmed SF, et al. Prevalence and associated risk indicators of retinopathy in a rural Bangladeshi population with and without diabetes. Ophthal Epidemiol. 2013;20:220–7.
85. Billah MM, Rahim MA, Rahman MA, et al. Pattern and risk factors of diabetic retinopathy among type 2 diabetic patients: experience in a tertiary care hospital. J Med. 2016;17:17–20.
86. Rai BB, Morley MG, Bernstein PS, et al. Pattern of vitreo-retinal diseases at the national referral hospital in Bhutan: a retrospective, hospital-based study. BMC Ophthalmol. 2020;20:1. https://doi.org/10.1186/s12886-020-01335-x.
87. Chhetri V, Pokhrel HP, Zangmo L, et al. Diabetes case burden at central regional referral hospital, Gelephu, Bhutan; a retrospective study. Int Healthcare Res J. 2020;4:38–43.
88. Agrawal RP, Ranka M, Beniwal R, et al. Prevalence of diabetic retinopathy in type 2 diabetes in relation to risk factors: hospital based study. Int J Diabetes Dev Ctries. 2003;23:16–9.
89. Rema M, Deepa R, Mohan V. Prevalence of retinopathy at diagnosis among type 2 diabetic patients attending a diabetic centre in South India. Br J Ophthalmol. 2000;84:1058–60.
90. Rema M, Premkumar S, Anitha B, et al. Prevalence of diabetic retinopathy in urban India: the Chennai Urban Rural Epidemiology Study (CURES) eye study, I. Invest Ophthalmol Vis Sci. 2005;46:2328–33.
91. Raman R, Rani PK, Rachepalle SR, et al. Prevalence of diabetic retinopathy in India: Sankara Nethralaya diabetic retinopathy epidemiology and molecular genetics study report 2. Ophthalmology. 2009;116:311–8.
92. Namperumalsamy P, Kim R, Vignesh TP, et al. Prevalence and risk factors for diabetic retinopathy: a population-based assessment from Theni District, South India. Br J Ophthalmol. 2009;93:429–34.
93. Raman R, Ganesan S, Pal SS, et al. Prevalence and risk factors for diabetic retinopathy in rural India. Sankara Nethralaya Diabetic Retinopathy Epidemiology and Molecular Genetic Study III (SN-DREAMS III), report no 2. BMJ Open Diabetes Res Care. 2014;2:e000005. https://doi.org/10.1136/bmjdrc-2013-000005.

94. Jonas JB, Nangia V, Khare A, et al. Prevalence and associated factors of diabetic retinopathy in rural central India. Diabetes Care. 2013;36:e69. https://doi.org/10.2337/dc12-2377.
95. Ramavat PR, Ramavat MR, Ghugare BW, et al. Prevalence of diabetic retinopathy in Western Indian type 2 diabetic population: a hospital–based cross–sectional study. J Clinic Diagnost Res. 2013;7:1387–90.
96. Gadkari SS, Maskati QB, Nayak BK. Prevalence of diabetic retinopathy in India: the All India Ophthalmological Society Diabetic Retinopathy Eye Screening Study 2014. Indian J Ophthalmol. 2016;64:38–44.
97. Rajalakshmi R, Behera UC, Bhattacharjee H, Das T, Gilbert C, Murthy GV, et al. Spectrum of eye disorders in diabetes (SPEED) in India. Report # 2. Diabetic retinopathy and risk factors for sight threatening diabetic retinopathy in people with type 2 diabetes in India. Indian J Ophthalmol. 2020;68:S21–S6.
98. 2016. www.who.int/diabetes/global-report.
99. Sasongko MB, Widyaputri F, Agni AN, et al. Prevalence of diabetic retinopathy and blindness in Indonesian adults with type 2 diabetes. Am J Ophthalmol. 2017;181:79–87.
100. World Health Organization. Diabetes Programme: country and regional data on diabetes. Geneva: World Health Organization; 2012.
101. Thoufeeq U, Das T, Limburg H, et al. First rapid assessment of avoidable blindness survey in the Maldives: prevalence and causes of blindness and cataract surgery. Asia-Pacific J Ophthalmol. 2018;7:316–20.
102. Patel S, Klein RM, Patel A, et al. Diabetic retinopathy screening and treatment in Myanmar: a pilot study. BMJ Open Ophthalmol. 2017;1 https://doi.org/10.1136/bmjophth-2017-000084.
103. Latt TS, Zaw KK, Ko K, et al. Measurement of diabetes, prediabetes and their associated risk factors in Myanmar 2014. Diabetes Metabolic Syndrome Obes Targets Ther. 2019;12:291. https://doi.org/10.2147/DMSO.S156270.
104. Thapa R, Twyana SN, Paudyal G, et al. Prevalence and risk factors of diabetic retinopathy among an elderly population with diabetes in Nepal: the Bhaktapur Retina Study. Clin Ophthalmol (Auckland, NZ). 2018;12:561. https://doi.org/10.2147/OPTH.S157560.
105. Mishra SK, Pant BP, Subedi P. The Prevalence of diabetic retinopathy among known diabetic population in Nepal. Kathmandu Univ Med J (KUMJ). 2016;14:134–9.
106. Paudyal G, Shrestha MK, Poudel M, et al. Prevalence and severity of diabetic retinopathy among diabetic patients presenting to a tertiary eye hospital in Nepal. Middle East Afr J Ophthalmol. 2019;26:210–5.
107. Agarwal LT, Agrawal N. Prevalence of diabetic retinopathy among self-reported adult diabetics in districts of eastern Nepal in a community-based study. Nepalese J Ophthalmol. 2017;9:136–42.
108. Katulanda P, Ranasinghe P, Jayawardena R. Prevalence of retinopathy among adults with self-reported diabetes mellitus: the Sri Lanka diabetes and Cardiovascular Study. BMC Ophthalmol. 2014;14:100. https://doi.org/10.1186/1471-2415-14-100.
109. Ranasinghe P, Jayawardena R, Katulanda P. The facts, figures, and reality of the diabetes epidemic in Sri Lanka: a systematic review. Int J Diabetes Dev Ctries. 2015;35:501–13.
110. https://www.iapb.org/wp-content/uploads/Sri-Lanka-Action-Plan-2013-17.pdf
111. Chetthakul T, Deerochanawong C, Suwanwalaikorn S, et al. Thailand diabetes registry project: prevalence of diabetic retinopathy and associated factors in type 2 diabetes mellitus. J Med Assoc Thai. 2006;89(Suppl 1):S27–36.
112. Chetthakul T, Likitmaskul S, Plengvidhya N, et al. Thailand diabetes registry project: prevalence of diabetic retinopathy and associated factors in type 1 diabetes mellitus. J Med Assoc Thai Chotmaihetthangphaet. 2006;89(Suppl 1):S17–26.
113. Coverage of Diabetic Retinopathy Screening and Prevalence of Diabetic Retinopathy in Public Health Regional Service Provider 6th, Thailand 2016. 2018;35(2):April–June.
114. Jongsareejit A, Potisat S, Krairittichai U, et al. The Thai DMS diabetes complications (DD. Comp.) project: prevalence and risk factors of diabetic retinopathy in Thai patients with type 2 diabetes mellitus. J Med Assoc Thai. 2013;96:1476–82.
115. Phoksunthorn T, Thatsnarong D. Retinopathy and macro-albuminuria in type 2 diabetic patients. J Med Assoc Thai. 2007;90:684–7.
116. Sriwijitkamol A, Moungngern Y, Vannaseang S. Assessment and prevalence of diabetic complications in 722 Thai type 2 diabetes patients. J Med Assoc Thai. 2011;94:168. PMID: 21721443.
117. Silpa-Archa S, Sukhawarn R. Prevalence and associated factors of diabetic retinopathy in Chandrubeksa Hospital, Directorate of Medical services, Royal Thai Air Force. J Med Assoc Thai. 2012;95(Suppl 4):S43–9.
118. Dawkins RC, Oliver GF, Sharma M, et al. An estimation of the prevalence of diabetes mellitus and diabetic retinopathy in adults in Timor-Leste. BMC Res Notes. 2015;8:249. https://doi.org/10.1186/s13104-015-1171-3.
119. https://www.dhsprogram.com/publications/publication-fr329-dhs-final-reports.cfm
120. World Health Organization. Regional Office for South-East Asia. Strengthening diagnosis and treatment of Diabetic Retinopathy in SEA Region. 2020. https://apps.who.int/iris/handle/10665/334224. License: CC BY-NC-SA 3.0 IGO.
121. Jonas JB, George R, Asokan R, et al., Vision Loss Expert Group of the Global Burden of Disease Study. Prevalence and causes of vision loss in cen-

tral and south Asia: 1900-2010. Br J Ophthalmol. 2014;98:592–8.

122. Das T. Blindness and visual impairment profile and rapid assessment of avoidable blindness in South East Asia: analysis of new data. 2017 APAO Holmes Lecture. Asia-Pac J Ophthalmol. 2018;7:312–5.
123. VISION2020 Secretariat, Ministry of Health Sri Lanka. National survey of blindness, visual impairment, ocular morbidity and disability in Sri Lanka. A report (2014–2015). http://www.iapb.org/wp--content/uploads/National-Survey-of-Blindness-A-Report-2014-2015.pdf
124. Thoufeeq U, Das T, Limburg H, et al. First rapid assessment of avoidable blindness (RAAB) in Maldives: prevalence and causes of blindness and cataract surgery. Asia Pac J Ophthalmol (Phila). 2018. https://doi.org/10.22608/APO.2017332.
125. Correia M, Das T, Mango J, et al. Nation-wide rapid assessment of avoidable blindness (RAAB) in Timor-Leste: prevalence and causes of blindness, visual impairment and cataract surgery. Clin Ophthalmol. 2017;11:2125–31.
126. Rahman M, Nakamura K, Kizuki M. Socioeconomic differences in the prevalence, awareness, and control of diabetes in Bangladesh. J Diabetes Complications. 2015;29:788–93.
127. Ahmed KR, Jebunessa F, Hossain S, et al. Ocular knowledge and practice among type 2 diabetic patients in a tertiary care hospital in Bangladesh. BMC Ophthalmol. 2017;17:171. https://doi.org/10.1186/s12886-017-0560-x.
128. Fottrell E, Ahmed N, Shaha SK. J, et al. Diabetes knowledge and care practices among adults in rural Bangladesh: a cross-sectional survey. BMJ Glob Health. 2018;3:e000891. https://doi.org/10.1136/bmjgh-2018-000891.
129. Islam FMA, Kawasaki R, Finger RP. Factors associated with participation in a diabetic retinopathy screening program in a rural district in Bangladesh. Diabetes Res Clin Pract. 2018;144:111–7.
130. Zam K, Kumar AM, Achanta S, et al. A first country-wide review of diabetes mellitus care in Bhutan: time to do better. BMC Health Serv Res. 2015;15:389. https://doi.org/10.1186/s12913-015-1026-6.
131. Prabhu M, Kakhandaki A, Chandra KR, et al. A Hospital based study regarding awareness of association between glycosylated haemoglobin and severity of diabetic retinopathy in type 2 diabetic individuals. J Clin Diagn Res. 2016;10:NC01–NC4. https://doi.org/10.7860/JCDR/2016/15834.7014.
132. Venugopal D, Lal B, Fernandes S, Gavde D. Awareness and knowledge of diabetic retinopathy and associated factors in Goa: a hospital-based cross-sectional study. Indian J Ophthalmol. 2020;68:383–90.
133. Hussain R, Rajesh B, Giridhar A, et al. Knowledge and awareness about diabetes mellitus and diabetic retinopathy in suburban population of a south Indian state and its practice among the patients with diabetes mellitus: a population-based study. Indian J Ophthalmol. 2016;64:272–6.
134. Shah K, Gandhi A, Natarajan S. Diabetic retinopathy awareness and associations with multiple comorbidities: insights from DIAMOND Study. Indian J Endocrinol Metab. 2018;22:30–5.
135. Kulkarni S, Kondalkar S, Mactaggart I, et al. Estimating the magnitude of diabetes mellitus and diabetic retinopathy in an older age urban population in Pune, western India. BMJ Open Ophthalmol. 2019;4(1):e000201. https://doi.org/10.1136/bmjophth-2018-000201.
136. Rajalakshmi R, Shanthirani CS, Anandakumar A, et al. Assessment of diabetic retinopathy in type 1 diabetes in a diabetes care center in South India-Feasibility and awareness improvement study. Indian J Ophthalmol. 2020;68(Suppl 1):S92–5.
137. Lingam S, Rani PK, Sheeladevi S, et al. Knowledge, attitude and practices on diabetes, hypertension and diabetic retinopathy and the factors that motivate screening for diabetes and diabetic retinopathy in a pyramidal model of eye health care. Rural Remote Health. 2018;18:4304. https://doi.org/10.22605/RRH4304.
138. Rani PK, Raman R, Paul PG, et al. Use of eye care services by people with diabetes–South Indian experience. Br J Ophthalmol. 2005;82:410–4.
139. Widyahening IS, van der Graaf Y, Soewondo P, et al. Awareness, agreement, adoption and adherence to type 2 diabetes mellitus guidelines: a survey of Indonesian primary care physicians. BMC Fam Pract. 2014;15:72. https://doi.org/10.1186/1471-2296-15-72.
140. Sasongko MB, Wardhana FS, Febryanto GA, et al. The estimated healthcare cost of diabetic retinopathy in Indonesia and its projection for 2025. Br J Ophthalmol. 2020;104:487–92.
141. Arifin B, van Asselt ADI, Setiawan D, et al. Diabetes distress in Indonesian patients with type 2 diabetes: a comparison between primary and tertiary care. BMC Health Serv Res. 2019;19:773. https://doi.org/10.1186/s12913-019-4515-1.
142. Adriono G, Wang D, Octavianus C, et al. Use of eye care services among diabetic patients in urban Indonesia. Arch Ophthalmol. 2011;129:930–5.
143. Rudijanto A, Saraswati MR, Yunir E, et al. Indonesia Cohort of IO HAT Study to evaluate diabetes management, control, and complications in retrospective and prospective periods among insulin-treated patients with type 1 and type 2 diabetes. Acta Med Indones. 2018;50:26–37.
144. Aung WP, Bjertness E, Htet AS, et al. Trends in diabetes prevalence, awareness, treatment and control in Yangon region, Myanmar, between 2004 and 2014; two cross-sectional studies. Int J Environ Res Public Health. 2019;16:3461. https://doi.org/10.3390/ijerph16183461.
145. Muecke JS, Newland HS, Ryan P, et al. Awareness of diabetic eye disease among general practitioners

and diabetic patients in Yangon. Myanmar. Clin Exp Ophthalmol. 2008;36:265–73.
146. Gyawali B, Hansen MRH, Povlsen MB, et al. Awareness, prevalence, treatment, and control of type 2 diabetes in a semi-urban area of Nepal: findings from a cross-sectional study conducted as a part of COBIN-D trial. PLoS One. 2018;13:e0206491. https://doi.org/10.1371/journal.pone.0206491.
147. Thapa R, Joshi DM, Rizyal A, et al. Prevalence, risk factors and awareness of diabetic retinopathy among admitted diabetic patients at a tertiary level hospital in Kathmandu. Nepal J Ophthalmol. 2014;6. https://doi.org/10.3126/nepjoph.v6i1.10760.
148. Sapkota RP, Upadhyaya T, Gurung G, et al. Need to improve awareness and treatment compliance in high-risk patients for diabetic complications in Nepal. BMJ Open Diabetes Res Care. 2018;6:e000525. https://doi.org/10.1136/bmjdrc-2018-000525.1.
149. Thapa R, Poudyal G, Maharjan N, et al. Demographics and awareness of diabetic retinopathy among diabetic patients attending the vitreoretinal service at a tertiary eye care center in Nepal. Nepal J Ophthalmol. 2012;4:10–6.
150. Dahal P, Adhikari H. Diabetic retinopathy awareness among diabetic patients attending COMS-TH. Kathmandu Univ Med J (KUMJ). 2017;15(57):79–83.
151. Wijesinghe MK, Liyanarachchi KD, Somasundaram NP, et al. Knowledge of patients with type 2 diabetes mellitus about their condition – a descriptive analysis original study. Sri Lanka J Diab Endocrinol Metab. 2016;6. https://doi.org/10.4038/sjdem.v6i1.7298.
152. Piyasena MMPN, Zuurmond M, Yip JLY, et al. Process of adaptation, development and assessment of acceptability of a health educational intervention to improve referral uptake by people with diabetes in Sri Lanka. BMC Public Health. 2019;19:614. https://doi.org/10.1186/s12889-019-6880-4.
153. Perera DP, De Silva RE, Perera WL. Knowledge of diabetes among type 2 diabetes patients attending a primary health care clinic in Sri Lanka. Eastern Mediterranean Health J. 2013;19:644–8.
154. Seneviratne B, Shamini P. Knowledge on diabetic retinopathy among diabetes mellitus patients attending the Colombo South Teaching Hospital, Sri Lanka. J US-China Med Sci. 2016;13:35–46.
155. Herath HMM, Weerasinghe NP, Dias H, et al. Knowledge, attitude and practice related to diabetes mellitus among the general public in Galle district in Southern Sri Lanka: a pilot study. BMC Public Health. 2017;17:535. https://doi.org/10.1186/s12889-017-4459-5.
156. Porapakkham Y, Pattaraarchachai J, Aekplakorn W. Prevalence, awareness, treatment and control of hypertension and diabetes mellitus among the elderly: the 2004 National Health Examination Survey III, Thailand. Singapore Med J. 2008;49:868–73.
157. Tiptaradol S, Aekplakorn W. Prevalence, awareness, treatment and control of coexistence of diabetes and hypertension in Thai population. Int J Hypertens. 2012;386453 https://doi.org/10.1155/2012/386453.
158. Ramke J, Maher L, Lee L, et al. Diabetes and its ocular complications: awareness among adults aged 40 years and older in Timor-Leste. Clin Exp Optom. 2012;95:377–81.
159. Ramke J, Lee L, Brian G. Prevalence of diabetes among adults aged ≥40 years in Timor-Leste. J Diabetes. 2012;4:392–4.
160. Afroz A, Alam K, Ali L, Karim A, et al. Type 2 diabetes mellitus in Bangladesh: a prevalence- based cost-of-illness study. BMC Health Serv Res. 2019;19:601. https://doi.org/10.1186/s12913-019-4440-3.
161. Dineen BP, Bourne RR, Ali SM, et al. Prevalence and causes of blindness and visual impairment in Bangladeshi adults: results of the National Blindness and Low Vision Survey of Bangladesh. Br J Ophthalmol. 2003;87:820–8.
162. Wangdi K, Jamtsho T. Risk factors for self-reported diabetes among Bhutanese adults: a nationally representative survey data analysis. PLoS One. 2018;13:e0206034. https://doi.org/10.1371/journal.pone.
163. Raman R, Gella L, Srinivasan S, et al. Diabetic retinopathy: an epidemic at home and around the world. Indian J Ophthalmol. 2016;64:69–75.
164. Pradeepa R, Rajalakshmi R, Mohan V. Use of telemedicine technologies in diabetes prevention and control in resource-constrained settings: lessons learned from emerging economies. Diabetes Technol Ther. 2019;21(S2):9–16. https://doi.org/10.1089/dia.2019.0038.
165. Raman R, Mahajan S, Padmaja RK, et al. Tele-health program for diabetic retinopathy in rural South India: a pilot study. E-Health Int. 2005;2:13–8.
166. Murthy GV, Sundar G, Gilbert C, et al. Operational guidelines for diabetic retinopathy in India: Summary. Indian J Ophthalmol. 2020;68:S59–62.
167. Ramasamy K, Raman R, Tandon M. Current state of care for diabetic retinopathy in India. Curr Diabetes Rep. 2013;13:460–8.
168. Rudijanto A, Soewondo P, Waspadji S, et al. The Indonesian society of endocrinology's summary article of diabetes mellitus national clinical practice guidelines. J ASEAN Fed Endocrine Societies. 2011;26:17–9.
169. Aboobakur M, Latheef A, Mohamed AJ, et al. Surveillance for non-communicable disease risk factors in Maldives: results from the first STEPS survey in Male. Int J Public Health. 2010;55:489–96.
170. Majeed NA, Shiruhana SA, Maniam J, et al. Incidence, prevalence and mortality of diabetes in children and adolescents aged under 20 years in the Republic of Maldives. J Paediatr Child Health. 2020;56:746–50.
171. https://www.worlddiabetesfoundation.org/projects/maldives-wdf10-53
172. Aye TT, Aung MW, Oo ES. Diabetes mellitus in Myanmar: socio-cultural challenges and strength. J Soc Health Diabetes. 2014;2:9–13.

173. Gyawali B, Ferrario A, van Teijlingen E, et al. Challenges in diabetes mellitus type 2 management in Nepal: a literature review. Glob Health Action. 2016;9:31704. https://doi.org/10.3402/gha.v9.31704.
174. WHO Diabetes Programme. Facts and figures about diabetes. 2017.
175. Arambewela MH, Somasundaram NP, Jayasekara HBPR, et al. Prevalence of chronic complications, their risk factors, and the cardiovascular risk factors among patients with Type 2 Diabetes attending the Diabetic Clinic at a tertiary care hospital in Sri Lanka. J Diabetes Res. 2018;4504287 https://doi.org/10.1155/2018/4504287.
176. Katulanda P, Rathnapala D, Sheriff R, et al. Province and ethnic specific prevalence of diabetes among Sri Lankan adults. Sri Lanka J Diab Endocrinol Metab. 2012;1:2–7. https://doi.org/10.4038/sjdem.v1i1.4180.
177. Reutrakul S, Deerochanawong C. Diabetes in Thailand: status and policy. Curr Diab Rep. 2016;16:28. https://doi.org/10.1007/s11892-016-0725-7.
178. Pongmesa T, Li SC, Wee HL. A survey of knowledge on diabetes in the central region of Thailand. Value Health. 2009;12(Suppl 3):S110–3.
179. Silpa-archa S, Ruamviboonsuk P. Diabetic retinopathy: current treatment and Thailand perspective. J Med Assoc Thai. 2017;100(Suppl 1):S136–47. PMID: 29927326.
180. Ruamviboonsuk P, Krause J, Chotcomwongse P, et al. Deep learning versus human graders for classifying diabetic retinopathy severity in a real-world nationwide screening program. NPJ Digit Med. 2019;2:1–9. https://doi.org/10.1038/s41746-019-0099-8.
181. Beede E, Baylor E, Hersch F, et al. A human-centered evaluation of a deep learning system deployed in clinics for the detection of diabetic retinopathy. In: Conference on Human Factors in Computing Systems – Proceedings. Association for Computing Machinery; 2020. https://doi.org/10.1145/3313831.3376718.
182. Kumluang S, Ingsrisawang L, Sangroongruangsri S, et al. A real-world study of effectiveness of intravitreal bevacizumab and ranibizumab injection for treating retinal diseases in Thailand. BMC Ophthalmol. 2019;19(1). https://doi.org/10.1186/s12886-019-1086-1.
183. https://www.iapb.org/wp-content/uploads/Timor-National-Plan.pdf
184. Scanlon PH. Update on screening for sight-threatening diabetic retinopathy. Ophthalmic Res. 2019;62:218–24.
185. Scanlon PH. Article Commentary: The English national screening programme for sight-threatening diabetic retinopathy. J Med Screen. 2008;15:1–4.
186. Hautala N, Aikkila R, Korpelainen J, et al. Marked reductions in visual impairment due to diabetic retinopathy achieved by efficient screening and timely treatment. Acta Ophthalmol. 2014;92:582–7.
187. Olafsdottir E, Andersson DK, Stefánsson E. Visual acuity in a population with regular screening for type 2 diabetes mellitus and eye disease. Acta Ophthalmol Scand. 2007;85:40–5.
188. Piyasena MM, Murthy GV, Yip JL, et al. Systematic review and meta-analysis of diagnostic accuracy of detection of any level of diabetic retinopathy using digital retinal imaging. Syst Rev. 2018;7:182. https://doi.org/10.1186/s13643-018-0846-y.
189. Wilkinson CP, Ferris FL III, Klein RE, et al. Proposed international clinical diabetic retinopathy and diabetic macular edema disease severity scales. Ophthalmology. 2003;110:1677–82.
190. Dutt S, Sivaraman A, Savoy F, et al. Insights into the growing popularity of artificial intelligence in ophthalmology. Indian J Ophthalmol. 2020;68:1339–46.
191. http://www.icoph.org/downloads/ICOGuidelinesforDiabeticEyeCare.pdf
192. American Diabetes Association. Standards of medical care in diabetes-2019 abridged for primary care providers. Clin Diabetes. 2019;37:11–34.
193. Gulshan V, Peng L, Coram M, et al. Development and validation of a deep learning algorithm for detection of diabetic retinopathy in retinal fundus photographs. JAMA. 2016;316:2402–10.
194. Rajalakshmi R, Subashini R, Anjana RM, et al. Automated diabetic retinopathy detection in smartphone-based fundus photography using artificial intelligence. Eye. 2018;32:1138–44.
195. Mohan V, Prathiba V, Pradeepa R. Tele-diabetology to screen for diabetes and associated complications in rural India: The Chunampet Rural Diabetes Prevention Project Model. J Diabetes Sci Technol. 2014;8:256–61.
196. Murthy KR, Murthy PR, Rao S, et al. A novel model to deliver advanced eye care for people with diabetes living in resource-poor settings: results of care provided to date. Diabetes Care. 2012;35:e31. https://doi.org/10.2337/dc11-2098.
197. Murthy KR, Murthy PR, Kapur A, Owens DR. Mobile diabetes eye care: experience in developing countries. Diabetes Res Clin Pract. 2012;97:343–9.
198. https://www.worlddiabetesfoundation.org/projects/bangladesh-wdf10-494
199. https://www.worlddiabetesfoundation.org/projects/bangladesh-wdf17-1541
200. https://www.worlddiabetesfoundation.org/projects/nepal-wdf16-1380
201. https://www.worlddiabetesfoundation.org/projects/indonesia-wdf13-828
202. https://www.worlddiabetesfoundation.org/projects/maldives-wdf10-537
203. https://www.worlddiabetesfoundation.org/projects/wdf18-1634
204. https://www.worlddiabetesfoundation.org/projects/bhutan-wdf10-493

205. https://www.lionsclubs.org/en/give-our-focus-areas/vision/sightfirst. Accessed 15 Oct 2020.
206. https://temp.lionsclubs.org/EN/pdfs/lcif/LCIF_diabetic_retinopathy.pdf
207. Namperumalswamy P, Nirmalan PK, Ramaswamy KM. Developing a screening program to detect sight threatening retinopathy in south India. Diabetes Care. 2003;26:1831–5.
208. https://www.iapb.org/news/orbis-international-scaling-up-to-meet-the-rising-tide-of-diabetic-retinopathy-world-wide/
209. Diabetic retinopathy initiative – sight for all. https://sightforall.org/diabetic-retinopathy-initiative/. Accessed 20 Oct 2020.
210. https://www.hki.org/our-stories/hki-helps-streamline-vision-screenings-people-diabetes-indonesia/
211. https://www.hki.org/our-stories/working-combat-blindness-diabetes-bangladesh/
212. Gilbert C, Murthy GV, Cooper A. The Queen Elizabeth Diamond Jubilee Trust's avoidable blindness programme. Indian J Ophthalmol. 2020;68:S1–2.

Neglected Tropical Diseases and Trachoma

13

Sunu Dulal, Sailesh Kumar Mishra, and Hugh R. Taylor

Key Points

- Trachoma, caused by *Chlamydia trachomatis*, is a neglected tropical disease (NTD) that affects the eye.
- It causes inflammatory conjunctivitis in young children, and if left untreated, leads to conjunctival scarring, and in turning of eyelashes and eyelids to cause irreversible corneal opacity and blindness.
- The disease is more prevalent in poor and crowded communities with unhygienic practices.
- Trachoma is a priority disease for World Health Organization (WHO); the WHO aims to eliminate trachoma blindness by 2030, an objective that is aligned with the sustainable development goals (SDGs).
- WHO has suggested SAFE (surgery, antibiotic application, facial cleanliness, and environmental improvement) and WASH (water, sanitation, and hygiene) to effectively prevent and treat trachoma and many other NTDs.
- Several programs and organizations, such as GET2020 (Global Elimination of Trachoma) and ITI (International Trachoma Initiative), are working together to achieve the goal of trachoma elimination
- Due to global efforts, trachoma prevalence has reduced from 1.5 billion cases in 2002 to 137 million cases in 2020.
- Currently, trachoma is a public health problem in 43 countries, and hyperendemic in 14 countries.
- The WHO has certified 10 countries as trachoma-free; this includes 2 South-East Asian countries, Myanmar and Nepal.

Neglected Tropical Diseases (NTDs) are a diverse set of communicable diseases that are usually prevalent in tropical and subtropical areas of 149 countries (Fig. 13.1) [1]. One in five people worldwide is at risk of NTDs. These diseases generally affect the poorest—approximately 1.6 billion people living in the most marginalized communities. In addition to the deaths they cause, NTDs also cause substantial disability, stigma, and loss of livelihood [2]. People living in poverty without adequate sanitation and in close contact with infectious vectors, domestic animals, and livestock are those worst affected (Fig. 13.1).

The World Health Organization (WHO) states that NTDs are "...chronically endemic and epidemic-prone tropical diseases, which have a very significant negative impact on the lives of

S. Dulal
Karnali Academy of Health Sciences, Jumla, Nepal

S. K. Mishra
Nepal Netra Jyoti Sangh, Kathmandu, Nepal

H. R. Taylor (✉)
Melbourne School of Population and Global Health, University of Melbourne, Melbourne, VIC, Australia
e-mail: h.taylor@unimelb.edu.au

T. Das, P. D. Nayar (eds.), *South-East Asia Eye Health*,
https://doi.org/10.1007/978-981-16-3787-2_13

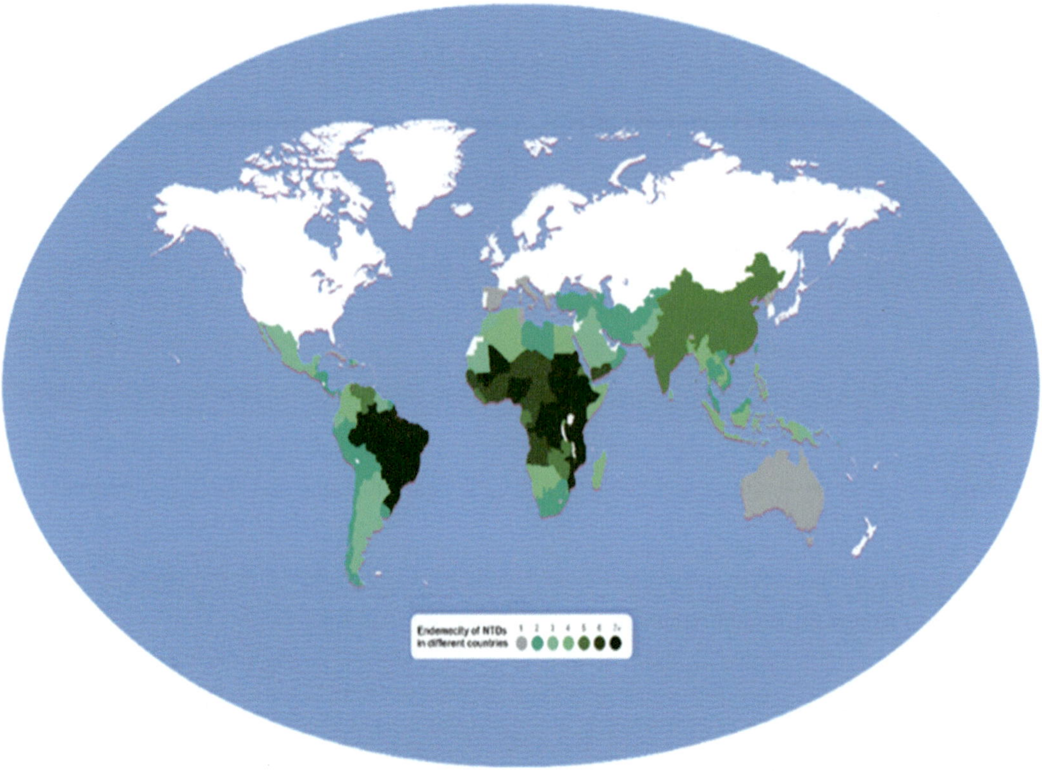

Fig. 13.1 Endemicity of neglected tropical disease in the world

poor populations [and] remain critically neglected in the global public health agenda" [3].

The diseases included in the NTD group are shown in Table 13.1.

The last three conditions, namely ectoparasitic infections (chromoblastomycosis and other mycoses), scabies, and snakebite envenoming, were added by the 10th meeting of the Strategic and Technical Advisory Group for Neglected Tropical Diseases in 2017 [4].

13.1 Global Initiatives

In 1996, in partnership with several non-government organizations, the WHO established the Global Alliance for the Elimination of Trachoma as a public health problem by 2020 (GET2020) [5]. In 2005, WHO established the Department of Control of Neglected Diseases, which focused its attentions on NTDs. Effective preventive chemotherapy (PCT) programs were started for five NTDs—onchocerciasis, lymphatic filariasis (LF), trachoma, schistosomiasis, and soil-transmitted helminths—that account for about 1 billion people at risk for at least one of these five diseases. In 2006, the United States Agency for International Development (USAID) launched the "NTD Control Program" for PCT for these five NTDs. It has three phases. Phase I with a budget of USD70 million was used for an "Integrated NTD Program" in 12 countries for 4 years (from 2006 to 2010); Phase II (Expansion Phase) was for 5 years (2010–2015), had a budget of USD516 million, and supported 31 countries. The emphasis during this phase was on developing methods for planning and management to scale up the coverage. Currently, Phase III (Acceleration phase) is for 4 years (2016–2020) and has a budget of USD100 million/year [4].

Studies have shown that clean water, sanitation, and hygiene (WASH) are critical for preventing and treating most NTDs, especially soil-transmitted helminthiasis, trachoma, schis-

Table 13.1 Twenty NTDs recognized by the WHO

Category	Disease
Protozoan infections	1. Chagas disease 2. Human African trypanosomiasis 3. ***Visceral leishmaniasis (kala-azar)***
Helminth infections	4. ***Taenia solium (neuro) cysticercosis/taeniosis*** 5. *Dracunculiasis (guinea worm disease)*[a] 6. ***Echinococcus*** 7. Foodborne trematodes 8. ***Lymphatic filariasis*** 9. Onchocerciasis 10. Schistosomiasis 11. ***Soil-transmitted helminthiases (ascariasis, hookworm diseases, trichuriasis, strongyloidiasis)***
Bacterial infections	12. Buruli ulcer 13. ***Leprosy*** 14. ***Trachoma*** 15. ***Yaws***
Viral infections	16. ***Dengue and chikungunya fevers*** 17. ***Rabies***
Fungal infections	18. Mycetoma, chromoblastomycosis, deep mycosis
Ectoparasitic infections	19. ***Scabies, myiasis***
Venom	20. ***Snakebite envenoming***

Source: World Health Organization. Neglected Tropical Diseases 2017 [1]

Diseases highlighted with bold and italicized text are prevalent in South-East Asia

[a]*Dracunculiasis (guinea worm disease)* has been eliminated

tosomiasis, lymphatic filariasis (LF), and guinea worm disease. The WHO highlighted the need for WASH and NTD collaboration in the Global Strategy document (2015–2020) on "Water, Sanitation, and Hygiene for accelerating and sustaining progress on Neglected Tropical Diseases" [6].

In 2020, tackling NTDs has been formally recognized as a target for global action towards attaining the Sustainable Development Goals (SDGs). Agenda 3.3 of SDG 3 states, "By 2030, end the epidemics of AIDS, tuberculosis, malaria and neglected tropical diseases and combat hepatitis, water-borne diseases and other communicable diseases." [7] The road map for NTD 2021–2030 sets out global targets for 2030 as well as milestones to prevent, control, eliminate, and eradicate a diverse set of 20 diseases and disease groups. The road map also addresses cross-cutting targets aligned with the WHO's Thirteenth General Program of Work (2019–2023) and the SDGs. It also proposes strategies for attaining these targets over the next decade [8].

Three of the 20 NTDs mentioned in this program have ophthalmic significance. These are trachoma, onchocerciasis, and leprosy; the first two directly affect the eye, and the ocular complications of leprosy can lead to severe visual impairment and blindness [9].

13.1.1 Neglected Tropical Diseases in South-East Asia

Among the six WHO regions (seven IAPB (International Agency for the prevention of blindness) regions), the South-East Asian region bears the highest burdens of leprosy, LF, and visceral leishmaniasis (kala-azar). Besides, the region also bears a significant proportion of the burden of soil-transmitted helminthiasis. Other NTDs prevalent in this region are yaws, taeniasis, scabies, myiasis, fungal infections, and snakebite [10]. Since leprosy, LF, kala-azar, yaws, and trachoma are targeted for elimination, significant progress has been made towards this goal [10].

13.1.2 Trachoma

Trachoma is a disease of the eye caused by an infection with the bacterium *Chlamydia trachomatis*. It is the leading cause of infectious blindness worldwide. Blindness from trachoma is irreversible [11].

13.1.3 Pathophysiology

Chlamydia trachomatis is an ancient organism that evolved with the dinosaurs [12]. It is an obligate intracellular gram-negative bacterium with a single chromosome of about 1 Mbp and a multicopy plasmid that functions as a virulence factor

[13]. Chlamydiae have a unique biphasic life cycle and can adapt to both intracellular and extracellular environments. In an extracellular environment, Chlamydiae are small, hard, and metabolically inactive and are known as elementary bodies. These organisms transform into larger metabolically active reticulate bodies called inclusion bodies that multiply by binary fission inside susceptible host cells. The nonhuman reservoirs for the chlamydia strains that infect humans are not known [14].

Endemic trachoma is caused by *C. trachomatis* serotypes A, B, Ba, and C. Infections of the genital tracts are generally caused by serotypes D to K, which can also infect the eye, causing ophthalmia neonatorum in infants, or inclusion conjunctivitis in adults [14]. Inclusion conjunctivitis may be clinically indistinguishable from trachoma; it manifests as follicular conjunctivitis with pannus, but rarely leads to conjunctival scarring. Genital serovars of *C. trachomatis* usually do not enter stable transmission cycles in communities and are not involved in the genesis of trachoma blindness [14].

Infection with *C. trachomatis* causes inflammation, with predominantly lymphocytic and monocytic infiltrates containing plasma cells and macrophages inside the follicles. The follicles are typical germinal centers with islands of intense B-cell proliferation surrounded by a sea of T-cells. Infection is recurrent, and prolonged inflammation due to conjunctival reinfection leads to conjunctival scarring. Conjunctival scarring is associated with atrophy of the conjunctival epithelium, loss of goblet cells, and replacement of the normal, loose, vascular subepithelial stroma with thick compact bands of type IV and type V collagen. The clinical changes are a delayed-type hypersensitivity reaction to chlamydial antigens (one of them is thought to be heat shock protein (HSP)-60). The chlamydial antigens induce immune responses with germinal centers (seen as follicles) and intense inflammatory infiltrates and papillae formation. Over time, this intense inflammation leads to scar formation, which, in turn, causes contraction and buckling of the tarsal plate of the upper lid, producing entropion and trichiasis [15].

The infection spreads through personal contact via hands, fomites including clothes (towels, bedding), and eye-seeking flies. With repeated infection episodes over several years, the conjunctival scars contract and distort the upper tarsus. This causes the eyelashes drawn in and rub on the cornea, causing pain, discomfort, and permanent damage to the cornea [11]. Eye and nose discharges are principal reservoirs of infection in young children who harbor the organism in their eyes and noses. Prognosis depends on the severity of the disease at the time of diagnosis, the appropriateness of treatment, and the risk of reinfection. Prognosis is good in people diagnosed early and treated appropriately. Reinfection worsens the prognosis [11]. Nearly 150 episodes of reinfection are required for prolonged and intense inflammation to cause lid scarring and trichiasis [16]. Severe disease may be stabilized, but the patient's vision may not be restored once corneal scarring develops, unless the diseased cornea is surgically replaced.

13.1.4 Epidemiology

Trachoma is a leading cause of infectious blindness worldwide. It is highly correlated with poverty, limited access to healthcare services, and water scarcity [15]. Trachoma persists in areas with poor personal and community hygiene, as well as in the hot, dry, and dusty climates of Africa, the Middle East, Asia, Latin America, the Pacific Islands, and remote aboriginal communities in Australia [17]. Based on the WHO March 2020 data, trachoma is a public health problem in 44 countries, and 137 million people living in areas where trachoma is endemic are at risk of trachoma-related blindness; and 1.9 million people have visual impairment or blindness [11].

In hyperendemic areas, active (inflammatory) trachoma is common among preschool children, with prevalence rates as high as 60–90%. Active disease clusters occur in families when the overall community prevalence decreases to around 20%. Infection is usually acquired when living in close proximity to others with active disease, and the family is the primary setting for transmission

[11]. The infection becomes less frequent and shorter in duration with increasing age. Severe blinding trachoma may be nearly twice as common in women than in men; this is believed to be related to women taking more childcare responsibilities and their proximity to young infected children [17].

The active disease most commonly occurs in preschool children; the highest prevalence is in children aged 3–5 years. Rarely, children younger than 10 years can manifest trichiasis in highly endemic areas. Typically, young children exhibit follicular trachoma with intense conjunctival inflammation, young adults exhibit trachomatous scarring, and middle-aged and older individuals exhibit trichiasis and corneal opacity. However, these signs are not mutually exclusive. Individuals may have follicular trachoma episodes with intense conjunctival inflammation even after cicatricial complications develop; therefore, follicles, scarring, and trichiasis may all be present in the same patient [17].

13.1.5 Histopathology

Active trachoma in children is characterized by a hyperplastic conjunctival epithelium and widespread inflammatory infiltrates of T- and B-lymphocytes, macrophages, plasma cells, and neutrophils [18]. In some places, this is organized into B-cell follicles. In adults with trachomatous scarring, the conjunctival epithelium is atrophic and goblet cells are lost. The loose subepithelial stroma is replaced with a thick scar of type V collagen. These new vertically orientated fibers are firmly attached to the tarsal plate and distort it [19]. Conjunctival inflammation in the presence of scarring and trichiasis is often observed and is associated with a T-cell infiltrate [19].

13.1.6 Immunopathology

The mucosal response to *C. trachomatis* infection involves several components of the immune system, although all the features of protective and pathological responses are still unclear [12].

Depending on the severity of inflammation, clinically active trachoma can persist for months after chlamydial infection becomes undetectable. Chronic severe conjunctival inflammation leads to scarring, probably through the activation of fibrogenic pathways [18]. Active trachoma is accompanied with increased expression of pro-inflammatory cytokines (IL-1 β) and tumor necrosis factor (TNF-α) and influx of macrophages into the infected area [19]. TNF-α has been found more frequently in the tears of individuals with trachomatous scarring [20]. A single nucleotide polymorphism (SNP) in the TNF-α promoter region, TNFA-308A, leads to increased TNF-α levels associated with increased risk of trachomatous scarring and trichiasis [21]. The anti-inflammatory cytokine IL-10 also influences the outcome of trachoma. Trachomatous scarring can result from a T-cell-mediated immune response to repeated chlamydial antigen exposure [22] or an innate pro-inflammatory response from the infected epithelium [23].

13.1.7 Diagnosis and Grading

Trachoma is usually diagnosed clinically. Slit-lamp or magnifying loupe (generally used during community and field screenings) can help detect early lesions. There are no visible signs in the early stage of the disease. Repeated infections cause conjunctival scarring; eye irritation is a prominent symptom during this phase [24].

The WHO has identified a simplified grading system for trachoma [24] based on independently scored clinical signs. This grading system can also be used by non-specialists such as nurses or eye health workers, to rapidly assess the prevalence of trachoma in a community. Each clinical sign has implications for understanding the epidemiology of the disease and the interventions used for treatment. Since active trachoma is most prevalent in young children, screening for active trachoma (trachomatous inflammation—follicular, TF, and trachomatous inflammation—intense, TI) is mostly restricted to children aged 1–9 years. Adults (older than 15 years) are generally screened for trachomatous trichiasis (TT) [12] (Table 13.2; Fig. 13.2).

Table 13.2 Simplified grading of trachoma (WHO) [24]

Stage	Description	Ocular findings	Treatment
TF	Inflammation—follicles	Beginning of infection. Five or more follicles—small bumps that contain lymphocytes are visible with magnification on the upper eyelid conjunctiva.	Topical antibiotics
TI	Inflammation—intense	Highly infectious stage. The eye is irritated, with a thickening of the upper eyelid.	Topical and systemic therapy
TS	Scarring and entropion	Repeated infections lead to scarring of the inner eyelid. The scars often appear as white lines when examined with magnification. Entropion could occur.	Lid surgery
TT	Trichiasis	As scarring of the inner lining of the eyelid continues, deformation occurs and causes trichiasis.	
CO	Corneal opacity	The cornea is affected, and repeated rubbing of the cornea by the in-turned eyelashes leads to corneal clouding.	Keratoplasty in extreme cases

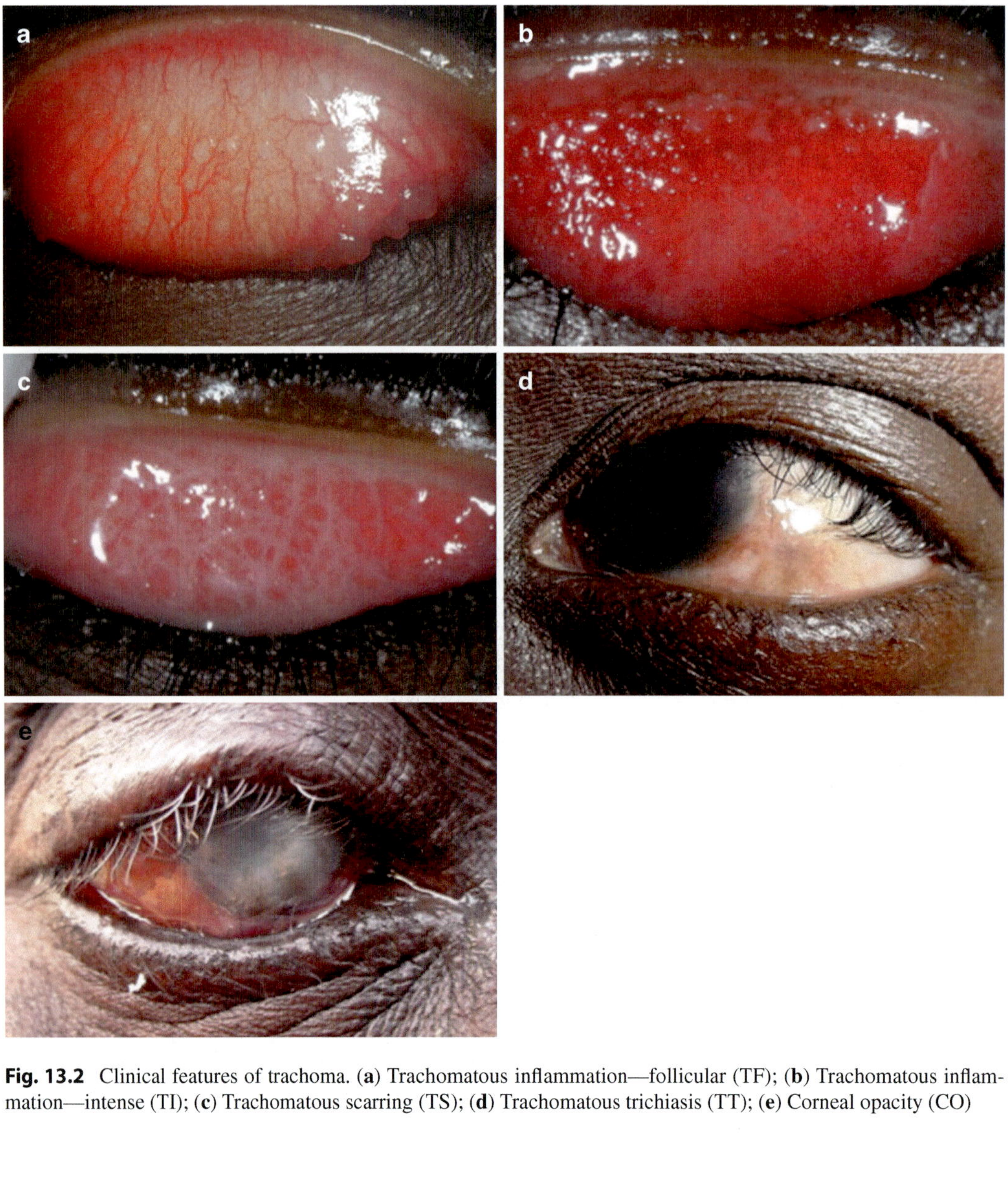

Fig. 13.2 Clinical features of trachoma. (**a**) Trachomatous inflammation—follicular (TF); (**b**) Trachomatous inflammation—intense (TI); (**c**) Trachomatous scarring (TS); (**d**) Trachomatous trichiasis (TT); (**e**) Corneal opacity (CO)

13.2 Management and Prevention of Trachoma

13.2.1 The GET2020 Program and the SAFE Strategy

13.2.1.1 The WHO Alliance for Global Elimination of Trachoma by 2020 (GET2020)

The GET2020 program was launched in 1996. It is a partnership that supports the country's implementation of the SAFE strategy and strengthening of national healthcare capacity through epidemiological assessment, monitoring, surveillance, project evaluation, and resource mobilization. It is open to all parties—governments, international organizations, and non-governmental organizations (NGOs)—willing and ready to contribute to global efforts [25].

In 1998 (at the 51st World Health Assembly), the WHO passed a resolution to eliminate trachoma as a public health problem by 2020 (WHA 51.11). The SAFE strategy goes beyond medical and surgical interventions and focuses on addressing behavioral and environmental aspects in countries where the disease is endemic [26]. Globally, there has been remarkable improvement in trachoma blindness prevention since the formation of GET2020. The number of people at risk of blindness from trachoma has reduced from 1.5 billion in 2002 to under 137 million in May 2020—a 91% decrease. In 2002, there were an estimated 7.6 million people with TT; but by May 2020, this had decreased by 74% to 2 million [27]. These achievements and progresses can be attributed to the following factors:

- SAFE Strategy
- Development of a clinical grading scheme
- Setting targets that define elimination of disease
- Building an evidence base for trichiasis surgery
- Azithromycin donation program
- The Global Trachoma Mapping Project

The SAFE Strategy

In 1996, the WHO recommended the "SAFE" strategy for tackling trachoma. It comprises three elements of primary, secondary, and tertiary prevention, but for the sake of an acceptable acronym, they are placed in the reverse order (Table 13.3) [28].

Table 13.3 Actions and levels of care in SAFE strategy

Acronym	Action	Level of care
S	Surgery to prevent blindness in those who have trichiasis/entropion	Tertiary
A	Antibiotics to clear ocular *C. trachomatis* infection	Secondary
F	Facial cleanliness to reduce transmission of ocular *C. trachomatis*	Primary
E	Environmental improvement, improved access to water, and good sanitation	Primary

The environment plays a crucial role in trachoma prevention. Improvement of the environment contributed significantly to the disappearance of trachoma in high-income countries, even in the absence of other specific interventions. A key sanitation intervention for trachoma control is promoting locally appropriate hygienic disposal methods of solid human waste. This is important, because female eye-seeking flies preferentially lay their eggs on human feces left exposed on the soil and act as mechanical vectors of *C. trachomatis* [28]. There have been suggestions that the "E" in SAFE could be E3 for environmental improvement, education, and economic development [29].

Setting Targets That Define Elimination

The third WHO Global Scientific Meeting and subsequent amendments provided the specific criteria for trachoma elimination using two measurable objectives: (1) reduction in the prevalence of trachoma infection to less than 5% among children aged 1–9 years in every endemic district; and (2) reduction of TT to less than 2 per 1000 population aged 15 years and older [30].

The WHO has set a process for validating a country as having eliminated trachoma [31]. The method of validating district-level data is as follows: (1) once a district (administrative unit for health management, with a population of 100,000–250,000) has achieved the objectives outlined above, then mass drug administration (MDA) ceases; (2) a period of at least 2 years must elapse during which there is no mass provision of antibiotics followed by a population-based survey to ensure that trachoma has not re-emerged; (3) an outside review group must evaluate the evidence and recommend either validation of elimination or further information/work. This is a critical process to objectively measure the gains and attendant costs to achieving the GET2020 goal of trachoma elimination [11].

Building an Evidence Base for Trichiasis Surgery

Bilamellar tarsal rotation surgery clinical trial in Oman resulted in the lowest recurrence rates of TT after surgery as compared to other conventional methods [32]. A review of 13 similar studies in the Cochrane database found a similar outcome [33]. These findings were the basis for the WHO's advocacy for this technique (trichiasis surgery for trachoma) [34]. Further refinements to improve surgical outcomes include posterior lamellar tarsal rotation, intraoperative use of a tarsal clamp, placement of the incision through the tarsus's length, and one-time use of 1 g of azithromycin immediately after surgery [35, 36]. Ideally, the recurrence rate after TT surgery should be no higher than 20% [37].

Azithromycin Donation Program

The long-acting oral antibiotic, azithromycin, is as effective in a single dose as 6 weeks of daily tetracycline ointment. Therefore, the single-dose azithromycin (Zithromax) treatment has much greater patient compliance than the tetracycline ointment that must be applied twice a day for 6 weeks. Additionally, single-dose treatments are more convenient and cost-effective for mass treatment at the community level [38]. In November 1998, Pfizer Inc., together with the Edna McConnell Clark Foundation, established the International Trachoma Initiative (ITI) to test the SAFE strategy using Zithromax in 5 of the 16 WHO trachoma priority countries. These countries were Ghana, Mali, Morocco, Tanzania, and Vietnam [39]. Since 1999, the ITI has approved and shipped over 876 million doses of azithromycin to trachoma-endemic countries and has massively scaled up its operations over the last few years with help from the Global Trachoma Mapping Project. ITI also houses the Global Trachoma Atlas, a real-time display of trachoma prevalence at the district level and worldwide changes in trachoma prevalence over time [38].

The Global Trachoma Mapping Project

To eliminate trachoma by 2020, it was essential for proper planning and intervention to know the extent of the area burdened with the disease. In 2012, the Global Trachoma Mapping Project was launched to complete the global trachoma map by conducting population-based surveys in 34 countries (1238 districts). This project required the participation of over 53 organizations and was the largest infectious disease survey ever undertaken [40].

13.2.1.2 Achievements

In the year 2002, there were an estimated 7.6 million people with TT; but by May 2020, this was reduced to 2 million—a decrease by 74%. As of 10 September 2020, 14 countries have reported trachoma elimination. The WHO has validated ten of these countries: seven countries in Asia (Cambodia, China, Islamic Republic of Iran, Lao People's Democratic Republic, Myanmar, Nepal, and Oman); two countries in Africa (Ghana and Morocco); and one country in Latin America (Mexico). At the time of writing, Gambia, India, Iraq, and Togo are waiting for validation [41, 42].

Despite these achievements over the past two decades, the GET2020 program will not be able to meet its target of eliminating trachoma by December 2020 [43]. Currently, there are 35 countries where trachoma is still endemic. Therefore, the Alliance has extended its overall target date to 2030, in line with the targets for several other NTDs, and the 2030 agenda for the SDGs. To expedite the process, the Alliance has set targets to eliminate trachoma in 20 countries by 2023 and in the remaining 15 countries by 2025. This revision is included in the draft of the NTD roadmap, 2021–2030 (Fig. 13.3).

The NTD roadmap 2021–2030 includes a call for a strategic shift from disease-specific per-

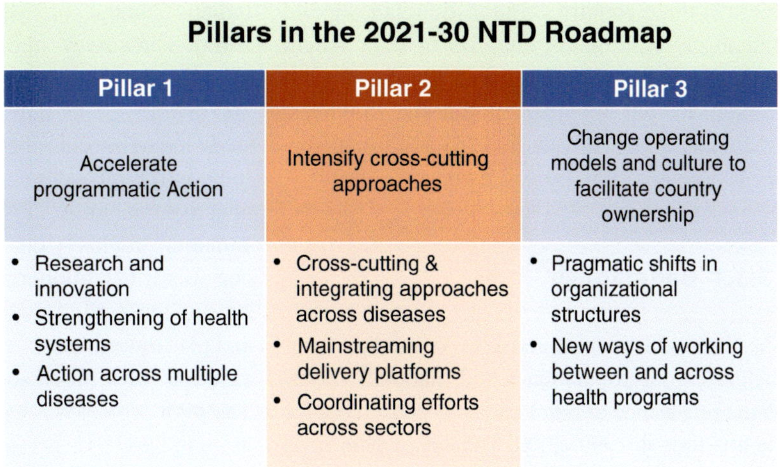

Fig. 13.3 The NTD roadmap (2021–2030)

Table 13.4 Number of TT in 2007 and 2020 and the status of elimination of trachoma [45, 46]

	2007		2020		
Country	Pop m	TT	Pop m	TT	Status of elimination of trachoma as a public health problem
Bangladesh					Thought, intervention required
Bhutan					Thought, intervention required
India	1087.12	443.0	1352.6	28	Known, intervention required
Indonesia					Thought, intervention required
Maldives					Thought, intervention not required
Myanmar	50.00	65.8	53	2	Validated, eliminated
Nepal	26.59	138.8	28	0	Validated, eliminated
Sri Lanka					Thought, intervention not required
Thailand					Thought, intervention not required
Timor-Leste					Investigated, intervention not required

Pop m population in millions, *TT* trachomatous trichiasis cases in thousands

spectives to a holistic approach based on universal health coverage (UHC) [27]. The three pillars of the NTD roadmap are: (1) accelerating program action, (2) intensifying cross-cutting approaches, and (3) changing the operating models and ownership culture (Fig. 13.3).

13.3 Trachoma in South-East Asia

Trachoma in South-East Asia has been known from ancient times as a blinding eye disease. Knowledge of trachoma dates as far back as the twentieth century BC to reports about Emperor Huang Ti Nei Ching who underwent surgery for trichiasis in China. Trachoma also appeared in the small farming communities developing in the Euphrates valley in Mesopotamia, along the Nile valley in Egypt, and along the Indus and Ganges rivers in South Asia [44]. It was widespread around the world in the 1920s and began to disappear in more developed countries as living conditions improved during the first half of the twentieth century. The advent of sulfonamides in the 1930s and the development of tetracycline in the 1940s accelerated this process. However, trachoma continued to be a public health problem in low- and middle-income countries. A summary of the current status of efforts in trachoma elimination is shown in Table 13.4.

The status of trachoma in 10 WHO South-East Asia Regions (excluding the Democratic People's Republic of Korea) is as follows: (1) two countries, Myanmar and Nepal, are declared trachoma free; (2) three countries, India, Bangladesh, and Bhutan are waiting for analysis of their recent studies; (3) it is not considered a public health problem in four countries, Indonesia, Maldives, Sri Lanka, and Thailand; and (4) additional survey is not needed in Timor-Leste.

13.3.1 Bangladesh

The National Blindness and Low Vision Survey of Bangladesh, a population-based, national survey on the prevalence of blindness, was carried out for the first time in 1999–2000. The age-standardized prevalence of bilateral blindness was 1.5% among people aged 30 years or older. Cataract was the predominant cause (79.6%) of bilateral blindness. Other causes were uncorrected aphakia (6.2%); macular degeneration (3.1%); optic atrophy, phthisical eye, and other posterior segment disorders (2.5% each); refractive error and glaucoma (1.2% each), and chorioretinitis (0.6%). Trachoma was not a cause of blindness or visual impairment in the survey [47].

13.3.2 Bhutan

The Royal Government of Bhutan, similar to all basic health services, provides eye care free of charge to all people. The primary eye care program was started in Bhutan in 1987. The first systematic survey carried out to assess the prevalence of blindness and visual impairment was a rapid assessment of avoidable blindness (RAAB) survey conducted in 2009 and repeated in 2018 [48]. A comparison of these two surveys shows that the prevalence of blindness and moderate-to-severe visual impairment (MSVI) has decreased, and the prevalence of refractive error (in the category of early visual impairment) and cataract has increased. In either survey, there were no reported cases of blindness or MSVI due to trachoma.

13.3.3 India

India conducted the first study on trachoma prevalence in 1956 (Trachoma Control Pilot Project, Indian Council of Medical Research, 1956–1963). The survey studied a rural population of over 177,000 people residing in 2494 villages in 302 districts of 15 states. The results of the pilot study led to the classification of different areas of India into three categories based on the presence of active trachoma (TF/TI), these being: (1) "high endemic" region (four states—three north and one west); (2) "moderate endemic" region (four states—one central, two east, and one northeast); and (3) "low endemic" region (seven states—two east, one west, three south, and one north) [49]. The pilot project was extended to a national program in 1963.

The program's three phases consisted of an "attack period" for 2 years, a "consolidation period" for 1.5 years, and a "maintenance period" for 2 years or more. It relied predominantly on mass treatment with tetracycline ointment [50]. By 2006, the prevalence of active trachoma (TF/TI) had reduced from over 70% in three northern Indian states to below 10%. There was no reduction in trachoma prevalence in the southern island of Nicobar. A survey in 2010 recorded that the prevalence of active disease in school children in Nicobar island was 50% and required three cycles of MDA of azithromycin to reduce the prevalence to below 10% by 2013.

In 2012, India further decided to conduct a rapid trachoma assessment in 15 districts and a prevalence study in 10 districts [51]. The National Program for Control of Blindness and Visual Impairment (NPCBVI) conducted the survey in the period 2015–2019 to generate new data on blindness and visual impairment in India. The large RAAB study, which assessed 85,135 people of age 50 years and above in 31 districts in 24 states, reported the prevalence of blindness at 0.36% in all age groups and 1.99% in the population aged 50 years or older. Major causes for blindness among people aged 50 years or older were cataract (66.2%), posterior segment disease including diabetic retinopathy and age-related macular degeneration (7.8%), non-trachomatous corneal opacity (7.4%), and glaucoma 5.5%. Trachomatous corneal opacity caused blindness in 0.8% of the tested population and severe visual impairment in 0.1% of this population [52]. The government of India has declared that active trachoma among children has been eliminated, but the prevalence of TT is still above the WHO elimination criteria [53].

13.3.4 Indonesia

Indonesia is not on the list of trachoma-endemic countries of the WHO South-East Asia Region. In a RAAB survey in west Java, age and sex-adjusted prevalence of blindness among people aged 50 or above was 2.8%. Untreated cataract was the most common cause of blindness. Trachomatous corneal opacity caused blindness and severe visual impairment in 1.1% and 2.6% of this population, respectively [54]. This study recommended a trachoma prevalence study although trachoma is not thought to be endemic in Indonesia.

13.3.5 Maldives

The first population-based visual impairment and blindness prevalence survey in the Maldives was the RAAB in 2016. The age and sex-adjusted prevalence of blindness and severe visual impairment in the Maldives was 2% and 1.9%, respectively. The leading cause of blindness was cataract (51.4%), followed by posterior segment anomalies (27.8%). Non-trachomatous scars were responsible for 5.6% of bilateral blindness in the country. Trachomatous corneal lesions were not detected [55].

13.3.6 Myanmar

Trachoma was identified as the single most important cause of blindness in central Myanmar (then Burma) during the 1960s. The Trachoma Control Project was established in 1964 by the Ministry of Health with support from the WHO and the United Nations Children's Fund (UNICEF). Nationwide surveys identified 11 districts and 14 townships, home to 6.2 million people, in Myanmar's central regions as the trachoma-endemic area [42]. Intervention programs in these 11 endemic districts consisted of TT surgery, topical treatment with tetracycline eye ointment for active trachoma, and health education. These programs also included educating school children on face, hands, and feet cleanliness. In the late 1990s, the Ministry of Health shifted their strategy for trachoma eradication from an active, vertical program to an integrated program in which trachoma screening and treatment were included in routine primary eye care activities. The SAFE strategy was also followed in all endemic districts [42].

The Meikhtila Eye Study (2005) showed that trachoma was responsible for 4.7% of all blindness cases in Myanmar. Annual prevalence data from 2010 to 2015 showed a decline in active trachoma infections in children under 10 across all regions (trachoma prevalence ranged from 0% to 0.05%). The RAAB 2018 reported that blindness attributable to trachoma had reduced to 0.01% in Myanmar [41, 56]; and this was confirmed by the survey in 2019. The WHO South-East Asia Regional Office (WHO SEARO) declared Myanmar as a trachoma-free country on 10 September 2020. It is now the second trachoma-free country, after Nepal, in the WHO South-East Asia Region [42, 56].

13.3.7 Sri Lanka

The National Blindness, Visual Impairment, and Disability Survey in Sri Lanka (2014–2015) was the first-ever national-level study on blindness and visual impairment in Sri Lanka. According to this survey, among people aged 40 years and older, the prevalence of blindness was 1.7%, severe visual impairment was 1.6%, and moderate visual impairment was 15.4%. Cataract was the most common cause of blindness (66.7%), followed by uncorrected refractive errors (12.5%) [57]. There were no reported cases of blindness or visual impairment due to corneal scars either trachomatous or non-trachomatous.

13.3.8 Thailand

The first RAAB in Thailand was conducted in 2014. In this study, the age and sex-adjusted prevalence of blindness among people aged 50 years and older was 0.6% [58]. Cataract was the leading cause of blindness (69.7%). Refractive errors, diabetic retinopathy, glaucoma, and non-trachomatous corneal opacities were responsible for 6.0%, 5.1%, 4.0%, and 2.0% of blindness, respectively. Trachoma lesions were not detected.

13.3.9 Timor-Leste

The first RAAB in Timor-Leste was conducted in 2016. The study reported an overall age and sex-adjusted prevalence of blindness among people aged 50 or older of 2.8%. Cataract was the most common cause of blindness (79.4%); other causes included posterior segment disorders (6.2%), glaucoma (5.2%), and unspecified corneal opacities (2.1%) [59]. There was no evidence of trachoma-related corneal scars in this study or in an earlier study [60]. Further analysis of published literature from Timor-Leste did not specify trachoma as a public health problem for which the costs of conducting a formal population-based trachoma prevalence survey could be justified [61].

Trachoma-free Nepal (Fig. 13.4)

The National Blindness Survey in Nepal, 1981 identified trachoma as a major cause of blindness. The reported prevalence of trachoma was 6.5% [62]. A non-governmental organization, Nepal Netra Jyoti Sangh (NNJS, established in 1978) initiated community-based trachoma control programs in endemic areas of Nepal in 1990 [63]. The National Trachoma Programme (NTP) with the objective of eliminating trachoma from all 20 endemic districts by 2017 was launched by NNJS and the Ministry of Health and Population. The program adopted the SAFE strategy which was rolled out in 5 endemic districts and involved 18 eye hospitals, 80 eye care centers, and 38 district branches affiliated to the NNJS [64].

Multisectoral engagement and an integrated approach to trachoma eradication was adopted, as additional partners joined the effort. While NNJS and the Ministry of Health and Population jointly implemented the strategy relating to provision of antibiotics and conducting surgeries for trichiasis, the Department of Water Supply and Sewerage (DWSS) worked to improve environmental conditions to limit transmission. The program was supported by the ITI and Research Triangle Institute (RTI) International/ENVISION [65]. The main goals of the program were to: (1) reduce the prevalence of active trachoma to less than 5% in children aged 1–9 years and (2) reduce prevalence of TT to less than 0.2% in people aged 15 years and older, in each of the previously endemic districts [11].

Using the WHO's simplified system for grading clinical trachoma, impact surveys were conducted after completion of required MDAs in endemic districts. Pre-validation surveillance surveys were conducted in 2017 to identify any re-emergence of the disease. With a successful outcome, Nepal submitted the required evidence and dossier to the WHO in 2018 claiming that trachoma had been eliminated as a public health problem. Nepal was certified as trachoma-free in May 2018 and was the first country to achieve this status in the WHO South-East Asia Region.

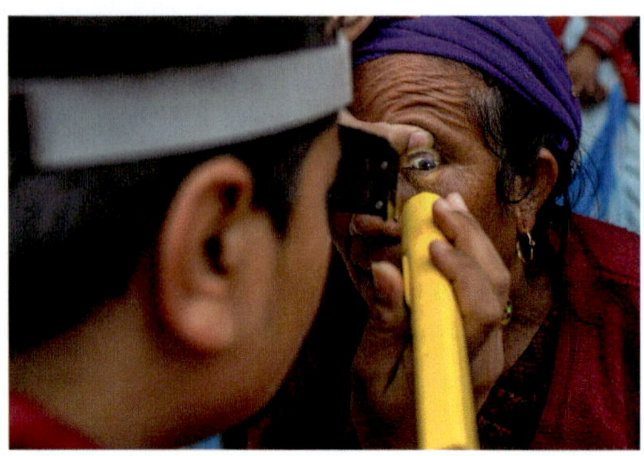

Fig. 13.4 Screening for trachoma in the community

13.4 Trachoma in the Rest of the World

Trachoma is the leading cause of infectious blindness in the world. Currently, it is the eighth-most common disease blinding disease in the world. It mainly affects people living in the most impoverished areas [11]. Trachoma is a public health problem in 43 countries and is responsible for the blindness or visual impairment of about 1.9 million people. It is hyperendemic in 14 countries, which include the impoverished and most rural areas of Africa, Central, South America, Asia, Australia, and the Middle East. It is responsible for ~1.4% of all cases of blindness worldwide. Africa remains the most affected continent and has received the most intensive efforts to control this disease. Due to global initiatives, the number of people affected by trachoma has reduced by 91%—from 1.5 billion in 2002 to 142 million in 2019 [66]. The current status of trachoma in the world is shown in Table 13.5.

WHO March 2020 data indicate that 137 million people live in trachoma-endemic areas and are at risk of trachoma blindness. In 2019, 92,622 people received surgical treatment for the advanced stage of the disease, and 95.2 million people were treated for trachoma with antibiotics. Global-level antibiotic coverage in 2019 was 57%. According to the GET2020 report, as of 1 May 2020, there was a backlog of over 1.95 million people with trichiasis in 1583 districts requiring "S" interventions; over 136.8 million people in 1255 districts needed "A," "F," and "E" interventions. Trachoma is suspected to be a public health problem in 187 districts, which covers approximately 35.5 million people [68]. As of 1 May 2020, according to the GET2020 database, trachoma is still a public health problem in some parts of 43 countries [69]. As of 15 September 2020, 14 countries have declared themselves trachoma-free, and the WHO has validated this claim in 10 of these countries.

Table 13.5 Trachoma-endemic countries showing the burden of trachoma [67]

Characteristics	High burden countries	Other countries	Validated for elimination
Countries	Burkina, Ethiopia, Faso, Guinea, Kenya, Mozambique, Niger, Nigeria, Pakistan, Senegal, Sudan, South Sudan, Tanzania, Uganda, Zambia	Afghanistan, Australia, Benin, Botswana, Burundi, Cameroon, Central African Republic Chad, Côte d'Ivoire Djibouti, Egypt, Eritrea, Fiji, Guatemala, Guinea Bissau, Kiribati, Mali, Malawi, Mauritania, Namibia, Nauru, Papua New Guinea, Solomon Islands, Somalia, Vanuatu, Yemen, Zimbabwe	Cambodia China Iran Laos Ghana Mexico Morocco Nepal[a] Oman Myanmar[a] ***Validation awaited:*** Gambia India[a] Iraq Togo
No. of Countries	14	29	14
% of the endemic population	83	17	0
% of TT burden	71	29	0

[a]WHO SEARO

References

1. World Health Organization. Neglected Tropical Diseases. www.who.int/neglected_diseases/diseases/en/. Accessed 12 Sept 2020.
2. Editorial. Lancet. 2019;394:2126. www.thelancet.com/pdfs/journals/lancet/PIIS0140-6736(19)33069-7.pdf
3. World Health Organization. Global plan to combat neglected tropical diseases 2008–2015. Geneva: World Health Organization; 2007.
4. Report of the Tenth Meeting of the WHO Strategic and Technical Advisory Group for Neglected Tropical Diseases, 29–30 March 2017, WHO. www.who.int/neglected_diseases/NTD_STAG_report_2017.pdf
5. World Health Organization. The WHO Alliance for GET2020. www.who.int/trachoma/partnership/en/. Accessed 12 Sept 2020.
6. Engels D. Neglected tropical diseases in the Sustainable Development Goals. Lancet. 2016. https://doi.org/10.1016/S0140-6736(16)00043-X.
7. World Health Organization, Brochure. Ending the neglect to attain the Sustainable Development Goals; A road map for neglected tropical diseases 2020-2031.
8. World Health Organization and Neglected Tropical Disease NGO Network. www.who.int/wash-health-toolkit/index.html. Accessed 12 Sept 2020.
9. Hogeweg M. Leprosy and the eye. Commun Eye Health J. 2001;14:32.
10. Narain JP, Dash AP, Parnell B, et al. Elimination of neglected tropical diseases in the South-East Asia Region of the World Health Organization. Bull World Health Organ. 2010;88:206–10.
11. World Health Organization. Fact Sheets. Trachoma 11 Aug 2020. https://www.who.int/news-room/fact-sheets/detail/trachoma. Accessed 12 Sept 2020.
12. Taylor HR, Burton MJ, Haddad D, et al. Trachoma. Lancet. 2014;384:2142–52. https://doi.org/10.1016/S0140-6736(13)62182-0.
13. Clarke IN. Evolution of Chlamydia trachomatis. Ann N Y Acad Sci. 2011;1230:E11–8.
14. Carlson JH, Porcella SF, McClarty G, et al. Comparative genomic analysis of Chlamydia trachomatis oculotropic and genitotropic strains. Infect Immun. 2005;73:6407–18.
15. Mariotti SP, Pascolini D, Rose-Nussbaumer J. Trachoma: global magnitude of a preventable cause of blindness. Br J Ophthalmol. 2009;93:563–8.
16. Gambhir M, Basáñez M-G, Burton MJ, et al. The development of an age-structured model for trachoma transmission dynamics, pathogenesis and control. PLoS Negl Trop Dis. 2009;3:e462. https://doi.org/10.1371/journal.pntd.0000462.
17. Lee AG. Trachoma; e medicine. Medscape. Updated July 24, 2019. https://emedicine.medscape.com/article/1202088-overview#a6. Accessed 12 Sept 2020.
18. Abu el-Asrar AM, Geboes K, Tabbara KF, et al. Immunopathogenesis of conjunctival scarring in trachoma. Eye. 1998;12:453–60.
19. Rajhi AA, Hidayat A, Nasr A, et al. The histopathology and the mechanism of entropion in patients with trachoma. Ophthalmology. 1993;100:1293–6.
20. Burton MJ. Trachoma: an overview. Br Med Bull. 2007;84:99–116.
21. Conway DJ, Holland MJ, Bailey RL, et al. Scarring trachoma is associated with polymorphism in the tumor necrosis factor alpha (TNF-alpha) gene promoter and with elevated TNF-alpha levels in tear fluid. Infection Immunity. 1997;65:1003–6.
22. Hu VH, Weiss HA, Massae P, et al. In vivo confocal microscopy in scarring trachoma. Ophthalmology. 2011;118:2138–46.
23. Reacher MH, Peer J, Rapoza PA, et al. T-Cells and trachoma – their role in cicatricial disease. Ophthalmology. 1991;98:334–41. https://doi.org/10.1016/s0161-6420(91)32290-5.
24. Stephens RS. The cellular paradigm of chlamydial pathogenesis. Trends Microbiol. 2003;11:44–51.
25. World Health Organization. What is trachoma. https://www.who.int/trachoma/disease/en/. Accessed 12 Sept 2020.
26. World Health Organization. Trachoma, global partnership for trachoma elimination. https://www.who.int/trachoma/partnership/en/. Accessed 12 Sept 2020.
27. World Health Organization. Fifty-first World Health Assembly Meeting Resolutions and Decisions, Geneva, 11–16 May 1998. www.who.int. Accessed 12 Sept 2020.
28. World Health Organization, the London School of Hygiene & Tropical Medicine, and the International Trachoma Initiative. Trachoma control. A guide for programme managers. www.who.int. Accessed 12 Sept 2020.
29. World Health Organization. Trachoma, strategy. https://www.who.int/trachoma/strategy/en/. Accessed 12 Sept 2020.
30. Emerson PM, Bailey RL. Trachoma and fly control. J Commun Eye Health. 1999;12:57.
31. World Health Organization. Validation of elimination of Trachoma as a Public Health Problem. World Health Organization Press; 2016. https://www.who.int. Accessed 12 Sept 2020.
32. World Health Organization. Report of the Third Global Scientific Meeting on Trachoma Report. World Health Organization 2010 July 19–20, 2010. www.who.int. Accessed 12 Sept 2020.
33. Reacher MH, Muñoz B, Alghassany A, et al. A controlled trial of surgery for trachomatous trichiasis of the Upper Lid. Arch Ophthalmol. 1992;110:667–74.
34. Burton MJ, Habtamu E, Gower EW. Interventions for trachoma trichiasis. Cochrane Database Syst Rev. 2015:CD004008. https://doi.org/10.1002/14651858.CD004008.pub3.
35. Habtamu E, Wondie T, Aweke S, et al. Posterior lamellar versus bilamellar tarsal rotation surgery for

trachomatous trichiasis in Ethiopia: a randomised controlled trial. Lancet Glob Health. 2016; https://doi.org/10.1016/S2214-109X(15)00299-5.
36. Merbs SL, Oktavec KC, Munoz BE, et al. Lower postoperative scar height is associated with increased postoperative trichiasis 1 year after bilamellar tarsal rotation surgery. Ophthalmic Epidemiol. 2015;22:200–7.
37. World Health Organization. Report of the 4th Global Scientific Meeting on Trachoma, Geneva, 27–29 November 2018. Geneva. www.who.int. Accessed 12 Sept 2020.
38. West SK. Milestones in the fight to eliminate trachoma. Ophthalmic Physiol Opt. 2020;40:66–74.
39. Kumaresan J. What is new in trachoma control? Commun Eye Health J. 2004;17:49.
40. World Health Organization. Eliminating trachoma: WHO announces sustained progress with hundreds of millions of people no longer at risk of infection. www.who.int. Accessed 12 Sept 2020.
41. World Health Organization. Trachoma. www.who.int. Accessed 12 Sept 2020.
42. Terminating trachoma. How Myanmar eliminated blinding trachoma. New Delhi: World Health Organization, Regional Office for South-East Asia; 2020. www.who.int. Accessed 12 Sept 2020.
43. World Health Organization. Amid continued progress, trachoma elimination programmes set their sights on 2030. www.who.int. Accessed 12 Sept 2020.
44. Taylor HR. Trachoma in Asia-A disappearing scourge. Taiwan J Ophthalmol. 2016;6:55–7.
45. World Health Organization. Status of elimination of trachoma as a public health problem Data by country, Global Health Observatory data repository. www.who.int. Accessed 12 Sept 2020.
46. World Health Organization. WHO Alliance for the Global Elimination of Trachoma by 2020. Weekly Epidemiological Rec. 2020;95:349–60. www.who.int. Accessed 12 Sept 2020.
47. Dineen BP, Bourne RRA, Ali SM, et al. Prevalence and causes of blindness and visual impairment in Bangladeshi adults: results of the National Blindness and Low Vision Survey of Bangladesh. Br J Ophthalmol. 2003;87:820–8.
48. Lepcha NT, Sharma IP, Sapkota YD, et al. Changing trends of blindness, visual impairment and cataract surgery in Bhutan: 2009–2018. PLoS One. 2019;14:e0216398. https://doi.org/10.1371/journal.pone.0216398.
49. Gupta UC, Preobragenski VV. Trachoma in India-endemicity and epidemiological study. Indian J Ophthalmol. 1964;12:39–49.
50. Preobragenski VV, Gupta UC. The National Trachoma Control Programme in India. Indian J Ophthalmol. 1964;12:68–73.
51. World Health Organization. Report of the 17th Meeting of the WHO Alliance for The Global Elimination of Blinding Trachoma, Geneva, 22–24 April 2013. www.who.int. Accessed 12 Sept 2020.
52. The National Blindness and Visual Impairment Survey 2015-2019. A summary report. National Programme for Control of Blindness &Visual Impairment, Directorate General of Health Services, Ministry of Health & Family Welfare, Government of India, New Delhi. www.npcbvi.gov.in. Accessed 12 Sept 2020.
53. Kumar A, Vashist P. Indian Community Eye Care in 2020: achievements and challenges. Indian J Ophthalmol. 2020;68:291–3.
54. Syumarti, Rini M, Ratnanina N, et al. Prevalence and causes of blindness in people age 50 years and above, the Intervention category and Action required reducing blindness in West Java province Indonesia. J Ophthalmol Clin Res. 2017;1(1):1–4. Research Article.
55. Ubeydulla T, Das T, Limburg H, et al. First rapid assessment of avoidable blindness survey in the Maldives: prevalence and causes of blindness and cataract surgery. Asia Pac J Ophthalmol (Phila). 2018;7:316–20.
56. Prevention of blindness in Myanmar: situation analysis and strategy for change. IAPB. www.iapb.org. Accessed 12 Sept 2020.
57. Banagala C, Gilbert C, Murthy GVS, et al. Prevalence, causes, magnitude, and risk factors of visual impairment and blindness in Sri Lanka. Ceylon Med J. 2018;63(s2):s10–7. https://doi.org/10.4038/cmj.v63i5.8735.
58. Isipradit S, Sirimaharaj M, Charukamnoetkanok P, et al. The first rapid assessment of avoidable blindness (RAAB) in Thailand. PLoS One. 2014;9:e114245. https://doi.org/10.1371/journal.pone.0114245.
59. Correia M, Das T, Magno J, et al. Prevalence and causes of blindness, visual impairment, and cataract surgery in Timor-Leste. Clin Ophthalmol. 2017;11:2125–31.
60. Ramke J, Palagyi A, Naduvilath T, et al. Prevalence and causes of blindness and low vision in Timor-Leste. Br J Ophthalmol. 2007;91:1117–21. https://doi.org/10.1136/bjo.2006.106559.
61. Correia M, Brunner D, Sharma M, et al. A search for trachoma in Timor-Leste: no evidence to justify undertaking population-based prevalence surveys. Ophthalmic Epidemiol. 25(Suppl 1):131–7. https://doi.org/10.1080/09286586.2018.1545037.
62. Brilliant LB, Pokhrel RP, Grasset NC, et al. Epidemiology of blindness in Nepal. Bull World Health Organ. 1985;63:375–86.
63. Mishra SK. Nepal eliminates Trachoma. IAPB; 2018. www.iapb.org. Accessed 16 Sept 2020.
64. Nepal eliminates trachoma as a public health problem. International Coalition for Trachoma Control; 2018. www.trachomacoalition.org. Accessed 16 Sept 2020.
65. National Trachoma Program. Nepal Netra Jyoti Sangh. https://www.nnjs.org.np/national-trachoma-program. Accessed 16 Sept 2020.

66. World Health Organization. Weekly epidemiological record. 26 SEPTEMBER 2014, 89th year; No. 39. 2014;89:421–8. www.who.int. Accessed 12 Sept 2020.
67. International Coalition for Trachoma Control, 2020 INSight, July 2011. www.trachomacoalition.org. Accessed 12 Sept 2020.
68. WHO Alliance for the Global Elimination of Trachoma by 2020 GET2020 Database as of 1 May 2020. www.trachomacoalition.org. Accessed 12 Sept 2020.
69. World Health Organization. Weekly epidemiological record. 24 July 2020. www.who.in. Accessed 12 Sept 2020.

14 Glaucoma: Burden, Practices, and Challenges

Mehal Rathore, Ronnie George, M. Baskaran, Rashima Asokan, Sunee Chansangpetch, and Lingam Vijaya

Key Points

- Glaucoma is a major cause of ocular morbidity and blindness in the South-East Asia region.
- The majority of glaucoma cases are undetected.
- There is an urgent need to improve case detection and management to minimize the projected increase in glaucoma caseloads as populations age.
- There are an inadequate number of glaucoma specialists, and they are often urban-centric.
- Teaching and training glaucoma specialists in residency programs needs strengthening.
- Most population-based studies in glaucoma have been conducted in India.
- Countries with poor awareness rates have a higher proportion of undetected disease.

Glaucoma is a neurodegenerative disorder characterized by typical degenerative structural changes of the retinal ganglion cells in the optic nerve head and produces corresponding visual field defects [1]. The pathophysiology of the condition is still unclear, but the condition is diagnosed by morphological changes in the optic disc. As the changes advance, the axonal death of the retinal ganglion cells causes permanent glaucomatous visual field damage. Elevated intraocular pressure is known to contribute further to the damage. Glaucoma is broadly classified as primary or secondary based on the cause of the disease.

14.1 Prevalence and Burden of Glaucoma

According to the World Health Organization (WHO), glaucoma is the second leading cause of blindness after cataract. In 2014, the reported global prevalence of glaucoma was 3.54% [2]. It is projected to affect 76 million people in 2020, increasing to 111.8 million people by 2040 (Fig. 14.1) [2]. Primary open-angle glaucoma (POAG) is more prevalent than primary angle-closure glaucoma (PACG) globally including Asia though there is a higher proportion of PACG

M. Rathore
Elite School of Optometry, Chennai, India

R. George (✉) · M. Baskaran · L. Vijaya
Smt Jadhavabai Nathmal Singhvee Glaucoma Services, Sankara Nethralaya, Chennai, India
e-mail: drrg@snmail.org; drmb@snmail.org; drlv@snmail.org

R. Asokan
Occupational Optometry Services, Medical Research Foundation, Sankara Nethralaya, Chennai, India
e-mail: rashima@snmail.org

S. Chansangpetch
Department of Ophthalmology, Faculty of Medicine, Chulalongkorn University and King Chulalongkorn Memorial Hospital, Thai Red Cross Society, Bangkok, Thailand
e-mail: sunee.ch@chula.ac.th

T. Das, P. D. Nayar (eds.), *South-East Asia Eye Health*,
https://doi.org/10.1007/978-981-16-3787-2_14

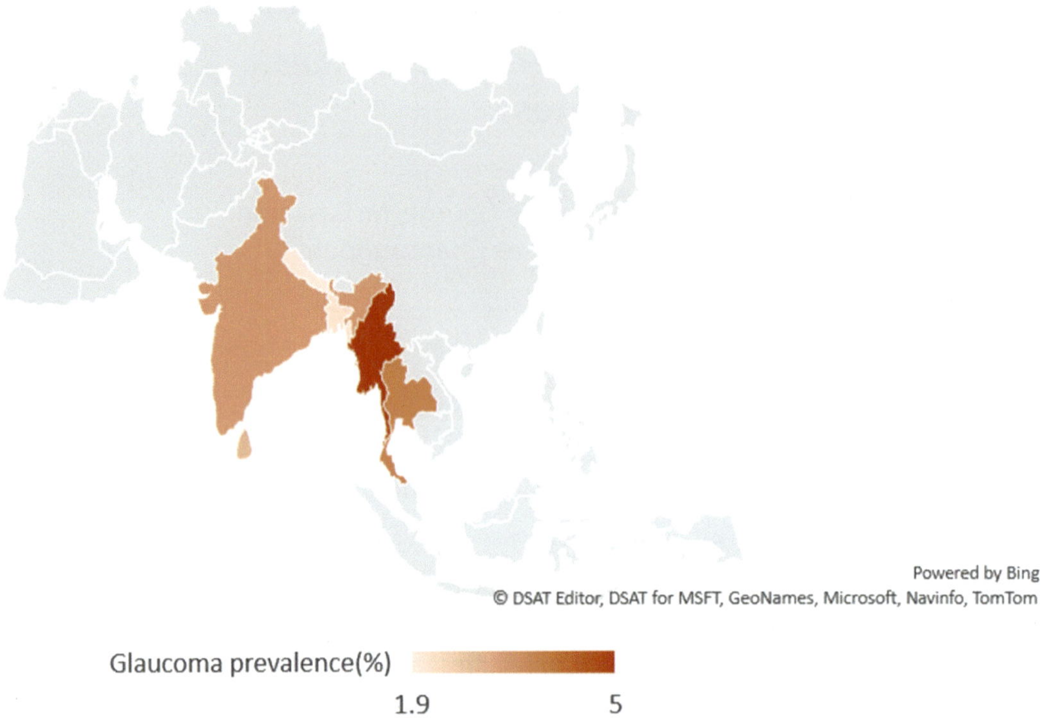

Fig. 14.1 Global prevalence of primary open-angle glaucoma. Source: Nature Review 2016; doi:10.1038/nrdp.2016.67. (Weinreb, R., Leung, C., Crowston, J., et al. Primary open-angle glaucoma. *Nat Rev Dis Primers* **2,** 16067 (2016). https://doi.org/10.1038/nrdp.2016.67)

in Asia than other continents of the world (Table 14.1) [2]. As of 2010, the pooled estimate of glaucoma in India was 11.2 million in people aged 40 years and above [20]. As the population ages, the prevalence of the disease is expected to increase with time. India alone is estimated to account for 20% of the total number of glaucoma patients worldwide by 2020 [21]. Besides the insidious nature of the disease, its late presentation in the clinic adds to the burden of the disease. As the disease progresses, it affects the individual's functional independence and social life [22, 23].

Globally, 1 in 15 blind person and 1 in 45 visually impaired person is due to glaucoma [24]. The Vision Loss Expert Group (VLEG) estimated that glaucoma remained the third most common cause for blindness (after cataract and uncorrected refractive error) both in 1995 and 2010 in Central and South Asia. The impact of aging and its effect on the absolute numbers of blind individuals in this relatively young population is striking. The estimated 250,000 blind persons due to glaucoma in 1990 nearly doubled to 499,000 in 2015 in a period of just 15 years [25].

Unlike a cataract, glaucoma does not have a one-time solution. Ideally, glaucoma must be diagnosed before it causes any functional damage [26]. However, this is often not possible because it is asymptomatic in most individuals until advanced damage occurs. By this point, there is a significant impact on the quality of life of the person. Once diagnosed, it requires regular monitoring and treatment modifications. If diagnosed in time, the visual prognosis is much better. According to a German study, an early diagnosis and immediate treatment reduces the chances of blindness occurring 20 years later by 50% [27]. Furthermore, missed visits to an ophthalmologist increase incidences of undiagnosed glaucoma sixfold; the type of eye care provider (ophthalmologist versus optometrist) consulted also increases the undiagnosed glaucoma rates [28–30]. The late diagnosis of the condition also

Table 14.1 Prevalence of glaucoma reported from population-based studies in the region [3–19]

Racial/Ethnic group and study location/year of study	Age (years)	Number of participants	All types of glaucoma (%)	POAG (%)	PACG (%)	Secondary glaucoma
Vellore, India, 1995 [3]	30–60	972	4.7	0.4	4.3[a]	–
Madurai, India, 1997 [4]	≥40	5150	2.5	1.7	0.5	0.3
West Bengal, India, 1999 [5]	≥50	1269	2.0	1.7	0.2	0.1
Andhra Pradesh, India, 2000 [6]	≥40	3724	3.1	2.2	0.9	–
Chennai, India (rural) 2004 [7, 8]	≥40	3924	4.3	1.6	0.9	1.8
Chennai, India (urban) 2008, 2013 [9, 10]	≥40	3850	4.6	3.5	0.9	0.2
Central India 2008 [11]	≥30	4711	2.7	1.9	0.2	
Kolkata, India, 2014 [12, 13]	>40	7128	3.2	2.1	1.0	0.2
Hooghly, India, 2014 [12, 13]	>40	6964	2.7	1.5	1.2	0.1
Kandy, Sri Lanka, 2007 [14, 15]	≥40	1375	2.9	2.3	0.6	–
Dhaka, Bangladesh,1998 [16]	≥40	2347	2.1	2.5	0.4	0.2
Meiktila, Myanmar, 2005 [17]	≥40	2076	5.0	2.0	2.5	0.5
Nepal; Bhaktapur Glaucoma study, 2010 [18]	≥40	4003	1.9	1.2	0.4	–
Rom Klao district, Thailand, 1999 [19]	≥50	701	3.8	2.3	0.9	–

PACG primary angle-closure glaucoma, *POAG* primary open-angle glaucoma
[a]Includes primary angle-closure and PACG

adds to the economic burden of treatment. Once the patient becomes symptomatic, it is often too late to reverse damage.

A poll of ophthalmologists attending the annual meeting of the Glaucoma Society of India provides interesting insights into glaucoma care patterns in India [31]. About 40% were self-reported glaucoma specialists, 50% were general ophthalmologists interested in glaucoma, and 10% were general ophthalmologists. There were wide variations in the responses among the three groups. Routine gonioscopy was performed more commonly in all glaucoma suspects or glaucoma patients by glaucoma specialists (83%) compared to non-glaucoma specialists (46%) and general ophthalmologists (48%) [31]. Indentation gonioscopy was less likely to be performed by non-glaucoma specialists (50%) and general ophthalmologists (42%) than glaucoma specialists (66%) [31]. More than 90% of glaucoma specialists performed yttrium-aluminum-garnet (YAG) laser peripheral iridotomy (LPI) as primary treatment for the angle-closure disease. Close to 20% of non-specialists only prescribed medical therapy [31]. Post-iridotomy assessment of the angle by gonioscopy was less common among non-specialists and general ophthalmologists (38–40%) than in glaucoma specialists (70%) [31]. Only a third of glaucoma specialists performed both trabeculectomy and glaucoma drainage services in this survey [31]. This could be related to a lack of training or cost considerations, but has implications on access to the appropriate management of the disease.

The Asia Pacific Glaucoma guidelines recommend certain standards for glaucoma evaluation. These include Goldmann applanation tonometry, indentation gonioscopy, and stereoscopic optic disc evaluation [32]. Surprisingly a fairly large proportion of glaucoma specialists (28%) routinely used non-Goldmann-style applanation tonometers, including non-contact tonometry (NCT) [31].

Intraocular pressure (IOP) is the only modifiable risk factor in glaucoma. The clinical decisions in glaucoma dependent on IOP measured by a non-Goldmann-style applanation tonometer have a significant impact on the management of patients with glaucoma. In the setting of population-based studies from India, most reported that a large proportion of those with POAG at presentation had IOP readings that were in the statistically normal range [8, 9]. The overdependence on IOP measurements for glaucoma diagnosis is a challenge [33]. IOP measured with non-standard techniques (Schiotz tonometry, non-contact tonometer, NCT, etc.) will further reduce its diagnostic importance. In one of the referral service care systems setup by optometrists, 67% of the referrals were due to overestimation of IOP by NCT [34]. The economic burden of wrong referrals may impact genuine glaucoma patients to delayed appointments or misdiagnoses in these situations.

14.2 Challenges

The challenges in detecting and managing glaucoma include access to care, inadequate training of ophthalmologists, and poor awareness.

The burden of glaucoma is further heightened in South-East Asia by the lack of trained ophthalmologists. As of 2005, there were 232,866 ophthalmologists in the world [35]. They were mostly concentrated in developed countries, leaving developing countries with a severe lack of experts [36]. In India, there were 17,000 ophthalmologists in 2015 [20, 35], and only a fraction of them were involved in glaucoma care. While this number has increased in the last 5 years, most ophthalmologists prefer to serve in urban localities, and access to eye care, specifically glaucoma care, is limited in the rural population. Since more than 70% of the Indian population resides in villages where only 25% of ophthalmologists practice, the 1:100,000 ophthalmologist: population ratio for India is much lower in rural India [20]. The Aravind Comprehensive Eye Survey conducted in the rural population of south Tamil Nadu (South India) reported that only one third of the people in this area had undergone an eye examination at any time in their lives, and three-fourths of the population aged 40 years or older required eye care services [37]. In a study among children in blind schools in rural Java (Indonesia), only 20% of congenital glaucoma patients had undergone glaucoma surgery; the remaining untreated patients were totally or near blind. Most pediatric ophthalmologists work in urban centers in Java; lack of access and poor socioeconomic conditions limit access to care [38]. In a glaucoma blindness survey, Baluchistan (the poorest province in Pakistan where 89% of the rural population live in highly deprived districts with limited access to eye care services) was found to have the highest prevalence of blindness [39]. There is a disconnect between need, availability, and access to eye care in many countries in this region.

Three other factors impact glaucoma care: gender inequity, quality medicine, and access to care. Women have poorer access to eye care services, in at least some parts of India [40]. While men are slightly more likely to have POAG in India, angle-closure disease was more common in women, i.e., 17 million vs 11 million in men [20]. Since PACG is a more blinding disease than POAG, such disparities in eye care access could result in greater visual morbidity from glaucoma among women [20]. Treatment of POAG is primarily medical therapy with surgery reserved for those who do not respond adequately to medication or in conjunction with cataract extraction [41]. Medically, low-cost generic glaucoma medications are widely available [41]. The use of glaucoma medications is steadily increasing. Cost considerations and government regulations often mandate the use of lower-cost brands. But there are concerns about the sub-optimal concentrations of antibiotics in eye drops and unacceptable environmental conditions for their storage [42, 43]. Generic glaucoma medications have been shown to have less IOP lowering effects in some studies [44]. Sleath et al. [45] reported that 20% of glaucoma patients in South India had to travel for at least half an hour, and 9% of glaucoma patients had to travel more than 2 h to purchase their medication. The access to glaucoma medications is likely to be worse in rural India and other parts of the country, since this study was done in the most urbanized state in India.

In most cases, glaucoma care involves the lifelong application of anti-glaucoma medication as topical drops. These medications have been shown to take up only 0.3% of the income in high-income groups but tend to take up as high as 137% of the income in the low-income group, and this cost further increases with age [46]. The never-ending expenses of glaucoma medications and lack of government subsidies lead to poor adherence to medication use and, in the long term, poor visual outcomes. Besides this, the availability of medicines in rural areas is important for good compliance to treatment. Also, the patient has to bear the indirect costs of transportation, lost wages, lodging, and diagnostics for his/her treatment. This was considered an important reason for the higher prevalence of blindness due to glaucoma among poor people in a report on the association between socioeconomic status and blindness in Pakistan [47]. Among those with established glaucoma, in a clinic-based study, Lee et al. [48] found that knowledge and perceptional barriers among glaucoma patients in South India were the main reason for missed visits in nearly 40% of those with poor follow-up. Thus awareness levels among those without the established disease could be worse [49].

Population-based studies from Chennai [Chennai Glaucoma Study (CGS)] and Andhra Pradesh [Andhra Pradesh Eye Disease Study (APEDS)] highlighted another issue in patients with PACG. According to the CGS, 40% (two out of five) of the people being treated for glaucoma at presentation had PACG [9]. The APEDS study reported similar misdiagnosis rates in their cohort. This is a serious cause for concern. Since a laser iridotomy is the first line of treatment for PACG, by not performing the laser iridotomy at diagnosis, these eyes are at a greater risk of progression despite medical therapy. PACG being a more aggressive blinding condition than POAG [9], the burden of misdiagnosis can be grave. The most likely reason for this misdiagnosis could be lack of routine practice of gonioscopy or due to incorrectly performed gonioscopy [50].

Other regions show differences based on their health care models. In Thailand, 39% of all secondary and tertiary hospitals (including university-based hospitals) are government-run, and 61% are privately run. Government hospitals mostly provide glaucoma care due to the reimbursement policy of the country. At the tertiary level, both government and private sectors are well equipped to manage glaucoma. At the secondary level, tonometry and gonioscopy are almost always available. Optic disc photography is now mostly available. Visual field and OCT (optical coherence tomography) are not yet generally available.

14.3 Awareness

In a clinic-based study from South India, knowledge and perceptional barriers were identified as the main reasons for missed visits in nearly 40% of patients with established glaucoma and poor follow-up (Table 14.2) [18, 48, 49, 51–60]. If we

Table 14.2 Awareness of glaucoma in studies from the region [18, 48, 49, 51–60]

Author	Year	Country	Study population	Glaucoma awareness %
CGS [49]	2004	India	Urban—adults above 40 years	3.3
Dandona et al. [51]	2001	India	Urban—above 15 years	2.3
Krishnaiah et al. [52]	2005	India	Rural—above 15 years	0.3
Gasch et al. [53]	2000	USA	General eye service patients—all ages	72.0
Attebo et al. [54]	1996	Australia	Community—adults above 49 years	93.0
Livingston et al. [55]	1995	Australia	Community—adults above 40 years	70.0
Michielutte et al. [56]	1984	USA	Community—above 14 years	81.0
Saw et al. [57]	2003	Singapore	Tertiary eye hospital—adults 35 years and above	23.0
Lau et al. [58, 60]	2002	Hong Kong	Community—adults above 40 years	78.4
Gyawali et al. [59]	2014	Nepal	"Free eye clinic"—adults of age 35 years and above	60.6
Thapa et al. [18]	2011	Nepal	Community—adults above 40 years	2.4
Islam et al. [48]	2015	Bangladesh	Community—adults of age 30 years and above	7.0

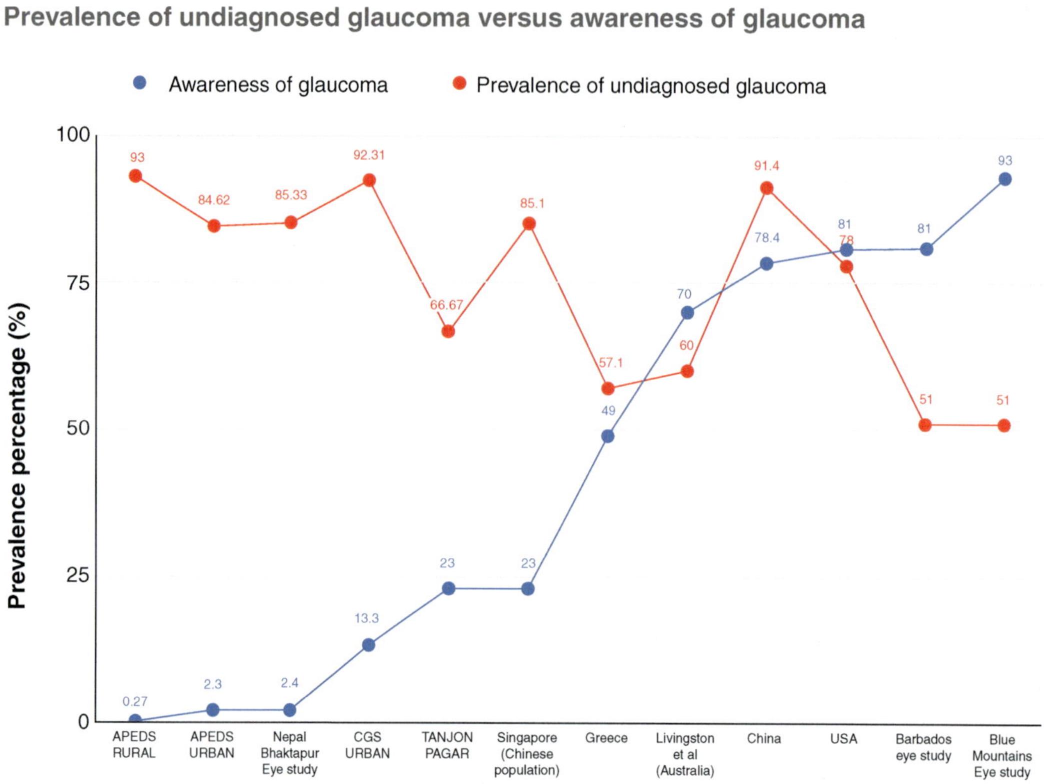

Fig. 14.2 Awareness versus prevalence of undetected glaucoma [29, 61–71]

compare awareness rates for glaucoma in a country versus the proportion of undetected disease, an inverse trend is seen. Countries with poor awareness rates have a higher proportion of undetected disease (Fig. 14.2) [29, 61–71].

14.4 Challenges in Training During and Post-residency

There are an estimated 1500 ophthalmology residency positions in India (1173 in 3-year Masters programs, and 355 in 2-year Diploma programs) [72]. In 2005, a questionnaire was administered to three-fourths of the residents in these programs [73]. From this questionnaire, it was found that there were postgraduate medical schools without functional slit lamps, indirect ophthalmoscopes, or operating microscopes. Among all medical schools, 25% did not have applanation tonometers, 34% did not have YAG lasers, and 45% did not have Goldmann perimeters (we assume that automated perimeters were not available). Although the mean numbers of new cases seen in the outpatient departments annually were 31,000, these numbers was as low as 778 cases annually in one center. A third of all glaucoma centers examined an average of 50 patients/day. The annual numbers of glaucoma surgeries performed in each center ranged from 2 to 115 with a mean of 74 surgeries annually; the lowest being 2 surgeries/year.

With such low caseload exposure to surgery, adequate outpatient exposure will be challenging. This lack of exposure leads many to apply for fellowships or observerships of 1 week to 2 years in duration. Participants who completed a 4-week intensive hands-on supervised training program were administered a questionnaire to assess their skills in multiple areas with each question graded from 0 to 4 [23]. The trainees were from different parts of India, Ghana, Vietnam, Bangladesh, Sri Lanka, Saudi Arabia, and Paraguay. Of these, 57% were trainee residents, and 43% were ophthalmologists with 1–15 years of experience. Pretraining mean scores were <1 (never done or occasionally done) for four-mirror gonioscopy and less than 2 (done, but not comfortable) for applanation tonometry (1.55). Pretraining scores for interpretation of Humphrey visual fields was 1.32, and assessment of the disc with a 78/90D lens was 2.11.

In a more recent survey, over 500 ophthalmologists were interviewed on their residency training, 2–10 years after they completed the program. They graded their skills in basic diagnostic skills from 0 to 10, with 10 being the highest skill level. Their perception of training in applanation tonometry and gonioscopy had reasonable mean scores of 6 and 5.7, respectively. But, close to 30% of the respondents had rated their skills in these techniques as 0 (no skill at all). Over half had done only one trabeculectomy [60]. These findings are not surprising in the context of the earlier survey. There are huge variations in the quality of training. Some centers with very high patient load and state-of-the-art equipment and facilities offer outstanding training to their residents and fellows, but these appear to be the exception rather than the rule.

In summary, glaucoma accounts for a large proportion of ophthalmic morbidity in the South-East Asian countries. There are wide variations in facilities and care across the country and region. In most countries, undetected glaucoma proportions are high, and awareness rates are poor. These could be addressed by strengthening residency training programs and improving awareness of the disease. There is an urgent need to address these issues since these are young populations; with aging and increased life expectancies, the numbers of those with glaucoma and glaucoma-related blindness are set to increase.

References

1. Nitta K, Sugiyama K, Wajima R, et al. Associations between changes in radial peripapillary capillaries and occurrence of disc hemorrhage in normal-tension glaucoma. Graefe's Arch Clin Exp Ophthalmol. 2019;257:1963–70.
2. Tham YC, Li X, Wong TY, et al. Global prevalence of glaucoma and projections of glaucoma burden through 2040: a systematic review and meta-analysis. Ophthalmology. 2014;121:2081–90.
3. Ramakrishnan R, Nirmalan PK, Krishnadas R, et al. Glaucoma in a rural population of southern India: the Aravind comprehensive eye survey. Ophthalmology. 2003;110:1484–90.
4. Raychaudhuri A, Lahiri SK, Bandyopadhyay M, et al. A population-based survey of the prevalence and types of glaucoma in rural West Bengal: the West Bengal Glaucoma Study. Br J Ophthalmol. 2005;89:1559–64.
5. Garudadri C, Senthil S, Khanna RC, et al. Prevalence and risk factors for primary glaucomas in adult urban and rural populations in the Andhra Pradesh Eye Disease Study. Ophthalmology. 2010;117:1352–9.
6. Vijaya L, George R, Arvind H, et al. Prevalence of angle-closure disease in a rural southern Indian population. Arch Ophthalmol. 2006;124:403–9.
7. Vijaya L, George R, Paul PG, et al. Prevalence of open-angle glaucoma in a rural south Indian population. Invest Ophth Vis Sci. 2005;46:4461–7.
8. Vijaya L, George R, Baskaran M, et al. Prevalence of primary open-angle glaucoma in an urban south Indian population and comparison with a rural population: the Chennai Glaucoma Study. Ophthalmology. 2008;115:648–54.
9. Vijaya L, George R, Arvind H, et al. Prevalence of primary angle-closure disease in an urban south Indian population and comparison with a rural population: the Chennai Glaucoma Study. Ophthalmology. 2008;115:655–60.
10. Nangia V, Jonas JB, Matin A, et al. Prevalence and associated factors of glaucoma in rural central India. The Central India Eye and Medical Study. PLoS One. 2013;8:e76434. https://doi.org/10.1371/journal.pone.0076434.
11. Paul C, Sengupta S, Banerjee S, et al. Open-angle glaucoma in a rural and urban population in Eastern India—the Hooghly river glaucoma study. Indian J Ophthalmol. 2020;68:371–4.
12. Paul C, Sengupta S, Banerjee S, et al. Angle closure glaucoma in rural and urban populations in eastern India—The Hooghly River Glaucoma Study. Indian J Ophthalmol. 2018;66:1285–090.
13. Casson RJ, Baker M, Edussuriya K, et al. Prevalence and determinants of angle closure in central Sri Lanka: the Kandy Eye Study. Ophthalmology. 2009;116:1444–9.
14. Sia DI, Edussuriya K, Sennanayake S, et al. Prevalence of and risk factors for primary open-angle glaucoma in central Sri Lanka: the Kandy eye study. Ophthal Epidemiol. 2010;17:211–6.
15. Rahman MM, Rahman N, Foster PJ, et al. The prevalence of glaucoma in Bangladesh: a population-based survey in Dhaka division. Br J Ophthalmol. 2004;88:1493–7.
16. Casson RJ, Newland HS, Muecke J, et al. Prevalence of glaucoma in rural Myanmar: the Meiktila Eye Study. Br J Ophthalmol. 2007;91:710–4.

17. Thapa SS, Berg RV, Khanal S, et al. Prevalence of visual impairment, cataract surgery and awareness of cataract and glaucoma in Bhaktapur district of Nepal: the Bhaktapur Glaucoma Study. BMC Ophthalmol. 2011;1 https://doi.org/10.1186/1471-2415-11-2.
18. Bourne RR, Sukudom P, Foster PJ, et al. Prevalence of glaucoma in Thailand: a population-based survey in Rom Klao District, Bangkok. Br J Ophthalmol. 2003;87:1069–74.
19. Choudhari NS, Pathak-Ray V, Kaushik S, et al. Prevalent practice patterns in glaucoma: poll of Indian ophthalmologists at a national conference. Indian J Ophthalmol. 2016;64:715–21.
20. George R, Ramesh SV, Vijaya L. Glaucoma in India: estimated burden of disease. J Glaucoma. 2010;19:391–7.
21. Quigley HA, Broman AT. The number of people with glaucoma worldwide in 2010 and 2020. Br J Ophthalmol. 2006;90:262–7.
22. Dubey S, Bedi H, Bedi M, et al. Impact of visual impairment on the wellbeing and functional disability of patients with glaucoma in India. J Curr Ophthalmol. 2019;32:14–8.
23. Bourne RRA, Taylor HR, Flaxman SR, et al. Number of people blind or visually impaired by glaucoma worldwide and in world regions 1990-2010: a meta-analysis. PLoS One. 2016; https://doi.org/10.1371/journal.pone.0162229.
24. Jonas JB, George R, Asokan R, et al. Prevalence and causes of vision loss in Central and South Asia: 1990–2010. Br J Ophthalmol. 2014;98:592–8.
25. Thomas R. Glaucoma in developing countries. Indian J Ophthalmol. 2012;60:446–50.
26. Michelson G, Hornegger J, Wärntges S, et al. The papilla as screening parameter for early diagnosis of glaucoma. Deutsches Aerzteblatt Int. 2008;105:583–9.
27. Topouzis F, Harris A, Coleman AL, et al. Factors associated with undiagnosed open angle glaucoma. The Thessaloniki Eye Study. Am J Ophthalmol. 2008;145:327–35.
28. Wong EY, Keeffe JE, Rait JL, et al. Detection of undiagnosed glaucoma by eye health professionals. Ophthalmology. 2004;111:1508–14.
29. Weih LM, Nanjan M, McCarty CA, et al. Prevalence and predictors of open-angle glaucoma: results from the visual impairment project. Ophthalmology. 2001;108:1966–72.
30. Jacob A, Thomas R, Koshi SP, et al. Prevalence of primary glaucoma in an urban south Indian population. Indian J Ophthalmol. 1998;46:81–6.
31. Asia Pacific Glaucoma Guidelines. South East Asian Glaucoma Interest Group. September 14, 2008. http://www.seagig.org/guidelines1.php. Accessed 28 Sept 2020.
32. Thomas R, Paul P, Rao GN, et al. Present status of eye care in India. Surv Ophthalmol. 2005;50:85–101.
33. Kamel K, Dervan E, Falzon K, et al. Difference in intraocular pressure measurements between non-contact tonometry and Goldmann applanation tonometry and the role of central corneal thickness in affecting glaucoma referrals. Ir J Med Sci. 2019;188:321–5.
34. Resnikoff S, Lansingh VC, Washburn L, et al. Estimated number of ophthalmologists worldwide (International Council of Ophthalmology update): will we meet the needs? Br J Ophthalmol. 2020;104:588–92.
35. Rao GN. Ophthalmology in India. Arch Ophthalmol. 2000;118:1431–2.
36. Robin AL, Nirmalan PK, Krishnadas R, et al. The utilization of eye care services by persons with glaucoma in rural south India. Trans Am Ophthal Soc. 2004;102:47–56.
37. Sitorus RS, Abidin MS, Prihartono J. Causes and temporal trends of childhood blindness in Indonesia: study at schools for the blind in Java. Br J Ophthalmol. 2007;91:1109–13.
38. Dineen B, Bourne RR, Jadoon Z, et al. Causes of blindness and visual impairment in Pakistan. The Pakistan national blindness and visual impairment survey. Br J Ophthalmol. 2007;91:1005–10.
39. Finger RP, Ali M, Earnest J, Nirmalan PK. Cataract surgery in Andhra Pradesh state, India: an investigation into uptake following outreach screening camps. Ophthal Epidemiol. 2007;14:327–32.
40. Thomas R, Sekhar GC, Kumar RS. Glaucoma management in developing countries: medical, laser, and surgical options for glaucoma management in countries with limited resources. Curr Opin Ophthalmol. 2004;15:127–31.
41. Weir RE, Zaidi FH, Charteris DG, et al. Variability in the content of Indian generic ciprofloxacin eye drops. Br J Ophthalmol. 2005;89:1094–6.
42. Aboshiha J, Weir R, Singh P, et al. To what extent does a lack of refrigeration of generic chloramphenicol eye-drops used in India decrease their purity and what are the implications for Europe. Br J Ophthalmol. 2008;92:609–11.
43. Narayanaswamy A, Neog A, Baskaran M, et al. A randomized, crossover, open label pilot study to evaluate the efficacy and safety of Xalatan® in comparison with generic Latanoprost (Latoprost) in subjects with primary open angle glaucoma or ocular hypertension. Indian J Ophthalmol. 2007;55:127–31.
44. Sleath BL, Krishnadas R, Cho M, et al. Patient reported barriers to glaucoma medication access, use, and adherence in southern India. Indian J Ophthalmol. 2008;57:63–8.
45. Nayak B, Gupta S, Kumar G, et al. Socioeconomics of long-term glaucoma therapy in India. Indian J Ophthalmol. 2015;63:20–4.
46. Gilbert CE, Shah SP, Jadoon MZ, et al. Poverty and blindness in Pakistan: results from the Pakistan national blindness and visual impairment survey. BMJ. 2008;336:29–32.
47. Lee BW, Parthasarathi S, John RK, et al. Predictors of and barriers associated with poor follow-up among

glaucoma patients in south India. Arch Ophthalmol. 2008;126:1448–54.
48. Ramesh SVe, Pradeep GP, George R, et al. Determinants of glaucoma awareness and knowledge in urban Chennai. Indian J Ophthalmol. 2009;57:355–60.
49. Thomas R, Muliyil J, George R. Glaucoma in southern India [letter]. Ophthalmology. 2001;108:1173–5.
50. Dandona R, Dandona L, John RK, et al. Awareness of eye diseases in an urban population in southern India. Bull World Health Organ. 2001;79:96–102.
51. Krishnaiah S, Kovai V, Srinivas M, et al. Awareness of glaucoma in the rural population of Southern India. Indian J Ophthalmol. 2005;53(3):205.
52. Gasch AT, Wang P, Pasquale LR. Determinants of glaucoma awareness in a general eye clinic. Ophthalmology. 2000;107:303–8.
53. Attebo K, Mitchell P, Cumming R, et al. Knowledge and beliefs about common eye diseases. Aust N Z J Ophthalmol. 1997;25:283–7.
54. Livingston PM, Lee SE, Paola CD. Knowledge of glaucoma, and its relationship to self-care practices, in a population sample. Aust N Z J Ophthalmol. 1995;23:37–41.
55. Michielutte R, Diseker RA, Stafford CL, et al. Knowledge of diabetes and glaucoma in a rural North Carolina community. J Commun Health. 1984;9:269–84.
56. Saw SM, Gazzard G, Friedman D, et al. Awareness of glaucoma, and health beliefs of patients suffering primary acute angle closure. Br J Ophthalmol. 2003;87:446–9.
57. Lau JTF, Lee V, Fan D, et al. Knowledge about cataract, glaucoma, and age-related macular degeneration in the Hong Kong Chinese population. Br J Ophthalmol. 2002;86:1080–4.
58. Gyawali R, Sarkar N. Glaucoma awareness in a hospital presenting population in Eastern Nepal. J Glaucoma. 2014;23:594–8.
59. Thapa SS, Berg RV, Khanal S, et al. Prevalence of visual impairment, cataract surgery and awareness of cataract and glaucoma in Bhaktapur district of Nepal: The Bhaktapur Glaucoma Study. BMC Ophthalmol. 2011;11 https://doi.org/10.1186/1471-2415-11-2.
60. Islam FM, Chakrabarti R, Islam SZ, et al. Factors associated with awareness, attitudes and practices regarding common eye diseases in the general population in a Rural District in Bangladesh: the Bangladesh population-based diabetes and eye study (BPDES). PLoS One. 2015;10:e0133043. https://doi.org/10.1371/journal.pone.0133043.
61. Foster PJ, Oen FT, Machin D, et al. The prevalence of glaucoma in Chinese residents of Singapore: a cross-sectional population survey of the Tanjong Pagar district. Arch Ophthalmol. 2000;118:1105–11.
62. Baskaran M, Foo RC, Cheng C, et al. The prevalence and types of glaucoma in an urban Chinese population: the Singapore Chinese Eye Study. JAMA Ophthalmol. 2015;133:874–80.
63. Konstas AG, Maskaleris G, Gratsonidis S, et al. Compliance and viewpoint of glaucoma patients in Greece. Eye. 2000;14:752–6.
64. Topouzis F, Wilson MR, Harris A, et al. Prevalence of open-angle glaucoma in Greece: the Thessaloniki Eye Study. Am J Ophthalmol. 2007;144:511–9.
65. Livingston PM, McCarty CA, Taylor HR. Knowledge, attitudes, and self-care practices associated with age related eye disease in Australia. Br J Ophthalmol. 1998;82:780–5.
66. Song W, Shan L, Cheng F, et al. Prevalence of glaucoma in a rural northern china adult population: a population-based survey in Kailu county, inner Mongolia. Ophthalmology. 2011;118:1982–8.
67. Shaikh Y, Yu F, Coleman AL. Burden of undetected and untreated glaucoma in the United States. Am J Ophthalmol. 2014;158:1121–9.
68. Leske MC, Connell AM, Schachat AP, et al. The Barbados Eye Study. Prevalence of open angle glaucoma. Arch Ophthalmol. 1994;112:821–9.
69. Mitchell P, Smith W, Attebo K, et al. Prevalence of open-angle glaucoma in Australia. The Blue Mountains Eye Study. Ophthalmology. 1996;103:1661–9.
70. Gupta A. Ophthalmology postgraduate training in India: stirring up a Horner's nest. Indian J Ophthalmol. 2017;65:433–4.
71. Murthy GV, Gupta SK, Bachani D, et al. Status of specialty training in ophthalmology in India. Indian J Ophthalmol. 2005;53:135–42.
72. Tejwani S, Murthy SI, Gadudadri CS, et al. Impact of a month-long training program on the clinical skills of ophthalmology residents and practitioners. Indian J Ophthalmol. 2010;58:340–3.
73. Gogate P, Biswas P, Natarajan S, et al. Residency evaluation and adherence design study: young ophthalmologists' perception of their residency programs – clinical and surgical skills. Indian J Ophthalmol. 2017;65:452–60.

Corneal Blindness and Eye Banking in South-East Asia

15

Anurag Taneja, Murugesan Vanathi, Alisha Kishore, Josie Noah, Shubhi Sood, Patrick Emery, Samara Andrade, Shaifali Sharma, and Sunita Chaurasia

Key Points

- Corneal blindness is the second most common cause of blindness in South-East Asia, second only to cataract.
- Corneal opacities account for 4.67% of total blindness in the South-East Asia region.
- The existing eye banking infrastructure in South-East Asia has been growing, but gaps remain in supply and demand.
- Except for India, Nepal, and Sri Lanka, eye banking in the other countries of the region is either inadequate or is still evolving.
- The main hurdles in eye banking are due to low social awareness of eye donation and the lack of an efficient eye banking network for cornea retrieval, tissue processing, distribution, and training of eye health personnel.
- The 2019 COVID pandemic has led to a slowdown in eye banking activities, adding to the existing challenges.

A. Taneja · J. Noah · S. Sood · P. Emery · S. Andrade
S. Sharma
SightLife, New Delhi, India
e-mail: anurag.taneja@sightlife.org; josie.noah@sightlife.org; shubhi.sood@sightlife.org; patrick.emery@sightlife.org; samara.andrade@sightlife.org; shaifali.sharma@sightlife.org

M. Vanathi · A. Kishore
RP Center, New Delhi, India

S. Chaurasia (✉)
The Cornea Institute, L V Prasad Eye Institute, Hyderabad, India
e-mail: sunita@lvpei.org

T. Das, P. D. Nayar (eds.), *South-East Asia Eye Health*,
https://doi.org/10.1007/978-981-16-3787-2_15

Blindness and visual impairment affect the quality of life of the affected individual and their family; it also impacts the socio-economic order of the country in many ways. A prevalence study in 2015 showed that of the 4.2 million blind people, 2.6 million people lived in East-, South-, and South-East Asian countries [1]. Corneal diseases are significant causes of blindness worldwide, second only to cataract [1, 2]. Many times, corneal blindness is treated by corneal grafting. Hence, corneal transplantation statistics are a proxy by which a country's ability to address corneal blindness can be measured. This chapter discusses the important causes of corneal blindness in the South-East Asia region and the available infrastructure to deal with these.

15.1 Epidemiology, Etiology, and Risk Factors

Globally in 2015, 253 million people were blind and/or visually impaired; of these, 6.17 million (2.4%) people had impaired vision due to corneal causes [3]. The prevalence of blindness (presenting visual acuity (VA) <3/60 in the better eye) and of moderate to severe visual impairment (MSVI: presenting VA <6/18 but ≥3/60 in the better eye) was highest in South Asia. [2] South Asia includes 32.65% of the world's blind individuals, 28.25% of the world's individuals with MSVI, and 26.73% of the world's individuals with mild vision impairment (VA between 6/12 and 6/18) [4]. A recent meta-analysis reported the estimated prevalence of cornea-related MSVI and blindness in Asia due to corneal diseases was 0.38% (95% CI: 0.30–0.46); the highest prevalence was in India (0.88%; 95% CI: 0.38–1.57) and lowest prevalence was in Sri Lanka (0.05%; 95% CI: 0.00–0.11) [5]. Regions with a higher prevalence of corneal blindness also have other health issues related to poverty, water scarcity, poor sanitation, harsh climate, and inhospitable geography. The lack of studies in the higher income regions likely reflects lower prevalence and better access to eye care. The age-standardized prevalence of blindness and MSVI is lower for men than women, probably due to gender inequity, differential access to medical services, and possibly, women's longevity [4].

A wide variety of infective and non-infective diseases that essentially lead to scarring cause cornea-related blindness. The Chennai Eye Disease Incidence Study, in rural and urban South India, reported a 6-year incidence for people >40 years of age; this study reported that the incidence of blindness was 0.48%, and that of monocular blindness was 3.2%. The incidence of monocular blindness was higher in rural than in urban populations. In this study, 3% of monocular blindness was due to corneal pathologies. Post-cataract surgery corneal decompensation accounted for 9.5% of blindness and 4.5% of monocular blindness. The leading risk factors for corneal blindness were age, rural residence, and cataract surgery [6]. The Corneal Opacity Rural Epidemiological (CORE) study in Northern India [7] reported a corneal disease prevalence of 3.7% and corneal blindness prevalence of 0.12%. The leading cause of bilateral corneal blindness was post-cataract surgery and psuedophakic bullous keratopathy (46.2%). The recent report of the national blindness and visual impairment survey (Rapid Assessment of Avoidable Blindness, RAAB, survey) showed that corneal blindness was the second leading cause of blindness in India. Trachoma, a leading cause of blindness in India in the past, is no longer a public health problem [8]. Most reports on corneal blindness occur in people >40 years of age; there is an under-representation of corneal diseases in children and young adults. The primary causes of corneal blindness in children are xerophthalmia, ophthalmia neonatorum, herpes simplex keratitis, and occasionally, chemical keratitis.

The management of corneal blindness primarily revolves around corneal transplantation, either partial or full-thickness, based on the clinical condition. Anterior corneal scarring/opacities are managed by anterior lamellar keratoplasty. The lesions selectively localized to the posterior membrane of the cornea are managed by posterior lamellar keratoplasty. Full-thickness transplants are needed for conditions that involve all layers of the cornea. Partial/selective keratoplasty techniques have been increasingly used in the last few decades. This has improved the utilization of the harvested cornea since the donor corneas with lower endothelial counts could also be differentially utilized. Despite these advances in techniques, there is a large unmet need for donor corneas in several countries in the South-East Asian region. The countries with the greatest need for corneal transplantation have fewer resources available for proper execution, such as eye banks, appropriate surgical facilities, and skilled human resources.

The etiology of corneal blindness and indications of transplants are often related, though, these must be assessed independently. In countries with well-established eye banks such as the USA and in many countries in Europe, the indications of corneal transplantation data may provide a sound measure of corneal disease burden amenable to transplants. But this measurement may not present an accurate assessment of corneal blindness burden in countries with inadequate eye banking facilities.

15.2 Eye Banking Infrastructure

With appropriate care and intervention, more than 80% of corneal blindness is either treatable or preventable. The standard of care for treating corneal blindness is a sight-restoring transplant that replaces the diseased or injured cornea with a healthy donor cornea. And yet, the world's eye banking infrastructure is not sufficiently equipped to meet the rising demands for healthy donor corneal tissue. Gaps in supply and demand are even more acute in South-East Asia, where non-trachomatous corneal opacities account for 4.67% of total blindness [9].

15.2.1 Gaps in Supply

India is the largest country in the South-East Asia region and has a somewhat different problem. By current demand, India may have a nearly sufficient supply of corneal tissue [10], but access to healthcare and paying capacity remain challenging (Figs. 15.1 and 15.2). In 2019, India collected just under 60,000 corneas yet less than 28,000 corneas were transplanted [11, 12]. The estimated demand for cornea in India is as high as 100,000 per annum or up to 70 per million people [11, 13].

India has over 740 registered eye banks [11]. But, only ~100 eye banks consistently report their data and 21 eye banks account for nearly 70% of the country's annual corneal transplants. Nepal has one thriving eye bank that supplies corneas in the country using an innovative recovery model and shares surplus tissue internationally [14]. The eye banking infrastructure in other countries in South-East Asia is less developed. For instance, Myanmar, the second-largest country in South-East Asia by area, has only two eye

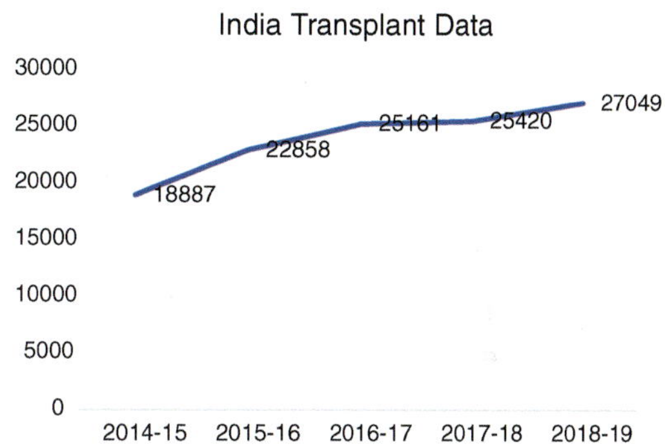

Fig. 15.2 Corneal transplantation data from India (Source: Eye Bank Association of India)

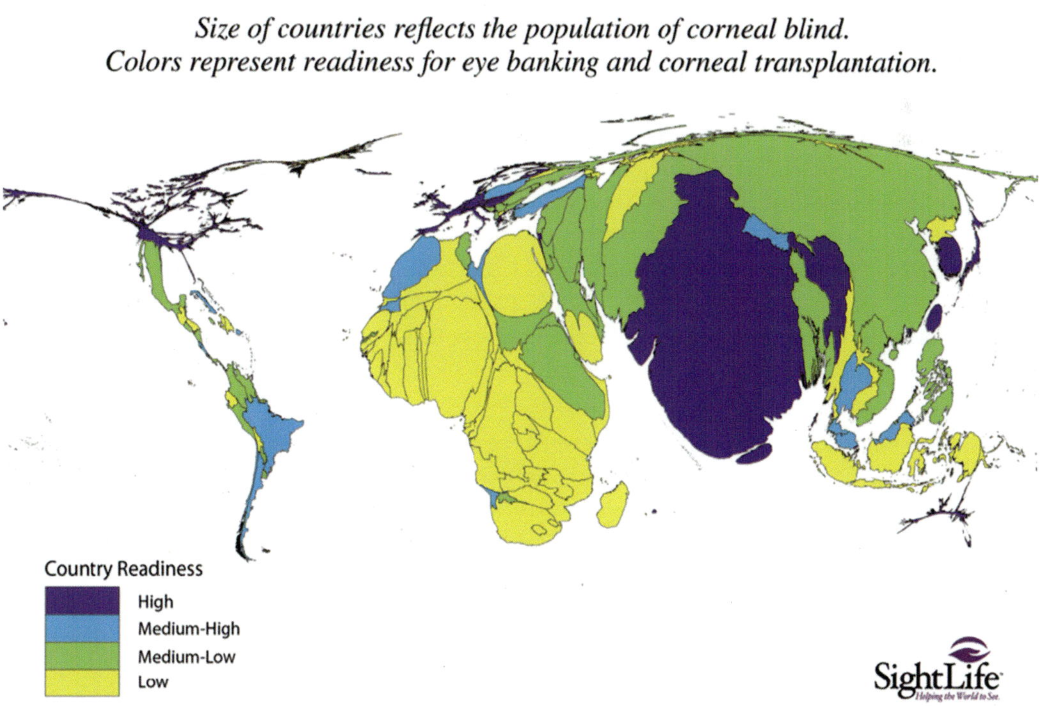

Fig. 15.1 World corneal blindness and readiness for corneal transplantation surgery. (Reproduced with permission from: Oliva MS, et al. Indian J Ophthalmol 2012; 60:423–7)

banks and only 150 cornea are collected annually [15]. Bangladesh has one functioning eye bank that is unable to recover enough corneas to meet the local demand.

15.2.2 Technical and Product Quality Standards in Eye Banking

In India, the eye donation is on the rise. But, the quality of eye banking in some regions of the country does not meet the recommended international standards; this results in low utilization of collected tissue for transplant. India has a National Program for Control of Blindness and Visual Impairment (NPCBVI), which defines technical standards for eye banks [16]. Since it is not mandatory to follow the standards set by the NPCBVI, eye banks have little incentive to adopt quality norms. The outcome is that only 44% of all collected corneas are utilized (Unpublished data from the Eye Bank Association of India, EBAI).

15.2.3 Public Funding and Effectiveness (Table 15.1)

The Indian Government incentivizes eye bank infrastructure development as a one-time grant benefit for equipment and cornea collections. However, there is no continuing benefit that promotes the quality and utilization of collected corneas [17].

Other South-East Asian countries like Nepal, Bangladesh, and Sri Lanka do not have formal eye banking guidelines or standards. The Sri Lankan eye bank is government-sponsored, and hence all resources are provided by the Government. Other countries in the region do not have a national policy.

15.2.4 Tissue Sharing

The eye banking status in South-East Asia countries does not meet its regional needs; eye transplantation is made even more difficult by a restrictive export-import policy on corneal tissue or lack thereof. For example, India does not allow the export of corneas outside of the country, but Sri Lanka has been a significant exporter of corneas globally for decades [18]. Recently, Nepal has also emerged as an exporter of corneas, with more than 30% of corneas recommended for transplant, distributed to Bangladesh and the Middle-East.

None of the South-East Asian countries have reached a state of absolute self-sufficiency. There are relative levels of self-sufficiency in countries like India, Nepal, and Sri Lanka. These countries collect enough corneas to meet their people's needs; however, the collections only meet the needs of those who have access to treatment and those who can pay for it, either out-of-pocket or through government schemes. In India, some of these are met through an innovative distribution system, such as the EBAI-SightLife Cornea Distribution System; this enables eye banks to provide excess corneas to surgeons across the country once local requirements have been met.

Table 15.1 Eye bank policy issues in selected South-East Asian countries compared with those of the UK and the USA

Country	Opt-in/out	Eye donation law	National Donor Registry/first-person consent	Mandatory death notification	Access to medical records before consent	Non-physician recovery	Processing fee
India	In	x	–	–	x	x	x
Nepal	In	x	–	–	–	x	x
Sri Lanka	In	x	–	–	–	x	x
UK	In	x	x	x	x	x	x
USA	In	x	x	x	x	x	x

15.2.5 Unique Models of Eye Banking in South-East Asia

15.2.5.1 Nepal: Cornea Collection at Temple

In 1998, the Nepal Eye Bank worked on a new strategy for cornea collection. The cornea procurement center was relocated to the Pashupati Temple, at the banks of the Bagmati River. The temple-based referral system resulted in a massive increase—a nearly 160% increase in 1998 and a 494% increase in 1999, compared to the earlier hospital referral system. The recovered corneas were also of high quality. This helped Nepal reduce patient waiting time for corneal transplants [19].

15.2.5.2 India: Cornea Distribution System

In 2012, the EBAI and SightLife initiated the unique cornea distribution system (CDS) to create a network between eye banks and cornea surgeons to increase access to tissues at the national level. Through this unique program (Fig. 15.3) the CDS has been distributing 30% more tissues year-on-year since 2012 and has been able to connect seven eye banks to surgeons in 50 cities. Many eye banks have set up remote recovery centers to increase the collection of quality corneas. For example, Ramayamma International Eye Bank (RIEB, Hyderabad, India), the 10th biggest eye bank in the world (as per numbers of cornea collections), has more than 30 recovery centers throughout the Indian state of Telangana and has met with great success in its efforts by ensuring that the eye donation counselors and technicians in such centers are thoroughly trained [12].

15.2.6 Eye Banking Classification in South-East Asia

The eye banking system has developed properly only in three countries of the region, India, Nepal, and Sri Lanka. These three countries can be considered adequate, but understandably, not all corneal blind individuals who may benefit from a corneal transplant are able to seek treatment. Figure 15.4 highlights some of the critical differences in the eye banking systems between South-East Asia and the ones in the western world.

Eye banking in the USA is an ideal example. All eye banks, irrespective of size, employ dedicated people for all required tasks. These eye banks have a structured governing board consisting of technical and non-technical people

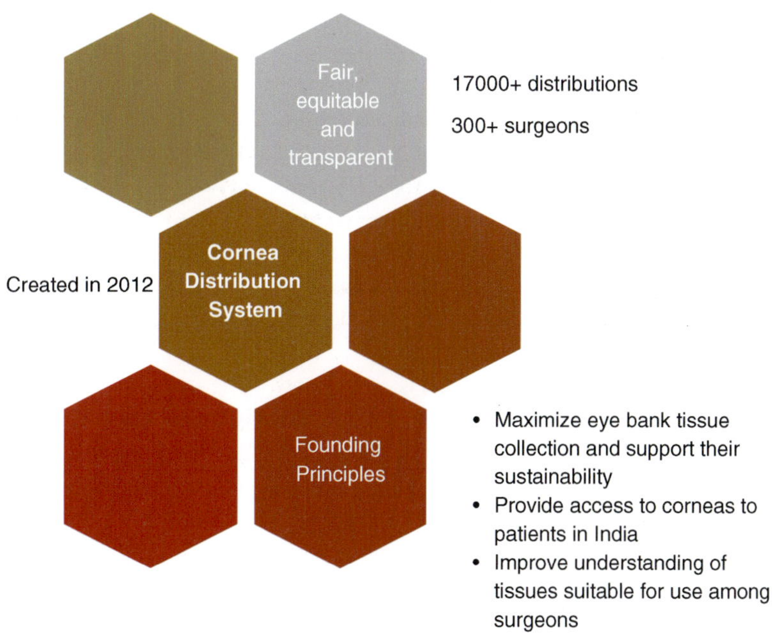

Fig. 15.3 Remote recovery centers for corneas in India

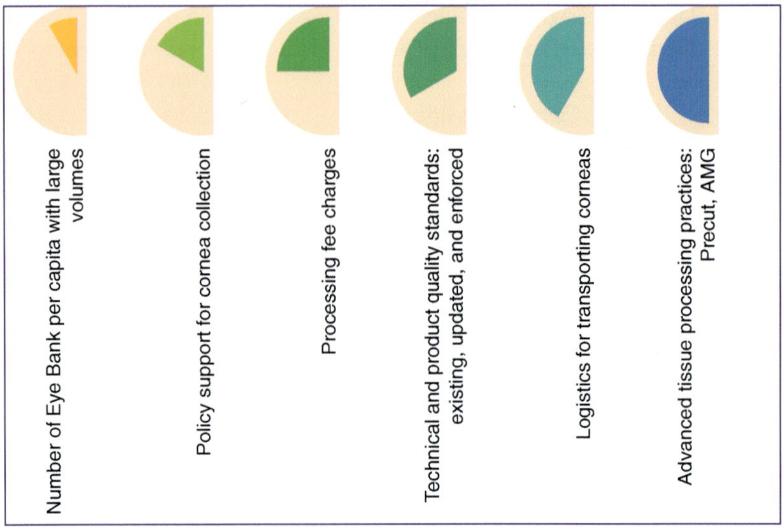

Fig. 15.4 Differences in eye banking in the western world compared to South-East Asia. *AMG* amniotic membrane graft

Table 15.2 Impediments to the eye banking system in South-East Asia region

Factors	India	Nepal	Bangladesh	Indonesia
Non-issue of mandatory death notification	x	x	x	x
Non-rigorous surveillance	x	x	x	–
No rigor for financial sustainability	x	x	x	x
Poor capacity building	x	x	x	x
No national governing body	–	x	x	x
Poor advocacy	–	–	x	x
High tissue processing fee	–	–	–	x

and adhere to the standards set by the Eye Bank Association of America (EBAA). The EBAA and other professional bodies, such as the American Academy of Ophthalmology (AAO) and the Food and Drug Administration (FDA), audit the eye banks. Most eye banks process the tissue to provide pre-prepared corneas for DSAEK (Descemet's stripping automated endothelial keratoplasty) and DMEK (Descemet's membrane endothelial keratoplasty) surgeries; some eye banks also use special procedures to provide preloaded keratoplasty grafts [20].

Eye banking in South-East Asia is an eclectic mix of characteristics. While it lacks most of the above-mentioned structural elements, there is a welcome change in some countries. India is slowly beginning to adopt supportive policies and collecting tissue processing fees, though the current collection does not even cover the actual costs. Some eye banks in India are beginning to supply precut tissue and AMGs (amniotic membrane grafts) [13]. Recently, the NPCBVI in India released updated eye banking standards; this is likely to promote quality practices across the eye banks.

15.2.7 Challenges for the Eye Banking System in South-East Asia

The impediments to the growth of a quality eye banking system are manifold, from policy to advocacy—some of these challenges in the South-East Asian region have been listed below in Table 15.2. In this region, India is comparatively more mature in eye banking.

15.3 Major Challenges in Eradicating Corneal Blindness

The key to eradicating corneal blindness in developing countries is to bridge the gap between the demand for and supply of donor corneal tissue [21]. The four essential components of donor tissue procurement of any eye banking system are: (1) approach and consent of potential donor family; (2) tissue recovery; (3) tissue processing; and (4) tissue distribution.

There are several challenges to successful implementation of these four keystones of procurement [12, 22]. Poor retrieval rates of eye banks with low procurement primarily center around ill-trained/poorly committed eye bank staff, recovery technicians, and grief counselors. Inefficient operation protocols in eye bank functioning involving the initial steps of approaching donor family and tissue retrieval results in poor harvesting despite the availability of potential donors. Insufficient advocacy and poor socio-cultural perceptions of the society toward organ/eye donation must be addressed consistently and at frequent intervals throughout the year. This is likely to increase awareness and social responsibility toward organ/eye donation. Restrictive regulations on organ donation tend to decrease the yield of donor tissue. Optimal tissue processing requires excellent logistics, such as good eye bank equipment, storage media, serology testing kits, good documentation, and tissue evaluation protocols. Tissue distribution is still plagued by the lack of an effectively functioning network balancing the demand and the supply. Adherence to medical standards for all these processes can only be ensured when the guidelines are uniformly implemented and religiously followed across the country and the region by all component eye banks.

Challenges in eye banking may be categorized into the following concerns:

1. Challenges with social awareness
2. Challenges with creating an efficient eye banking network
   (a) Tissue procurement
   (b) Tissue processing
   (c) Tissue distribution networking
   (d) Finance
   (e) Human resources training
   (f) Expansion in eye banking
3. Challenges with the healthcare delivery system

1. **Challenges with Social Awareness**

The socio-cultural behavior needs a more positive outlook toward eye donation, an attitude change to organ/eye donation as a "social responsibility" from a "request-response obligation." A year-round public awareness program on eye donation, supported by the Government or other financial institutions, is likely to enhance voluntary donation. "Required request" laws (such as those in the USA and Brazil) and "Presumed consent" laws (such as those in the USA and the Philippines) will help overcome difficulties in approaching and gaining the consents of donor families in practical situations [22]. Such laws will also help to improve public awareness and acceptance of eye donation.

2. **Challenges with creating an efficient eye banking network**

(a) Tissue Procurement:

The constant challenge that most eye banks face is in maximizing the collection of utilizable donor corneal tissue. This calls for adequate training of the procurement personnel to identify and differentiate donors and donor tissues with a high probability of utilization.

(b) Tissue Processing:

Tissue Evaluation:
The current technique of corneal tissue harvesting has shifted to in situ corneoscleral rim excision. The tissue evaluation relies on visual inspection by slit-lamp biomicroscopy and specular micrography at the eye bank, and slit-lamp biomicroscopy by the transplanting surgeon. Corneal physicians/eye bank technicians evaluating the tissue must be familiar with optimal evaluation techniques before distribution. A useful technique is dark field bio-micrography of eye

bank donor corneas; this allows assessment of the entire corneal surface area to detect localized lesions of varying brightness and a better understanding of tissue clarity. Besides, digital imaging allows better documentation. Most importantly, it enables eye banks to identify corneas with previous refractive surgeries, such as the laser in situ keratomileuses (LASIK) and photorefractive keratectomy, likely to be missed on a slit-lamp examination alone [23]. In the recent past, an examination of donor corneal tissue in vitro by anterior segment optical coherence tomography is also recommended to detect prior refractive surgery procedures [24, 25].

Advanced eye banking equipment:
With the continuing rise in refractive surgeries, eye banks have a new challenge in detecting refractive corneal surgery during tissue processing. The resultant corneal structural alterations in such donor corneas can negatively influence clinical results in recipients. Low coherence interferometry techniques using a broadband continuum source has been described as being able to detect interfaces due to prior LASIK surgeries in the donor corneas [26]. Investment in automated lamellar keratoplasty equipment for performing donor tissue lamellar cuts to enable eye banks to provide precut tissue for endothelial keratoplasty is a new requirement. Equipment such as deep-freeze storage, higher-end eye banking refrigerators, serology kits, and specular microscopes are also required for high performing eye banks. All eye bank personnel must be trained in using these equipment.

The availability of low-cost donor corneal tissue preservation-storage media is limited. Donor preservation media used in recent times include McCarey–Kaufman (MK) medium (Bausch & Lomb), Optisol GS (Bausch & Lomb), LIFE 4°C (Numedis Inc), and Cornisol (Aurolab). Although MK medium is less expensive, it allows for a relatively shorter storage time of only 4–6 days. Except for Cornisol, all other longer time storage preservation media are expensive.

The COVID19 pandemic has significantly impacted eye banks' performance, further increasing difficulties in logistics such as usage of special personal protective equipment and the likelihood of mandatory serology testing for the corona SARS-2 virus in the donors before cornea recovery.

Donor tissue preparation for precut tissue for lamellar corneal surgeries:
Only very few eye banks in Asia are competent to provide precut tissue for lamellar endothelial surgeries. Eye bank technicians competent in donor tissue preparation for customized corneal lamellar surgeries can encourage the use of these new procedures by corneal surgeons. This will also reduce corneal blindness since endothelial keratoplasty is known to outperform penetrating keratoplasty in those patients where it can be done.

There are several places where corneal surgeons lack the adequate logistics to prepare endothelial donor tissue and hence opt to perform penetrating keratoplasty instead. With the surgeons transiting to DMEK, eye banks have to equally rise to the challenge of preparing and transporting these tissues safely and in adequate numbers [27]. Preoperative endothelial cell count, graft detachment, graft infection, surgical expenses, and surgical time and effort significantly influence endothelial keratoplasty performance. Hence, eye banks must validate and standardize the donor tissues distributed for endothelial keratoplasty procedures [28, 29].

(c) Distribution networking:

Tissue distribution is still plagued by poorly functioning networking and regional connectivity. This impacts the distribution of surplus donor corneas to areas and surgeons in need; this denies care to those in need of the tissue and at the same time reduces the utilization of the procured corneas. Regional regulations governing tissue distribution must be re-examined to ensure maximum utilization of harvested and utilizable donor tissue. A novel innovation in tissue transportation is the reusable passive thermal container for donor corneal tissue that can maintain a stable and appropriate temperature for 60–71 h even in challenging hypo- and hyperthermic environments. This can help maintain the viability of transported corneal tissues for longer durations of time [30].

(d) Financial concerns in eye banking:

Eye banking is mostly seen as a not-for-profit endeavor the world over and does not encourage many to invest. The economic problems of India's functioning eye banks include support for training, logistics, and human resource costs. These constraints make eye banks function more like eye donation centers. The essential equipment for a basic eye bank are specular microscopes and slit lamps. A higher order eye bank will mandate additional equipment such as optical coherence tomography and extended period corneal storage media. To meet additional expenses and make eye banking sustainable, eye banks must explore legitimate means of achieving financial sustainability. One such means is to collect the processing fee for donor corneas, at least from all high volume keratoplasty centers. Collection of processing fees is possible when a uniform protocol and policy across the country are developed and implemented. Other costs are the expenses incurred at awareness and promotional campaigns. Currently, most of these expenses are borne by non-governmental agencies but should gradually shift to health planning programs for long-term system management.

(e) Human resources training

Successful retrieval of donor corneas involves the grief counselors' coordinated functioning with the recovery technician and eye bank manager. Training also includes sensitization of the staff to the working conditions, mostly dealing with people in grief. Their approach to the potential donor family plays a massive role in securing a positive family response. Experienced grief counselors achieve a high consent rate. Retaining trained eye bank staff is a huge challenge where career growth is limited.

(f) Expansion in eye banking

An established eye bank's dynamic and efficient functioning indicates a successful eye banking network rather than the mushrooming of several smaller eye banks across the country. Many such small eye banks spread across India (more than 700 such eye banks) seem to be contributing poorly to eye banking progress [12]. The lack of a proactive eye banking approach by such small eye banks results in poor tissue utilization and a low yield of transplantable corneas. These also compromise the standards of eye banking and can drain existing resources with duplication of many eye-banking-related activities.

Regulatory standards toward essential infrastructure and equipment, trained human resources, documentation, record keeping, donor corneal tissue evaluation protocol, and eye banking accreditation guidelines are major challenges in establishing a good eye banking system. An appropriate strategy of a comprehensive and self-sustaining model functioning from a regional/territorial system under the jurisdiction of amicable team leadership is one that incorporates hospital cornea retrieval program (HCRP) practices with voluntary retrieval, develops effective training modules of eye banking personnel, and designs a seamless logistical system of tissue procurement, processing, preservation, and distribution.

3. **Challenges with the healthcare delivery system**

Eradication of corneal blindness rests on optimal eye care delivery to those in need. This requires an integrated approach, from identifying and referring appropriate patients from the primary/secondary level for corneal grafting surgery at the tertiary care centers. Tertiary care centers are usually equipped with adequate medical and surgical expertise to handle corneal transplantation procedures. Expansion of eye banking services also needs expanded training programs to new regions and more cornea surgeons. This ensures that corneal grafting expertise is accessible to even those serving in remote areas in developing countries.

15.4 Preventive Aspects of Management

Nearly half of corneal blindness can be prevented [31]. The leading causes are infectious keratitis, vitamin A deficiency, and trachoma. Ocular trauma and corneal ulceration are often underreported but may be responsible for 1.5–2.0 million new cases of monocular blindness every year. Infectious keratitis is a leading cause of corneal blindness, with a disproportionate burden in developing countries like Nepal and India. While total blindness in Nepal and India has reduced significantly over the past 20 years, the relative prevalence of blindness caused by corneal scarring, trauma, and infection has doubled [32]. Traditional eye medicines have also been implicated as a significant risk factor for corneal ulceration in developing countries. Prevention of coreal diseases is more cost-effective because of difficulties in treating corneal infection/injury and uncertainties in treatment outcomes.

15.4.1 Existing Cornea Blindness Prevention Efforts and Evidence of Success

The burden of blindness from eye injuries is high in low- and middle-income countries, particularly those with large agricultural industries and those with legacies of war and civil unrest [15]. In South-East Asia, agriculture is one of the common livelihoods in rural areas; but access to eye care is minimal in these areas.

The prevention of infectious keratitis and ulcer has focused on: (a) early, effective treatment of ocular trauma, including abrasions; (b) education of local village doctors against the use of herbal medicines to treat eye trauma; (c) scientific management of corneal ulcers; (d) increase in protective equipment for at-risk industries (e.g., agriculture and heavy metal industries); and (e) better control of fireworks and other common causes of trauma (e.g., landmines in Cambodia) [15].

In 2013, the Proctor Foundation (University of California, San Francisco, USA) recommended prophylactic topical antibiotics as a cost-effective and practical approach to preventing corneal infection-related blindness. SightLife piloted the Corneal Blindness Prevention program in 2017 in Nepal and 2018 in India, in partnership with different eye hospitals. One such program worked with the available female Community Health Workers (CHWs) after a short specialized training in eye care and treatment of corneal abrasions. CHWs acted as the first aid responders in their community. At the time of writing, these CHWs have seen nearly 23,000 people (India and Nepal); approximately 14,000 had corneal abrasions. The CHWs were successful in treating all but 425 people referred to secondary and tertiary care hospitals for further care. This program was considered significantly cost-effective, scalable, and structured. The cost of diagnosis and preventive treatment per patient was low (INR 70 or NPR 100 100, equivalent to USD1).

Successful prevention programs for vitamin A deficiency, rubella, and measles have centered on vitamin A supplementation, nutrition education, food enrichment, and vaccines. Widespread vitamin A supplementation for school-age children, specifically in areas with a high prevalence of vitamin A deficiency, has proven effective, particularly when combined with food fortification programs that ensure longer-term prevention measures. Helen Keller International began research on food security in Nepal in 2007 and quickly identified crop interventions required to combat Vitamin A deficiency. They supported communities in farming orange-fleshed sweet potatoes rich in Vitamin A and highly nutritious vegetables. These were complemented with nutrition education. Widespread adoption of these programs in Nepal has had substantial success in preventing new cases of blindness.

Efforts on prevention of trachoma have been centered on acceptable practices, from environmental improvements (such as improved access to clean water and sanitation to prevent transmission) to antibiotics and facial cleanliness in communities where trachomatous inflammation is prevalent (follicular trachoma >5%) [31]. WHO has declared two countries in the South-East Asian region, Nepal and Myanmar, as trachoma-free countries.

15.4.2 Future Outlook for Corneal Blindness Prevention

Preventive care is a critical public health initiative and long-term solution to preventing corneal blindness. There is a need to expand existing successful interventions to more geographies to combat corneal blindness. Efforts should be made to integrate preventive interventions with the existing government-run programs to ensure sustainability and strengthening local eye health infrastructure. Mass advocacy and awareness on eye safety in partnership with local stakeholders and the Government, more often for the people who work in agricultural fields, or for those in high-risk occupations, can reduce instances of eye trauma to a great extent.

15.5 Future Directions

Progress toward the elimination of corneal blindness in South-East Asia will require significant public-private leadership and collaboration. Governments must develop favorable policies to enable early detection and treatment of corneal opacities, enable eye banks to legally operate, and maximize donation opportunities, and also work toward financial sustainability. Clinicians will require government support to ensure adequate access to training and reimbursement. The policies behind these initiatives are well-proven across geographies as they have consistently resulted in a much higher return on health system development investment than in geographies where policy enablers are lacking.

While global eye health leaders have taken an interest in South-East Asia health system development, many countries lack formal assessments and strategies to address the issue of corneal blindness. The policy enablers required for health system development are typically similar across geographies, but intensive evaluations must be completed before developing country- or region-specific strategies.

References

1. Flaxman SR, Bourne RRA, Resnikoff S, et al. Global causes of blindness and distance vision impairment 1990-2020: a systematic review and meta-analysis. Lancet Glob Health. 2017;5:e1221–34. https://doi.org/10.1016/S2214-109X(17)30393-5.
2. Jonas JB, George R, Asokan R, et al. Prevalence and causes of vision loss in Central and South Asia: 1990-2010. Br J Ophthalmol. 2014;98:592–8. https://doi.org/10.1136/bjophthalmol-2013-303998. Epub 2014 Jan 23.
3. GBVI: Global Cause Estimates. IAPB Vision Atlas; 2018. http://atlas.iapb.org/global-burden-vision-impairment/gbvi-global-cause estimates/. Accessed 31 Mar 2019.
4. Nangia V, Jonas JB, George R, et al. Vision Loss Expert Group of the Global Burden of Disease Study. Prevalence and causes of blindness and vision impairment: magnitude, temporal trends and projections in South and Central Asia. Br J Ophthalmol. 2019;103(7):871–7. https://doi.org/10.1136/bjophthalmol-2018-312292. Epub 2018 Nov 8.
5. Tran TM, Duong H, Bonnet C, et al. Corneal blindness in Asia: a systematic review and meta-analysis to identify challenges and opportunities. Cornea. 2020;39(9):1196–205. https://doi.org/10.1097/ICO.0000000000002374.
6. Vijaya L, Asokan R, Panday M, et al. Baseline risk factors for incidence of blindness in a South Indian population: the Chennai eye disease incidence study. Invest Ophthalmol Vis Sci. 2014;55:5545–50. https://doi.org/10.1167/iovs.14-14614.
7. Gupta N, Vashist P, Tandon R, et al. Prevalence of corneal diseases in the rural Indian population: the Corneal Opacity Rural Epidemiological (CORE) study. Br J Ophthalmol. 2015;99:147–52. https://doi.org/10.1136/bjophthalmol-2014-305945. Epub 2014 Nov 13.
8. Kumar A, Vashist P. Indian Community eye care in 2020: achievements and challenges. Indian J Ophthalmol. 2020;68:291–3. https://doi.org/10.4103/ijo.IJO_2381_19. PMID: 31957710; PMCID: PMC7003597.
9. Bourne RRA, Flaxman SR, Braithwaite T, et al. Magnitude, temporal trends and projections of the global prevalence of blindness and distance and near vision impairment: a systematic review and meta-analysis. Lancet Glob health. 2017;5:e888–97. https://doi.org/10.1016/S2214-109X(17)30293-0.
10. Gain P, Jullienne R, He Z, et al. Global survey of corneal transplantation and eye banking. JAMA Ophthalmol. 2016;134:167–73. https://doi.org/10.1001/jamaophthalmol.2015.4776.
11. Eye Bank Association of India Data 2018-19. www.ebai.org.
12. Oliva MS, Schottman T, Gulati M. Turning the tide of corneal blindness. Indian J Ophthalmol. 2012;60:423–7. https://doi.org/10.4103/0301-4738.100540. PMID: 22944753; PMCID: PMC3491269.
13. Chaurasia S, Mohamed A, Garg P, et al. Thirty years of eye bank experience at a single centre in India. Int Ophthalmol. 2020;40:81–8. https://doi.org/10.1007/s10792-019-01164-y. Epub 2019 Aug 22.
14. Bajracharya L, Bhandari SK, Twyana SN. Donor profile, tissue evaluation and comparison of voluntary and motivated corneal donation in Nepal Eye

Bank. Clin Ophthalmol. 2020;14:95–101. https://doi.org/10.2147/OPTH.S225922. PMID: 32021073; PMCID: PMC6969692.
15. Whitcher JP, Srinivasan M, Upadhyay MP. Corneal blindness: a global perspective. Bull World Health Organ. 2001;79:214–21. Epub 2003 Jul 7. PMID: 11285665; PMCID: PMC2566379.
16. Standards of EyeBanking in India. www.npcbvi.gov.in.
17. Sangwan VS, Gopinathan U, Garg P, et al. Eye banking in India: a road ahead. JIMSA. 2010;23(3):197–9.
18. The Barcelona principles: an agreement on the use of human donated tissue for ocular transplantation, research, and future technologies©. Cornea. 2018;37(10):1213–7. https://doi.org/10.1097/ICO.0000000000001675.
19. Ruit S, Tabin G, Gurung R, et al. Temple eye banking in Nepal. Cornea. 2002;21:433–4. https://doi.org/10.1097/00003226-200205000-00025.
20. Lambert LG, Chamberlain WD. The structure and evolution of eye banking: a review on eye banks' historical, present, and future contribution to corneal transplantation. J Biorepo Sci Appl Med. 2017;5:23–40.
21. Pineda R. Corneal transplantation in the developing world: lessons learned and meeting the challenge. Cornea. 2015;34(Suppl):S35–40. https://doi.org/10.1097/ICO.0000000000000567.
22. Franzco DR, Fanzco SW. Corneal blindness: a global problem. Clin Exp Ophthalmol. 2014;42:213–4.
23. Merin LM, Brown MF. Darkfield biomicrography of eye bank donor corneas. Cornea. 2001;20:210–3. https://doi.org/10.1097/00003226-200103000-00021.
24. Wolf AH, Neubauer AS, Priglinger SG, et al. Detection of laser in situ keratomileusis in a postmortem eye using optical coherence tomography. J Cataract Refract Surg. 2004;30:491–5. https://doi.org/10.1016/j.jcrs.2003.06.007.
25. Lin RC, Li Y, Tang M, et al. Screening for previous refractive surgery in eye bank corneas by using optical coherence tomography. Cornea. 2007;26:594–9. https://doi.org/10.1097/ICO.0b013e31803c5535.
26. Verrier C, Veillas T, Lépine F, et al. Interfaces detection after corneal refractive surgery by low coherence optical interferometry. Biomed Optics Express. 2010;5:1460–71. https://doi.org/10.1364/BOE.1.001460. PMID: 21258562; PMCID: PMC3018127.
27. Boynton GE, Woodward MA. Eye-bank preparation of endothelial tissue. Curr Opin Ophthalmol. 2014;25:319–24. https://doi.org/10.1097/ICU.0000000000000060. PMID: 24837574; PMCID: PMC4131679.
28. Parekh M, Baruzzo M, Favaro E, et al. Standardizing Descemet Membrane Endothelial Keratoplasty graft preparation method in the eye bank—Experience of 527 Descemet Membrane Endothelial Keratoplasty tissues. Cornea. 2017;36:1458–66. https://doi.org/10.1097/ICO.0000000000001349.
29. Parekh M, Salvalaio G, Ruzza A, et al. Posterior lamellar graft preparation: a prospective review from an eye bank on current and future aspects. J Ophthalmol. 2013;2013:769860. https://doi.org/10.1155/2013/769860. Epub 2013 May 30. PMID: 23819041; PMCID: PMC3683473.
30. Shachar TS, Bowman J, Bango J, et al. Precise temperature control of donor cornea tissue with reusable passive thermal container. Cornea. 2011;30:977–82. https://doi.org/10.1097/ICO.0b013e318206862a.
31. World report on vision. Geneva: World Health Organization; 2019. www.who.int. Accessed 1 Dec 2020.
32. Sapkota YD, Limburg H. Epidemiology of blindness in Nepal: 2012. https://doi.org/10.3126/nepjoph.v4i2.6545.

Low Vision, Vision Rehabilitation, and Assistive Technology

16

Patanjali Dev Nayar, Suraj Singh Senjam, Beula Christy, Sara Varughese, G. V. S. Murthy, Praveen Vashist, and Vivek Gupta

Key Points

- Low vision is an important cause of visual disability.
- The World Health Organization estimates that globally more than 1 billion people with disabilities will require one or more assistive products.
- Around 91 million people with visual impairment live in the South-East Asia Region, and ~20 million have low vision.
- In South-East Asia, very few centers provide inclusive low vision services.
- Most low vision services are monodisciplinary; consist of clinical diagnosis and dispensing of low vision aids. Disability-inclusive low vision services that include habilitation with rehabilitation within an integrated approach are required.
- The loss of binocular vision, particularly in students, can be categorized as best-corrected visual acuity as less or better than 1/60. These students should be encouraged to use vision-based assistive technologies for education.
- The Global Cooperation on Assistive Technology (GATE) is a global commitment to improving access to assistive products.
- To improve access to high quality and affordable assistive products in all countries, the WHO has introduced the *Priority Assistive Products List* (APL); the APL includes 16 devices for people with visual disabilities.
- The five interlinked areas of assistive technology, five Ps are: People, Policy, Products, Personnel, and Provision.
- The World Health Organization is developing three additional tools to assist the Member States in developing national assistive technology policies and programs.

The World Health Organization (WHO) estimates that more than 1 billion people live with some degree of health impairment and compro-

P. D. Nayar (✉)
Regional office for South East Asia,
World Health Organization - India,
New Delhi, India
e-mail: nayarp@who.int

S. S. Senjam · P. Vashist · V. Gupta
Community Ophthalmology, Dr. Rajendra Prasad Centre for Ophthalmic Sciences, All India Institute of Medical Sciences, New Delhi, India

B. Christy
Institute for Vision Rehabilitation, L V Prasad Eye Institute, Hyderabad, India
e-mail: beula@lvpei.org

S. Varughese
CBM India, New Delhi, India
e-mail: sara.varughese@cbm.org

G. V. S. Murthy
Indian Institute of Public Health, Hyderabad, India
e-mail: Murthy.Gvs@iiphh.org

T. Das, P. D. Nayar (eds.), *South-East Asia Eye Health*,
https://doi.org/10.1007/978-981-16-3787-2_16

mised functionality (disabilities) that restrict and limit their activity and participation in the events of daily life. This number is likely to be doubled by 2030 due to aging populations and debilitating non-communicable diseases and continuing demographic and epidemiological transition [1]. People with blindness and visual impairments comprise a significant proportion of this population; they often suffer from a lack of access to services and opportunities and live a compromised quality of life.

Assistive technologies (ATs) can improve functioning, enhance daily living activities, and allow people with visual disabilities to live independently (Fig. 16.1). These play a key role in social inclusion and participation, thereby enabling people to be active and productive members of society. ATs can also reduce the burden of care on caretakers or family members of persons with disabilities. Additionally, increasing awareness regarding AT products and enhancement of the rights-based approach is likely to positively impact the hitherto skewed "need–demand–supply" triad for these devices for low vision. Currently, only 1 of 10 people in need has access to assistive products (APs) globally; this need is higher in South-East Asia. Low income, patchy industrialization, inadequate education and awareness, and resource-deficiency in this region contribute to this gap. People with low vision, including children and older people, have weak voices. Only a few countries have developed policies and responses to address their needs.

Access to good quality and affordable ATs is one of the key components of the United Nations (UN) Convention on the Right of Persons with Disabilities (Article 20) [2]. In the context of eye health, one of the key functions of Universal Health Coverage (UHC) is the provision of rehabilitative care and appropriate assistive health technology for people with vision loss. At the heart of the Sustainable Development Goals (SDGs) is the pledge that "no-one is left behind." People with disabilities, especially women and older people, are among the population groups frequently left behind.

The *World Report on Vision* (WHO 2019) seeks to stimulate action to meet these challenges in countries by proposing integrated people-centered eye care (IPCEC) to strengthen the health system [3]. The IPEC can help address significant challenges faced by those with low vision and visual disabilities. The IPCEC adopts a health system perspective with four strategies: (1) engaging and empowering people and communities; (2) reorienting the model of care to a strong primary care system; (3) coordinating services within and across sectors; and (4) creating an enabling environment. The 71st World Health Assembly adopted a resolution (WHA 71.8) urging the Member States to develop, implement, and strengthen policies and programs to improve access to ATs [4]. The adoption of the resolution represents a milestone in ensuring access to ATs for everyone, everywhere, to help progression towards UHC, the 2030 agenda for the SDGs, and in realizing the Convention on the Rights of Persons with Disabilities.

The present chapter attempts to bring out the magnitude and impact of low vision in South-East Asia and the status of low vision rehabilitation services encompassing ATs and community-based rehabilitation.

Resolution 71.8 of World Health Assembly on Assistive Technology

The World Health Assembly Resolution 71.8 in May 2018 recalled the United Nations Convention on the Rights of Persons with Disabilities, under which 175 Member States have committed, *inter alia*, to ensure access to quality assistive technology at an affordable cost (Article 20) and recognize that the inclusion of assistive technology, in line with countries' national priority and context, into health systems is essential for realizing progress towards the targets in the SDG relating to Universal Health Coverage called upon Member States to improve access to assistive technology for all types.

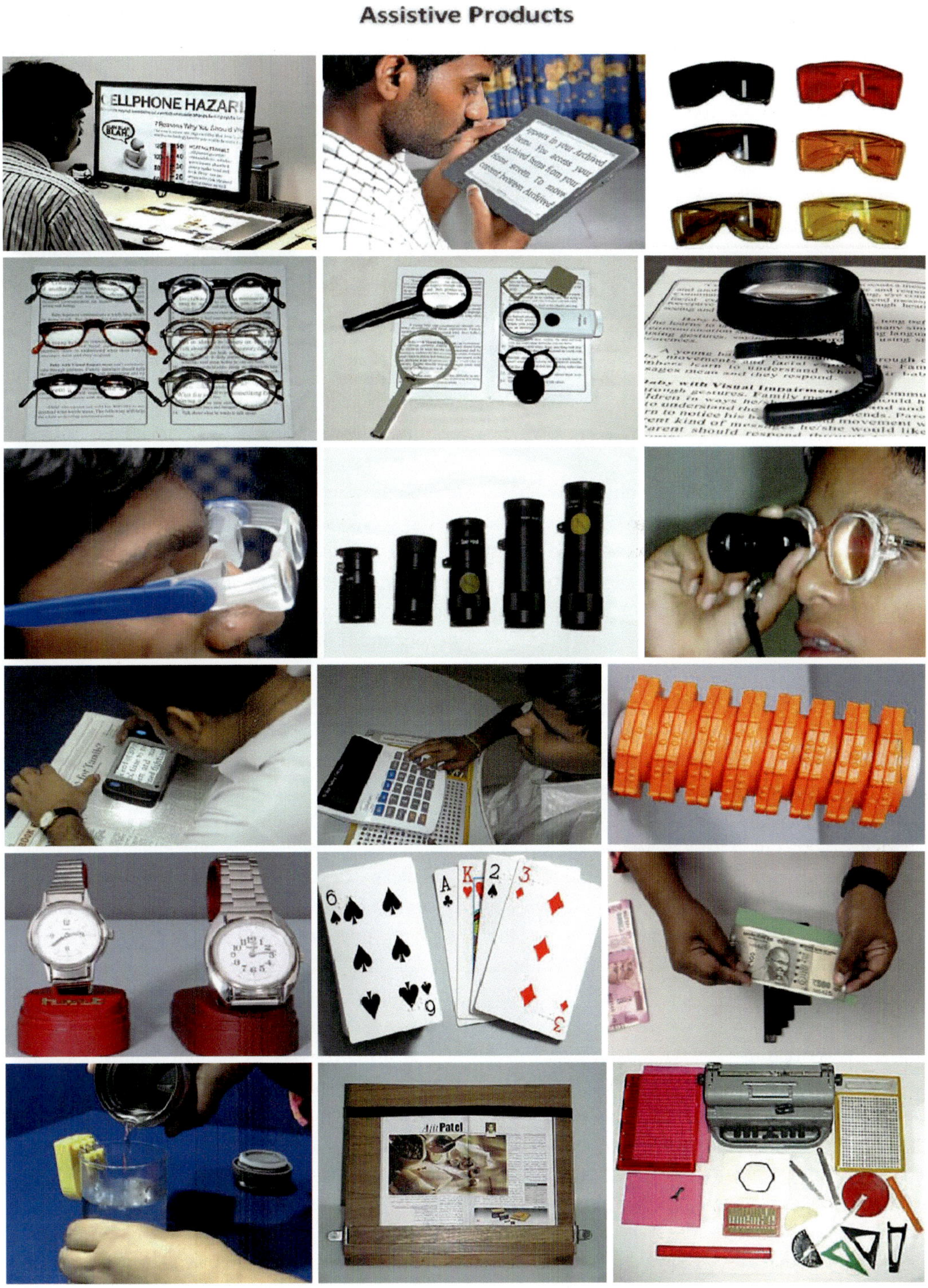

Fig. 16.1 Assistive devices for low vision and vision rehabilitation. First row: left—CCTV, middle—large e-prints, right—filters; Second row: left—spectacles (magnifiers), middle—hand-held and pocket magnifiers, right—stand magnifiers; Third row: left—See TV glasses, middle and right—telescopes; Fourth row: left—video magnifier, middle—talking calculator, right—Braille puzzles toys; Fifth row: left—tactile watch, middle—large print cards, right—Notex; Sixth row: left—liquid sensor, middle—reading stand, right—Braille educational materials

16.1 Low Vision, Functional Low Vision, and Blindness: Definitions

Measuring visual acuity

An important measure of visual function is the distance visual acuity (VA). This measure is based on assessing the ability to discern letters on an eye chart at specified distances. Normal vision is usually defined as a VA of 6/6 or 20/20. This means that a person with normal vision can see at a distance of 6 m (20 ft in imperial) with both eyes, a letter (called an optotype), on an eye chart designed to be seen at 6 m or 20 ft.

Visual impairment

Globally, the definitions of blindness have changed over the years [5]. Since October 2006, the WHO definition of blindness, adopted under the International Classification of Diseases-10 (ICD 10) using presenting visual acuity (PVA) is as follows:

1. **Mild visual impairment**—PVA for distance <6/12, but ≥6/18 in the better eye
2. **Moderate visual impairment**—PVA for distance <6/18 but ≥6/60 in the better eye
3. **Severe visual impairment**—PVA for distance <6/60, but ≥3/60 in the better eye or visual field <20°, but ≥10° around central fixation
4. **Blindness**—PVA for distance <3/60 in the better eye or visual field <10° around a central fixation

The WHO defines low vision in two ways. From an epidemiological perspective, the WHO's 10th revision of "The International Statistical Classification of Diseases, Injuries, and Causes of Death" defines low vision as VA < 6/18 but ≥3/60 in the better eye with the best possible correction [6]. However, from a service provider's perspective at the 1993 Bangkok meeting, the WHO redefined a functional definition of low vision as "a person who has impairment of visual functioning even after treatment and/or standard refractive correction, and has a VA < 6/18 to LP (light perception), or a visual field of less than 10° from the point of fixation, but who uses or is potentially able to use vision for the planning and/or execution of a task" [7].

In the USA, a visual field of less than 20° from the point of fixation is also considered low vision. In India, the percentage of vision loss based on best-corrected vision acuity (BCVA) and field of vision from the center of fixation is shown in Figs. 16.2 and 16.3. The major advantage of this functional definition is that it enlarges the range of persons with low vision. As per this criterion, only people with no LP are considered "blind." This revised definition focuses on "functionality" and thereby increases the scope of planning low vision services to maximize the functional use of residual vision for day-to-day activities to the extent possible. Other important considerations for low vision management are low contrast sensitivity and loss of dark adaptation.

16.2 Impact of Low Vision

Low vision is not only a chronic health problem, it also impacts a person's quality of life. Therefore, the health consequences associated with low vision can extend much beyond the eye and visual system. It impedes an individual's social integration and functionality, ability to learn or perform normal daily tasks, and employment and educational opportunities. Besides, people with low vision are also more prone to accidents and falls, and at a higher risk of mental health problems such as depression and anxiety. Low vision also significantly impacts families, caregivers, communities, and nations [8]. In the UK, the value of losing a healthy life associated with sight loss and blindness was estimated at GBP 19.5 billion [9]. Globally, the DALY (disability-adjusted life years) lost due to visual impairment has increased by 47%, from 12.8 million to 18.8 million between 1990 and 2010 [10].

Right Eye Vision [Best Corrected Visual Acuity – BCVA]

	6/6 to 6/18	6/24	6/36	6/60	3/60	2/60	1/60	HMCF to PL-
6/6 to 6/18	0%	10%	10%	10%	20%	30%	30%	30%
6/24	10%	40%	40%	40%	50%	60%	60%	60%
6/36	10%	40%	40%	40%	50%	60%	60%	60%
6/60	10%	40%	40%	40%	50%	60%	60%	60%
3/60	20%	50%	50%	50%	70%	80%	80%	80%
2/60	30%	60%	60%	60%	80%	90%	90%	90%
1/60	30%	60%	60%	60%	80%	90%	90%	90%
HMCF to PL-	30%	60%	60%	60%	80%	90%	90%	100%

Fig. 16.2 Percentage of visual disability based on the best-corrected visual acuity (Source: Ministry of Social Justice & Empowerment, India)

Fig. 16.3 Percentage of visual disability based on field of vision (Source: Ministry of Social Justice & Empowerment, India)

Left Eye

Right Eye

	<40° to 20°	<20° to 10°	<10°
<40° to 20°	40%	50%	60%
<20° to 10°	50%	70%	80%
<10°	60%	80%	100%

16.3 Magnitude of Visual Disabilities

The World

The Vision Loss Expert Group (VLEG) periodically reports magnitude of global blindness and MSVI (moderate to severe visual impairment). The VLEG estimated that in 2015, globally, there were 36 million blind and 217 million people with MSVI; in 2019, these numbers have increased to 43.2 and 295.3 million, respectively [11, 12]. Around 90% of these people live in low- and middle-income countries (LMICs). Besides, an estimated 1.4 million children around the world become or are born blind and need vision rehabilitation interventions for the rest of their lives [13].

South-East Asia

The South-East Asia Region (SEAR) contributes 62% of the world's visual impairment. SEAR is home to ~91 million people with visual impairment, and 79 million people live with low vision or MSVI [14]. Around 20 million people in SEAR live with functional low vision. The common causes of low vision, as per a 2002 study in

India, are retinal diseases (37%), amblyopia (27%), optic atrophy (15%), glaucoma (12%), and corneal diseases (9%) [15].

16.4 Examination and Referral for Low Vision and Rehabilitation Services

The four key elements for an effective low vision examination are: (1) review of medical records, (2) observation, (3) assessment of functional need, and (4) assessment of the visual system.

(1) **Review of medical records:** Reviewing previous medical and surgical records of the patient serves as the starting point for eye examination, including refraction.
(2) **Observation:** Observations on visual functioning can provide valuable information on an individual's functional abilities and limitations (for example, increased head and eye movement can indicate progressive visual field loss; head-turning while reading can be the results of scotomas, etc.)
(3) **Assessment of functional needs:** Limitations in functional activities such as home management, schoolwork, computer work, glare issues, mobility issues, etc. can be assessed through careful and comprehensive notes.
(4) **Assessment of capabilities and limitation of the visual system:** The clinical measures of this evaluation include: VA measurements for distance and near-subjective and objective, contrast sensitivity, color vision, visual field, glare testing, binocularity, and comprehensive eye examination.

The impact of vision loss in children is complex. A multidisciplinary, holistic approach and coordinated effort can maximize their residual vision for enhancing their participation in educational, recreational, and social activities. Unlike adults, specific expertise, methodologies, and tools are required to evaluate and manage low vision in children. There should be flexibility in conducting tests in more than one session to obtain better results. Children, in general, are less vocal and non-advocate.

In adults, in addition to the clinical examination procedures, it is strongly recommended that functional vision assessments (FVAs) also be conducted to observe the effects of low vision and assess the visual skills used for functional vision (Table 16.1).

Referral

Referral to low vision rehabilitation service is often decided on visual acuity threshold and visual field loss criteria. But, the criteria based on these two visual functions alone is insufficient for referral as other factors equally impact the visual functioning and quality of life [16]. The following are the guidelines for identifying people who may potentially need a referral for low vision services [17–21].

- Vision loss which cannot be corrected through optical/medical/surgical intervention
- BCVA <6/18 in the better eye after correction
- Visual field loss, central or peripheral
- Contrast sensitivity loss
- Scotoma in the visual fields
- Color deficiency
- Children with developmental delays and disabilities
- Diplopia
- Acute monocular vision loss
- Photophobia (cone dystrophies, achromatopsia, aniridia, oculocutaneous albinism, etc.)
- Night blindness
- Hemianopia
- Acquired brain damage (stroke, tumor, cerebral contusion, etc.)
- Functional complaints such as frequent bumping into objects, problems in near work

Table 16.1 The tools and methodologies used in clinical measurement of low vision

Examination	Recommendation	Tools
Distance vision	logMAR (Minimum Angle of Resolution) test charts provide a high contrast, geometric progression of size differences between lines and proportional spacing	Bailey-Lovie logMAR, Lighthouse (Sloan letters), Feinbloom chart, Lea symbols chart
Near vision	Graded continuous text materials	Bailey-Lovie word reading chart, Lighthouse "NUMBER" card, Lighthouse near VA test chart, Lea symbols
Refraction	Objective refraction—retinoscopy with a wide-aperture trial lens, Subjective refraction—adjustable trial frame and wide-aperture loose lenses	–
Color vision	For red, green, and blue, at least	Ishihara chart Farnsworth dichotomous test (D-15).
Visual field	Peripheral and central visual field	Manual/Automated perimeter Amsler grid
Glare testing	Subjective—brightness acuity tester (BAT) Objective—effect of filters to relieve the glare on a bright sunny day	–
Binocularity	Stereo-tests	Stereo fly test, Reindeer test.
Comprehensive eye exam	Rule out gross pathologies of the eye	Slit-lamp exam for anterior segment tonometry, Direct and indirect ophthalmoscopy
Children	Lea assessment tools for VA—symbols/gratings Lea assessment tools for contrast sensitivity (CS)—Hiding Heidi, symbols Visual fields: Lea flickering wand Stereopsis: Stereo smiles, Randot stereo test Color vision: Color vision testing made easy Dorsal stream function: Lea mailbox Ventral stream function: Heidi expressions test Therapeutic/diagnostic tool: Sanet vision integrator (for eye-hand coordination, dynamic visual processing, visual attention, balancing, visual memory, etc.)	

16.5 Status of Low Vision and Vision Rehabilitation Services in South-East Asia Region: The Need–Demand–Supply Triad

The current need-demand-supply triad for low vision services points to a yawning gap. Though significant by themselves, the large unmet "needs" in the populations are not fully reflected in the unmet "demand" for low vision services and aids. Additionally, the inadequate "supply" of services, even for the current demand level, compounds the problem for a variety of reasons. A global survey on low vision services reported that seven South-East Asia countries had some form of low vision service but with less than 10% coverage among people in need [18]. Some of the barriers are lack of trained people, preoccupation of professionals in curative (medical and surgical) ophthalmic care, and lack of facilities (diagnostic or corrective equipment and assistive devices); at some centers, these barriers are non-utilization of available technologies, high out-of-pocket spending, and poor support for repair and maintenance of expensive devices. A national survey on low vision service in India reported that merely 48 of 701 (7%) eye care institutions had dedicated low vision service centers. Most others work predominantly with clinical orientation for prescribing near and distance optical magnifiers alone (unpublished data). Most of these centers do not practice a person-centric care and do not have community activites.

The SWOT (strengths, weaknesses, opportunities, and threats) analysis on South-East Asia is an apt description of the present status on low vision and rehabilitation activities and provisions. This could also help plan future strategic planning for better services (Table 16.2).

Table 16.2 The regional perspective of low vision and rehabilitation care in South-East Asia

Strengths (S)	Weaknesses (W)
• Availability of low vision and rehabilitation services • Adequacy of human resources for care • Inclusion of low vision care in some professional training courses • Existence of Centers of Excellence with rehabilitation facilities • Linkages between ophthalmology services and primary rehabilitation • Low vision is defined as an area of interest by social services departments	• The magnitude of the issue is not fully understood by Ministries of Health • Low vision rehabilitation is not a health system priority • The organization of low vision care is particularly complex • Systems are not target driven • Funding is not adequately coordinated • Inadequate and poor data collection and monitoring • Poor collaboration between care providers • Poor continuity of care
Opportunities (O)	**Threats (T)**
• Adequate human resources in countries with the largest populations • VISION 2020 initiatives in all countries • Country-specific strategies for low vision care • Awareness of the rights of persons with disabilities • Active participation of NGOs in promoting low vision care	• Lack of standardized protocol for training professionals on low vision rehabilitation care • Vision rehabilitation is not given priority in overall eye care • Lack of collaboration among sectors • Insufficient funding allocations • Low vision care is not included in care management strategies

NGOs non-government organizations

16.6 Barriers and Challenges in Accessing Services

Early referral to low vision services can optimize the ability to maintain independence, and rehabilitation can yield major quality-of-life benefits. These interventions can potentially benefit up to 90% of people with low vision; however, except for a few high-income countries, less than 10% of people with low vision have access to specialist services in most LMICs. Besides, many people do not access services until their vision loss is severe, and quality of life is grossly affected.

The major challenge in delivering low vision services is identifying key people and organizations within each country who can lead low vision programs, advocate for change, and coordinate the efforts of primary, secondary, and tertiary healthcare facilities. Creating referral linkages among professionals (ophthalmologists, optometrists, rehabilitation counselors, and special educators) for appropriate services will help individuals gain timely access to appropriate services. There is a persistent need for high-quality outcomes research in nearly all areas of low vision services to identify the effectiveness of specific services. Quantitative and qualitative studies of populations, interventions, service delivery, and outcomes of public policies are essential to identify improved methods of service delivery.

(a) **Barriers related to service providers**

The shortage of professionals with specialized training in low vision rehabilitation limits low vision care delivery in many countries. Lack of training of the eye care professionals and ignorance of the benefits of low vision services are important factors for delayed referrals. Early referral maximizes the benefits of low vision and rehabilitation intervention. But the referral criteria should not be limited to visual acuity; instead, it should encompass all functional low vision parameters described earlier. Failing to explain the purpose of making a referral to low vision care may set an unrealistic expectation on the rehabilitation outcome, resulting in disappointments and dissatisfaction. The prevailing misconception that low vision care is time-consuming and not lucrative limits the number of professionals interested to work in this field.

(b) **Barriers related to service models**

In LMICs, the low vision and rehabilitation services are either unavailable or inadequate to meet all needs, including those for children with special needs. There is a lack of inter-disciplinary or "integrated" care that incorporates input from a range of professionals (optometrists, ophthalmologists, low vision consultants, rehabilitation therapists, special educators, social workers, etc.), and often services are fragmented without intersectoral consultation. The geographic barrier to access low vision services is another major challenge since it is available mostly only in major cities. Significant deficits in the provision of care include the size of the healthcare workforce (eye care professionals) and the training it receives.

(c) **Barriers related to demand**

The causes of reduced uptake and non-acceptance of low vision services are many. These are low awareness of availability of assistive devices, improper understanding of the benefits of the services, lack of felt need, denial of the problems among patients, out-of-pocket spending to procure devices, opportunity costs for patient and family, social stigma on devices, fear of losing employment, and lack of referral services. All of these result in reduced *said* and *unsaid* needs and underutilization ("low demand") of low vision rehabilitation services [19, 20]. Besides, the absence of these services in most eye care facilities and skewed/urban dominated distributions of facilities are also the other reasons for poor demand and utilization [21, 22]. Inadequate transport systems, especially from rural areas, mobility issues, and non-availability of physical assistance, are other related deterrents to accessing care [23]. Psychological factors like denial and depression among patients may also prevent them from availing of low vision and rehabilitation services [24].

With the global increases in life expectancy and chronic diseases, there will be more people with low vision globally. Failure to provide appropriate low vision services to these growing numbers of people may prevent many individuals from achieving full social inclusion and optimal quality of life. This failure also deprives society of the human and economic contributions of many individuals, thereby increasing the costs to society.

16.7 Strategies and Models to Strengthen Services for Low Vision Services

Anecdotal evidence shows that most low vision services are predominantly clinical and are provided by tertiary eye care facilities in India. They conform solely to the provision of optical and non-optical aids without addressing vision rehabilitation or community care. This nature of practice is suboptimal in managing individuals with visual disabilities. One needs a holistic approach.

Disability-Inclusive Low Vision Services

In 1980, the International Classification of Impairments, Disabilities, and Handicaps (ICIDH-I) and the WHO defined disability as "any restriction or lack of ability, resulting from an impairment, in performing any activity within the range considered normal for a human being" [25]. In 2001, the ICIDH-II, now named ICF (The International Classification of Functioning, Disability, and Health) recommended that disability should no longer be viewed as merely the result of anatomical impairment or diseases; it should instead be viewed as the interaction between a medical condition and the person's environment [26]. By this new definition, both low vision and unavoidable blindness are visual disabilities in the context of ocular health.

Multidisciplinary Approach

Low vision management is an extended and long-term process that needs a multidisciplinary approach, including clinical and rehabilitation services for visual disabilities (low vision and unavoidable blindness) operating in a dynamic complex system that requires a broader consideration than clinical practices. In South-East Asia, the current practices for low vision management focus exclusively on clinical aspects or diseases without many rehabilitation components such as education, mobility, assistive products, vocational training, social welfare, etc. While all efforts must be made to manage low vision clinically, it is also important to improve the quality of life, independence, and daily living activities of people with low vision. Other important elements for low vision management are accessible environment and treating people with dignity, respect, and positive attitudes.

Clinico-Socio Model for Low Vision Service

Clinical diagnosis and dispensing of low vision aids constitute only one part of managing low vision and visual disability. The other part is the care tailored to specific needs as assessed by a team of low vision-oriented professionals, the ophthalmologists, optometrists, orthoptists, special educators, occupational therapists, orientation and mobility trainers, social workers, and counselors. A clinico-social low vision services model (Fig. 16.4) builds services in-line with person-centered care principles by working together with hospital and community-based organizations [27]. It is developed after identifying the gaps in the current practices, literature reviews (narrative), and critical analysis, including the national action plan report on low vision and rehabilitation services conducted in tertiary eye care centers. Networking with various NGOs (non-governmental organizations) optimizes the services components and draws closer to the person-centered approach [3]. In this approach, the healthcare provider and the challenged individual collaborate, and the caregivers and the family members develop a good partnership to arrive at a solution tailored for the individual.

Adopting the Integrated Approach

Low vision services could be offered at all levels of care [28]. In many countries, there is inadequate integration of low vision care between these service levels; this leaves a vast majority of

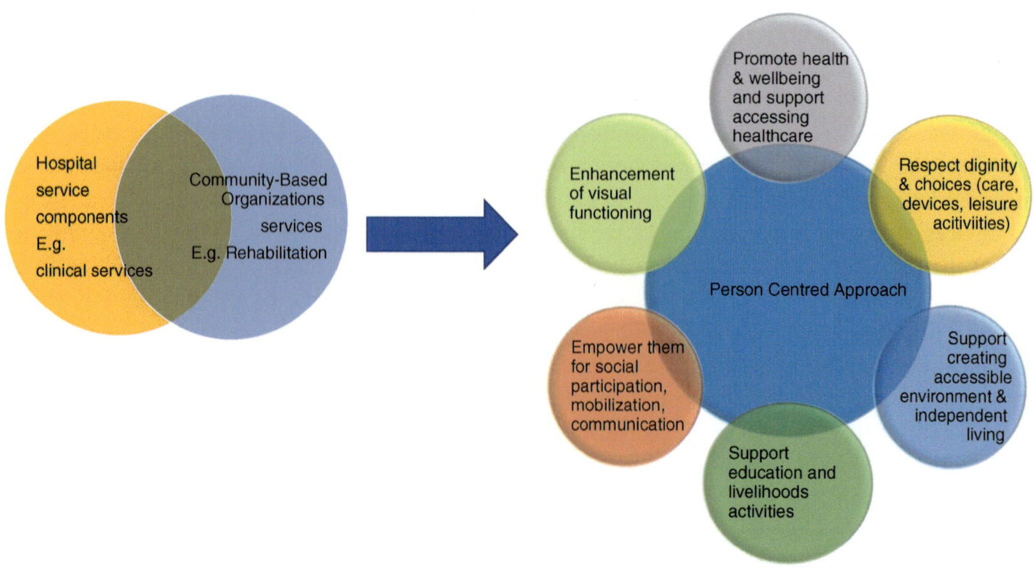

Fig. 16.4 The Clinico-Social Model of Low Vision Service [27]

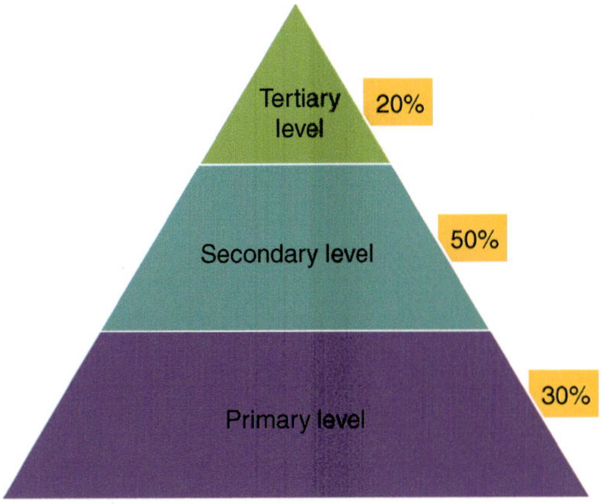

Fig. 16.5 Quantum of people with low vision benefiting at different levels of care [28]

people with low vision with no service or poor service. The American Academy of Ophthalmology recommends that 30% of the low vision population be appropriately served at a primary level, 50% at a secondary level, and 20% at the tertiary level of care (Fig. 16.5) [29].

Strengthening services at all levels are important and necessary. The WHO has defined international standards for effective service delivery at each level of care. The essential elements include guidelines for human resources, equipment, service needs, and place of service. A set of optional components is added as "plus" services for primary and secondary levels to broaden and strengthen vision rehabilitation at the community and district levels (annexures). In 2020, the ongoing COVID-19 pandemic has further laid bare gaps and challenges in the healthcare services.

16.8 Assistive Technology for Visual Impairment

Assistive Technology (AT)

AT is an umbrella term that includes assistive, adaptive, and rehabilitative devices for people with disabilities and also includes the process used in selecting, locating, and using them. AT promotes greater independence by enabling people to perform tasks that they were formerly unable to accomplish or had great difficulty accomplishing them.

The WHO defines the meaning and purpose of AT through the following terminologies [30]:

- Assistive Technology, AT, is applying organized knowledge and skills related to assistive products, including systems and services. It is a subset of health technology.
- Assistive Products, APs, are external products (including devices, equipment, instruments, or software), the primary purpose of which is to maintain or improve an individual's functioning and independence. APs are also used to prevent impairment and secondary health conditions.
- Priority APs are those products that are essential to maintain or improve an individual's functioning and be available at a price that the community/state can afford [31].

Traditionally, ATs for visually impaired and blind people are often built on the sense of touch, vibration, hearing, and smell. These devices enhance body functionality and improve daily performance, thus promoting independent living and ensuring better quality of life. The wide range of ATs, from low technology devices such as mobility canes, braille slates, typoscopes, etc. to highly sophisticated technology such as computer software, electronic gadgets, mobile software, etc., can meet the unique requirements of people of all ages related to mobility, daily living, education, employment, leisure activities, personal safety, and many more. The UHC includes quality rehabilitation and appropriate AT for people with visual loss as one of its key components. Table 16.3 lists APs built on body sense and activity [32–34].

A person with functional low vision or blindness can use either visual-based assistive devices (e.g., magnifiers) or visual substitution assistive devices (e.g., Braille materials) (Table 16.3). However, in practice, the focus wherever possible should be on improving the functionality of the person rather than sticking to definitions. It is necessary that low vision specialists and vision rehabilitation professionals encourage and moti-

Table 16.3 Types of assistive technologies based on body sense and human activities

Type	Element	Assistive Technology (AT)
Body sense	Visual	Large print books, optical and non-optical magnifiers
	Tactile	Braille reading books, mobility or smart canes
	Sound	DAISY (digital accessible information system), liquid sensor, color detector, notetaker
Activity	Education	Pre-academic learning—Embossed print or sound toys Reading—Optical magnifiers (near/distance) Writing—Typoscope (multiple window), Brailler Mathematics—Braille compass, Brailler ruler Science—Tactile maps/tactile anatomy charts
	Orientation and mobility	Long walking cane, Guide cane
	Games and leisure	Braille cube, Braille chess
	Daily living activities	Notex, talking watch

Table 16.4 Visual loss categorization and use of assistive technologies [31, 32]

Visual loss ranges	<6/18 up to 3/60	<3/60 up to 1/60	<1/60 to LP & NLP
WHO	Low vision	Blindness	
	Functional low vision (<6/18 up to LP)		
AT potential beneficiaries	Low vision to 1/60		<1/60 Blindness

Courtesy: Senjam SS 2018, New Delhi
LP/NLP light perception/no light perception

vate their visually challenged patients to use their residual vision to the maximum in performing daily activities, including the students using their residual vision in their education activities. Functional low vision has a wide range, from <6/18 to LP. But a student with LP cannot use ATs (large print books, typoscope, magnifiers), whereas one with vision of <3/60 can use either vision-based ATs (magnifiers, typoscope, large print books) or tactile-based ATs (Braille, audio devices) [35, 36]. Thus choice of the ATs has to be individualized.

To avoid this dilemma, a simplified classification of visual loss is designed as a guide to choosing the preferred type of AT for students with vision loss [35]. This simplified vision loss classification uses a benchmark cut-off of best-corrected binocular visual acuity lesser or better than 1/60 (Table 16.4). Any residual vision function of <1/60 becomes an adjunct to the use of blind skills. Such people must preferably rely on visual substitution ATs or non-visual or haptic devices. This classification is a guide to the preferential choice of ATs without discouraging cross use of devices since the use of combined techniques maximizes benefits.

Some of the recommended uses of ATs for students are as follows [34]:

- Low vision, <6/18 to 1/60: Visual skill ATs such as magnifiers, typoscopes, and large print books.
- Vision <1/60 to blind: Visual substitution ATs such as Braille books or keyboards, DAISY books.

Students with visual disabilities need ATs for a wide range of activities. Studies in schools for the blind in Delhi have shown that students could not access appropriate ATs for their education [34]. Screen readers such as non-visual desktop access (NVDA) are freely available online, but awareness about them and their uses were poor. Educating caregivers is as important as educating patients in the acceptance and use of these devices. A similar recommendation was made in a hospital-based study; in this case, patients attending visual rehabilitation clinics could be triaged into two categories based on presenting vision of <6/18 to 1/60 and <1/60, for appropriate low vision and rehabilitation services [37].

16.9 Improving Access to Assistive Technology

There are multiple challenges in accessing ATs. In many countries, access to APs, particularly in the public sector, is poor or non-existent; this leads to high out-of-pocket spending. The major reasons for this are: non-availability of AT products for demonstration/purchase at district/state level rehabilitation centers and hospitals; inadequate funding; inefficient service delivery; poor monitoring of quality and safety standards; and lack of trained personnel for prescription, fitting, user training, and follow-up care.

Affordable and appropriate access requires government commitment to adequate and sustained financing, including efficient procurement and delivery systems of products listed in the WHO assistive products list (APL). Inclusion of ATs, aligned with different countries' national priorities and contexts, into health systems is essential for realizing progress towards the targets in the SDGs relating to UHC (inclusive and equitable quality education, inclusive and sustainable economic growth, full and productive employment, and decent work for all). It may be recalled that the United Nations Convention on the Rights of Persons with Disabilities, under which 175 Member States have committed, *inter alia*, asks to ensure access to quality ATs at an affordable cost (Article 20) [2].

To improve access to high quality, affordable APs in all countries, the WHO has introduced the *Priority Assistive Products List* (APL). The APL is the first stage of implementing a global commitment to improving access to APs—the Global Cooperation on Assistive Technology (GATE). The APL includes 50 priority APs, selected on the basis of widespread need and impact on a person's life. The APL aspires to follow in the footsteps of the WHO Model *List of Essential Medicines*, which creates awareness among the public, mobilizes resources, and stimulates competition. Similar to the WHO *List of Essential Medicines*, the APL is intended to be a catalyst in promoting access to AT everywhere and for everyone.

Access to APs for low vision cannot improve in a silo; it will improve only when the access to APs as a whole improves. Thus, relevant Ministries must: (1) pay attention to policies and programs to facilitate access to these products within UHC; (2) encourage international and/or regional collaboration for the manufacturing, procuring, and supply of priority APs; (3) build a cadre of trained human resources for the provision and maintenance of APs; (4) develop a national list of APLs; (5) promote research and development to make existing APs affordable; (6) use new technology to create unique and user-friendly products; (7) collect population-based data on the needs of AT that helps for advocacy and evidence-based strategies; (8) and promote inclusive barrier-free environments so that all people who need AT devices can make optimum use of them for independent living and safe participation in society.

Integration at Community Eye Care Delivery System

The fundamental component of the WHO Global Disability Action Plan 2014–2021 is to enhance the quality of life and improve access to ATs for persons with disabilities, including those with visual disabilities. The WHO Rehabilitation 2030: A Call for Action, a comprehensive and quality rehabilitation service including equitable access to healthcare services, is an important guide for actions [38].

Most of the SEAR countries belong to LMICs with limited resources. Therefore, to be cost-effective, the low vision rehabilitation (LVR) programs in this region should focus on providing devices through a country-specific eye health delivery system. Each SEAR country has a national healthcare infrastructure system, from primary to tertiary healthcare facilities. Appropriate LVR programs should be available at each health facility and must be expanded to the community. Integration with the existing healthcare delivery system will improve the accessibility of and help sustain the LVR program, including improved access and use of the required AT products. The integrated model of LVR and primary eye care services with the general healthcare system is cost-effective, brings in many collateral benefits, and is most suited for developing countries.

In general, SEAR countries, including India, face a huge lag in the development of adequate eye care infrastructure and human resources for low vision and ATs at all levels; and when and where these exist, are unable to deal with the growing need for such services. For example, in India, only around 4000 vision centers have been built, against the target requirement of 20,000 vision centers by 2020. Besides, most of these centers do not cater to low vision needs.

16.10 Community-Based Inclusive Development in Low Vision

Community-Based Inclusive Development (CBID, formerly known as Community-Based Rehabilitation) is an approach to enable inclusion of people with disabilities on the ground—to ensure that people with disabilities have access to the same opportunities as their peers. CBID begins in the everyday lives of people and aims at achieving sustainable change. Together, people analyze and address the issues that contribute to or hinder the inclusion of people with disabilities in their community. CBID is founded on self-empowerment and participation of people with disabilities and their communities. This is the basis of collective action to build resilient, equitable, and inclusive communities.

The outcomes of CBID should result in the communities that are proactive and aware of the needs of persons with disabilities. In such communities, efforts are made to ensure that local services are accessible, available, affordable, and of high quality. Services in such communities are non-discriminatory, and people with disabilities have the capacity and confidence to participate in community life.

How does this translate into the practice for those with low vision?

1. Communities are aware of low vision; they understand that low vision is different from blindness, with specific accessibility and inclusion requirements. This awareness reduces stigmatization. It is particularly important for children who are often stigmatized as lazy or blind.
2. Teachers, rehabilitation providers, and community workers receive specific training on low vision. They understand the needs of children and adults with low vision and possess the know-how to address those needs.

Case Study

CBM has been successful in providing Community-Based Rehabilitation programs with center-based and outreach services in Indonesia, Thailand, Vietnam, and the Philippines. A project in Indonesia on providing low vision services identified distance and cost as two key barriers: The study found that children up to 6 or 7 years of age with vision problems and those with disabilities may be best identified and referred by community volunteers and key informants. Networking with key people in the community and their networks, grassroots organizations and primary health services, is the first step in systematically detecting children in need of vision checks. Follow-up on the use of spectacles and low vision-related interventions can also be done at the community level with the help of caregivers and community volunteers.

CBM, Bangalore, India

3. There is provision for testing, fitting, and dispensing appropriate low vision aids close to the communities where such people live.

Role of Community-Based Inclusive Development in Low Vision Rehabilitation

Some of the following activities could make CBID a success in the community:

1. Referrals: Referrals are a two-way process.
   (a) CBID projects can identify those with low vision in the community and refer them to low vision services. They can also periodically arrange for low vision services at a convenient location for the ease of people who are unable to travel to a town or city for the service.
   (b) Eye health service providers can collaborate with CBID providers to ensure that people identified with low vision receive support in the community.
2. Education

(a) Support education for children and students with visual impairment at all levels of education.
(b) Advocate for these children to receive education in mainstream schools instead of "special schools" with reasonable accommodation. The schools can extend simple supports, such as seating the children in the first row, improving contrast on boards, etc.
(c) Help mainstream teacher understand the needs of children with low vision.
(d) Ensure that families of those with low vision understand the needs of their children and are aware of available resources to manage low vision.

3. Focus on communities
   (a) The powerful agents of change and motivators are those people with low vision and visual impairment when they are CBID workers themselves.
   (b) The CBID community workers can help people with visual impairment overcome barriers in the community and help them identify livelihood opportunities

16.11 WHO Global Cooperation on Assistive Technology

The WHO estimates that more than 1 billion people with disabilities will require one or more APs. The number is likely to be doubled by 2030 because of the increasing numbers of aging populations. However, currently, only 1 in 10 people in need has access to APs due to high costs, limited availability, and poor awareness. Hence, there is a substantial gap between the demand for and provision of APs in many LMICs; this can potentially limit educational and work opportunities for younger people, and independent living for older people with low vision.

With an aim to facilitate that high-quality and affordable APs could be available to everyone in need, the WHO initiated a flagship program in 2011—GATE-in partnership with other UN agencies, international organizations, donor agencies, professional organizations, academia, and organizations of/for persons with disabilities. The overarching objectives of GATE are: (1) access to education, (2) to earn a living, (3) overcome poverty, (4) participate in all societal activities, and (5) live with dignity.

Under this global initiative, in 2016, the WHO published the APL. This is the first stage of implementing a global commitment to improving access to APs. The WHO acknowledges that improving access to ATs requires a people-centered ecosystem between the five Ps—people, policy, products, personnel, and provision (Fig. 16.6). An overarching policy is crucial across all proposed areas supported by comprehensive data collection and effective financing mechanisms. Through national AT policies, an effective governance could ensure an adequate supply of quality, affordable products, and appropriately trained personnel for service provision.

The APL has 50 APs for people with disabilities, a selection based on the need and impact on a person's life. This list has been drawn up after an extensive consultation process among users, service providers, and other stakeholders from across the world. This list includes 16 APs, specific to people with visual impairment, based on the senses of touch, vibration, and sound (Table 16.5).

The GATE list of APs is the baseline on which each Member State could further develop a national priority list of APs according to its need and available resources. The Member States could also use the GATE list to develop policies, design service delivery, market-sharing, procurement, reimbursement, and insurance coverage.

APs will have maximum impact when their use is supported with national policies and legislations integrated into the existing health services. Towards this end, the WHO is developing three additional tools to assist the Member States in developing national AT policies and programs as an integral component of UHC. These tools include:

- Policy—The AT policy framework will include financing mechanisms (health and welfare insurance programs), guidance on implementing the APL, standards, training, and service delivery systems.

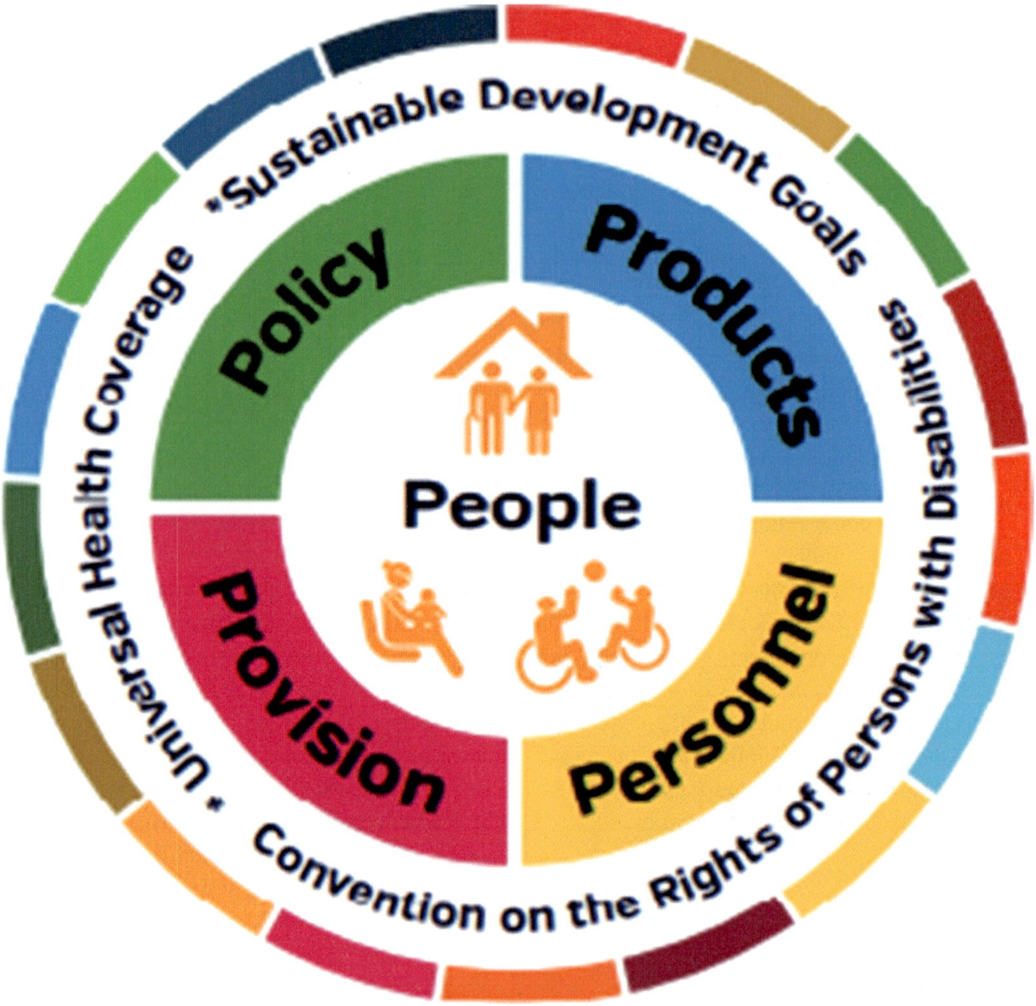

Fig. 16.6 The five interlinked areas of assistive technology (five Ps of AT)—People, Policy, Products, Personnel, and Provision (Source: WHO) [36]

Table 16.5 Global Cooperation on Assistive Technology (GATE) list of Assistive Products for people with visual impairment

1	Alarm signalers with light/sound/vibration	9	Digital hand-held magnifiers
2	Audio players with DAISY capability	10	Optical magnifiers
3	Braille displays (note-takers)	11	Recorders
4	Braille writing equipment/Braillers	12	Screen readers
5	Canes/sticks	13	Simplified mobile phones
6	Deaf-blind communicators	14	Spectacles; low vision, short distance, long-distance, filters and protection
7	Handrails/grab bars	15	Talking/Touch-sensitive watches
8	Keyboard and mouse emulation software	16	White canes

- Personnel—The APs training package will include four essential service provision steps, assessment, fitting, training, and follow-up and repair. This will add to the health and rehabilitation personnel's skillset to provide a range of APs at the primary and community level.
- Provision of APs service delivery model that is best suited for the specific needs of the Member State which would enable people to access APs for all their functional needs from a single point source.

Annexure

1. **Large print books**—Individuals with low vision have difficulty in reading small and usual print size text (N 6-8). Large size print text (N 20) with font size of 16–18 helps in reading.
2. **Typoscope**—It can be used for either reading guide (one window) or writing guide (multiple windows) according to the design being made. Single window typoscope is useful for albinism individuals.
3. **Reading stands**—It helps in avoiding from bending over the surfaces while viewing texts. It also helps to Braille readers.
4. **Low vision lamps**—Enhance lighting may help people with low vision to read easier, thereby, improving the reading performance. For example, compact fluorescent (CFL), incandescent lamps, light emitting diode, and halogen lamps, etc. with different luminosity will be of help in reading. Objective measurement of the reading ability as well as subjective ratings of visual comfort with lighting preference should be considered in assessing the suitability.
5. **Optical magnifiers**—Optical magnifiers (near and distance), for example, hand-held magnifiers, dome, stand and pocket magnifiers, telescopes are task-specific optical aids that enlarge the image formed on the retina.
6. **Electronic Magnification Aids** (EMA)—Electronic magnifiers are usually termed as electronic vision enhancement system (EVES). The devices range in size from large desktop units (Closed Circuit Televisions—CCTV) to hand-held video magnifiers with different size.
7. **Braille Reading Materials (BRM)**—Braille is a tactile system of raised dots that enables students with visual impairment to access the information by touching. Learning Braille reading with fingers is one of the oldest techniques to route for literacy among the visually impaired and blind people. Braille codes used worldwide has a standard rectangular cell, which contains up to six dots in a 2 by 3 grid. Reading materials are typically available in three encoding levels. Grade 1, in which words are fully spelled; Grade 2, which uses abbreviations and contractions, and Grade 3, which involves authors' personal and nonstandard shorthand.
8. **Refreshable Braille Display (RBD)**—Refreshable Braille Display works with a screen reader and enables the user to read what's on the computer screen by touch on Braille display. A Braille display has a different size from 12 to 80 Braille cells, each cell has six or eight pins which are connected electronically to the computer to be able to move up and down when type on Perkins style key pad and to display a Braille version of characters on the computer screen. The price of Braille displays is very expensive depending on the number of characters displayed.
9. **Braille Translator Software** (BTS)—Braille Translation Software translates electronic documents into Braille codes and sends it to a Braille embosser (special Braille printer—Braille embosser) which produces a hard copy of the original text. BTS recognizes a variety of digital text file formats, e.g. MS Word, PDF, HTML, etc. The common translation software includes Duxbury Braille Translator, Braille 2000, etc.
10. **Audio Format Materials** (AFM)—AFM is beneficial for many students with low vision and blind. It enables students to read or access information through hearing, e.g. Digital Accessible Information System

(DAISY), Book Port Plus, etc. There may be dedicated audio players, e.g. Booksense; device that displays text and play, e.g. Victor Reader Stream; multipurpose audio devices, e.g. I Pod, or computer software, e.g. Easy Reader.

11. **Screen Reader Software**—This software allows people or students with low vision and blind to convert text on a computer screen and in documents to synthetic speech, i.e. audio output as well as keystrokes entered on the keyboard, and navigational information. Screen readers require the use of keyboard shortcuts, most of which the user must memorize the keys. Many screen readers work with multiple programs, but some screen readers are specific to certain programs, e.g. JAWS, NVDA, COBRA, SuperNova, etc. NVDA is freely available online.
12. **Braille slate and stylus**—This is a low cost, portable low-technique writing tool. It is like a pencil and paper concept. The slate is usually made from two panels that stabilizes the paper and while the stylus is used to punch through the holes in one of the panels to create the Braille dots.
13. **Jot a Dot**—It is also a low-tech writing tool made of lightweight plastic material that is small and easily portable. It is useful for taking quick and short notes by students.
14. **Braille typewriter (Perkins Brailler)**—It is a portable low-tech writing tool with six keys corresponding to each of the six Braille dots. There are many models of the Perkins Brailler that suit according to the needs.
15. **Braille computer keyboards**—This is a specially designed computer keyboard which corresponds to Braille code on its keys.
16. **Large computer keyboards**—This is a keyboard with 2.5 M notation print size.
17. **Digital audio recorder**—The non-displayed digital recorder is specially designed for persons with visual impairment which can record teachers' lectures to replace writing notes, e.g., PlexTalk.
18. **Braille electronic note taker**—It is a small and portable device for storing information with the use of the Braille or typewriter keyboards. The stored information can be accessed through an inbuilt speech synthesizer or a Braille or both.
19. **Walking or long cane**—It is designed primarily for mobility tool to identify objects in the path of the users. The length of the cane depends upon the height of the user, and usually, it extends from the floor up to between sternum and under the chin when user is standing upright.
20. **Children's walking cane**—This cane works same as long walking cane but designated for use by children. It is shorter than long cane.
21. **Symbol or identification cane**—Symbol cane is primarily used to notify the general public that the person has a visual impairment or low vision. It is often shorter and lighter than others. It intends not to be used as a body support or to detect obstacles on the floor or as a mobility tool. Red and white color banded symbol cane highlight both visual and hearing impairment. Sometimes, a long symbol can be used for mobility to detect any kerbs, doorways, or obstruction in low contrast. Such canes are intended to be used for persons with some residual visual function.
22. **Guide cane**—This is a short and thin cane but longer than symbol cane usually extending from the floor to the user's waist when standing upright with more limited mobility function. The guide cane is used to scan for kerbs and steps by individual with some residual visual function. It is usually used diagonally across the body for protection and warning the user of obstacles in low contrast or in dark or nighttime.
23. **Support cane**—The white support cane is designed to offer physical support to the user. This tool is heavier and stronger and has a very limited role as a mobility device.
24. **Green cane**—It is used in some countries to designate that the user has low vision while the white cane designates that the user is blind.

25. ***GPS Devices*—**GPS hardware and software enable navigation to a desired destination. Some GPS based devices detect objects in the user's path and alert the user by vibrating or chirping as the person approaches the object. Some GPS software provide information on points of interest, altitude, and speed. (Example: Kapten PLUS GPS, Miniguide, Wayfinder Access, Mobile Geo, etc.)
26. **Liquid level sensor**—It is a specially designed device which alerts visually impaired students by monitoring the level of liquid in a cup or glass either a sound or vibration or both as liquid touches at the tip of device.
27. **Talking color detector**—This device can differentiate a variety of colors with a voice once it touches on the surface.
28. **Talking watch or alarm clock**—This talking device clearly announces the time and can be used for alarm.
29. **Pill organizer**—This device is particularly useful for low vision or blind individuals who need to consume multiple medications every day. It has a separate compartment for pills taken in the different time of the day. Color code lids or Braille markings box are available.
30. **Simplified mobile phone**—This is a simple basic phone which makes easier to feel and navigate. Features like the adjustable or large font or screen magnifiers, adjustable screen contrast and brightness or Braille entry may have in the phone.
31. **Mobile Applications**—The smart phone accessibility has increased significantly in recent years. Specialized accessibility applications (screen reading or screen magnification software) that work on smartphones and tablets. Many mobile applications will have in-built accessibility features such as: optical character recognition (OCR), object recognition, global positioning system (GPS), and route finding. (Example: Be My Eyes, TapTapSee, KNFB Reader, Color ID, etc.)
32. **Talking money identifier**—It helps visually impaired individuals to identify money with a voice function. Other tactile note identifier is a money organizer wallet, notex, NoteChecker, etc.
33. **Household, personal, and other independent living products**—A variety of household items, independent living products are available with large print, tactile markings or audible speech. (Example: Kitchen—Liquid level indicator, measuring cups, braille label. Personal—wrist watches in braille and large print, magnifying mirror, travel organizer. Health products—Talking weighing scale, thermometer, large print insulin syringe, braille medicine pill organizer
34. **Virtual assistants**—Voice assistants perform tasks or services for users based on spoken commands or questions, read information out loud or perform tasks without requiring the user to look at a screen. (Example: Amazon Alexa, Apple Siri, Android's Google)

Other Useful Resources:

1. https://iapb.standardlist.org/essential-lists/essential-list-low-vision/
2. https://www.iapb.org/news/low-vision-curriculum/
3. https://www.iapb.org/learn/work-groups/low-vision/
4. https://www.who.int/classifications/icf/en/
5. https://www.who.int/disabilities/technology/gate/en/
6. https://www.who.int/publications/i/item/9789241548052
7. https://www.lighthouseguild.org/
8. https://enviter.eu/members/the-netherlands/royal-dutch-visio

References

1. World Health Organization. Summary world report on disability. WHO; 2011. p. 1–24.
2. Article 20 – Personal mobility | United Nations Enable. https://www.un.org/development/desa/disabilities/convention-on-the-rights-of-persons-with-disabilities/article-20-personal-mobility.htm
3. WHO. World Report on Vision. 2019. https://www.who.int/publications/i/item/world-report-on-vision

4. WHO. Improving access to assistive technology for everyone, everywhere. 2016. https://apps.who.int/iris/handle/10665/207694
5. Leat SJ, Legge GE, Bullimore MA. What is low vision? A re-evaluation of definitions. Optom Vis Sci. 76:198–211.
6. WHO | Priority eye diseases. https://www.who.int/blindness/causes/priority/en/index4.html
7. Pararajasegaram R. Low vision care: the need to maximise visual potential. Community Eye Heal. 2004;17(49):1–2.
8. Köberlein J, Beifus K, Schaffert C, et al. The economic burden of visual impairment and blindness: a systematic review. BMJ Open. 2013; https://doi.org/10.1136/bmjopen-2013-003471.
9. Pezzullo L, Streatfeild J, Simkiss P, et al. The economic impact of sight loss and blindness in the UK adult population. BMC Health Serv Res. 2018;18:63. https://doi.org/10.1186/s12913-018-2836-0.
10. Salomon JA, Haagsma JA, Davis A, et al. Disability weights for the Global Burden of Disease 2013 study. Lancet Glob Heal. 2015;3:e712–23. https://doi.org/10.1016/S2214-109X(15)00069-8.
11. Bourne RRA, Flaxman SR, Braithwaite T, et al. Magnitude, temporal trends, and projections of the global prevalence of blindness and distance and near vision impairment: a systematic review and meta-analysis. Lancet Glob Heal. 2017;5:e888–97. www.thelancet.com/pdfs/journals/langlo/PIIS2214-109X(17)30293-0.pdf
12. Bourne R, Adelson J, Flaxman S, et al. Trends in prevalence of blindness and distance and near vision impairment over 30 years and contributed to the global burden of disease in 2020. SRN Electronic J. 2020; https://doi.org/10.2139/ssrn.3582742.
13. Gilbert C, Foster A. Childhood blindness in the context of VISION 2020 – the right to sight. Bull World Health Organ. 2001;79:227–32.
14. Murthy G, Malhotra S. Status of eye care in South-East Asia Region. Delhi J Ophthalmol. 2013;24:114–8.
15. Dandona R, Dandona L, Srinivas M, et al. Planning low vision services in India. Ophthalmology. 2002;109:1871–8.
16. Sapkota YD, Limberg H, Pokhrel RP, et al. Epidemiology of blindness in Nepal 2012 Report. 2012. https://www.researchgate.net/publication/236308859_Epidemiology_of_Blindness_in_Nepal_2012
17. Thapa R, Bajimaya S, Paudyal G, et al. Prevalence and causes of low vision and blindness in an elderly population in Nepal: the Bhaktapur retina study. BMC Ophthalmol. 2018;18:42. https://doi.org/10.1186/s12886-018-0710-9.
18. Casson RJ, Newland HS, Muecke J, et al. Prevalence and causes of visual impairment in rural Myanmar. The Meiktila Eye Study. Ophthalmology. 2007;114:2302–8.
19. Dineen BP, Bourne RRA, Ali SM, et al. Prevalence and causes of blindness and visual impairment in Bangladeshi adults: results of the National Blindness and Low Vision Survey of Bangladesh. Br J Ophthalmol. 2003;87:820–8.
20. De Boer MR, Langelaan M, Jansonius NM, et al. Evidence-based guidelines on the referral of visually impaired persons to low vision services. Eur J Ophthalmol. 2005;15:400–6.
21. Low vision: why and when to recommend. www.reviewofoptometry.com/low-vision-why-and-when-to-recommend
22. Lim YE, Vukicevic M, Koklanis K, et al. Low vision services in the Asia-Pacific region: models of low vision service delivery and barriers to access. J Vis Impair Blind. 2014;108:311–22.
23. O'Connor PM, Lamoureux EL, Keeffe JE. Predicting the need for low vision rehabilitation services. Br J Ophthalmol. 2008;92:252–5.
24. Pollard TL, Simpson JA, Lamoureux EL, et al. Barriers to accessing low vision services. Ophthalmic Physiol Opt. 2003;23:321–7.
25. WHO | International classification of functioning, disability and health (ICF). WHO; 2019. www.who.int/classifications/icf/en/
26. World Health Organization. How to use the ICF: a practical manual for using the International Classification of Functioning, Disability and Health (ICF). WHO. https://www.who.int/classifications/drafticfpracticalmanual.pdf. Accessed 4 Dec 2020.
27. Senjam SS. Developing a disability inclusive model for low vision service. Indian J Ophthalmol. 2020; (in press).
28. Ryan B. Models of low vision care: past, present and future. Clin Exp Optom. 2014;97:209–13.
29. American Academy of Ophthalmology. Low vision: levels of care – American Academy of Ophthalmology [Internet]. [cited 2020 Nov 30]. https://www.aao.org/disease-review/low-vision-levels-of-care. Accessed 4 Dec 2020.
30. World Health Organization. Global Cooperation on Assistive Technology (GATE). 2016. https://www.who.int/disabilities/technology/gate/en/. Accessed 4 Dec 2020.
31. World Health Organization. Priority assistive products list. 2017. https://www.who.int/phi/implementation/assistive_technology/global_survey-apl/en/. Accessed 4 Dec 2020.
32. Senjam SS. Assistive technology for education of students with visual disability: classification matters. Kerala J Ophthalmol. 2019;31:86–91.
33. Senjam SS, Gupta V, Vashsit P. A handbook of assistive technology for people with visual disability. New Delhi: Century Publication; 2019. http://centurypublications.co.in/a-handbook-of-assistive-technology-for-people-with-visual-disability. Accessed 4 Dec 2020.

34. Senjam SS, Foster A, Bascaran C, et al. Assistive technology for students with visual disability in schools for the blind in Delhi. Disabil Rehabil Assist Technol. 2019; https://doi.org/10.1080/17483107.2019.1604829.
35. Senjam SS, Foster A, Bascaran C. Assistive Technology for visual impairment and trainers at Schools for the Blind in Delhi. https://doi.org/10.1080/10400435.2020.1839144.
36. Senjam SS, Foster A. Situation analysis on the awareness, utilization and barriers to access of assistive technology among children with visual imparment in schools for the blind Delhi [Master's thesis]. International Centre for Eye Health, London School of Hygiene & Tropical.
37. Senjam SS, Foster A, Covadonga B, Vashist P. Awareness, utilization and barriers in accessing assistive technology among the young patients attending in low vision rehabilitation clinic of a tertiary eye care centre in Delhi. Indian J Ophthalmol. 2019;67:1548–54.
38. Rehabilitation 2030: a call for action. www.who.int/disabilities/care/Rehab2030MeetingReport_plain_text_version.pdf

Part IV

Human Resource for Health

Ophthalmology in South-East Asia: Practices and Priorities

17

B. R. Shamanna, Rolika Bansal, and Santosh G. Honavar

Key Points

- Globally, there is a shortage of ophthalmologists; this shortage is especially critical in the South-East Asian region. The distribution of ophthalmologists between urban and rural areas is also unequal.
- In 2015, there were an estimated 232,866 ophthalmologists in 194 countries catering to 7.4 billion people with a mean of 31.7 ophthalmologists/million population.
- The WHO South-East Asia Region, with an estimated global population share of 38.4% in 2020 and 44.3% in 2030, will face a consequent increase in the number of visually impaired people; therefore, this region will need more eye care professionals, including ophthalmologists.
- Residency training in ophthalmology must be redesigned in each country to include a uniform basic module based on contextual local needs.
- Unsupervised programs are a grave issue; only a few institutes offer standard and world-class sub-specialty training in ophthalmology in the South-East Asian region.
- Lack of exposure to newer diagnostic modalities, few opportunities to practice surgery during the residency program, and therefore, a low capacity to deal with complications during surgery are common problems in training.
- Lately, professional bodies have partnered with international organizations and eminent institutes to improve the standards of ophthalmic education and training programs.

In 2019, an estimated 2.2 billion people around the world were visually impaired [1], and in at least 1 billion people, the vision impairment could have been prevented or treated. Inadequate access to eye care contributes to a major part of the inequity and inequality in eye care services in most countries. System weaknesses across many countries, including high-income countries, have seen that trained and capacitated human resources contribute to this uneven distribution. While the integrated people-centered eye care (IPCEC) team approach is the foundation for rectifying this inequality, ophthalmologist-led referral networks have to meet the service needs of the population.

The report unequivocally admits that the shortage of trained human resources is one of the greatest challenges and significant barrier to increasing the availability of eye care services for prevention and treatment of eye problems. Globally, most eye care services are driven and delivered by ophthalmologists, whether it is per-

B. R. Shamanna (✉)
School of Medical Sciences, University of Hyderabad, Hyderabad, India

R. Bansal · S. G. Honavar
Centre for Sight, Hyderabad, India
e-mail: brsham@gmail.com

T. Das, P. D. Nayar (eds.), *South-East Asia Eye Health*,
https://doi.org/10.1007/978-981-16-3787-2_17

forming eye surgeries, treating common eye conditions, or handling sight-threatening conditions like glaucoma, diabetic retinopathy, and age-related macular degeneration.

17.1 Ophthalmology: A Global Picture

A recent study on the ophthalmology workforce in 198 countries has shown that practicing ophthalmologists are unequally distributed between urban and rural areas. The study further shows that not only is this distribution inequitable, but that there are fewer practicing ophthalmologists than those predicted by earlier projections (Fig. 17.1). In 2015, there were an estimated 232,866 ophthalmologists in 194 countries catering to 7.4 billion people with a mean number of 31.7 ophthalmologists/million population [2]. This publication also estimated that the number of ophthalmologists is growing annually at a rate of 2–3%. While training more ophthalmologists is important, an assessment of the contextual needs is also required. The recommendation of the study was to also focus on the appropriate distribution of ophthalmologists to ensure equity of eye care services and coverage for vulnerable groups to achieve universal eye and healthcare.

17.2 Ophthalmology: South-East Asia Region

The World Health Organization (WHO)–IAPB (International Agency for the Prevention of Blindness) South-East Asia Region includes 11 countries: Bangladesh, Bhutan, Democratic People's Republic (DPR) of Korea, India, Indonesia, the Maldives, Myanmar, Nepal, Sri Lanka, Thailand, and Timor-Leste [3]. The South-East Asia, East Asia, and Oceania Region as well as the South Asia Region are home to the greatest number of people who have vision loss (Fig. 17.2) [4]. These two regions are also home to 52% of the global population. The current numbers and densities of ophthalmologists in these regions are shown in Table 17.1 [5].

It is estimated that the WHO South-East Asia Region's share of the world population is likely to increase from 38.4% in 2020 to 44.3% in 2030, and so, this region will also face an increase in the number of visually impaired people. A projection made to achieve IPCEC in this region

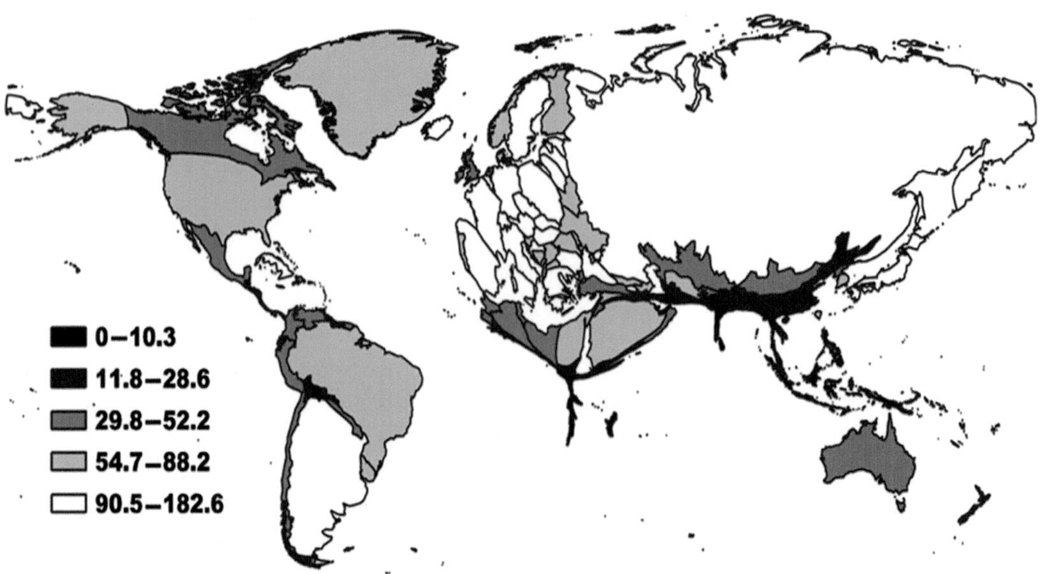

Fig. 17.1 Global distribution of ophthalmologist density (the number of ophthalmologists per million population) (Source: with permission from British Journal of Ophthalmology, 2020; doi: 10.1136/bjophthalmol-2019-314336)

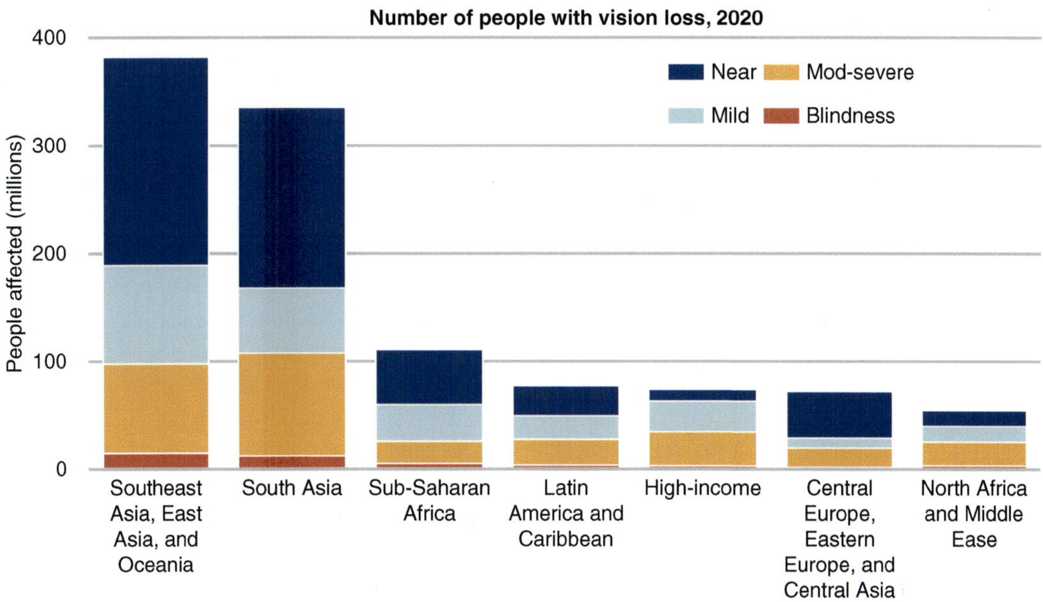

Fig. 17.2 Global burden of disease: region-specific vision loss in 2020 (Source: Vision Atlas 2020)

Table 17.1 Distribution of ophthalmologists in South-East Asia [5]

Country	Population (thousands)	Reported number of ophthalmologists	Ophthalmologists per million population
Bangladesh	160,996	1000	6.2
Bhutan	775	8	10.3
DPR Korea	25,155	1230	48.9
India	1,311,051	17,000	13.0
Indonesia	257,564	1300	5.0
Maldives	364	19	52.2
Myanmar	53,897	312	5.8
Nepal	28,514	240	8.4
Sri Lanka	20,715	104	5.0
Thailand	67,959	1300	19.1
Timor-Leste	1185	5	4.2

indicates that at least 429,802 community workers, 164,784 allied ophthalmic personnel (AOP), and 10,744 ophthalmologists will be required in public facilities by 2030 [6].

Due to unavailability of complete data sets on all cadres of eye health workers in all countries, it is difficult to accurately gauge the numbers of eye health workers in the South-East Asian region. However, since 2010, the numbers of ophthalmologists in this region have increased in all countries except probably Timor-Leste. But, some countries still rely on teams of service providers from other countries to meet their eye health needs. The ideal density of ophthalmologists is 1 per 100,000 people; this density has been achieved in only a few countries in the South-East Asian region, namely, Bhutan, India, the Maldives, and Thailand, but there is a gross urban–rural divide in the distribution of ophthalmologists. Additionally, the difficult terrain in three countries, namely, Bhutan, Nepal, and the Maldives, are important factors in the maldistribution of ophthalmologists, infrastructure, and delivery of eye care in these countries [7]. There is also a need for capacity building and proportionate distribution of human resources, including ophthalmologists for adequate rural reach and poverty alleviation. This is key to Universal Eye Health Coverage and charting the progress towards sustainable development goals.

17.3 Training and Education

"The goal of education is understanding, and the goal of training is performance" is a sentiment perfectly articulated by Frank Bell. A precise blend of the two, understanding and training, is mandatory for optimum output. Considering the integral role of this amalgam in the overall development of a budding ophthalmologist, regulatory associations have always emphasized the requirement for comprehensive training and education to residents. To deliver standardized care to patients, future generations of ophthalmologists must be trained and educated with well-equipped institutions functioning as per the guidelines set by regulatory bodies.

During this stage of transformation, residents need to catalogue their strengths and weaknesses and assume responsibility for patient care and active decision making, which must be an integral part of a well-structured educational system. Timor-Leste does not offer either a Bachelor's program in medicine or a Residency program in ophthalmology. Amongst those who provide training, several programs in many countries lack appropriate facilities and adequate funding. It becomes challenging to work with optimal proficiency without compromising on the quality of training and patient care. These countries also run on the concept of meritocracy, and there is a significant disparity in the training standards and exit criteria [8].

The two main perspectives of learning—behaviorism and constructivism (psychological and social)—are the pillars of growth for any resident and mold them into becoming more organized physically, emotionally, and intellectually. The concept of "*see one, do one, teach one*" has now been transformed into "*see many and learn from the outcome, do many under supervision and learn from the outcome, and finally, teach many with supervision and learn from the outcome*" [9]. Even though the Halstedian concept holds true for years together, in the current scenario, it is practical to be able to critically dissect one's own untoward outcomes and embrace what each surgical experience has to offer for successful evolution.

Plato was mentored by Socrates through incessant questioning and debate by which his perceptions of the universe were tested. Therefore, mentors play the most important roles in an ophthalmologist trainee's life [10]. Mentors motivate, empower, encourage, and nurture self-confidence; they teach, offer wise counsel, and raise the mentee's performance bar [11].

The primary aim of general ophthalmic education is to inculcate knowledge of appropriate examination techniques and basic principles mandatory for providing primary care [12]. With limited resources and an abundant need for optimal care, can it be possible to train, educate, and transform budding surgeons into independent and conscientious specialists with adequate skills, knowledge, and attitude? This usually depends on the basic module of training followed in the country based on individual needs and requirements in that region. With a well-crafted system set in place by regulatory authorities and state-of-the-art equipment, a holistic approach towards patient care without inexcusable errors is very much possible.

17.4 Curriculum and Competency

Medical academicians and specialists have been working tirelessly to provide a well-structured system and curriculum in different South-East Asian countries. A well-designed curriculum across several institutes of postgraduate excellence, training in research and ethics, appropriate selection of assessment tools, and promotion of teamwork and management skills are mandatory for collating existing knowledge and creating new paradigms. But the current educational systems in these countries demand that residents put in long hours in highly variable training programs in ill-defined accreditation standards [13]. Standardization is imperative for assuring competence amongst graduates so that they can render a consistent quality of service [14]. The

Table 17.2 Ophthalmology training in South-East Asian countries (2019)

	Countries	Number of years Masters	Diploma	End evaluation	Regulatory body
1	Bangladesh	3	2	Continuous assessments	Bangladesh Medical and Dental Council (BMDC)
2	Bhutan	2	NA	Continuous assessments	Bhutan Medical and Dental Council (BMDC)
3	DPR Korea	NA	2	NA	NA
4	India	3	2	Continuous assessments, Term-end examination	National Medical Commission (NMC) for Master of Science & Doctor of Medicine degrees; National Board of Examinations (for Diplomate of National Board or DNB)
5	Indonesia	4	–	Institution specific	Indonesia Medical Council
6	Maldives	3	–	Continuous assessments	Maldives Medical and Dental Council (MMDC)
7	Myanmar	2	2	NA	Myanmar Medical and Dental Council (MMDC)
8	Nepal	3	–	Term-end examination	National Academy of Medical Sciences
9	Sri Lanka	4	2	Progress reports, Peer team ratings, Continuous assessments	Sri Lankan Medical Council
10	Thailand	3	–	Continuous assessments, Term-end examination	The Medical Council of Thailand
11	Timor-Leste	NA	NA	NA	NA

NA not available

ophthalmology curricula currently offered in different South-East Asian countries are enlisted in Table 17.2.

India has taken initiatives to meet the challenges of disparate training systems and maintain standards by inviting examiners from the United Kingdom Royal Colleges [13]. Bangladesh is making efforts to ensure quality control for all postgraduate courses at state medical schools. The lack of revalidation and lack of a system to provide credits for educational activities in several South-East Asian countries leave professional colleges unsupervised. The scattered educational system in several countries poses a major challenge to eye care service.

Keeping in mind the required knowledge and skills for effective and safe practice in ophthalmology, and taking into account the social milieu and disease patterns specific to India, a detailed preferred curriculum has been outlined. This curriculum also enlists the minimum infrastructure required for mandatory diagnostic and therapeutic procedures needed for optimal training. Suggestions for the inclusion of an overview of hospital management, practice management, and financial management in the curriculum have also been suggested to ensure professionalism in medical graduates from the grassroots training level. These aspirational guidelines were designed based on the assessment of surgical skills (Ophthalmology Surgical Competency Assessment Rubric, OSCAR) and Ophthalmic Clinical Evaluation Exercise (OCEX), as adapted from the curriculum of the International Council of Ophthalmology (ICO) [15]. An integrated curriculum must include knowledge about basic medical sciences, clinical skills, optics and refraction, super-specialties, ophthalmic pathological/microbiological/biochemical sciences, community ophthalmology, research approach, medical ethics, management, and communication skills [16].

Establishing national and centralized sources and transitioning to a competency-based education system with optimized resources and faculty support should be of great help. Incorporating the six Accreditation Council for Graduate Medical Education (ACGME) competencies—patient care and procedural skills, medical knowledge, system-based practice, practice-based learning and improvement, professionalism, and interpersonal and communication skills [17]—will further enhance ophthalmology education.

17.5 Sub-specialty Training

An excellent foundation of comprehensive ophthalmology is essential to build sub-specialty skills further. As a resident masters the fundamentals of the subject, it becomes easier for him/her to think and work independently. In India, the NMC (National Medical Commission) and the NBE (National Board of Education) have introduced recognized fellowship programs and Master of Chirurgiae (MCh) degrees in several institutes; this is a welcome step towards progress in encouraging ophthalmology as a sub-specialty for specialized and categorized care.

Various studies have highlighted that immediately after completing a fellowship, several trainees from different sub-specialties were not confident in using their newly acquired skills and expressed the need for restructuring in the programs. There were varied opinions among faculty within any given institution [18]. However, there was a satisfactory increment in the research projects undertaken and publications by such fellows as compared to those who did not pursue such programs. The trainees also expressed the need for additional knowledge about trade and industry to be able to choose the equipment and consumables required in their practice [18]. It is mandatory to encourage independent thinking, networking, technical training, critical thinking, creative imagination, and attendance in various national and international conferences and webinars at the sub-specialty level. There is a need for exchange of knowledge between students of developed and developing countries to promote the import of high-end technology and preferred practice patterns.

Apprenticeship-based training encourages professionalism and helps in acquisition of standard and transferable skills for the progression of a career. It helps build the next generation of reliable ophthalmologists. The appraisal-based training programs, followed in many developed countries, also seem promising. In such programs, mentors make every effort to unmask the untapped potential of the mentee. It is the last step of training before the mentees begin their independent careers and transform into researchers, teachers, and leaders [19].

17.6 Harmonization

In India, the recent shift of regulation between regulatory bodies (from the MCI (Medical Council of India) to NMC) is believed to have brought a significant change in how medical professionals, government officials, and various medical institutions provide standardized and high-quality medical education and adequate infrastructure [20]. It is hoped that the collective wisdom of the parliamentarians, medical professionals, governments, and professional medical organizations will prevail. The deficiencies in the current form of the NMC Bill will be addressed sufficiently to help provide standardized and high-quality medical education at all levels. This may aid in neutralizing the healthcare paradox in India.

17.7 Barriers and Solutions

The All India Ophthalmology Society (AIOS), with a member strength of over 17,000 ophthalmologists, conducted a survey to collect data on how young ophthalmologists viewed their own professional competence and the limiting factors in their pursuit for patient care. The survey revealed that several residents were not exposed to the latest diagnostic modalities. The residents had some of the best theoretical knowledge, but they lacked confidence in dealing with surgical complications. This was partly due to a lack of modern instrumentation and training [21]. Residents were also less inclined to take on research, publish papers, and undertake wet laboratory workups even though a dissertation had been a part of their training schedule [22].

Over the last few decades, with the advent of advanced technology and emphasis on rehabilitation and disease management, postgraduate training in ophthalmology has improved in various countries in the South-East Asian region [23]. Despite ongoing efforts by the governments, regulatory bodies, medical college authorities, and international organizations, only a few reports have highlighted the opinions and feedback of medical postgraduate students. Studies have indicated a low level of satisfaction in residents; this could be related to the lack of supervision and relatively few chances for surgical training, especially in procedures like phacoemulsification and non-cataract surgery [24]. Even though their knowledge about refraction was appropriate, the residents' exposure to low-vision aids and their skills in writing up prescriptions remained grossly inadequate. Most residents felt the need for regular performance evaluations, further training in basic examination techniques, use of advanced equipment, wet lab training, and regular access to internet facilities [25–28]. Understandably, the residents-in-training are not considered appropriate critics of what is best for them as their perspectives and outlooks are limited, and they could have unrealistic expectations [14].

The lack of uniformity in the assessment patterns in different institutions in the same region cannot be ignored. Several countries also must address the deficiency of dedicated curricula or teaching hours for public health ophthalmology. With most of the world's population living in South-East Asian countries, community eye care cannot be ignored. The residents must also learn to assess patients' psychological and social problems. It is encouraging that the faculty-to-student ratio has improved significantly in the past few years; this will enhance mentor–mentee relationships and add to the apprenticeship pool in this region.

VISION 2020 by the WHO has escalated the acceptance of several productive national-level programs and involvement of non-governmental organizations (NGOs) in eye care service training in these countries. However, the maldistribution of available resources at the central level has proven to be a prime obstacle in the path of eye care training development.

17.8 Partnerships, Professional Bodies, and Progress

The International Council of Ophthalmology (ICO), a global organization, has been working in partnership with supranational and ICO member societies to ensure high-end education and quality patient care worldwide. With the concept of "World Alliance for Sight" and the initiative of "Refocusing Ophthalmic Education," ICO has been successfully redefining teaching tools, educational residency and fellowship programs, conferences, team training models, web-based teaching courses, webinar network, and communication technologies for teaching and learning in multiple languages to ensure collaborations and exchanges of ideas and outlooks between professionals [29].

Accreditation is essential. Accreditation in Indonesia and Thailand is based on the regulations laid down by the Indonesia Medical Council and the Medical Council of Thailand, respectively [30]. The College of Ophthalmologists of Sri Lanka, established in 1991 (continuation of the Ophthalmological Society of Sri Lanka, founded in 1957), is the only professional body of ophthalmologists in the country [31]. The Sri Lankan Medical Council is responsible for protecting healthcare workers and maintaining academic and professional standards in the country [32]. Regulatory bodies in India like the MCI (now replaced by the NMC) and the National Board of Examinations for the DNB have been keeping the ophthalmology curriculum for training at par with developed countries over the decades with the best possible regulations along with the mindful contributions of the national ophthalmology professional body (All India Ophthalmological Society) [33]. Bhutan (Medical and Health Council Act 2002), Bangladesh, the Maldives, and Myanmar have their respective Medical and Health Councils to regulate postgraduate courses [34, 35]. These countries have established MoUs (memorandums of understanding) with international institutions for specialty training. Bangladesh follows the regulations and curriculum designed by regulatory bodies like the ICO and the Royal College of Ophthalmologists. The Government of Nepal has established the National Academy of Medical Sciences (NAMS) to provide trained professionals, high-quality health services, and conduct research in specialty health services [36].

A need for individualized, region-specific curricula in various countries is highly recommended to overcome deficiencies in expertise and ensure that eye care providers receive high standards of training, regulation, and certification.

17.9 Health Systems Approach in the South-East Asian Region

South Asia, South-East Asia, East Asia, and Oceania, where 52% of the world's population live, are also home to an estimated 64% of all people with vision loss (Vision Atlas 2020; *www.iapb.org*). This is in contrast to the high-income regions, which have 14% of the global population, and only bear 7% of the worldwide burden of vision impairment [1].

The solutions to help the visually challenged in South-East Asia region are:

- Eye care treatments are available and cost-effective: Trained ophthalmologists are critical to addressing the cataract-related vision impairment burden in the region.
- Increasing access to eye care services will prevent vision loss: IPCEC (Integrated People-Centered Eye Care) requires a continuum of health interventions that can address the full spectrum of eye conditions according to people's needs and throughout their life course; this depends on leveraging the role of ophthalmologists in the chain of service delivery efficiently.
- Affordable eye care services are required to meet demands: Under the UHC (Universal Health Coverage), everyone should receive the full spectrum of essential, quality health services they need, including eye care, without suffering financial hardship; the role of the ophthalmologist in this system is crucial.

A health system consists of all organizations, institutions, resources, and people whose primary purpose is to improve health. The health system delivers preventive, promotive, curative, and rehabilitative interventions through a combination of public health and healthcare facilities, providing healthcare by both state and non-state actors. The WHO framework structures health systems in terms of six core components or "building blocks," which are: (1) leadership and governance, (2) financing, (3) health workforce, (4) service delivery, (5) access to essential medicines, and (6) health information systems. Strengthening health systems involves strengthening each of these areas.

Many countries in the South-East Asian region have an established health system. The region has demonstrated very significant and visible leadership and governance for service delivery initiatives by establishing national eye care programs and health policies several decades ago (for example, the National Blindness and Visual Impairment Program, 1976, in India). Also, there is ample evidence that these countries invest in health workforce and education improvements. Financial commitments for eye programs and leveraging information technology for communication have also seen rapid growth in this region. Indigenization and local production of medicines, consumables, and even fabrication of equipment have given a boost to many eye care programs in this region.

Many countries in the region have well-trained ophthalmologists, but their distribution and other enabling factors hinder their service initiatives. Deficiencies exist in exposure to diagnostic and surgical methods. Certification and validation procedures are not universal; clinical audits are still not standard practice. These aspects impact quality. With improved access to information technology, innovations in capacity building and education are needed within the region. While it reduces the cost of care, it also helps with the standardization of service delivery norms and fostering the best-practice models.

17.10 Moving Towards Universal Eye Health in the South-East Asia Region

It is estimated that if the WHO South-East Asia Region adopts the IPCEC system, it would require at least 429,802 community workers, 164,784 allied ophthalmic personnel, and 10,744 ophthalmologists in public eye care facilities by 2030 [6]. The region has also witnessed improved cataract surgical rates and quality of cataract surgery over the past two decades. The gains in the region have reduced the global magnitudes of blindness and vision impairment. Nevertheless, eye care infrastructure and the availability of appropriate human resources for eye care vary considerably across this region [37]. Adequate focus on health systems strengthening, boosting primary eye care, and generating evidence of progress made through monitoring and evaluation mechanisms will be imperative for realizing the goal of eliminating avoidable blindness from the region in coming years [38, 39].

The WHO Global Action Plan for eye health 2014–2019 [40] which focused on universal access to eye care emphasized that health systems strengthening and integrating eye care into the health system delivery were of prime importance. Countries in the region have worked towards universalizing eye care for all by strengthening health systems and developing human resources with an eye care team approach, financial allocation, setting up infrastructure, and making available affordable medicines and supplies. The augmented management information systems have substantially aided in improving service delivery and patient care. Sustained efforts through motivational leadership and governance have been hallmarks in the South-East Asia Region programs. Of particular note are the investments in quality-driven service delivery, which have been central to local eye care needs, coupled with monitoring and evaluation mechanisms to track the region's overall eye health progress. Strengthening eye care through concerted action involving multiple stakeholders and fostering long-term partnerships with multiple players will be critical in realizing the goal of eliminating avoidable blindness in the South-East Asian region and charting the progress towards the SDGs [37].

17.11 The Way Forward

Currently, consideration of equity is weak in the eye health plans of the South-East Asia Region countries. There is a need for disaggregated data that will help shape priorities and address the most marginalized people's eye care needs in the context of the IPCEC system. Promoting universal eye health is central to achieving UHC. Countries in this region and their development partners should work collectively to advocate for and achieve improved outcomes for preventable and treatable conditions [41]. The role of the ophthalmologist as a "5 star" professional (care provider, decision-maker, communicator, community leader, and manager) [42] in the regional eye health programs will now become even more critical. Grillo's historical review about the developments in residency training and improvements in the standard of care in South-East Asian countries is an inspiring account that can encourage people to resolve major lacunae in the system and address current issues dogging the eye care delivery system [43].

It is mandatory to encourage and train ophthalmologists to make timely diagnoses, develop and reformat treatment plans specific to patients, and critically assess outcomes. The cyclic nature of institutional virtue has to be kept in mind while breaking the aforementioned barriers; this entails the acceptance that the current system had probably been part of considerable controversy in the past [44, 45].

The way forward is to resolve our current problems by assessing existing protocols and curricula and updating them in a timely manner to ensure attainment of greater heights. Ultimately, there is a need to ensure that eye care workforce planning is an integral part of health workforce planning in the South-East Asian region, with the roles and responsibilities of the ophthalmologist factored into the milieu.

RECOMMENDATIONS

- A comprehensive registry to document all available human resources for health, including ophthalmologists who practice surgery or only provide consultation. Periodic updating of this registry is critical.
- Designing a uniform and basic ophthalmologist training module aligned to contextual country/ region specific needs.
- Establishment of surgical wet labs.
- Uniformity in the quality of the ophthalmologist, standards of curricula, and accreditation with systems of trained supervision.
- At least one center of excellence that can train a specialist for every 0.5 million population is needed; this center must also be enabled to address specialty needs in ophthalmology.
- Ophthalmologists must receive training in newer diagnostic modalities, be offered enough surgical opportunities, and have mentorship that will allow them to develop the capacity to deal with surgical complications independently.
- Create an enabling environment for research.
- Professional bodies should continue to invest time and effort in the South-East Asian region through partnerships with international organizations and eminent institutes to improve the standards of ophthalmic education and training programs.

References

1. World report on vision. Geneva: World Health Organization; 2019.
2. Resnikoff S, Lansingh VC, Washburn L, et al. Estimated number of ophthalmologists' worldwide (International Council of Ophthalmology update): will we meet the needs? Br J Ophthalmol. 2020;104:588–92.
3. Vision Atlas. www.iapb.org/learn/vision-atlas. Accessed 16 Oct 2020.
4. Bourne R, Jaimie A, Seth F, et al. Trends in prevalence of blindness and distance and near vision impairment over 30 years and contribution to the Global Burden of Disease in 2020. Lancet Glob Health. 2020. Advanced online publication. https://doi.org/10.2139/ssrn.3582742.
5. Resnikoff S, Lansingh VC, Washburn L, et al. Estimated number of ophthalmologists' worldwide (International Council of Ophthalmology update): will we meet the needs? Br J Ophthalmol. 2020;104-4-588-inline-supplementary material-1.
6. Das T, Keeffe J, Sivaprasad S, et al. Capacity building for universal eye health coverage in South East Asia beyond 2020. Eye (London). 2020;34:1262–70.
7. Sapkota YD. Human resources for eye health in South Asia. Community Eye Health J. 2018;31:S1–2.
8. Honavar SG. Ophthalmology residency training in India: Quo vadis? Indian J Ophthalmol. 2017;65:427–8.
9. Rohrich RJ. "See one, do one, teach one": an old adage with a new twist. Plastic Reconstructive Surg. 2006;118:257–8.
10. Assael LA. Every surgeon needs mentors: a Halsteadian/Socratic model in the modern age. J Oral Maxillofacial Surg. 2010;68:1217–8.
11. Honavar SG. Mentoring is a serious business. Indian J Ophthalmol. 2019;67:1915–7.
12. Shuttleworth GN, Marsh GW. How effective is undergraduate and postgraduate teaching in ophthalmology? Eye (Lond). 1997;11:744–50.
13. Mendis L, Adkoli BV, Adhikari RK, et al. Postgraduate medical education in South Asia. Br Med J. 2004;328:779. https://doi.org/10.1136/bmj.328.7443.779.
14. Gogate P, Biswas P, Natarajan S, et al. Residency evaluation and adherence design study: young ophthalmologists' perception of their residency programs – clinical and surgical skills. Indian J Ophthalmol. 2017;65:452–60.
15. Grover AK, Honavar SG, Azad R, et al. A national curriculum for ophthalmology residency training. Indian J Ophthalmol. 2018;66:752–83.
16. Honavar SG. Steps to standardize ophthalmology residency programs in India. Indian J Ophthalmol. 2018;66:733–9.
17. Golnik KC, Lee AG, Wilson MC. A national program director survey of the shift to competency-

based education in ophthalmology. Ophthalmology. 2008;115:1426–30.
18. Narayanan R, Gupta SR, Honavar SG. Fellowship training in India: how to produce leaders? Indian J Ophthalmol. 2018;66:1671–2.
19. Pandey SK, Sharma V. Ophthalmology training and teaching in India: how these young ophthalmologists can become leaders of tomorrow? Indian J Ophthalmol. 2018;66:1517–8.
20. Honavar SG. National Medical Commission Bill, 2019 – Good intent but unmet expectations. Indian J Ophthalmol. 2019;67:1259–60.
21. Thomas R, Dogra M. An evaluation of medical college departments of ophthalmology in India and change following provision of modern instrumentation and training. Indian J Ophthalmol. 2008;56:9–16.
22. Gogate PM, Biswas P, Natarajan S, et al. Residency evaluation and adherence design study: young ophthalmologists' perception of their residency programs II: Academics and research dissertation. Indian J Ophthalmol. 2017;65:12–8.
23. Biswas P, Gogate PM, Maskati QB, et al. Residency Evaluation and Adherence Design Study III: Ophthalmology residency training in India: then and now–improving with time? Indian J Ophthalmol. 2018;66:785–92.
24. Young AL, Jhanji V, Liang Y, et al. A survey of perceived training differences between ophthalmology residents in Hong Kong and China. BMC Med Educ. [Internet]. 2015 [cited 2020 Oct 31];15. https://www.ncbi.nlm.nih.gov/pmc/articles/PMC4587816. https://doi.org/10.1186/s12909-015-0440-0.
25. Gogate P, Deshpande M, Dharmadhikari S. Which is the best method to learn ophthalmology? Resident doctors' perspective of ophthalmology training. Indian J Ophthalmol. 2008;56:409–12.
26. Ajay K, Krishnaprasad R, Divya DS. Ophthalmic surgical training in Karnataka and Southern India: present status and future interests from a survey of final-year residents. Indian J Ophthalmol. 2015;63:306–11.
27. Ajay K, Krishnaprasad R. Feedback of final year ophthalmology postgraduates about their residency ophthalmology training in South India. Indian J Ophthalmol. 2014;62:814–7.
28. Murthy GVS, Gupta SK, Bachani D, et al. Status of speciality training in ophthalmology in India. Indian J Ophthalmol. 2005;53:135–42.
29. Golnik K, Mayorga E, Spivey B, et al. International Council of Ophthalmology: Refocusing ophthalmic education in the Asia-Pacific Region and beyond. Asia Pac J Ophthalmol (Phila). 2012;1:255–8.
30. The Medical Council of Thailand. www.tmc.or.th/En/. Accessed 2 Nov 2020.
31. The College of Ophthalmologists of Sri Lanka. www.cosl.lk/. Accessed 2 Nov 2020.
32. SLMC Web Site – Sri Lanka Medical Council. www.srilankamedicalcouncil.org/. Accessed 2 Nov 2020.
33. Medical Council. www.srilankamedicalcouncil.org/. Accessed 2 Nov 2020.
34. National Board of Examination. https://www.natboard.edu.in/. Accessed 31 Oct 2020.
35. Bhutan Medical and Health Council. https://www.bmhc.gov.bt/. Accessed 2 Nov 2020.
36. Bangladesh Medical Research Council Bulletin. www.banglajol.info/index.php/BMRCB. Accessed 2 Nov 2020.
37. NAMS. https://nams.org.np/. Accessed 2 Nov 2020.
38. Murthy GVS. Eye care in South Asia, 1988–2018: developments, achievements and future challenges. Community Eye Health J. 2017;30:99–101.
39. Murthy GVS, Malhotra S, Vashist P. Status of eye care in South East Asia Region. Delhi J Ophthalmol. 2013;24:114–8.
40. Murthy GVS, Shamanna BR. Tackling the challenges of eye care in India. A roadmap to India's health. Independent Commission on Development & Health in India. Voluntary Health Association of India, New Delhi, India, 2018. p. 235–9.
41. WHO Report. Universal eye health: a global action plan 2014-2019. Geneva: WHO; 2013.
42. Ramke J, Zwi AB, Silva JC, et al. Evidence for national universal eye health plans. Bull World Health Organ. 2018;96:695–704.
43. Boelen C. From fragmentation to unity in health care: a challenging journey. Changing medical education and medical practice, June 1996:2. www.who.int/hrh/en/HRDJ_1_1_02.pdf. Accessed 2 Nov 2020.
44. Schwartz SI. The evolution of medical education. Surgery. 1999;125:17–8.
45. Ritchie WP. Graduate education: how we got to where we are. Surgery. 1999;125:15–6. https://doi.org/10.1016/S0039-6060(99)70281-3.

Optometry in South-East Asia

18

Kovin Naidoo, Anitha Arvind,
Carmen Abesamos-Dichoso, Kah Ooi Tan,
and Pirindha Govender-Poonsamy

Key Points

- There is significant variation in the level of training and scope of practice for optometrists in South-East Asia.
- The number of optometrists needed in the region is calculated based on an optometrist to population ratio of 1:10,000, a ratio where optometrists function in a primary care capacity.
- There is a substantial maldistribution of optometrists in the region, which contributes significantly to the paucity of this cadre even where the numbers of optometrists may satisfy the requirement (Fig. 18.1).

K. Naidoo (✉)
African Vision Research Institute: UKZN, Durban, South Africa

School of Optometry, University of New South Wales, Sydney, Australia
e-mail: kovin.naidoo@essilor.com

A. Arvind
Optometry Practitioner, Chennai, India

C. Abesamos-Dichoso
Asia Pacific Council of Optometry, Manila, Philippines

K. O. Tan
Asia Optometric Congress, Hong Kong, Hong Kong
e-mail: kahooi@nthalmic.com

P. Govender-Poonsamy
AVRI: University of KwaZulu-Natal, Global Ophthalmic Institute, Durban, South Africa
e-mail: govenderp@ukzn.ac.za

The World Council of Optometry (WCO) defines optometry as a healthcare profession that is autonomous, educated, and regulated (licensed/registered). Optometrists are the primary healthcare practitioners of the eye and visual system, who provide comprehensive eye and vision care that includes refraction and spectacle dispensing, detection/diagnosis and management of diseases of the eye, and the rehabilitation of conditions of the visual system [1]. Despite this definition, there is great variation in training and scope of practice for optometrists across the world; South-East Asia is no exception. The WCO has recognized these variations and developed a competency model to identify the level at which the optometrists practice in different situations. There are four categories of optometrists based on the scope of practice and competencies [2] (Table 18.1).

The role of optometry differs depending on the scope of practice. However, the aim is to upgrade all optometry functions to level 4 competency so that the profession can fully contribute to comprehensive eye health, especially at a time when human resources for eye care are inadequate.

The scope of practice has a significant impact on the integration of optometry into public health systems. In some instances, optometry is primarily, if not exclusively, confined to the private sector with limited articulation with public health systems. Optometry in South-East Asian countries is yet to attain its highest professional scope of practice compared to its western counterparts.

T. Das, P. D. Nayar (eds.), *South-East Asia Eye Health*,
https://doi.org/10.1007/978-981-16-3787-2_18

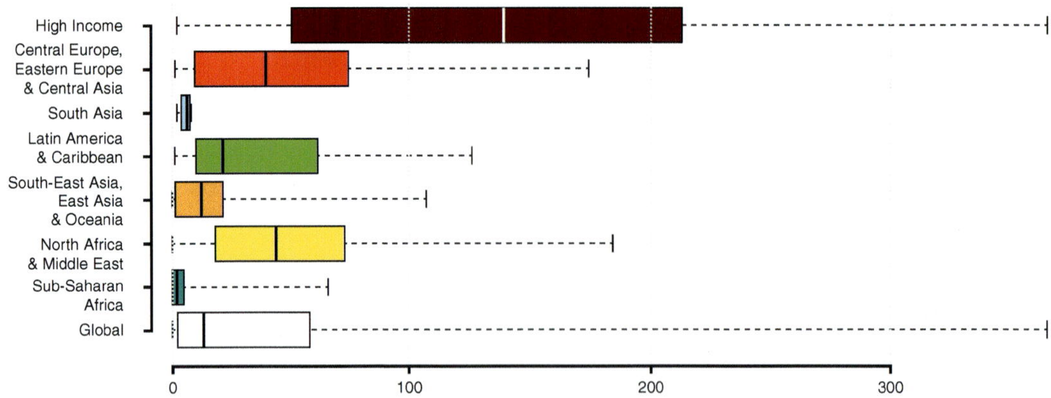

Fig. 18.1 The number of optometrists per million population in 128 countries for which data is available (Source: IAPB Vision Atlas 2017)

Table 18.1 Competency and scope of work at different levels of optometry service [2]

Competency level	Nomenclature	Capabilities
1	Optical Technology (OT) services	Management and dispensing of ophthalmic lenses, ophthalmic frames, and other ophthalmic devices that correct defects of the visual system.
2	Visual Function (VF) services	OT + Investigation, examination, measurement, recognition, and correction/ management of defects of the visual system (note: practitioners at Level 2 are considered to be optometrists).
3	Ocular Diagnostic (ODx) services	OT + VF + Examination and evaluation of the eye and adnexa, and associated systemic factors; to detect, diagnose, and manage the disease.
4	Ocular Therapeutic (OTx) services	OT+ VF + ODx + Use of pharmaceutical agents and other procedures to manage ocular conditions/diseases.

Optometry education, as well as the scope of practice, is varied in South-East Asia. Densely populated countries like India are yet to fully recognize optometry as a health profession. In absence of proper licensing system, regulation, and career development, the graduate optometrists in India have only a limited scope of practice despite the huge potential for development of this profession.

Different cadres of eye care practitioners exist in the South-East Asian region, offering different levels of service to the public. In the developed world, optometrists are primary eye care practitioners who are institutionally educated and clinically trained in the art and science of optometry [3]. They play a major role in preventive eye healthcare systems [4]. In the developing world, the optometrists function at either the primary level (mainly in the private sector) or the secondary level as a part of the eye health team.

Despite this variation in scope, optometry is the primary provider of refractive services. Globally, refractive error is the leading cause of vision impairment and the second leading cause of blindness [5]. Therefore, this elevates the role of optometry in addressing blindness and vision impairment in South-East Asia. Also, the myopia is fast emerging as a leading public health challenge of our time. The current prevalence of myopia in the South-East Asian region is expected to increase from 46.1% to 62% by 2050, when the global average will be around 50% [6]. The additional impact of myopia, particularly high myopia, on ocular diseases such as myopic macular degeneration, glaucoma, early-onset cataract, and retinal detachment, places a greater focus on the role of optometry in healthcare systems, at least insofar as diagnosing eye diseases are concerned. Therefore, the scope and level of training of these professionals have to be urgently addressed. But the numbers of optometrists in the South-East Asian region are inadequate to meet the needs of this region.

The World Health Organization (WHO) has suggested that there should be at least 1 optometrist for 100,000 people by 2010 and reach a ratio of 1:50,000 by the year 2020 in underserved populations [7]. However, in an optimal setting where optometrists serve as primary eye care practitioners, a ratio of approximately 1:10,000 is ideal [8]. To achieve such an optometrist to population ratio (1:10,000) in the major South-East Asian countries (India, Indonesia, Nepal, Sri Lanka, and Thailand) which have a collective population of 1773 million [9], at least 177,388 optometrists will be required. According to a study conducted by the WCO, African Vision Research Institute, and Brien Holden Vision Institute, these South-East Asian countries currently have only 82,581 optometrists (less than 50% of the required number). These numbers are obviously inadequate to meet the rising prevalence of myopia and the subsequent demand for clinical services. With the current training trajectory, the chances of the numbers of optometrists increasing in immediate future are very bleak. Hence, optometry must partner with other Primary vision care cadres to develop an ecosystem that ensures that refractive services reach the most vulnerable and underserved people in society. For example, in India, the Eye Mitra program (Essilor) has empowered primary vision care providers to provide eye care services in rural areas. Technology allows optometrists to link-up with such programs and provide oversight and mentoring, thus expanding the contribution that optometrists can make to strengthen such programs.

Optometry has not been central to blindness prevention efforts in this region. This includes involvement in organizations such as the International Agency for the Prevention of Blindness (IAPB). Given the prevalence of refractive error and its relative importance to blindness and vision impairment, this needs to be rapidly addressed. Appropriately addressing refractive error as a cause of blindness and vision impairment will make a huge contribution to blindness prevention efforts in the region. In this respect, greater involvement of national associations in national and regional IAPB structures is important.

Advocacy has to be a key aspect of optometry in South-East Asia. It should encompass efforts to engender support for the expansion of optometry training, development of regulatory frameworks for the profession, development of optometry posts in the public health system, and integration of optometry in blindness prevention efforts. Furthermore, optometry should play a central role in advocating government efforts to address uncorrected refractive error and access to affordable eye care.

The following is the state of optometry in the key countries of the South-East Asian Region:

Bangladesh

Optometry is an autonomous healthcare profession in Bangladesh. This is not a regulated profession; optometrists offer services to the public as allied eye care personnel. In this country, ophthalmologists currently carry the major burden of providing primary eye care services.

Optometry education

Optometry education is not uniform and may be offered as a 4-year program or even a 1- or 2-year diploma program in Bangladesh by private institutions. Several short-term courses ranging from 1 to 6 months are also offered across Bangladesh in refraction, orthoptics, and low vision correction. Optometry education is fragmented across the country.

Scope of practice of optometry

Due to an unregulated environment, the scope of practice of optometry is ill-defined, with optometrists primarily offering services such as refraction, low vision detection and correction, and orthoptics. The Bangladesh Optometric Society (BOS) is the professional body that represents optometrists in Bangladesh.

Distribution of visual impairment (VI) and uncorrected refractive error (URE)

Cataract is the leading cause of avoidable blindness in Bangladesh [10]. The national blindness and low vision survey reported that cataract (74%) and followed by refractive error (19%) were the leading causes of low vision [11]. A recent study on eye diseases among adults in an urban slum population in Bangladesh showed a high prevalence of refractive errors (63%) that calls to provide primary eye care to the population [12].

Shortage of personnel

There is an acute shortage of ophthalmic personnel in Bangladesh, with 1200 optometrists and ophthalmic technicians offering optometry services to the public at a ratio of 1:135,989 [13].

Bhutan

Eye care services are free for all citizens and are integrated at all levels of the healthcare system in Bhutan. Recently, the first eye hospital capable of providing specialized eye care services and subspecialization services in eye care was opened in Bhutan. It will be serving as the national referral center in Bhutan, supporting primary and secondary level eye care at the regional and district levels [14]. Optometrists are a recognized cadre of eye care professionals in Bhutan and are regulated by the Bhutan Medical and Health Council (BMHC).

Optometry education

There are no schools for optometry education in Bhutan. Interested students gain their optometry education overseas. Optometry posts are open for those having an undergraduate degree in optometry (Bachelor of Optometry) or a Doctor of Optometry (OD).

Scope of practice of optometry

The Quality Assurance and Standardization Division (QASD) and the Ministry of Health in Bhutan have laid down the standards of practice and delivery of eye care services for the Kingdom of Bhutan. Optometrists registered to practice and posted within Bhutan's healthcare system are permitted to use approved pharmaceutical agents for diagnostic and therapeutic purposes. No private practice of optometry is allowed in Bhutan. The job description for optometrists includes:

- Eye examination including diagnosis, treatment, and management of eye diseases, and referral of complicated cases to ophthalmologists for further treatment.
- Provision of non-surgical treatment for all eye problems including low vision rehabilitation, vision therapy, and provision of spectacle and contact lenses.
- Involved in teaching and training of technicians.
- Involved in planning, implementation, and monitoring of health activities in districts.
- Involved in conducting relevant research with the concerned authorities.

Distribution of VI and URE

A recent survey in Bhutan showed that untreated cataract was the most prevalent cause (54%) of blindness, 57% of severe vision impairment, and 65% of moderate visual impairment [15]. Uncorrected refractive errors were the main cause of early visual impairment (47%).

Shortage of personnel

Currently, eye care services for the entire population of Bhutan (773,278) are offered by 54 ophthalmic technicians, 9 ophthalmologists, and 9 optometrists [14]. To be able to reach the ideal optometrists to population ratio of 1:10,000, Bhutan would need 77 optometrists providing services. The Government of Bhutan has a goal to become the first country in the world to be free of uncorrected poor vision and has inked a partnership with Essilor to sustainably strengthen the country's vision care infrastructure through training and capacity building, philanthropic support, and awareness-raising.

India

Optometry in India is fragmented, although this country had opened its first school of optometry (offering a 2-year diploma program) in 1958. Optometry is not yet recognized as an independent healthcare profession in the country and remains unregulated. The government recognizes diploma and degree courses in optometry education (at the undergraduate, postgraduate, and doctoral levels) but does not define their entry and exit competencies, thereby resulting in a cadre with significant variations in knowledge and skills. Optometrists in the country mainly offer refractive services to the public, and their scope of practice is defined by the place of work. Ophthalmologists share the current burden of providing basic and comprehensive eye examinations to the public in the country.

Optometry education

The unregulated environment for optometry in India and the huge demand for meeting the eye care needs of the population have led to various training programs with multiple competencies which increase the possibilities for unethical practice. The Government of India recognizes optometry education offered either as a diploma by the State Medical Council or as a degree under the University Grants Commission (UGC). Optometry degree programs are currently offered as 4-year undergraduate programs and as 2-year masters programs at a few universities. Doctoral programs are also offered at a couple of universities across the country.

Scope of practice of optometry

The scope of practice of optometry in India is poorly defined (Indian Express, 2011). Different cadres of eye care providers conduct eye examinations, including refraction, with varying aptitudes and preparation programs. Optometrists are primarily involved in refractive services, followed by optical dispensing, contact lens dispensing, and low vision correction services. Optometrists' scope of practice is dictated by the place of practice with hospital-based optometrists being involved in diagnostic services and optical outlet-based optometrists being involved in optical dispensing and refractive services. Optometrists in India are placed at Level 2 of the WCO global competency-based model of the scope of practice as they do not have the legal rights to use pharmaceutical agents for diagnostic and/or therapeutic purposes.

Distribution of VI and URE

Blindness and VI are two of the most significant public health issues in India, which is home to 20.5% of the world's blind, 22.2% of the world's low vision population, and 21.9% of those with VI [16]. Cataract is the leading cause of avoidable blindness in India, followed by uncorrected refractive errors [16, 17].

Shortage of personnel

Currently, ophthalmologists in India shoulder most of the burden of providing basic and comprehensive eye care to the Indian population. The ophthalmologist to population ratio in urban India is 1:25,000, while in rural India, it is 1:219,000 [18, 19]. With respect to optometry and spectacle provision, published data show that India has 9000 optometrists who have undergone training for a minimum of 4 years and 40,000 ophthalmic technicians/assistants who have undergone training for 2 years (India Optometric Federation, 2010). In 2010, India required 115,000 trained optometrists to provide comprehensive vision care for all. A more recent estimation has shown that to serve a population of 1.3 billion people [9], 138,000 optometrists will be required. However, India has less than half that number, with only 64,000 optometrists functioning at various levels of competency.

Indonesia

Optometry is a recognized profession in Indonesia. All optometrists need to have a license to practice and renew their license every 5 years after fulfilling Continuous Professional Development (CPD) requirements. However, there is no formal legislation regulating the scope of practice of optometrists or opticians in the country. There are 8600 optometrists in Indonesia, the majority with a 3-year diploma. There is also a unique network of primary vision care providers, known as Optik Keliling (Mobile Optician) in Indonesia; these vision care providers travel on motorcycles to perform basic vision screenings and dispense glasses outside of the cities. Essilor is working to upskill these entrepreneurs with specialist training to continue to provide affordable and quality vision care across the semi-rural and rural Indonesia. Given the population of the country and the time taken to train optometrists, partnerships with such cadres and a link-up with tele-optometry need to be developed.

Optometry education

There are 11 schools at the diploma level, which produce approximately 40–50 students per year per school. The most established is the Academy of Optometry Leprindo. One program at Ukrida University (established in 2018/2019) offers a 4-year degree program in optometry.

Professional associations

Optometrists are represented by their professional association, the Ikatan Refraksionis Optisien Indonesia (IROPIN), the Indonesia Optometrists Association [20]. The association collaborates with the Department of Health to arrange vision screening in different provinces of Indonesia. Indonesia's population is 273.5 million [9]; there is a need for 27,352 optometrists to have an ideal optometrist to population ratio of 1:10,000. However, as of now, there are only 8600 optometrists in the county.

Challenges

Capacity building is necessary to improve the scope and quality of service. Furthermore, there is a need to upgrade the current practitioners with diploma qualifications to the degree level.

Myanmar

The Ministry of Health in Myanmar has proposed legislation governing optometrists, but enforcement is limited in absence of a structured optometry education and poorly defined scope of optometry practice. Currently, there are 46 optometrists in Myanmar. The majority are from the training center at Yangon Eye Hospital, the country's main eye hospital.

Optometry education

There is no formal diploma or degree program in optometry in Myanmar. The only course available is a 2-year course provided by the Yangon Eye Hospital which admits 50–60 students annually; ophthalmologists or senior optometrists train these students.

Professional associations

Optometrists in Myanmar are not represented by any professional association. Yangon Eye Hospital is the main lead in organizing vision and eye health screening, and eye care services are available at no cost for Myanmar residents at government eye hospitals. An estimated 17 million people need vision correction in Myanmar.

Challenges

A systematic optometry program integrated into the formal university education system is not in place. Once developed, this will then need support of a comprehensive legislation for optometrists. There is a need for the current optometrists in the country to upgrade their skills so that they could provide comprehensive eye care.

Nepal

Optometry is a recognized and regulated profession in Nepal. Ophthalmologists, optometrists, ophthalmic assistants, optical dispensers, and eye health workers fulfill Nepal's eye care needs with a current population of 30 million. But there is no independent optometry council.

Optometry education

Optometry education in Nepal began in 1998 to meet the shortage of eye health professionals in the country. Optometry education is offered as a 4-year undergraduate program (Bachelor of Optometry) and as a 2-year postgraduate program (Master of Optometry), which is approved and accredited by the Nepal Health Professional Council (NHPC). Currently, three institutes offer undergraduate programs, and two institutes offer postgraduate programs in optometry. The NHPC sets standards for the provision of optometry education in the country.

Scope of practice of optometry

Currently, the NHPC, the statutory body maintaining the register and granting practice certificates to those registered, regulates Nepal's optometry practice. The code of ethics issued by the NHPC allows registered optometrists to practice independently as primary eye care practitioners. Optometrists serve as the point of entry into the eye care system in the country and share the following responsibilities in healthcare delivery: preventive care; health education; health promotion; health maintenance; diagnosis; treatment and rehabilitation; counseling; and consultation. Optometrists in Nepal are permitted to use authorized pharmaceutical agents for diagnostic and therapeutic uses in practice.

Distribution of VI and URE

Prevalence of visual impairment is high among Nepal's elderly population, with low vision prevalence at 52.9%, and blindness at 1.94%; uncorrected refractive error was the major cause of low vision and VI [21].

Shortage of personnel

VISION 2020 recommends 1 optometrist for a population of 50,000 for under-developed countries, so based on this, there is a requirement of 600 optometrists for the current population of 30 million in Nepal. There are currently 350 optometrists in Nepal, according to published reports [21]. Inequality in the distribution of existing human resources and brain drain are the current challenges in Nepal, which, when overcome, could make Nepal self-reliant in ophthalmic human resources [22].

Sri Lanka

The eye care burden in Sri Lanka is managed mainly by ophthalmologists. The College of Ophthalmologists of Sri Lanka is the main training body for ophthalmologists, ophthalmic technicians, and nurses. The Sri Lanka Optometry Association (SLOA), established in 1961, was the first to offer a diploma in optometry in the year 1999. The SLOA currently has close to 500 members and allows its members to use "Optometrist (Opt)" as a prefix and protects its members' interests by introducing a code of ethics and organizing training programs. Despite these developments, Sri Lanka is yet to offer an undergraduate degree program in optometry or recognize optometry as an independent healthcare profession.

Optometry education

The SLOA offers two courses in optometry; one is a 1-year Diploma in Optometry program, and the other is a 2.5-year higher national diploma.

Scope of practice of optometry

The scope of practice of optometry is not defined in Sri Lanka as there are different cadres of eye care providers with varying degrees of knowledge and training offering eye care services. The optometrists offer services such as providing refractive correction through spectacles and contact lenses, low vision care, and vision therapy.

Distribution of VI and URE

In a recent study to estimate the prevalence of visual impairment in Sri Lanka among adults >40 years of age, the prevalence of blindness was 1.7% and low vision was 17% [23]. Cataract (67%) and uncorrected refractive errors (13%) were the most common causes of blindness; the most common causes of VI were uncorrected refractive errors (62%) and cataract (24%).

Shortage of personnel

Ophthalmologists provide primary and comprehensive eye care in Sri Lanka and currently, the country has a ratio of nine ophthalmologists per million population [24]. There are only 600 optometrists at competency level 3.

Thailand

Optometry is a recognized profession in Thailand. There are 250 optometrists licensed and registered by the Ministry of Public Health.

Legislation

All optometrists need to have a license to practice, and they need to renew every 2 years under the supervision of the sub-committee in the Ministry of Public Health. The optometrists are represented by a professional association, the Association of Thai Optometrists. Local or provincial administration offices of the Department of Health and local NGOs organize vision screenings from time to time in different provinces, reaching an average of 10,000 patients each year.

Optometry education

Optometry education is delivered through three Doctor of Optometry programs which are located at Ramkhamhaeng University, Rangsit University, and Naresuan University.

Challenges

The legislation needs to be reviewed to ensure that the full scope of optometry is reflected. Postgraduate or skill development courses for teaching faculty are required, so also public awareness about the optometry profession and services.

Summary

There is much variation in the level of training and scope of optometry practice in most countries of the South-East Asian region (Table 18.2). The low numbers of optometrists and their skewed distributions are probably the biggest problems in ensuring appropriate eye care for the entire population of each country. Extensive investment is required to expand the training and

Table 18.2 Optometry in South-East Asia

Country	Training			Legislation	Competency level	Professional body	Population[a]	Number needed[b]	Number available
	Masters	Degree	Diploma						
Bangladesh	None	1	Several[c]	No	Level 2	Yes	164,689,383	16,468	1200
Bhutan	None	None	None	Yes	Level 4	No	773, 278	77	63
India	30	119	80	No	Level 2 & 3	Yes	1,380,004,385	138,000	64,000
Indonesia	0	1	11	Yes	Level 2	Yes	273,523,615	27,352	8600
Myanmar	0	0	0	No	Level 1	No	54,045,420	54,045	46
Nepal	2	3	7	Yes	Level 4	Yes	29,136,808	2914	350
Sri Lanka	None	None	2	No	Level 2 & 3	Yes	21,413,249	2141	600
Thailand	3	3	0	Yes	Level 3	Yes	69,799,978	6980	250

[a]Population based on the "Asian Countries by Population in 2020" (www.worldometers.info)
[b]Number needed is based on the optometrist to population ratio of 1:10,000 with optometrists serving a primary care role
[c]Exact number is not known

administer appropriate regulations for acceptable optometry program and optometrists. Given the prevalence of refractive error in the region and the development of myopia as a major public health challenge, there is considerable growth potential for optometry in South-East Asia. Technology allows for this potential to be amplified via collaboration with other primary vision care providers and should be embraced to create greater access to eye care for the entire population of this region.

References

1. World Council of Optometry. WCO's concept of optometry. 2020. https://worldcouncilofoptometry.info/concept-of-optometry/. Accessed 20 Oct 2020.
2. World Council of Optometry. A global competency-based model of scope of practice in optometry. 2015. https://worldcouncilofoptometry.info/wp-content/uploads/2017/03/wco_global_competency_model_2015.pdf
3. Masnick K, Gavzey R. What is an optometrist? Optom Vis Sci. 2004;81:289–90.
4. De Souza N, Looi S, Shinde L, et al. The role of optometrists in India: an integral part of an eye health team. Indian J Ophthalmol. 2012;60:401–5.
5. Flaxman SR, Bourne RRA, Resnikoff S, et al. Global causes of blindness and distance vision impairment 1990–2020: a systematic review and meta-analysis. Lancet Glob Health. Epub ahead of print 2017. https://doi.org/10.1016/S2214-109X(17)30393-5.
6. Holden BA, Fricke TR, Wilson DA, et al. Global prevalence of myopia and high myopia and temporal trends from 2000 through 2050. Ophthalmology. 2016;125:1036–42.
7. World Health Organization. Global Initiative for the elimination of avoidable blindness. 2000. https://apps.who.int/iris/bitstream/handle/10665/63748/WHO_PBL_97.61_Rev.2.pdf?sequence=1. Accessed 25 Oct 2020
8. Aldebasi YI, Ahmed MI, Monaco WA. Are optometrists necessary in primary health care centres in Saudi Arabia? Afr Vis Eye Health. 2018;77:a402. https://doi.org/10.4102/aveh.v77I1.402.
9. Asian Countries by Population. 2020. Worldometer. www.worldometers.info. Accessed 20 Oct 2020.
10. Khan M. Bangladesh model of eye care (Modular Eye Care, MEC). Community Eye Heal. 2000;13:24–5.
11. Dineen B, Bourne R, Ali S, et al. Prevalence and causes of blindness and visual impairment in Bangladeshi adults: results of the National Blindness and Low Vision Survey of Bangladesh. Br J Ophthalmol. 2003;87:820–8.
12. Sutradhar I, Gayen P, Hasan M, et al. Eye diseases: the neglected health condition among urban slum population of Dhaka, Bangladesh. BMC Ophthalmol. 2019;19:38. https://doi.org/10.1186/s12886-019-1043-z.
13. Rai M. Challenges of optometry in SAARC. Acta Sci Ophthalmol. 2019;2(2):02–5.
14. International Agency for the Prevention of Blindness. First eye hospital in Bhutan. IAPB; 2019. https://www.iapb.org/news/first-eye-hospital-in-bhutan/. Accessed 20 Sept 2020.
15. Lepcha NT, Sharma IP, Sapkota YD, et al. Changing trends of blindness, visual impairment and cataract surgery in Bhutan: 2009-2018. PLoS One. 2019;14:e0216398. https://doi.org/10.1371/journal.pone.0216398.
16. Pascolini D, Mariotti SP. Global estimates of visual impairment: 2010. Br J Ophthalmol. 2012;96:614–8.
17. Neena J, Rachel J, Praveen V, et al. Rapid assessment of avoidable blindness in India. PLoS One. 2008;3:e2867. https://doi.org/10.1371/journal.pone.0002867.
18. Thomas R, Paul P, Rao GN, et al. Present status of eye care in India. Surv Ophthalmol. 2005;50:85–101.
19. Sight Savers International India. EYE CARE IN INDIA – a situational analysis. Hyderabad. https://www.sightsaversindia.in. Accessed 17 Nov 2020
20. IROPIN. Ikatan Refraksionis Optisien Indonesia. 2020. http://iropin.org/adart/. Accessed 20 Oct 2020.
21. Thapa R, Bajimaya S, Paudyal G, et al. Prevalence and causes of low vision and blindness in an elderly population in Nepal: the Bhaktapur retina study. BMC Ophthalmol. 2018;18:42. https://doi.org/10.1186/s12886-018-0710-9.
22. Singh SK, Thakur S, Anwar A. Nepal: self-reliant in ophthalmic human resources. Community Eye Heal. 2018;31:S9–S10.
23. Banagala C, Gilbert C, Murthy GVS, et al. Prevalence, causes, magnitude and risk factors of visual impairment and blindness in Sri Lanka. Ceylon Med J. 2018;63:s10–7.
24. Sapkota YD. Human resources for eye health in South Asia. Community Eye Heal. 2018;31:S1–2.

Allied Ophthalmic Personnel: Workforce, Education, and Training

19

M. Babar Qureshi, Lynn Anderson, Trupti Kulkarni, A. H. M. Enayet Hussain, Indra P. Sharma, Dhivya R. Ramasamy, Rohit C. Khanna, Aldiana Halim, Yuddha D. Sapkota, and Prut Hanutsaha

Key Points

- Allied ophthalmic personnel (AOP) are the key technical workforce in eye care.
- AOPs comprise opticians, ophthalmic nurses, orthoptists, ophthalmic and optometric assistants, ophthalmic and optometric technicians, vision therapists, ocularists, ophthalmic photographers/imagers, and ophthalmic administrators.
- Although there have been some notable achievements in formalizing the training curriculum for a few AOP cadres by some countries in South-East Asia, most countries in this region lack a uniform curriculum and accreditation of this cadre of eye care professionals.
- The International Joint Commission of Allied Health Personnel in Ophthalmology (IJCAHPO) is working with governments and national

M. B. Qureshi (✉)
Inclusive Eye Health (IEH) and Neglected Tropical Diseases, CBM, Cambridge, UK
e-mail: babar.qureshi@cbm.org

L. Anderson
International Joint Commission on Allied Health Personnel in Ophthalmology, St. Paul, MN, USA
e-mail: landerson@jcahpo.org

T. Kulkarni
Inclusive Eye Health, CBM, Cambridge, UK
e-mail: trupti.kulkarni@cbm.org

A. H. M. Enayet Hussain
Directorate General of Medical Education, Ministry of Health and Family Welfare, Dhaka, Bangladesh

I. P. Sharma
Gyalyum Kesang Choeden Wangchuck National Eye Center, Jigme Dorji Wanchuck National Referral Hospital, Thimphu, Bhutan
e-mail: ipsharma@jdwnrh.gov.bt

D. R. Ramasamy
LAICO, Aravind Eye Care System, Madurai, India
e-mail: dhivya@aravind.org

R. C. Khanna
Allen Foster Community Eye Health Research Centre, Gullapalli Pratibha Rao International Centre for Advancement of Rural Eye Care, L V Prasad Eye Institute, Hyderabad, India
e-mail: rohit@lvpei.org

A. Halim
Cicendo Eye Hospital, Bandung, Indonesia

Y. D. Sapkota
International Agency for the Prevention of Blindness South-East Asia Region, Hyderabad, Telangana, India
e-mail: ysapkota@iapb.org

P. Hanutsaha
Department of Ophthalmology, Ramathibodi Hospital, Mehidol University, Bangkok, Thailand
e-mail: prut.han@mahidol.ac.th

T. Das, P. D. Nayar (eds.), *South-East Asia Eye Health*,
https://doi.org/10.1007/978-981-16-3787-2_19

bodies to devise accredited national and international certification programs, including a uniform curriculum and training regimen, for a holistic framework to ensure AOP cadre quality and legitimization of the profession.

- The demand for all AOP cadres is expected to increase in coming years as the world adopts universal eye health coverage and delivers eye care through an integrated people-centered eye care model.

Globally, approximately 43 million people are blind and 295 million people are moderate to severe visually impaired. Therefore, the prevention of blindness is a high-priority global agenda. The "VISION 2020: The Right to Sight" global initiative was launched with the aim of eliminating avoidable blindness by the year 2020. This ambitious goal can only be achieved through strengthening of health systems with improved provision of eye care delivery at all levels. This, in turn, depends on the availability of appropriately trained eye care professionals, including the Allied Ophthalmic Personnel (AOP) (Fig. 19.1).

This chapter explores the role of the allied ophthalmic personnel (AOP) in South-East Asia in delivering eye care services. It looks at the workforce in general, and their education and training as seen through the layers of the health system, i.e. the AOP at a primary (where available, or cadres that support AOPs), secondary, and tertiary levels in Bangladesh, Bhutan, India, Indonesia, Nepal, and Thailand. It also explores gaps in the availability of AOPs and pressing challenges prevalent in the workforce. The common elements are presented within each level of the health system, with highlighted exceptions, where present.

19.1 Allied Ophthalmic Personnel

The allied ophthalmic personnel (AOP) comprise opticians, ophthalmic nurses, orthoptists, ophthalmic and optometric assistants, ophthalmic and optometric technicians, vision therapists, ocularists, ophthalmic photographers/imagers, and ophthalmic administrators [1]. Some countries have amended this list to include refractionists (Indonesia) and optometrists (Thailand); on the other hand, Bhutan does not explicitly recognize opticians as an AOP cadre. The differences seen in these three countries in the South-East Asian region are examples of differences in education, training, and roles and responsibilities in different countries across the health system.

Shortage of eye health workforce has been reported in most of the South-East Asian countries. This was highlighted in the World Health Report in 2006 [2]; thereafter, this issue gained sufficient momentum to merit widespread investigation and international action to bring about

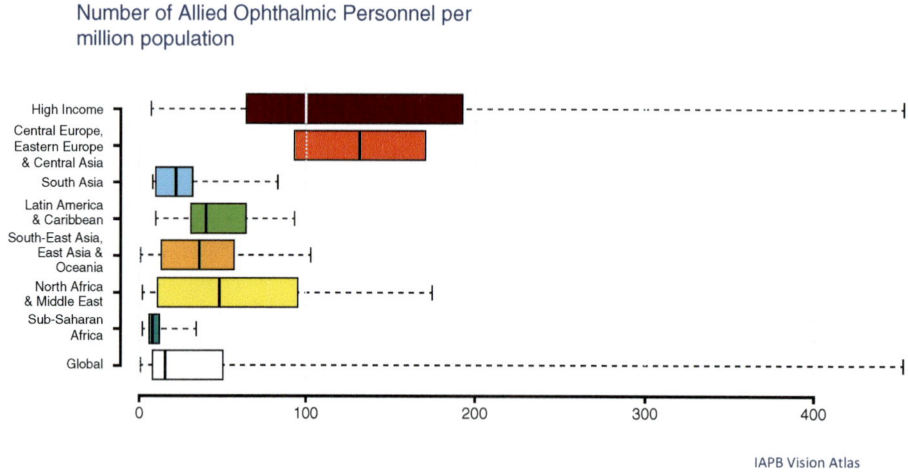

Fig. 19.1 Distribution of allied ophthalmic personnel per million population (Source: IAPB Vision Atlas, 2017)

changes. The report was a major driving force for the expansion of the health workforce in order to meet the health-related Millennium Development Goals (MDGs) and subsequently the Sustainable Development Goals (SDGs). The Global Health Workforce Alliance was established to accelerate progress towards the achievement of the global goals by identifying and implementing solutions to address health workforce shortages [3].

19.1.1 AOP in Different Levels of Healthcare

19.1.1.1 Primary Level

Workforce An explicit AOP cadre is rare in primary healthcare, many countries harness the skills of community health workers (often referred to as "informal eye care workers") in order to identify, diagnose, and manage common eye problems including referral to secondary health centers. Such personnel, trained in primary eye care, constitute an important part of identifying unmet needs within the community and are at the frontline in the fight against avoidable blindness.

In Indonesia, there is a two-tiered approach within primary healthcare, where community eye nurses (CEN) manage strategies for visual impairment control programs in the community, train community health workers to identify common causes of eye problems, and refer patients to higher eye care centers for further treatment. In Nepal, ophthalmic assistants functioning at secondary and tertiary levels play a key role in supervising primary eye care personnel at health post and community levels. Bhutan uses ophthalmic technicians, stationed at primary care centers and district hospitals to perform vision assessments, perform simple refraction, and plan and implement ophthalmic activities in the districts in coordination with local health authorities, administrative officials, and community leaders. The Indian healthcare system deploys a cadre called the paramedical ophthalmic assistant (PMOA) functioning at the primary level. These staff are responsible for community screening, referrals, and eye health education; they work at the Health and Wellness centers which provide comprehensive primary healthcare, including basic ophthalmology services. A similar model of providing primary eye care (PEC), i.e. vision centers, predominantly exists in the non-governmental sector and has demonstrated how primary eye care can successfully achieve coverage in a sustainable manner in India [4].

With the advent of telemedicine, the vision center model has brought sustainable comprehensive eye care to the primary level. These centers are manned by PEC technicians who receive in-house training by the respective base hospitals. They are trained to perform preliminary eye examinations and referrals, as well as in dispensing spectacles. Coupled with teleconsultations with the ophthalmologist at the base hospital, the PEC technicians are able to provide comprehensive primary eye care services. This vision center model has been successfully adopted by a few state governments, namely, Odisha and Tripura, in India [5]. More recently, over 3000 primary health centers have an integrated vision center manned by PMOAs [6].

Education and Training Bhutan has a formal training program to qualify as an ophthalmic technician; this includes a 2-year certificate program or a 3-year diploma, along with a short training session on community eye health, provided by the Khesar Gyalpo University of Medical Sciences of Bhutan (KGUMSB). First launched in 1987, the country's Primary Eye Care Program (PECP) commenced at the KGUMSB (the then Royal Institute of Health Science) [7]. The objective of training and inducting AOPs into the health system was to create a pool of dedicated professionals to improve primary eye care services in the country, as Bhutan only had a handful of trained medical and health professionals then. In most other countries, training of AOPs is limited or non-existent, leaving a gap in the requirement for and availability of qualified personnel to support the AOP cadre. Figure 19.2 shows this gap as it exists in Indonesia.

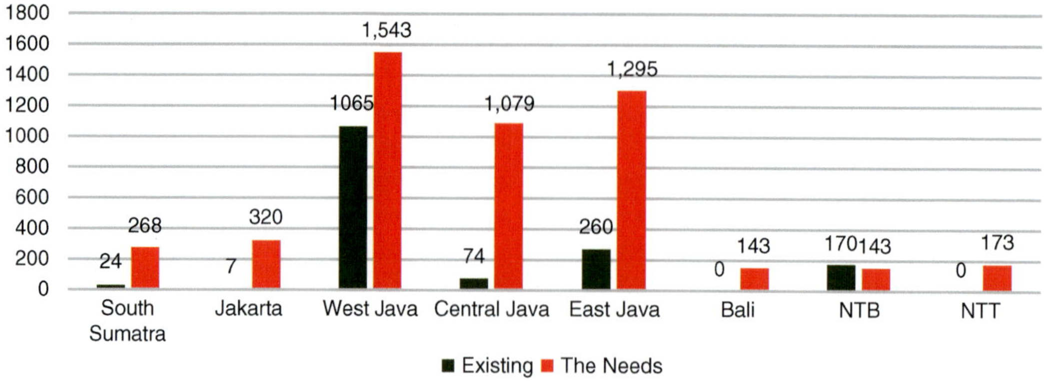

Fig. 19.2 The gap in existing versus required numbers of community eye nurses at the primary level of healthcare in eight provinces in Indonesia. *NTT* Nusa Tenggara Timur, *NTB* Nusa Tenggra Barat

19.1.1.2 Secondary Level

Workforce In most countries, AOPs are formally part of the secondary and tertiary levels of healthcare, while providing supervisory support (including training) to community health workers at the primary level. Therefore, it is fair to state that AOPs at the secondary level perform an important role in ensuring that community health workers at the primary level are adequately trained and supported to identify common vision problems and refer patients to the secondary level. In addition, AOPs assist specialists such as optometrists, cataract surgeons, etc., at the secondary levels in their clinical and surgical procedures. Once again, there are different AOP cadres at this level in different countries, with ophthalmic nurses and ophthalmic assistants being common across most South-East Asian countries. Notable exceptions of country-specific cadres are:

- Indonesia's refractionists perform simple refractive assessments and support quality checks in the production of spectacles.
- Bhutan's ophthalmic technicians, after extended experience at the primary level of healthcare, continue at the secondary level by supporting diagnostic and operating room procedures, including administration and monitoring of local anesthesia.
- Bangladesh's opticians and mid-level ophthalmic personnel are part of the Government's share in eye care provision (50% of the country's eye care); however, the quality and level of services provided by these personnel is quite disparate at different secondary healthcare facilities.
- India's optometrists and optometric assistants perform refractive assessments and support consultation for refractions. As a notable exception, registered general nurses, and not ophthalmic nurses, support cataract-related services in government hospitals. Many secondary eye care hospitals also have eye care counsellors to educate patients, and opticians to dispense spectacles, who, although not formally recognized in the AOP cadre, are crucial to supporting refraction services.

Education and Training Given the key role that AOPs play in eye care service delivery, several countries have worked on and are continuing to focus on education and further training for the cadres. Nepal's 3-year training course for ophthalmic assistants was launched in 1981, and the curriculum was formalized in 1989 after recognition of the course by the Skill Testing Department of the Government of Nepal/Council for Technical Education and Vocational Training (CTEVT) and the Nepal Health Professional Council (NHPC). Since then, more than eight training institutions enable accreditation of more than 300 ophthalmic assistants annually. The curricula at these institutions equip these assistants to diagnose, refer, and initiate treatment for most common eye problems; carry out basic low vision assessment; perform operative and post-operative patient management; impart primary eye health education on health promotion; and organize and run outreach activities such as screening camps and school health programs. The program is considered one of the strongest in the region.

Bhutan's 2-year certification program and 3-year diploma program for ophthalmic technicians are supported by additional training in diagnostic and clinical procedures.

Indonesia's refractionists must receive a 3-year diploma before being considered qualified enough to work at secondary hospitals.

Nurses in Thailand's community hospitals receive 1–4 years of training to gain a Bachelor of Nursing Science degree after qualifying as a practical nurse before they support the ophthalmologists in visual acuity measurements, basic eye treatments, diabetic retinopathy screening, detecting cataract cases, and referral of patients for higher level care.

19.1.1.3 Tertiary Level

Workforce AOP cadres at the tertiary level of healthcare are almost similar to those in the secondary level; however, AOPs at the tertiary level have higher skill sets and more knowledge and experience to support more advanced ophthalmic practices at the tertiary and specialty hospitals. Their responsibilities range from vision assessment to assisting ophthalmologists in surgical procedures, including wide-ranging administrative tasks such as outpatient and inpatient management and care, training or supervising other AOPs, and supporting advocacy on eye health. In India's private sector, AOPs at tertiary levels are trained to perform higher level tasks such as biometry, visual field evaluation, optical coherence tomography, fundus angiography, grading ophthalmic images, and assist in the operating room for more complex eye conditions.

Education and Training Most South-East Asian countries have at least some accredited courses for training of AOPs, with the exception of Bangladesh, which is yet to make notable strides in developing a nationally agreed course curriculum for AOPs. In Bangladesh, most AOPs are trained by private institutions or NGOs. At present, in Bangladesh, a range of eye hospitals and institutions are carrying out different AOP and ophthalmic paramedic training programs; however, these programs are designed to only fulfill their organizations' needs. A good number of organizations and hospitals/institutions also offer training programs for refractionists, ophthalmic assistants, orthoptic specialists, etc., in addition to courses on low vision and counselling. Despite these efforts, the annual enrolment of students in these courses is inadequate to meet the current needs of the country. The durations of these courses vary from 3 months to 2 years. Table 19.1 highlights the currently available courses offered for AOPs and ophthalmic paraprofessionals (mostly by private and NGO-run eye hospitals and institutions) in Bangladesh.

In Thailand, ophthalmic nurses take up a 4-month "Certificate of Ophthalmic Nurse" course and optometrists must take up a 6-year "Bachelor of Optometry" course.

The Government of India has adopted the strategy of competency-based assessment (CBA) to support and develop the AOP cadre by the National Skill Development Council's Health Sector Skill Council. This model has also been used by large eye care training institutions and the voluntary sector [8].

That being said, more needs to be done to bridge the gap in the availability of and need for qualified AOPs in many countries, which is only possible with strong initiatives from the government.

19.1.2 Public–Private Partnerships in Strengthening the AOP Cadre

Several countries have systems in place to support provision of eye care, including strengthening of the AOP workforce through training. The most successful of these are those supported by public–private partnerships, a joint effort by government health systems, the development sector,

Table 19.1 AOP training courses offered by private institutions and NGO-run eye hospitals in Bangladesh

Name of AOP training course	Number of organizations/ institutions offering the course	Couse duration	Annual enrolment numbers
Ophthalmic assistant/Mid-level Ophthalmic Personnel (MLOP) course	5	1–2 years	110
Ophthalmic technician	1	2 years	20
Ophthalmic paramedics	1	1 year	10
Refraction	5	1 year	35
Orthoptist	3	6 months	15–20
OT management	3	1–3 months	15–20
OPD management	2	1–3 months	20
Counselling	3	1–3 months	35–40
Low vision	2	3 months	30–40
Optical dispensing	2	3 months	2–5
Ophthalmology training for nurses[a]	1	3 months	20
Ophthalmic assistant nursing training	1	3 months	20

[a]This customized ophthalmology training is being offered to the diploma or graduate nurses who are involved in eye care service delivery

and private organizations. Optical shops and cadres within such systems are the most common examples. India's Eye Mitra rural optician program has taken a novel micro-entrepreneurial approach to address uncorrected refractive error in the community [9]. This program has trained over 400 opticians with skills to begin their own micro business. Such endeavors have immense potential to bridge the gap in the demand for and supply of consistent and continued service provision.

19.1.3 Challenges in Expanding the AOP Workforce and Their Training

19.1.3.1 Shortage of AOPs

The shortage of eye care professionals, including AOPs, exists in different severities and has different root causes, depending on the particular specialty, the country health systems, and context. Healthcare priorities therefore change from time to time. Thus, a country's health system should be restructured based on demand and supply to provide required levels of healthcare efficiently to all those who need it. In the Universal Eye Health: a Global Action Plan 2014–2019, the WHO recommended that the Ministries of Health (MoHs) should report the number of ophthalmologists and AOPs annually to measure a country's progress in creating enough workforce for its eye care needs [10]. The Global Human Resource Development Assessment for Comprehensive Eye Care (GHRDACEC) 2006 was the first of its kind to investigate specific workforce issues affecting the progress of the eye care profession as a whole internationally [11].

Indonesia conducted a comprehensive situational analysis in 2018 to identify gaps in the demand for and supply of AOPs in eight of its provinces (Figs. 19.3 and 19.4).

In Bangladesh, one of the critical impediments to providing high volumes and quality of cataract surgeries is the lack of AOPs in both, public and private sectors. The challenges include inadequate ophthalmologist-to-population and AOP-to-population ratios, and insufficient AOP skills training. Estimates suggest that Bangladesh had 626 ophthalmologists (1 per 222,388 people) and 471 AOPs (1 per 295,573 people) in 2006 [10]. Although more recent estimations suggest that these numbers have increased over time (about 1300 ophthalmologists and 900 AOPs), a significant shortage still persists. To meet workforce related VISION 2020 targets, Bangladesh requires about 1614 ophthalmologists (1 per 100,000 people) and over 3230 AOPs (1 per <50,000 people).

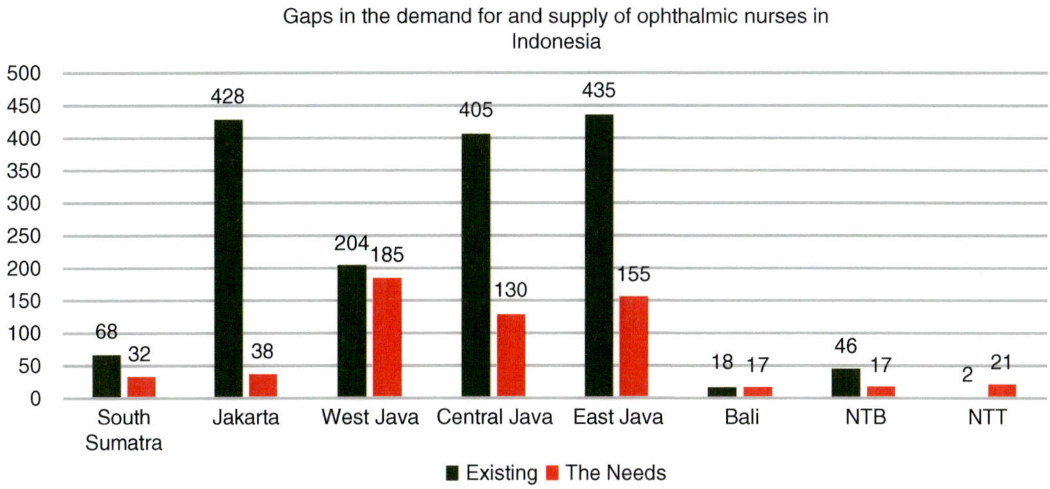

Fig. 19.3 The gap in existing versus required numbers of ophthalmic nurses at the primary level of healthcare in eight provinces in Indonesia. *NTT* Nusa Tenggara Timur, NTB Nusa Tenggra Barat

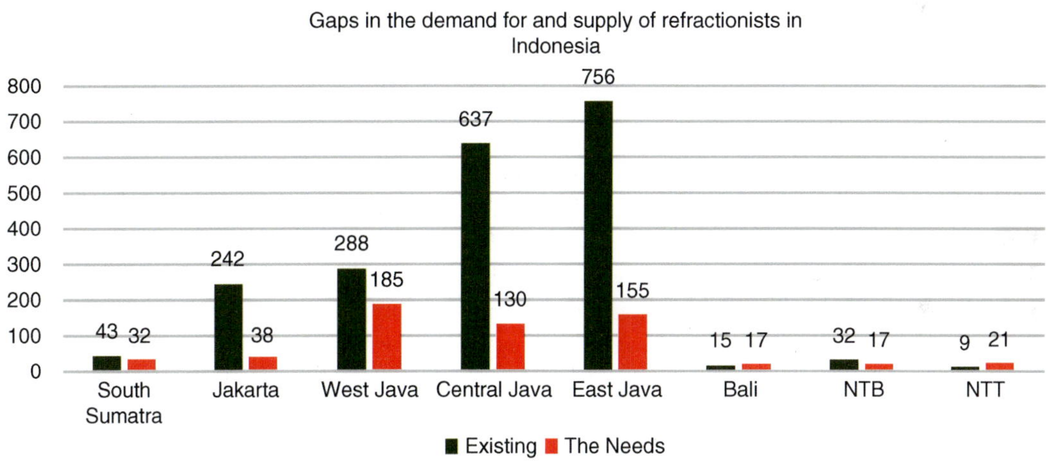

Fig. 19.4 The gap in existing versus required number of refractionists at the primary level of healthcare in eight provinces in Indonesia. *NTT* Nusa Tenggara Timur, *NTB* Nusa Tenggra Barat

19.1.3.2 Lack of Formalized Training Structures

Ophthalmic paraprofessionals are a crucial part of any eye care team and country-specific eye care programs; for example, cataract surgery performance is closely dependent on the availability of trained AOPs. Several countries in the South-East Asian region have disparate training facilities, most commonly a mix of formal and informal structures. There has been a conscious effort to harmonize training institutions and course curricula within each country as per their needs and health system setups.

Bangladesh's National Eye Health Plan 2014–2020 had recognized the need for strengthening the AOP workforce and had proposed the following strategies to address problems associated with the training of AOPs:

1. Establishing a national center for training of AOPs and other ophthalmic paraprofessionals at the National Institute of Ophthalmology and Hospital (NIO&H)
2. Developing standard curricula for AOP training in consultation with international training centers/institutions

India is working towards a more formalized training structure, and the advent of the Allied and Healthcare Professions Bill, which will mandate that these informal cadres are formally recognized, is a significant step in this direction [12]. In addition, formal continuous professional development of the AOP cadre is also an important aspect in the continuously evolving field of ophthalmology. While this structure exists for ophthalmologists, it must be structured for AOPs as well [13].

The aforementioned challenges also exist in other South-East Asian countries in some form or other, leading to continued disparities in AOP requirements and availability. Some other common challenges are:

- Unregulated AOPs' engagement in eye care services delivery
- Uneven distribution; availability of AOPs is concentrated mostly in cities and semi-urban areas.
- Lack of uniform curriculum in AOP training within countries, which is often coupled with non-accreditation of the courses.

Accredited courses have an important role in curriculum formalization and pave the way for harmonized approaches to synergizing qualifications across diverse AOP cadres, both, in numbers and qualification criteria of this workforce. Countries like Nepal and India are already working towards this; Bhutan has had good success in this aspect. It is equally important to periodically review the course content of different AOP cadres to address gaps in workforce availability and for regular assessment of the knowledge and skills of the cadre itself, as a means to ensure quality of the workforce.

In addition to training program accreditation, strategies like CBA and certification are emerging as ways to fast track and develop the AOP cadre. National and international certifications, such as those provided by the IJCAHPO, as well as government licensure or registration, also advance the development and legitimization of the AOP profession and cadres. However, there is need for a wider replication of these strategies across countries and regions in order to address the need for adequate numbers of skilled AOPs.

It will take a concerted effort for governments to tackle these challenges by spearheading initiatives such as public–private partnerships, establishing formal curricula, adequate training, equitable distribution, and even near-competitive pay scales to keep up with the demand for AOPs and fill the ever-widening gaps in this necessary workforce.

19.2 Conclusion

The importance of health workforce (including the AOPs) provision has gained significance and is considered one of the most pressing issues worldwide. Healthcare industry experts predict a promising future for those who are in the allied health and specialized nursing careers; employment of these groups is expected to grow by at least 20% by 2025. This surge in demand will continue to foster opportunities across a variety of specialties in the health workforce. During a time when employment opportunities are decreasing in many industries globally, employment opportunities in healthcare are and will continue to increase. To maintain and expand the eye care workforce for the future, increases in recruitment, training, and retention will be essential. Although recruiting and training more AOPs are important steps, overall eye care workforce availability and other health system factors may also play significant roles. However, scaling up the eye care workforce is a complex, multifactorial health system issue that requires coordinated action, availability of people with the appropriate skill-mix, and functional options for task-sharing and task-shifting to other categories of eye care and primary care providers. The repercussions of any changes made to the key eye care workforce must be considered carefully and optimal use of the current workforce should be made. Finally, focusing on an appropriate country-wise distribution of well-trained AOPs along with ophthalmologists will help ensure equity of services in terms of equal and increased access to eye care for vulnerable populations, so that eye care needs are universally met.

References

1. World Health Organization. Universal eye health: a global action plan 2014–2019. http://www.who.int/blindness/EyeHealthActionPlanWHA66.pdf. Accessed 29 Aug 2020.
2. World Health Organization. The World Health Report 2006: working together for health. http://www.who.int/whr/2006/en/. Accessed 29 Aug 2020.
3. World Health Organization. Global health workforce alliance strategic plan 2006. http://www.ghwa.org/. Accessed 29 Aug 2020.
4. Khanna RC, Sabherwal S, Sil A, et al. Primary eye care in India – the vision center model. Indian J Ophthalmol. 2020;68:333–9.
5. Tripura Vision Centre Project. https://health.tripura.gov.in/?q=teleopthalmology. Accessed 19 Oct 2020.
6. Rajshekhar V, Gupta P. National Programme for Control of Blindness (NPCB) in the 12th Five Year Plan: an overview. Delhi J Ophthalmol. 2017;27:290–2.
7. Primary Eye Care Program. A strategic plan: enhancing Bhutan eye health services. Department of Medical Services, Ministry of Health, Bhutan. 2017. (Unpublished).
8. Arora S, Mathur U, Datta P. Competency-based assessment as a reliable skill building strategy for allied ophthalmic personnel. Community Eye Health. 2018;31(102):S5–6.
9. Eye Mitra. https://www.essilorseechange.com/what-we-do/2-5-new-vision-generation/eye-mitra/. Accessed 19 Oct 2020.
10. Bourne RRA, Flaxman SR, Braithwaite T, et al. Magnitude, temporal trends, and projections of the global prevalence of blindness and distance and near vision impairment: a systematic review and meta-analysis. Lancet Glob Health. 2017;5:e888–97.
11. Human Resource Development Working Group. Global human resource development assessment for comprehensive eye care 2006. www.iapb.org/wp-content/uploads/Global-HR-Development-Assessment-for-Comprehensive-Eye-Care_2006.pdf. Accessed 9 Nov 2020.
12. The allied and healthcare professions bill, 2018. http://164.100.47.5/committee_web/BillFile/Bill/14/113/LX%20of%202018_2019_2_14.pdf. Accessed 19 Oct 2020.
13. Ramasamy D, Gilbert SS. How to 'do' CPD with your team (from the organisation's perspective). Community Eye Health. 2017;30(97):9–10.

Part V

International Organizations

CBM in South-East Asia

20

Striving for Excellent, Integrated, and Inclusive Eye Health Services

Harpreet Kapoor, Manfred Mörchen, M. Babar Qureshi, and Trupti Kulkarni

CBM is an international Christian development organization committed to improving the quality of life of people with disabilities in the world's poorest communities. The organization's work on eye health began in the 1960s, and the very first cataract surgery supported by CBM was conducted in Afghanistan in 1966. CBM is a founding member of VISION 2020 and has been extensively involved in the achievement of this global initiative. CBM has supported partner organizations in South-East Asia to effectively implement comprehensive and inclusive eye care services for more than 50 years. This includes multi-pronged interventions to prevent and treat avoidable blindness and improve the quality of life of those with permanent visual impairment. To effectively achieve the "Right to Sight" for all, CBM supports its partners in addressing all aspects of comprehensive eye care—including promotion, prevention, curative interventions, and rehabilitation—and ensuring that these initiatives reach even the most marginalized communities.

This chapter highlights CBM's work in delivering high-quality eye care in some of the South-East Asian countries.

20.1 Towards Strengthened Eye Health Systems in India

CBM has had a presence in India since 1967, and over the years, several of its programs have been implemented successfully across the country, enabling partner organizations to develop high-quality, affordable, and sustainable eye care services. The organization has been instrumental in nurturing several small eye care centers into established tertiary-level organizations such as the Poona Blind Men's Association (PBMA)'s H. V. Desai Eye Hospital (Pune), Joseph Eye Hospital (Trichy), and the Ophthalmology

H. Kapoor · M. Mörchen
Inclusive Eye Health—Asia, New Delhi, India

M. B. Qureshi (✉)
Inclusive Eye Health (IEH) and Neglected Tropical Diseases, CBM, Cambridge, UK
e-mail: Babar.Qureshi@cbm.org

T. Kulkarni
Inclusive Eye Health, CBM, Cambridge, UK
e-mail: Trupti.Kulkarni@cbm.org

T. Das, P. D. Nayar (eds.), *South-East Asia Eye Health*,
https://doi.org/10.1007/978-981-16-3787-2_20

Department of Christian Medical College (Ludhiana). These hospitals contribute to the five-tier pyramidal eye health model of LV Prasad Eye Institute (Hyderabad) that has been suggested for integrated people-centered eye care (IPCEC) in countries with populations exceeding 50 million people [1]. CBM has also partnered with LV Prasad Eye Institute in programs focusing on disability inclusion in providing comprehensive eye care services. In India, CBM reaches out to nearly 2.2 million people with visual impairments annually and provides free or subsidized surgery for more than 200,000 patients who have limited access to quality services due to financial, social, or geographical barriers.

For effective planning and implementation of evidence-based programs, CBM supports partner organizations in conducting cost-effective surveys, including Rapid Assessment of Visual Impairment (RAVI) and Rapid Assessment of Avoidable Blindness (RAAB) studies. CBM has supported the R.P. Centre for Ophthalmic Sciences (New Delhi) in conducting three RAVI studies in northern India in 2017. Partnership with this apex institute of ophthalmology was initiated in 2015 to develop a resource and training center for low vision and rehabilitation; the partnership also aimed to promote services for low vision across government health systems, which included Regional Institutes of Ophthalmology, as well as non-government eye care organizations. With CBM's support, the Joseph Eye Hospital at Trichy has also been developed into a training institute for other partner organizations to strengthen services for low vision in the region.

20.2 Improving the Quality of Cataract Surgical Services in Nepal

Cataracts and refractive errors remain the most common causes of blindness and visual impairment in the South-East Asian region [1]. One of the flagship programs of CBM has been the Eastern Regional Eye Care Program (EREC-P) in Nepal, which was initiated in 1982 as a response to the findings of the first nationwide blindness survey conducted in 1979–1980 jointly by the Government of Nepal and WHO. Nationally, the prevalence of bilateral blindness was 0.84%, and an alarming 8.58% of people over 60 years of age were blind. Cataracts accounted for 83.6% of avoidable blindness [2]. CBM, in collaboration with the Nepal Netra Jyoti Sangh, the central coordinating body for eye care in Nepal, established the Sagarmatha Choudhary Eye Hospital in Lahan to provide eye care services at an affordable cost to the underprivileged population of the East Terai region (Fig. 20.1). Over a short period of time, the Lahan Eye hospital gained popularity for its high-quality surgical services.

Newer disease continued to challenge the region. An inclusive tertiary eye care center, the Biratnagar Eye Hospital, was also established with CBM's support to provide standardized treatment for other emerging causes of blindness, including vitreoretinal disorders, glaucoma, and corneal and childhood blindness. Over 1 million patients are currently examined, and 120,000 eye surgeries are performed annually at these two hospitals under the EREC-P. Albrecht Hennig, the Founder-Director of the hospital, developed the innovative fish hook technique for cost-effective suture-less cataract surgery and suggested that "rapid recovery of good vision can be achieved with suture-less manual ECCE (extracapsular cataract extraction) surgery at low cost in areas where there is a need for high volume cataract surgery" [3].

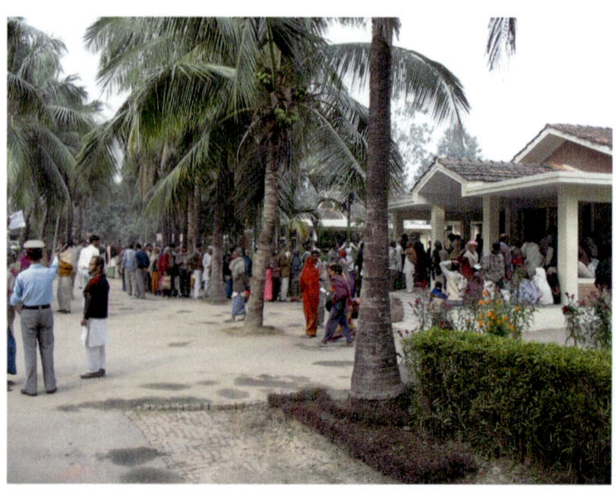

Fig. 20.1 Lahan Eye Hospital, Nepal (*Published with permission from CBM*)

20.3 Strengthening Human Resources for Efficient Service Delivery

Capacity building for effective delivery of inclusive and comprehensive eye health has been one of the priority areas of CBM's work in the South-East Asian region. Over the past few decades, CBM has supported the training of various cadres of mid-level ophthalmic personnel and upgrading of ophthalmologists' skills to create a more efficient workforce to tackle the ever-increasing demand for eye care services while ensuring that the benefits of technological advances are extended to the underserved population. CBM also strongly advocates the employment of people with disabilities in eye hospitals (Fig. 20.2).

Recognizing the deficiencies in postgraduate surgical training for ophthalmologists, and the growing demand for phacoemulsification surgery even in rural populations, CBM collaborated with ZEISS to set up phacoemulsification training centers to enhance the surgical skills of ophthalmologists and hence improve outcomes of cataract surgery. The first such center was established in Paraguay in 2018 and in India in 2019 (H. V. Desai Eye Hospital, Pune). The International Council of Ophthalmology (ICO) and CBM jointly developed the "ICO-CBM Phaco Surgeon Training Curriculum" which has been implemented in several institutes to ensure that all trainees achieve the desired level of competency in phacoemulsification surgery [4].

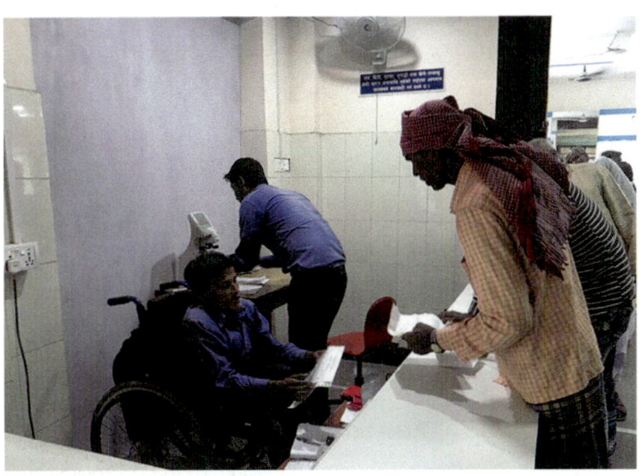

Fig. 20.2 Wheelchair-bound staff at the optical shop at Biratnagar Eye Hospital, Nepal (*Published with permission from CBM*)

20.4 Towards Inclusive Eye Health Services

CBM's work in the South-East Asian region is based on the "leave no one behind" agenda of the Sustainable Development Goals (SDGs) and the UN Convention on the Rights of Persons with Disabilities (UNCRPD). This is of utmost importance in a region where people from vulnerable groups, including people with disabilities, "are either denied or receive very little appropriate quality of health care, and eye care is no exception" [5]. The following sections highlight the contribution of CBM's work in delivering accessible and inclusive services.

20.4.1 Evidence

CBM has supported population-based surveys that have strived to increase the body of evidence regarding access barriers to eye health services [6]. For example, results from a cross-sectional survey from Telangana, India, suggested that people with visual impairments had a higher risk of poverty and unemployment than others. Also, among people with visual impairment, 15% had moderate or severe physical impairment or epilepsy, and 25% had a moderate or severe hearing impairment. Among those who were blind, 43% were also disabled in some other way [6]. This study concluded that "people with functional difficulties in multiple domains may find it difficult to access eye care services, highlighting the need for inclusive eye health" [6].

20.4.2 Implementation of Inclusive Eye Health Services in Indonesia

Indonesia has contributed significantly to the development of inclusive eye health services. An "Inclusive System for Effective Eye-care (I-SEE)" pilot program was initiated in 2013 in Bandung district, West Java, to strengthen existing health systems and improve access to eye health services for patients with disabilities.

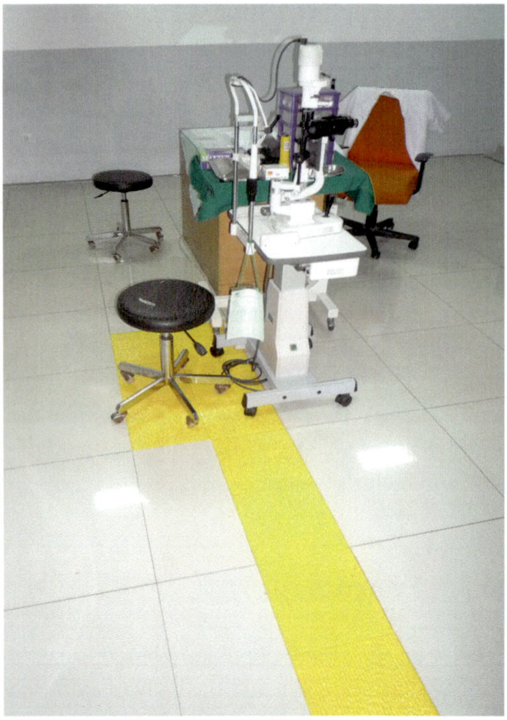

Fig. 20.3 Improving wayfinding at Cicendo Eye Hospital, Bandung, Indonesia (*Published with permission from CBM*)

The program included training eye health staff on the concepts of inclusive health, improving the physical accessibility of eye health facilities (Fig. 20.3), and improving referral pathways between the local Organization of People with Disabilities (OPD) eye health services.

Results from a qualitative study about the I-SEE program's implementation process suggested that "strategies for disability inclusion should be included from the planning phase of an eye health program and they are relatively simple and feasible to include" [7].

20.5 Challenges

Despite ongoing efforts to improve eye health service delivery in the South-East Asia region, this region has a long way to go before such services can become fully accessible, affordable, and available for all. Cultural or social challenges such as barriers to or stigmas against health-seeking behavior, mainstreaming inclusion for service delivery, lack of enough ophthalmic personnel to support growing needs, and even climate change have exacerbated problems in eye care delivery and threaten to shadow the achievements. Recent efforts to reduce access barriers to eye health services for vulnerable populations suffer from elusive data to document the impacts of targeted programs. It is unclear how far training on, for example, inclusive eye health results in more people with disabilities accessing eye health services. Eye health services supported by CBM have also intensified collaborations with the OPD to improve referral networks to and from eye health services; however, it is still difficult to quantify the impact of this change [8]. Currently, CBM also provides practical tips to improve the accessibility of eye health services for people with disabilities [9].

20.6 Conclusion

The aging populations of the South-East Asia region will substantially increase the absolute numbers of blind people or those who are visually impaired, in the next few decades. To achieve universal eye health coverage, more efforts are needed to achieve IPCEC, as recommended in the WHO World Report on Vision, and to ensure that vulnerable populations, including people with disabilities, can access eye health services of high quality. CBM will continue to strive for excellence and quality in strengthening health systems by working with government and other organizations to integrate eye care into general healthcare systems. This will aid in ensuring that avoidable visual impairment can be just that—avoidable—and that services can be delivered within a sustainable model of health systems.

References

1. Das T, Keeffe J, Sivaprasad S, et al. Capacity building for universal eye health coverage in South East Asia beyond 2020. Eye. 2020;34:1262–70.
2. Brilliant LB, Pokhrel RP, Grasset NC, et al. Epidemiology of blindness in Nepal. Bull World Health Organ. 1985;63:375–86.

3. Hennig A, Kumar J, Yorston D, et al. Sutureless cataract surgery with nucleus extraction: outcome of a prospective study in Nepal. Br J Ophthalmol. 2003;87:266–70.
4. ICO-CBM Phaco Surgeon Training Curriculum. http://www.icoph.org/downloads/ICO-CBM-Phaco-Curriculum.pdf. Accessed 07 Oct 2020.
5. Rao GN. The Barrie Jones Lecture—eye care for the neglected population: challenges and solutions. Eye. 2015;29:30–45.
6. Mactaggart I, Polack S, Murthy GVS, et al. A population-based survey of visual impairment and its correlates in Mahabubnagar district, Telangana State, India. Ophthalmol Epidemiol. 2017;25:238–45.
7. Marella M, Smith F, Lukman H, et al. Factors influencing disability inclusion in general eye health services in Bandung, Indonesia: a qualitative study. Int J Environ Res Public Health. 2018;16:23. https://doi.org/10.3390/ijerph16010023.
8. Mörchen M, Bush A, Kiel P, et al. Leaving no one behind: strengthening access to eye health programs for people with disabilities in 6 low- and middle-income countries. Asia Pac J Ophthalmol. 2018;7:331–8.
9. CBM. Inclusion made easy in eye health programs. https://www.cbm.org/fileadmin/user_upload/Publications/Inclusion_in_Eye_Health_Guide.pdf. Accessed 07 Oct 2020.

21 Combat Blindness International

Suresh R. Chandra and Reena Chandra Rajpal

Combat Blindness
INTERNATIONAL

Combat Blindness International (CBI) was founded in 1984 by Suresh Chandra, MD, now a professor emeritus with the Department of Ophthalmology and Visual Sciences at the University of Wisconsin-Madison School of Medicine and Public Health. CBI's primary mission is to eliminate preventable blindness worldwide, particularly in low-income nations, by providing sustainable and equitable solutions for problems of sight through partnerships and innovation. CBI has always focused on reaching the most vulnerable populations worldwide, bringing quality, and equitable eye care to those with poor or no resources.

S. R. Chandra (✉) · R. C. Rajpal
Combat Blindness International, Madison, WI, USA
e-mail: chandra@combatblindness.org; rchandrarajpal@combatblindness.org

CBI's work focuses on two major areas: (1) elimination and prevention of avoidable blindness and (2) building capacity and infrastructure for sustainable eye care. Rather than providing "top-down" solutions, CBI collaboratively works at the grassroots level, partnering with local eye hospitals and institutions to establish eye health programs for cataract and other conditions that directly impact adults and children. In addition, CBI also provides education and training to the eye health personnel working with their partner organizations to become self-sustainable. Finally, CBI supports the establishment of surgical centers in areas previously devoid of eye care or even medical care. It works to ensure that these centers are self-sustaining within 3–5 years of being built. By providing affordable and accessible care, ensuring that the right tools and supplies are available, and building surgical centers where they are needed, CBI ensures that equitable eye care is available to those who need it most.

21.1 Founder's Story

In the early 1980s, Dr. Chandra traveled to India, Africa, Thailand, and Indonesia to lecture on and demonstrate high-technology retinal and vitreous surgery techniques. During one of these trips, he realized that high-tech surgery was not the answer to the overwhelming number of cases

T. Das, P. D. Nayar (eds.), *South-East Asia Eye Health*,
https://doi.org/10.1007/978-981-16-3787-2_21

of avoidable blindness. In India, in 1983, when Dr. Chandra was walking to an operating room to perform a 4-h retinal surgery, he passed through a hallway with 50 patients waiting to receive cataract surgery. After completing the 4-h surgery, he walked back down the same hallway and noticed that all 50 patients were gone. This sparked Dr. Chandra's curiosity, prompting him to ask a nurse where all the patients had gone. She informed him that all the patients had been operated on and were recovering. Dr. Chandra realized that in the amount of time it took him to complete one retinal surgery, 50 patients had received cataract surgeries. The best possible outcome that his retinal surgery patient could hope for was 20/40 vision, while all those patients with cataracts would have 20/20 vision in 24 h. He saw, for the first time, a clear picture for the work and mission to which he would dedicate himself for decades to come.

Cataracts cause half of the world's blindness. The simple fact that one can correct half the world's vision problems quickly and inexpensively compelled Dr. Chandra to bring together friends and civic leaders to form CBI in 1984. Today, ophthalmologists and community leaders in Madison make up CBI's Board of Directors, and renowned ophthalmologists and chief executive officers (CEO)s from around the world serve on the advisory board of the organization.

21.2 CBI's Impact

CBI's focus has always been to eliminate cataract blindness (Fig. 21.1). CBI supported a single eye camp at Sitapur Eye Hospital (India) in its first year, by providing the necessary support for 300 cataract surgeries. In its early years, CBI also addressed xerophthalmia (due to vitamin A deficiency) and night blindness, both of which were major causes of blindness in children under 5. In collaboration with its partners, CBI was active in conducting malnutrition screening on children, and treating vitamin A-deficient children with vitamin A boosters (Fig. 21.2). Besides this, CBI also worked with community health workers to educate people on eye health and provide seeds

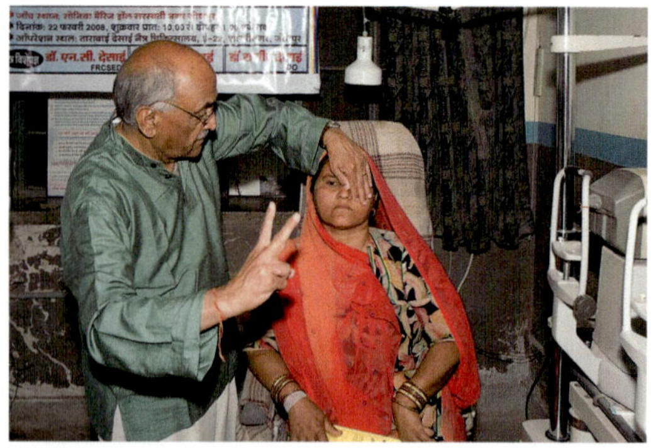

Fig. 21.1 Dr. Suresh Chandra examining a patient after cataract surgery in Jodhpur, India (Published with permission from Combat Blindness International)

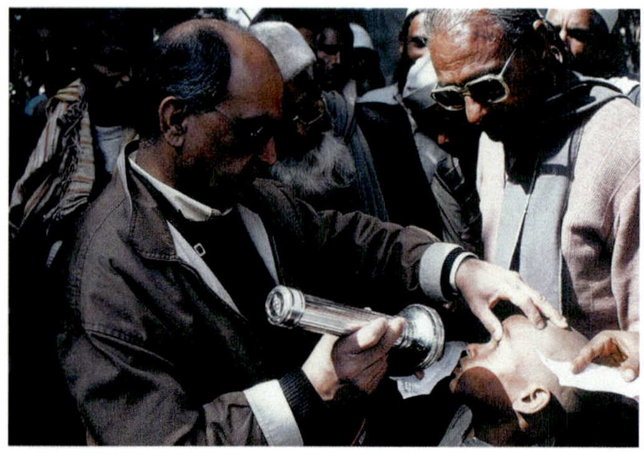

Fig. 21.2 Dr. Suresh Chandra examining a child with xerophthalmia (Published with permission from Combat Blindness International)

to grow vegetables rich in vitamin A in a community kitchen garden.

Since its inception, CBI has grown significantly and made remarkable impacts. To date, CBI has screened over 2.6 million people, including over 700,000 children, and provided for nearly 370,000 sight-saving surgeries for men, women, and children in 17 countries on 4 continents. In Asia alone, CBI has screened over 2.5 million people and provided for over 300,000 surgeries. CBI has also supported more than 500 young women in India to their efforts to become ophthalmic paramedical personnel and backed two surgical centers in India (Fig. 21.3). Today, CBI supports an average of over 280,000 screenings and 15,000 surgeries globally per year; of these, over 270,000 screenings and 14,000 surgeries are carried out in Asia alone.

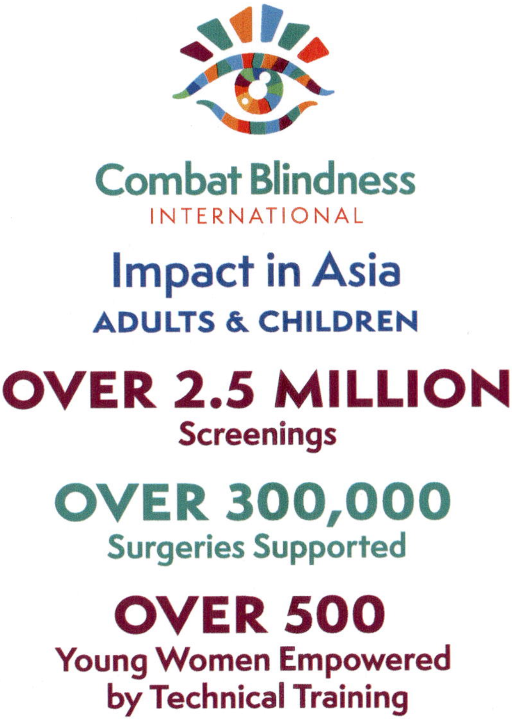

Fig. 21.3 Combat Blindness International (CBI) in Asia

Three accomplishments define CBI's success and its transformational impact on alleviating avoidable blindness around the world: (1) its ability to build strong partnerships with indigenous hospitals and institutions; (2) its commitment to equitable care by supporting the establishments of Aurolab at Arvind Eye Hospital in Madurai, India; and (3) its empowerment of young women through workforce generation in supporting the Certified Ophthalmic Paramedic Program at Dr. Shroff's Charity Eye Hospital in Delhi, India.

21.3 Partnership Building

Since its founding, CBI has built and leveraged partnerships to create sustainable methods to end avoidable blindness, both in South Asia and worldwide; in India, these efforts have been in partnership with the Aravind Eye Care System, L.V. Prasad Eye Institute, Dr. Shroff's Charity Eye Hospital, Sankara Nethralaya, and Sitapur Eye Hospital. CBI has always sought out organizations that share the same passion for aiding and empowering the world's most vulnerable; this outlook has been the bedrock of its many strong relationships with other organizations over the years.

Through these partnerships, CBI is able to promote sustainable methods to screen patients and provide cataract surgeries to eliminate backlogs, use local resources to improve access to eye care, and increase the capabilities of its partners through education and training. CBI also supports local ophthalmologists', technicians', and nurses' education, increasing their partners' ability to operate sustainably and independently. Through this partnership building, CBI is able to create the capacity to restore sight to patients who previously had no access to eye care or resources to pay for treatment, while also increasing their partners' ability to provide sustainable and equitable eye care services.

CBI has partnered with L.V. Prasad Eye Institute (LVPEI) since 1997 in a longstanding relationship of much success. CBI supported work in LVPEI's primary institutes in Hyderabad (Telangana) and Bhubaneshwar (Odisha) and the rural areas of Keonjhar (Odisha) in India. In Hyderabad, CBI provided funds for obtaining the operating equipment for four outreach programs in 1997 and supported 7694 cataract surgeries from 1997 to 2002. In Bhubaneswar, CBI sponsored the Community Comprehensive Eye Care Center to support the outreach activities of this new institute (established in 2006), provided a van to transport patients to the facility, funded 10,255 cataract surgeries since 2007, and financed the skill development for basic ophthalmic technicians and nurses. Through this project the CBI provided scholarships to local students for paramedical training from 2008 to 2011, after which these students were employed in vision centers or community surgical centers.

CBI also partnered with LVPEI, the Jack Deloss Charitable Trust, and the Bijayananda Patnaik Family to finance a building at Keonjhar in Orissa to serve as a surgical center serving 1 million people (Fig. 21.4). The Bijayananda

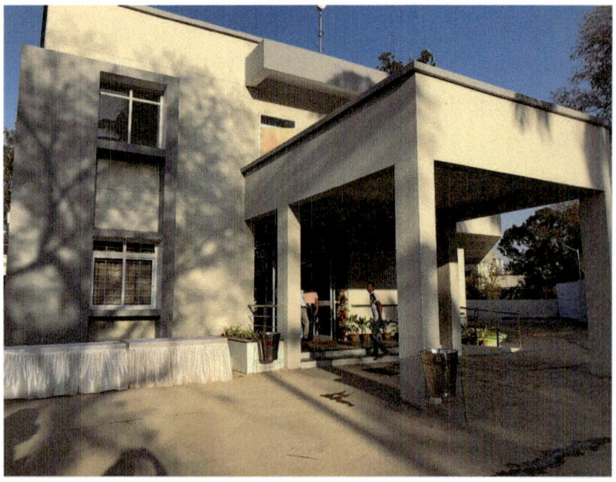

Fig. 21.4 Bijayananda Patnaik Eye Center, Keonjhar, Orissa (with permission from LV Prasad Eye Institute)

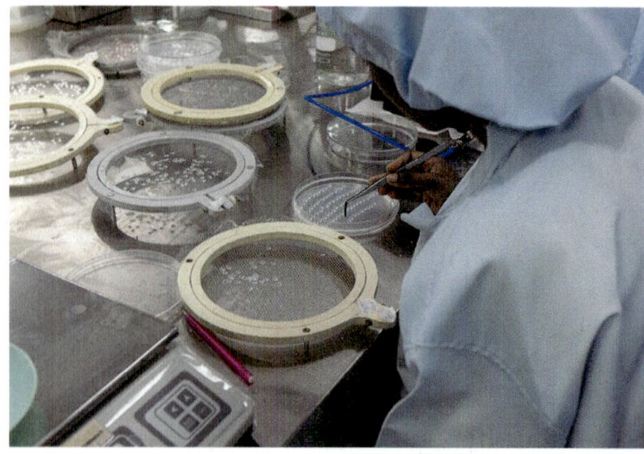

Fig. 21.5 Production of intraocular lenses at Aurolab, Madurai, India (with permission from Aurolab)

Patnaik Eye Center opened in March 2018; in its first year, 15,335 people were screened for vision problems, and 315 cataract surgeries were performed.

21.4 Equitable Care: Aurolab

In the early days of providing cataract surgery in low-income countries, patients were treated in large eye camps, where an assembly line approach was taken for surgical care. Patients with cataracts had their clouded lens removed and were given "coke-bottle" glasses. Although this was a good short-term approach, it was not a sustainable solution. If a patient returned to their home or work and broke or lost their glasses, they were blind again. Therefore, the solution was not equitable. Dr. Chandra felt strongly that a patient in a lower-income country should receive the same quality of care that one would expect in a higher-income country.

In 1992, CBI was one of three like-minded non-governmental organizations (NGOs) that supported the establishment of Aurolab at Madurai (Fig. 21.5). Aurolab is the manufacturing division of the highly respected Aravind Eye Hospital in Madurai, India. Aurolab began producing intraocular lenses (IOL) and provided those lenses to CBI at the cost of roughly USD 2 per lens. Today, Aurolab produces over 2 million IOLs annually and has expanded its range of products to include sutures and other ophthalmic consumables. Aurolab provides these ophthalmic consumables at low costs to NGOs in 120 countries.

With these low-cost lenses, CBI's medical partners provide the same surgeries to their poorest patients that were previously only available to those who could pay. This was a game-changer because it meant that more organizations could provide low-cost surgeries to reduce the backlog of cataract cases worldwide.

21.5 Empowerment Through Workforce Generation: Certified Ophthalmic Paramedic (COP) Program

The shortage of trained eye care professionals is one of the major obstacles facing eye care programs and global health worldwide, but nowhere more so than in the developing world—particularly India, which is home to one-third of the world's 36 million blind people. In partnership with Dr. Shroff's Charity Eye Hospital in India, CBI supports a training course for young women that trains them to become Certified Ophthalmic Paramedics (COPS) and educates them to become strong, empowered women (Fig. 21.6).

These young women complete their training to become mid-level professionals capable of fulfilling several vital functions of traditional oph-

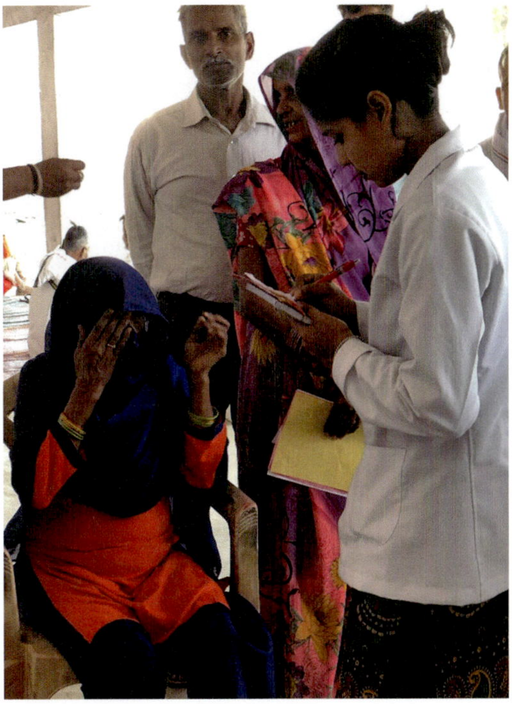

Fig. 21.6 Refraction exam by a COP student, Vrindavan, India (Published with permission from Combat Blindness International)

thalmologists. After just 2 years of training, the young women can perform the duties of vision technicians, nursing assistants, patient counselors, medical records personnel, and optical. These COPs reduce the strain on ophthalmologists so that the ophthalmologists can focus on sight-restoring procedures and surgeries.

Through this program, CBI helps build a trained medical workforce for rural regions where the need is great. The program also makes eye care delivery more efficient while empowering women and reducing poverty through education and employment. The COP program almost always chooses young women from surrounding rural areas of a community as candidates for training. These young women also play a critical role in in-patient education, such as counseling, motivation, and follow-up care in the community. What is equally important is that these young women achieve financial independence and develop important life skills, including those of critical thinking, self-awareness, and communication.

21.6 Conclusion

CBI was established due to one man's desire to give back to his people. Since 1984, CBI has flourished through its vital global partnerships and its determination to be an innovator in providing sustainable and equitable care to the most vulnerable men, women, and children in the world.

Alleviating avoidable blindness continues to be a challenge around the world. To meet this challenge, CBI will continue to expand its existing cataract and pediatric programs throughout Asia. Besides this, CBI is committed to helping the growth of the COP program at Dr. Shroff's Charity Eye Hospital to educate and empower more young women and increase the number of mid-level personnel who can help reduce avoidable blindness in India and beyond.

22 Essilor: Eliminating Uncorrected Refractive Errors by 2050

Anurag Hans

22.1 Addressing a Public Health Crisis

The World Health Organization (WHO) estimates 80% of visual problems can be prevented or treated [1]; so why can't everyone enjoy good vision? Four key barriers to the correction of refractive errors are:

- **lack of awareness** about the need to protect one's vision, that poor or deteriorating eyesight is not something that one has to live with and can be treated, and the need to visit an eye care practitioner regularly;
- **lack of access** to vision care since 90% of those without vision correction live in developing economies at the base of the pyramid [2], far away from an optician or optometrist;
- **lack of affordable solutions** to correct one's vision since these are traditionally developed for urban and affluent consumers; and
- **lack of acceptance** of the problem and adoption of the simplest solution—a pair of glasses. In some countries, there is still a stigma about wearing glasses. Or people simply fail to get into the habit of putting them on when needed.

The good news is that many actions are happening around the world to address these barriers. These efforts are being led by the public and private sectors and supported by multilateral organizations and donors.

At Essilor, we consider good vision is a basic human right and is driven by our mission to improve lives by improving sight. We have an ambition to eliminate uncorrected refractive errors from the world by 2050—to that end, we launched the landmark "Eliminating Poor Vision in a Generation" report in 2019. Supported by NGOs and governments, it offers a roadmap to achieving this ambition and proposes four areas of action to addressing the barriers.

1. **Creating sustainable access points**

Lack of access to vision care and a lack of universal eye health systems impact many countries. Hence, expanding sustainable access must be a priority. Our inclusive business "2.5 New Vision Generation" (2.5 NVG) continues to find new and sustainable ways to provide

A. Hans (✉)
Essilor, Singapore, Singapore
e-mail: anurag.hans@essilor.com.sg

T. Das, P. D. Nayar (eds.), *South-East Asia Eye Health*,
https://doi.org/10.1007/978-981-16-3787-2_22

vision care to underserved populations without access to conventional distribution channels. Through inclusive business programs like Eye Mitra (India), Eye Mitro (Bangladesh), Mitra Mata (Indonesia), and readers access points in Cambodia; we are training unemployed and underemployed people at the base of the pyramid to become primary vision care entrepreneurs for their communities, bringing vision care where it was unavailable before.

Partnering with governments, hospitals, and NGOs expands existing access or creates new access such as mobile vans, vision centers, and large-scale vision screening events that will help extend reach to more people. These partnerships have been successfully executed in many countries including India, Bhutan, and Nepal.

Case Story 1

Our inclusive business programs (Fig. 22.1)

Eye Mitra in India

The Eye Mitra (Hindi for "Friend of the Eye") program addresses three key issues: providing vision correction, developing skills, and creating jobs. First started in India in 2013, the program has since been adapted and expanded to Bangladesh, China, Indonesia, and Kenya. It is one of many inclusive business models Essilor has developed and deployed. Together all these business models represent the world's largest rural optical network with over 16,000 primary vision care entrepreneurs, serving more than 360 million people worldwide

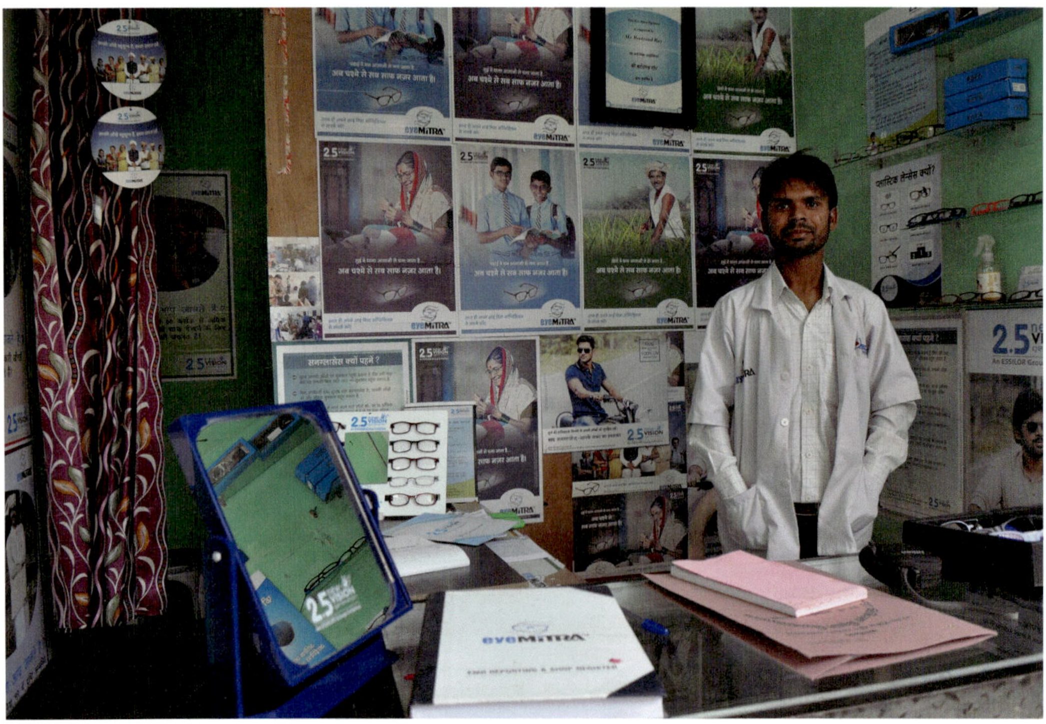

Fig. 22.1 The Eye Mitra program trains unemployed and underemployed youth from rural areas to become primary vision care entrepreneurs in their own communities. © *Essilor 2016. All Rights Reserved*

with sustainable access to vision care (figures quoted are accurate as of September 2020). An impact study of the India program involving nearly 400 Eye Mitras serving 70,000 wearers across six districts showed a total quantifiable impact of USD 4.4 million a year, including the economic impact of increased earnings and increased productivity of wearers. If scaled up to all districts in India, the Eye Mitra model will represent a total potential impact of USD 487 million a year for the country. A follow-up study on the model shows these entrepreneurs typically experience a three- to seven-times increase in lifetime earnings. The model's total quantified impact (social return-on-investment for entrepreneurs and beneficiaries) is 25–48 times.

A gender study is being undertaken to understand the impact of being a female Eye Mitra; the baseline results are promising. Females feel more empowered after becoming an Eye Mitra due to an increase in income, a higher propensity to save, and a greater ability to contribute to family income and decision-making. Besides, the model has a substantial impact across 7 of the 17 United Nations Sustainable Development Goals with a particularly high impact on gender equality and poverty reduction, apart from providing decent work and contributing to health and well-being.

Case Story 2

Partnering Bhutan to be the first country in the world free of uncorrected refractive errors (Fig. 22.2)

In 2018, Essilor formalized a partnership with the Royal Government of Bhutan and the Central Monastic Body to sustainably strengthen the country's vision care infrastructure and support it on its journey to becoming the first "uncorrected refractive errors-free country" in the world—through training and capacity building, philanthropic support, and awareness-raising.

To address the lack of skilled eye care professionals and access to eyewear in the country, we are working with the government to adapt the Eye Mitra program for Bhutan. Additionally, we are training existing government health assistants, village health workers, and monks from the Central Monastic Body to perform basic visual acuity tests, distribute simple reading glasses, and direct patients with refractive errors to eye health practitioners, if necessary.

To meet the immediate need for correction and protection, we support the Ministry of Health's Bhutan School Sight program (which offers free vision screening for all students aged 6–18) and an adult screening program with free glasses and screening events. This donation will be sufficient to provide first-time eyewear to all Bhutanese citizens with uncorrected refractive errors, around 25% of the population. We are also partnering with the Ministry of Health in its "National Eye Health Strategic Plan" (2018–2024) by contributing to the development of national guidelines and a legal regulatory framework for optical services and practice, as well as collaborating on a nation-wide awareness campaign on good vision.

2. **Philanthropy to help those most in need**

While the community-based inclusive business approach can solve 90% of the uncorrected refractive errors issue, the most vulnerable people will always need help through subsidized or free vision care services. For this segment, philanthropy will always play a role. Essilor's philanthropic strategy is embedded within our business strategy and involves different programs and approaches, all united in their goal to achieve long-term social impact. Essilor's Vision Foundations organize philanthropic programs

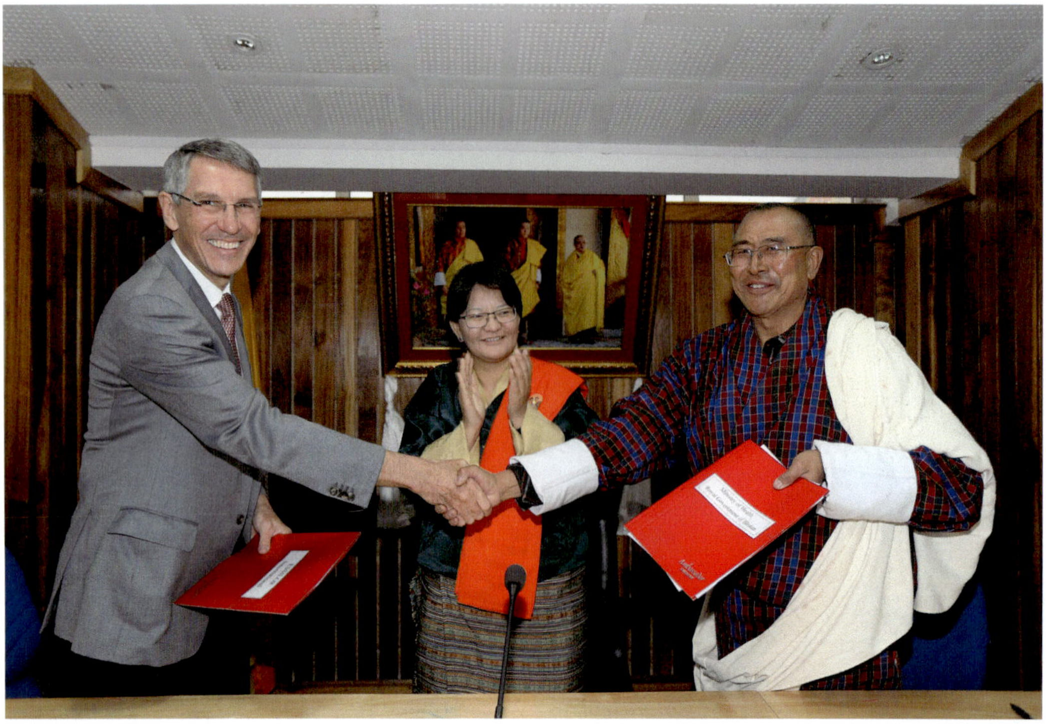

Fig. 22.2 (From left to right) Hubert Sagnières, Chairman of Essilor International shaking hands with Dr. Ugen Dophu, Secretary, Ministry of Health to formalize Essilor's partnership with the Royal Government of Bhutan as Bhutan's Minister of Health, Lyonpo Dechen Wangmo looks on. © *Essilor 2018. All Rights Reserved*

worldwide to provide free glasses to people most in need. Vision For Life, our social impact fund, supports all programs that address the needs of those with uncorrected poor vision and bring about socio-economic benefits for them and their communities. Our inclusive business models can also help us deliver philanthropy efforts through access points in a cost-effective manner.

Case Story 3

Doddaballapura, first India region free of uncorrected refractive errors (Fig. 22.3)

The completion of the Namma Kannu Namma Doddaballapura (NKND) project, scheduled for 2021, will lead to Doddaballapura, in the state of Karnataka, India, with nearly 330,000 residents, being declared the first region in India free of uncorrected refractive errors. A joint initiative by Essilor Vision Foundation India with the Ministry of Health and Family Welfare of the Government of Karnataka, Prerana Trust, a not-for-profit organization, and iDrishti Eye Hospitals, a social impact organization, the NKND project was launched in September 2018 and seeks to eliminate uncorrected refractive errors from Doddaballapura and bring sustainable access to vision care to the region.

The NKND project has extended vision screening services across Doddaballapura. A team of trained personnel visited each household in Doddaballapura to spread awareness of good vision, conduct vision screenings, and dispense glasses if needed. People with complex vision correction needs who cannot be equipped on the spot were referred to the nearest mobile eye camp equipped with mobile buses and qualified optometrists from iDrishti Eye Hospitals to provide them with a comprehensive eye examination. An impact study

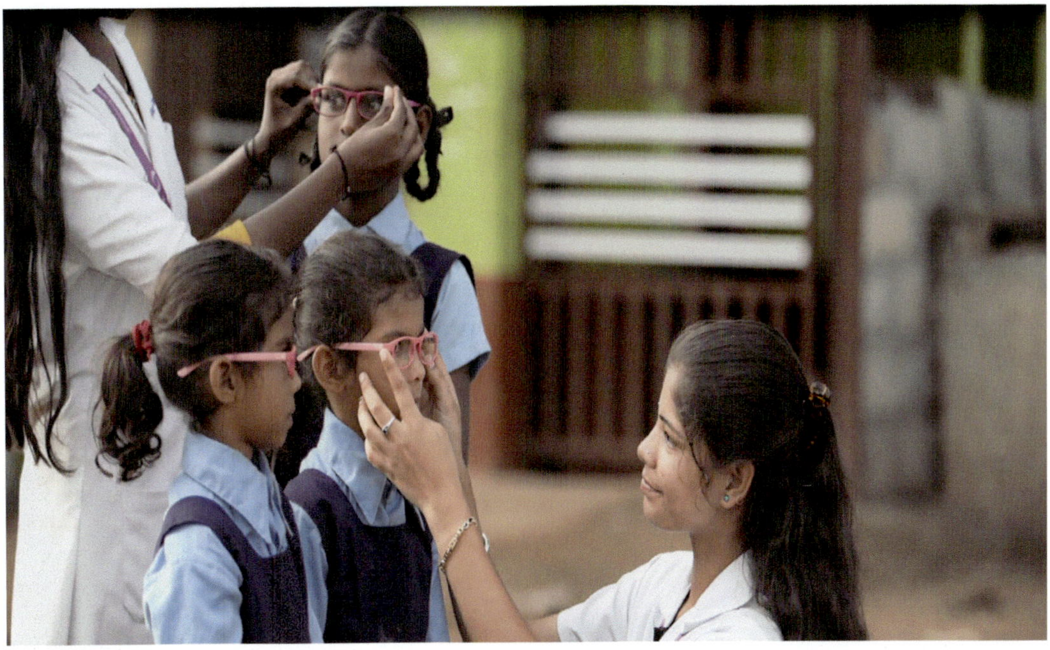

Fig. 22.3 The Namma Kannu Namma Doddaballapura project aims to make the Doddaballapura in Karnataka the first region in India to be free of uncorrected refractive errors. *© Essilor 2019. All Rights Reserved*

on the project found a substantial improvement in adults' and children's daily lives after vision correction.

3. **Raising awareness for vision care**

Raising awareness is a critical first step to embarking on a public health campaign because people can be misinformed, misled, or even completely unaware of the health challenges they face. Many do not know they can do something about uncorrected refractive errors. Building awareness is about sending impactful messages into communities to secure their attention and spread the message by word of mouth.

Awareness is also about advocacy with the governments and health organizations to prioritize vision care, as demonstrated by the work carried out by the Vision Impact Institute, an organization supported by our social impact fund. The Vision Impact Institute focuses on raising awareness about the importance of vision correction and protection to make good vision a global priority.

Case Story 4

See Now with international superstar, Amitabh Bachchan (Fig. 22.4)

See Now is a global campaign created by The Fred Hollows Foundation in partnership with Sightsavers, VISION 2020 India, and Vision For Life. Its objective is to increase awareness and drive public mobilization on ending avoidable blindness and vision impairment. In 2019, a pilot campaign was launched in Uttar Pradesh, North India, with celebrity ambassador Mr. Amitabh Bachchan. The campaign called for people to get their vision tested at existing eye care services. Targeted communications on eye health were delivered via social and traditional media. Using a free "call back" service, respondents were advised the location of their nearest eye health service. The campaign was conducted in five districts of Uttar Pradesh and reached over 32 million people, with over 9200 people participating in free vision screening programs.

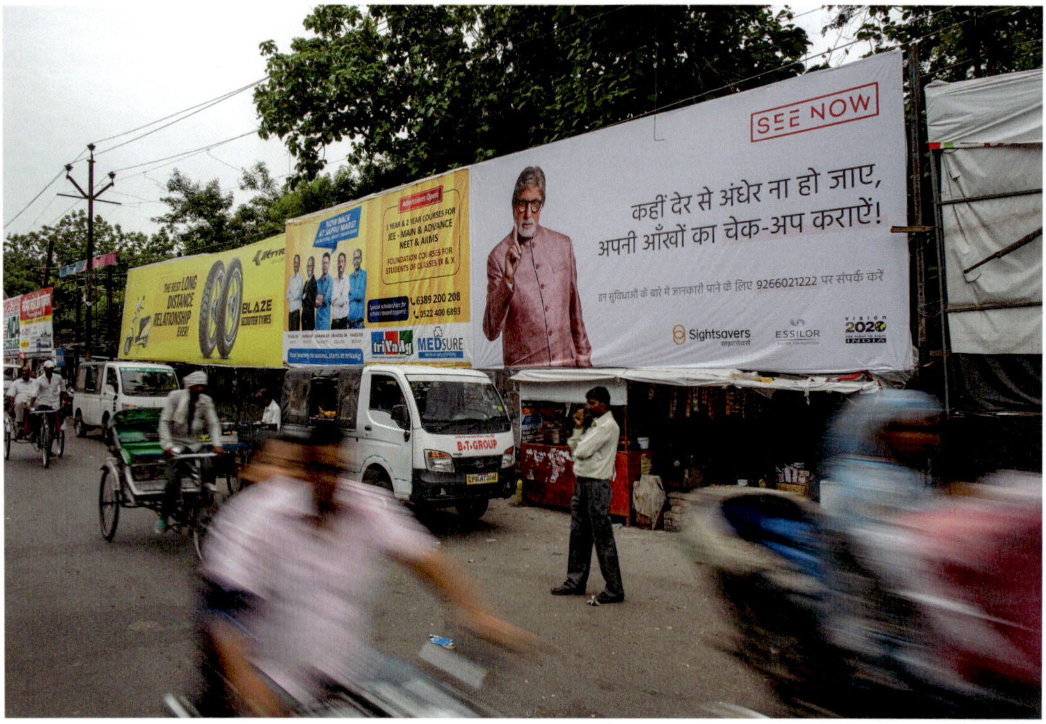

Fig. 22.4 Headlining the See Now campaign in Uttar Pradesh, India, celebrity ambassador Mr. Amitabh Bachchan encourages people to get their eyes checked (Published with permission from *Michael Amendolia, The Fred Hollows Foundation* 2019)

> Phase two of See Now was launched in February 2020, targeting 32 districts in Uttar Pradesh. Despite the impact of COVID-19, it reached over 49 million people, and over 87,000 people were screened.

4. **Innovation to create affordable products, screening tools, and service delivery models**

Innovation is needed across the entire vision care delivery chain, from screening tools and products to service delivery models, to fast-track access for people at the base of the pyramid (BoP). Our BoP Innovation Lab works with 2.5 New Vision Generation to incubate new inclusive business models and technology solutions to reach populations with no access to vision care, in partnership with corporates, startups, NGOs, foundations, or development funds.

Solutions must be affordable, such as our 2.5 New Vision Generation range of spectacles designed with the preferences and needs of BoP consumers in mind without compromising on quality standards. Screening tools must be accessible, scalable, and affordable, like our ClickCheck™, an easy-to-use tool to detect refractive errors. Service delivery must be efficient and adaptable to different environments, mainly post COVID-19. Our tele-refraction models use technology to remotely connect primary vision care providers and their customers to an urban optometrist to supervise the refraction process. Customers get high-quality care; primary vision care providers can offer an enhanced service, boosting their credibility and potential income, and optometrists can play a mentoring and supervisory role. To adhere to safe distancing measures, a home delivery model is piloted in India where customers can make appointments for at-home vision screenings, facilitated by tele-refraction.

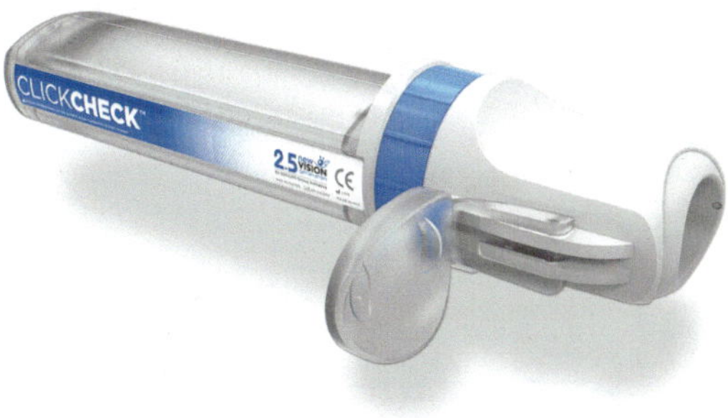

Fig. 22.5 The ClickCheck™ vision screening tool promises to make vision screening easy and affordable for primary vision care providers. © *Essilor 2019. All Rights Reserved*

Case Story 5

The ClickCheck™ Refraction Tool—Vision Screening Made Possible Anywhere (Fig. 22.5)

One of the key barriers to bringing vision care to the developing world is the lack of affordable testing tools—an autorefractor which tests for refractive errors can cost from USD 2000 to USD 20,000. Priced at a fraction of an autorefractor, the ClickCheck™ vision screening tool is an invaluable innovation; it is portable, easy-to-use, does not require electricity to operate, and is ideal for vision screening in all settings. Winner of our See Change innovation challenge in 2016, the ClickCheck™ vision screening tool was conceptualized by TEAMS Design, an award-winning design consultancy. After refinement and field testing by the teams from our BoP Innovation Lab, 2.5 New Vision Generation, and Center of Innovation and Technology, the ClickCheck™ vision screening tool is now available for use by all primary vision care providers and NGOs.

22.2 Partnerships

Partnership is key to accelerating change. We are a founding partner of the USD 1 billion Vision Catalyst Fund, a multi-stakeholder initiative to bring eye care to everyone in the Commonwealth and around the world. As founding partner, we will contribute specialist knowledge to raise awareness and create sustainable access to vision and have pledged to provide up to 200 million people with ophthalmic lenses by 2030. We are part of the EYElliance, a coalition to find solutions to the world's unmet need for glasses.

22.3 Establishing an Industry-First Universal KPI Template to Measure Success

Working with renowned global health experts and as part of the Eliminating Poor Vision report, we have developed a universal key performance indicator (KPI) template for the industry, the first of its kind, to determine if an area is free of uncorrected refractive errors. We are proactively encouraging our partners to use the template at <https://www.essilorseechange.com/elimination-in-a-generation/> to measure their programs (Fig. 22.6). So far, iDrishti Eye Hospitals in India have used it to measure the Essilor-partnered Namma Kannu Namma Doddaballapura program.

22.4 Collective Actions: The Way Forward

To date, Essilor has created sustainable access to vision care for over 360 million people in developing communities by establishing more than 16,000 access points and inclusive businesses (figures quoted are accurate as of September 2020). Through these and our philanthropic initiatives, we have helped over 37 million people around the world access their first pair of glasses (figure quoted is accurate as of September 2020). But there is still more to do until no one suffers the social, economic, and individual cost of uncorrected refractive errors. The "Eliminating Poor Vision in a Generation" report demonstrates that we have a once in a lifetime opportunity to end this universal healthcare crisis in a generation by working together.

	Financially sustainable access point	Affordable solutions	Funding for subsidized/free services and products	Awareness
Input KPIs Have the interventions been implemented?	100 percent of people have at least one access point within one day's return travel	Corrective lenses equal to three days wages or less are available to all people	Subsidized or free refractive error solutions are available for those living in extreme poverty for life and all children of the working poor before the age of 10, and provided when needed subsequently	All communities receive information about importance of vision care (including URE)
Intervention outputs Are the interventions reaching the required number of people?	95 percent of children aged 2-16 receives one eye exam per year✦ 95 percent of adults over the age of 16 receives one eye exam per two years✦	Number of corrective solutions distributed equals the projected RE population (95 percent)		100 percent of people were exposed to at least one message about vision care (including URE) in the last one year
Program outcomes Has success been definitively achieved?	95 percent of people with refractive errors have had their vision corrected			

✦Except when specific diseases are detected.

Fig. 22.6 Eliminating Uncorrected Poor Vision KPI Template that can be used to determine progress of any region toward become free of uncorrected refractive errors. © *Essilor 2019. All Rights Reserved*

References

1. World Health Organization. Visual impairment and blindness. World Health Organization; 2014. Fact Sheet N°282. https://web.archive.org/web/20150512062236/; http://www.who.int/mediacentre/factsheets/fs282/en/
2. World Health Organization. Universal eye health: a global action plan 2014–2019. World Health Organization; 2013, p. 4. https://www.who.int/blindness/AP2014_19_English.pdf

23 Embedding Equity, Innovation, and Partnerships into Eye Health

The Fred Hollows Foundation in Nepal, Bangladesh, and Myanmar

Jon Crail and Aildrene Tan

The **Fred Hollows** Foundation

In the early 1990s, the world's top ophthalmologists gathered at a conference in Nepal to discuss the future of cataract care [1]. Among them were Professor Fred Hollows, an Australian ophthalmologist known for his sight-saving work in Asia, Africa, and the Australian Outback. Accompanying him was Dr. Sanduk Ruit, a Nepalese eye doctor closely mentored by Fred (Fig. 23.1).

At the time, cataracts in Nepal were treated by Intracapsular Cataract Extraction, which often required patients to wear thick glasses after operation [2]. But Hollows and Ruit had a different vision. They presented their work on performing small-incision microsurgery; this less intensive procedure allowed them to implant a tiny intraocular lens (IOL) to replace the clouded lens of the eye. Despite its potential, the two doctors were met with strong opposition from the medical community, with fears that it was too complicated and too expensive. At the time, an IOL cost around US$ 200 each [3]. In response, Hollows stood up and did not mince his words: "You guys have no vision. There will be a time when you do surgeries, and you will provide IOL instead of these thick glasses." It was a turning point for Hollows and Ruit. They were compelled to prove that their idea would work if they could mass produce IOLs at a lower price.

Hollows passed away in 1993, just a few months after he founded The Fred Hollows Foundation, a non-profit organization dedicated to eliminating avoidable blindness. Ruit continued the work that he and Hollows started, and in 1994, with financial support from The Foundation, he co-founded the Tilganga Institute of Ophthalmology (TIO) in Kathmandu. The Foundation worked with TIO to build the Fred Hollows Intraocular Lens Laboratory in Kathmandu, which opened in 1994. With technical support from Australia and New Zealand, this world-class factory realized Hollows' and Ruit's dream of bringing down the cost of IOLs to just a few dollars. Today, the IOL factory profits support TIO to subsidize other activities such as outreach camps.

Now, almost three decades after it was founded, The Fred Hollows Foundation works in more than 25 countries with local partners to deliver programs that strengthen health systems and ensure equitable access to eye health services. In IAPB's South-East Asia Region, The Foundation has projects in Bangladesh, India, Indonesia, Myanmar, Nepal, and Timor Leste. In 2019, in these six countries, The Foundation's

J. Crail (✉) · A. Tan
The Fred Hollows, Sydney, Australia
e-mail: jcrail@hollows.org; atan@hollows.org

T. Das, P. D. Nayar (eds.), *South-East Asia Eye Health*,
https://doi.org/10.1007/978-981-16-3787-2_23

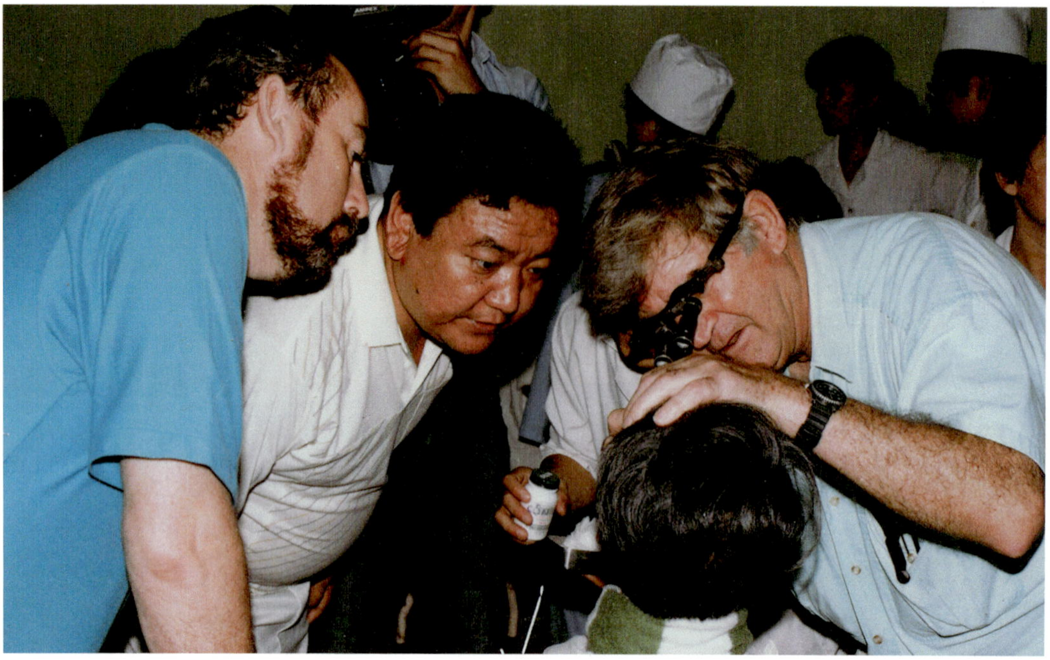

Fig. 23.1 Dr Sanduk Ruit (center) and Professor Fred Hollows (right) conduct cataract training workshops in Hanoi, Vietnam in 1992. Photo: Michael Amendolia/The Fred Hollows Foundation

support contributed to screening more than 1.8 million people, treatment of more than 140,000 patients, and training of more than 14,500 doctors, nurses, and teachers.

This chapter focuses on The Foundation's programs in Nepal, Bangladesh, and Myanmar and illustrates how through innovation and effective partnerships, we can address inequities and reach more people with high-quality eye care.

23.1 Nepal: Addressing Inequity Through Targeted Approaches

Nepal has one of the highest cataract surgical rates in the region, second only to India. A Rapid Assessment of Avoidable Blindness (RAAB) survey in Bagmati Province in 2019 showed a cataract surgical coverage rate of 95.9% among blind people [4]. This is a remarkable figure on par with many higher-income nations and well above the widely accepted target of 80% [5].

Despite the impressive numbers, there are still groups missing out on services, such as those in remote areas, women, and other marginalized groups. Nepal has a backlog of around 185,000 people requiring cataract surgery—most of whom live outside Kathmandu [6]. Nepal's geography contributes to inequity in access to eye health services. Of those living in remote and rural areas, 33% are multidimensionally poor, compared to 7% of their urban counterparts [7]. The rate of blindness among women from high altitude regions is twice the rate of men nationally (at 66.7% vs 33.3%) [8]. The recent RAAB survey found three times as many women as men blind from cataract [4]. Recognizing the need to address these inequities, The Foundation is shifting to a targeted programming approach.

The Foundation supports TIO to deliver Outreach Microsurgical Eye Clinics in rural and remote regions of Nepal, accommodating hundreds of patients at a time. Existing Community Eye Centers are extending even further into remote areas with a trial of remote clinics that target people who are too far from Community Eye Centers to access eye care services. Teleophthalmology services were established in 2019, making it possible for people living in the remote districts of Nuwakot and Dhading to access specialty services in Kathmandu. The timing of these services' establishment has proven to be very useful during the COVID-19 pandemic.

Special attention is now being directed toward Nepal's poorest province, Karnali. From 2011 to 2014, the province had the least improvement in development [7] and is underserved in eye care. This is a new region for The Foundation and TIO to work together. Issues affecting the availability of eye health services—such as the lack of equipment and insufficient trained ophthalmic staff—will be addressed initially to expand support over time.

To address gender inequities, The Foundation and TIO have implemented strategies to support better access to eye health care for women, such as bringing outreach camps close to people's homes, subsidizing surgeries, training and mobilizing female community health volunteers, and holding community awareness activities. Recognizing that gender inequity is multifaceted and requires more than a "quick fix", a research trial was undertaken recently to identify strategies more likely to impact women's access to and uptake of eye health services [9]. The ongoing trial will strengthen gender-equitable approaches to eye health throughout all future programming in Nepal.

23.2 Bangladesh: Continuously Innovating to Close the Gender Gap

Bangladesh has persistent gender inequities in eye health. Women in Bangladesh are more likely to be blind (2.7% compared to 1.6% of men) or vision impaired (4% of women compared to 2.9% of men) [10]. Some of the underlying barriers to accessing eye care include low-decision making power among women, limited gender-sensitive service delivery partly due to social stigma, limited access to information, difficulties traveling alone for services, financial constraints, and a low priority given to eye care [11]. The Foundation estimates that 15.3 women need to receive cataract surgery for every 10 men to make services equitable [12]. Gender-equitable eye care service delivery has been a key focus of The Foundation since it started working in Bangladesh in 2008.

Bangladesh is known for its thriving Ready-Made Garment industry that employs more than 4 million workers. The majority are women, and vision problems are among the top five priority health issues they face, partly due to the nature of the work. Based on The Foundation's research, more than 60% of garment workers report suffering from eye conditions. Factories are profit-oriented and time-conscious enterprises, and workers often do not have enough time or money to visit eye health services in their spare time. The Foundation has worked with 17 garment factories, 6 women's cafes, and 2 garment association hospitals to conduct awareness-raising activities and provide on-site eye care services. In most cases, medical centers within factories do not offer eye care, so The Foundation has trained factory medical staff and provided equipment to its partner factories. Women coordinators encourage the use of self-detection vision corners on factory floors.

The results are excellent, with garment workers taking regular breaks to rest their eyes, conducting self-checks, reporting eye health issues, and seeking treatment when necessary. As well as these health benefits, almost 90% of workers report needing less time to finish their work after being provided with eyeglasses. By demonstrating investment in eye health results in productivity gains, some of the best records for health intervention, factory owners are convinced that women's eye health should be prioritized. Cost-sharing models have also been implemented, where the patient and factory management contribute to the cost of glasses. The Foundation is now looking for ways to adopt these lessons in other settings, such as shoe and ceramic factories.

The Foundation has also made strides in reaching women outside industrial centers. According to the Bangladesh National Blindness and Low Vision Survey, the Division of Barisal recorded the country's highest prevalence of bilateral blindness. The Foundation's extensive research on gender inequities in eye care in Barisal showed women are much more likely to drop out of eye care referral systems because of financial and social reasons that include restrictions on traveling without male companions, dependence on male family members for treatment costs, less access to information, and privacy issues in health facilities. The Foundation's project in Barisal aimed to address these issues by delivering innovative approaches that fit the local culture. The Foundation has led the way by upgrading health facilities to include breastfeeding corners, separate toilets, and separate waiting areas for women. Digital token systems were also set-up to prevent men from pushing women out of the queue. Communication materials that promote equitable eye care services were developed. Communication activities such as courtyard meetings—locally known as Uthan Baithak—were carried out to reach women in their households.

To encourage women to seek medical attention, The Foundation has also trained more than 500 local pharmacists—community figures often regarded as a trusted source of information. Community health workers were trained to empower women and encourage them to take charge of their health. At the end of the project, more than 80% of female patients were satisfied with the health centers' services. More women also had access to eye health services, comprising 58% of people screened for eye diseases.

Aiming to reach a larger number of potential beneficiaries, The Foundation has also integrated eye care in Maternal and Child Health (MCH) clinics for the first time in Bangladesh. Clinics such as the Smiling Sun Clinic Network are well-known throughout the country, bringing eye health closer to more female patients. In 2016, The Foundation's Bangladesh Country Manager, Dr. Zareen Khair, was awarded L'Occitane Foundation's first Sight Award for Innovation, pioneering innovations that improve the sight of more than 135,000 women and children in rural Bangladesh.

With these gains, The Foundation in Bangladesh is working toward implementing strategies to improve eye health access for other marginalized groups such as people living with a disability, sex workers, transgender people, and Rohingya refugees, and occupational groups like tea garden workers and snake charmers.

23.3 Myanmar: Laying the Groundwork Through Strategic Partnerships

In September 2020, WHO declared Myanmar as having officially eliminated trachoma as a public health problem. In 2005, trachoma—the world's leading infectious cause of blindness—was responsible for 4% of all blindness in Myanmar. By 2018, trachoma prevalence had fallen below the threshold to a mere 0.008%. This achievement was made possible through the Trachoma Control and Prevention of Blindness Program (TC&PBL), a key partner of The Foundation in Myanmar. TC&PBL is the lead government agency responsible for blindness prevention programs in the Disease Control Department of the Ministry of Health and Sports.

The Foundation only established an office and partnership with the government in Myanmar in 2017, but it has made great inroads into supporting eye health by establishing and maintaining partnerships with government partners such as TC&PBL.

As a result of these partnerships, Myanmar launched its first National Eye Health Plan (NEHP 2017–2021). The Foundation conducted the situational analysis of the NEHP, which guides and aligns the planning and implementation of all eye health programs across the country. The Foundation then piloted an eye health model in Shan State. The Disease Control Department and other departments at the state and regional levels recognized its success, and it was expanded to Magway and Ayeyarwady. The Foundation's model is now being considered for national rollout.

The Foundation provided technical and financial support to review and revise existing primary eye care manuals and materials. The Foundation also worked with TC&PBL to finalize the components of primary eye care kits and source suppliers. Almost 4000 primary eye care kits were distributed to The Foundation's current project areas.

With these achievements, the government has recognized the importance of eye health and has included it for the first time in the National Health Policy draft.

23.4 Conclusion

Although Nepal, Bangladesh, and Myanmar comprise a small section of the region, our work in these countries reflects the urgent need to prioritize eye health globally. The 2019 WHO World Report on Vision predicts that eye care needs would increase dramatically in the coming decades. With at least 2.2 billion people worldwide who are blind or vision impaired, health systems need to be strong and capable of meeting the growing demand for eye care.

NGOs have a huge role to play to help governments strengthen their health systems. To be effective, organizations need to tailor programs to specific countries and communities. Ensuring equity and inclusion, introducing innovations, and maintaining strategic partnerships are crucial to creating and sustaining eye health programs that reach the poor and marginalized.

References

1. The friendship of two 'miracle workers': Fred Hollows and Sanduk Ruit. https://www.abc.net.au/radionational/programs/lifematters/barefoot-surgeon/10609654. Accessed 4 Aug 2020.
2. Hennig A. Cataract surgery in Nepal: then and now. Nepal J Ophthalmol. 2010;2(4):83–6.
3. 25 Dollars, 10 minutes, 1, life changed forever. https://www.cureblindness.org/our-story/innovative. Accessed 13 Sept 2020.
4. Gurung R, Thapa SS, Rai NK, Shrestha MK, Gurung K, Poudel M, Upreti R, Sapkota YD, D'Esposito F, Neupane A, Dahal A, Ruit S. Rapid Assessment of Avoidable Blindness (RAAB) survey in Bagmati Province of Nepal, 2020. Kathmandu: Tilganga Institute of Ophthalmology; 2019.
5. Gray Z, Ackland P. Cataract surgical coverage: an important indicator for eye health and for monitoring progress towards Universal Health Coverage. Int Agency Prevention Blindness. 2015.
6. Deloitte Touche Tohmatsu India LLP. Progress review of current strategic plan and recommendations for a 5 year future strategic plan and implementation road-map – Tilganga Institute of Ophthalmology. February 2018.
7. Government of Nepal National Planning Commission. Nepal's Multidimensional Poverty Index: analysis towards action. 2018.
8. National Research and Monitoring Department of Mepal Netra Jyoty Sangh and Survey Advisory Committee. The epidemiology of blindness in Nepal 2012. 2012.
9. Hazel YP, Malla C, Afford A, Hillgrove T, Gurung R, Dahal A, Shah S, Shrestha MK, Manandhar A. Continuous knowledge translation in action: designing a programmatic research trial for equitable eye health for rural Nepalese women. Int J Environ Res Public Health. 2020;17(1).
10. Muhit M, Wadud Z, Islam J, Khair Z, Shamanna BR, Jung J, Khandaker G. Generating evidence for program planning: rapid assessment of avoidable blindness in Bangladesh. Ophthal Epidemiol. 2016;23(3):176–84.
11. Mainuddin A, Ara Begum H, Rawal LB, Islam A, Shariful Islam SM. Women empowerment and its relation with health seeking behavior in Bangladesh. J Family Reprod Health. 2015;9(2):65–73. http://www.ncbi.nlm.nih.gov/pubmed/26175761
12. The Fred Hollows Foundation. Bangladesh Beneficiary Inequity Profile [2016–2019].

24 Helen Keller International's Eye Health Partnerships and Accomplishments in South-East Asia

Nick Kourgialis and Satyaprabha Kotha

Founded in 1915, Helen Keller International (HKI) is a non-profit organization working in 21 countries, primarily in Africa and Asia. HKI mission is to save and improve the sight and lives of the world's most vulnerable populations. We combat the causes and consequences of blindness, poor health, and malnutrition by establishing programs based on evidence and research in vision, health, and nutrition and by building the technical and operational capacity of local partners to provide services to those in need. We envision a world where no one suffers from preventable or treatable blindness or low vision, no one suffers from malnutrition, and fewer people suffer a loss of their productive years due to disability and premature death. To accomplish this, we work with local government, non-profit, and private sector systems and promote the development of sustainable, large-scale programs that deliver effective solutions to overcome preventable blindness and malnutrition.

HKI designs programs to be sustainable by building local ownership and capacity, strengthening existing systems, and focusing attention and resources on building resilience. Achieving sustainable development requires full partnerships with governments, communities, civil society, and the private sector that are based on a shared vision, open communication, and mutual accountability. We believe the most effective programs and operational systems are evidence-based and contextually relevant, and are rooted in state-of-the-art knowledge and local situational analysis. Therefore, we design and test innovative approaches to the current challenges and utilize rigorous evaluation to maximize impact and develop new knowledge. HKI has supported blindness prevention efforts in South-East Asia for over 50 years. A brief description of some of these accomplishments is provided below.

24.1 Nepal

In 2017, HKI received a grant from the USAID Child Blindness Program to establish a pilot retinopathy of prematurity (ROP) program in

N. Kourgialis (✉)
Helen Keller International, New York, NY, USA
e-mail: nkourgialis@hki.org

S. Kotha
Helen Keller International, Jakarta Selatan, Indonesia
e-mail: skotha@hki.org

T. Das, P. D. Nayar (eds.), *South-East Asia Eye Health*,
https://doi.org/10.1007/978-981-16-3787-2_24

Kathmandu, Nepal, in partnership with the Tilganga Institute of Ophthalmology and neonatal intensive care units within three hospitals. In developing this program model, we recognized that a fully integrated and complementary care system that focuses equally on prevention as well as identification and treatment of ROP was critical to reducing the incidence of vision loss among premature infants.

ROP programs have traditionally prioritized screening and treatment efforts focused solely on an infant's eyes while neglecting to make the critical investments needed to build the capacity of neonatal intensive care units and their staff, and to reduce the number of children placed unnecessarily at risk, for example, by inadequate monitoring and regulation of oxygen use. The key elements of HKI's ROP program included: (1) assessing current neonatal intensive care unit (NICU) practices and capacity, identifying gaps in equipment and training, and improving the level of care through the adoption of global NICU standards; (2) supporting the use of retinal cameras to conduct ROP screening and the adoption of a telemedicine-based approach to ROP management; and (3) educating parents regarding the risks posed by ROP and providing the necessary counseling and support to encourage compliance with recommended screening and treatment plans.

Based on the success of this initial pilot, a subsequent USAID Child Blindness Program grant was awarded in 2019 to support the replication and refinement of this model in the Mid-Western Terai district (Banke) in partnership with three additional hospitals/NICUs and the Fateh Bal Eye Hospital, Nepalgunj. Program refinements included the use of a mobile phone-based messaging system to improve parental awareness of ROP and compliance with recommended screening and treatment plans, and research into the use of low-cost retinal cameras and artificial intelligence software that automatically grades retinal images captured by screeners within the NICUs, immediately determines the presence of disease, and expedites the referral of infants requiring further examination and treatment.

Through these continued investments, we hope to further expand the evidence base regarding effective prevention and treatment strategies to address ROP in Nepal; to build a broad-based constituency of private and government medical institutions, clinicians, parents, and other key stakeholders advocating for governmental investments in ROP care; and to contribute to the establishment of national guidelines governing this care and the adoption of a coordinated national strategy to reduce vision loss due to ROP.

24.2 Indonesia

Over its ~50-year presence in Indonesia, HKI has made significant and varied contributions to the prevention of blindness and visual impairment and consistently advocated for the support of these efforts by the Indonesian Ministry of Health. These contributions include the support of national vitamin A supplementation campaigns that reduced the prevalence of childhood blindness and improved child survival; investments in cataract surgical training and community-based primary eye health services that facilitated the identification and restoration of sight for people blinded by cataract; an innovative diabetic retinopathy program that supported increased cooperation among the eye health and diabetes sectors, piloted the use of and supported the broader adoption of tele-ophthalmology-based diabetic retinopathy services in Jakarta, Bandung, and Yogyakarta, and successfully integrated diabetic retinopathy training within ophthalmology residency programs throughout Indonesia. HKI also supported the establishment of tele-ophthalmology-based ROP programs in Jakarta and Makassar.

HKI's pioneering work in inclusive education led to greater recognition of visually impaired children's educational needs as well as the educational needs of those with other forms of disability. Working in collaboration with the Government of Indonesia, HKI designed and implemented an inclusive education program, including the creation of early intervention centers for preschool-age children, that provided more than 30,000 children with disabilities an opportunity to learn, experience a sense of belonging, and to fulfill their potential. The resulting government policies and investments continue to provide significant societal benefit by reducing the isolation and stigmatization of children with disabilities, permitting them to enter mainstream schools and achieve their full educational potential. Beginning in 2017, HKI also sought to address the vocational needs of secondary school students with physical and intellectual disabilities by developing guidelines and curricula focused on developing vocational skills and the establishment of internship programs. This included training 30 inclusive education teachers from Jakarta and Depok to implement the curriculum and increase their overall capacity to serve their students.

Finally, HKI has sought to expand access to vision services for children by supporting the integration of pediatric eye health services within Indonesia's broader health and educational systems over the past decade. In Jakarta, this involved establishing school-based eye health programs that screened, provided eyeglasses to, and suggested referrals for further examination and treatment when required for hundreds of thousands of children (Fig. 24.1).

Similarly, in the city of Surabaya, an integrated system of care was developed that included the establishment of a dedicated pediatric eye health clinic, the training of a pediatric ophthalmologist capable of addressing complex disorders, and the training of community-based healthcare workers and teachers to conduct eye health screenings in schools and community-

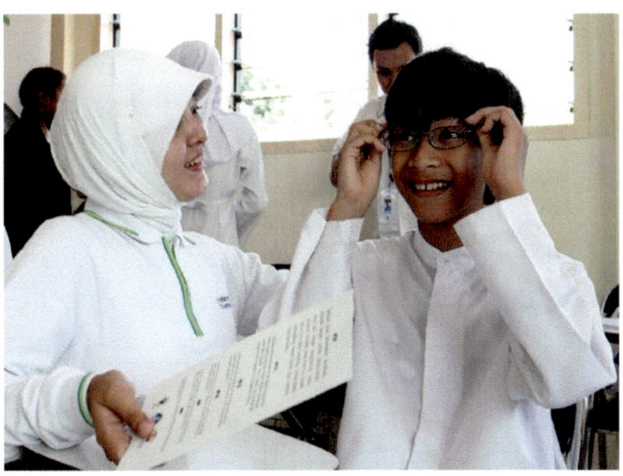

Fig. 24.1 Clear vision brings smiles to children in an Indonesia school. © HKI Intl

based health clinics, where preschool-age children with eye health disorders could also be identified. This approach was expanded upon in the Province of South Sulawesi and Nusa Tenggara Barat by a consortium of organizations that included CBM, Orbis, and the Fred Hollows Foundation, with support from Standard Chartered Bank's "Seeing is Believing" program. In South Sulawesi, investments in training and equipment provision were made at all levels of the health system. This included the training and equipping of staff in maternal-child health posts; developing and integrating vision centers within community health clinics; building secondary pediatric eye health capacity within district hospitals; establishing a dedicated pediatric eye health clinic at the Hasanuddin Hospital in Makassar; supporting sub-specialty training in pediatric ophthalmology; and significantly enhancing access to low vision services in the province. Through the collaborative efforts of HKI and its partner organizations, we sought to establish a fully integrated pediatric eye health system that could serve as a model for replication and be brought to scale throughout Indonesia.

24.3 Bangladesh

HKI's work in Bangladesh began in 1978, supporting the government's blindness prevention program, conducting the first National Nutritional Blindness survey, and assisting the Ministry of Health and Family Welfare to establish the national Vitamin A supplementation program. HKI has also made significant contributions to addressing the needs of visually impaired children in Bangladesh. Beginning in 1995, HKI initiated the Technical Assistance to the Education and Rehabilitation of the Blind (TAERB) project, which promoted integrated education for the visually impaired in 64 districts in Bangladesh. From the mid to late 1990s, the HKI also worked in partnership with the Chittagong Eye Infirmary and Training Complex (CEITC) to establish local manufacturing capacity for low vision assistive devices and develop pediatric eye health screening capacity within community health clinics in the Chittagong hill tracts. Through these efforts, access to primary eye care services was enhanced within these extremely isolated and underserved communities. The ability to identify and treat children with potentially blinding disorders also improved significantly.

More recently, HKI has sought to address the growing threat of diabetes-related vision loss in Bangladesh by successfully establishing dedicated diabetic retinopathy clinics in several regions of the country and advocating for increased governmental support for diabetes prevention and disease management efforts, diabetic retinopathy care, and increased integration of these services. Over 80,000 individuals have been screened, and more than 7000 have been treated over the past 8 years. Key partners have included the CEITC, the Feni Diabetes Hospital, the National Institute of Ophthalmology Hospital in Dhaka, the Mymensingh Medical College Hospital, and Shaheed Ziaur Rahman Medical College Hospital in Bogra, where diabetic retinopathy screening and treatment capacity were enhanced through the provision of state-of-the-art equipment and training. Critical investments in equipment, including state-of-the-art retinal cameras, monitors, data management systems/servers, and lasers, were made to support partner facilities. Equally important investments in training were also made. These included:

1. Educating diabetes healthcare providers and patients regarding the consequences of diabetic eye disease and the need for annual eye examination.
2. Educating mid-level health personnel to accurately photograph and grade images of the retina and to refer patients for further examination and treatment.
3. Adopting a systematic quality assurance regimen that demonstrated the relative quality and cost-efficiency of image grading conducted by mid-level health personnel rather than ophthalmologists helped identify individuals requiring further training or support.
4. Educating clinicians to treat patients effectively and to provide patients with education and counseling required to ensure compliance with recommended diabetic retinopathy treatment plans.

24.4 Myanmar

Beginning in 2001, HKI worked in close cooperation with the Trachoma Control and Prevention of Blindness Department at the Myanmar Ministry of Health to support the elimination of trachoma as a public health problem. This goal was finally achieved in September 2020 when the World Health Organization (WHO) validated the elimination of trachoma. HKI's contributions to this effort were noted in the WHO report, "*Terminating Trachoma: How Myanmar Eliminated Blinding Trachoma.*"

Equally important investments were made in building cataract surgical capacity in Myanmar, particularly in the central dry zone, where most of the trachoma control efforts were conducted initially. Through these efforts, 20 Secondary Eye Centers that primarily serve poor rural communities were provided with the necessary training, equipment, and consumables needed to establish high-quality, sustainable cataract services over the past 15 years. During this period, over 400,000 sight-restoring cataract surgeries were performed by these facilities. Besides these, critical investments in ophthalmology residency training were made at leading teaching hospitals in Yangon and Mandalay to address Myanmar's significant eye health human resources needs.

Over the past 5 years, the range of programs supported by HKI has expanded. It now includes integrating eye health services within school health programs and integrating diabetic retinopathy screening and referral capacity within noncommunicable disease clinics. The latter effort will include the testing and assessment of low-cost retinal cameras, paired with artificial intelligence software, and an examination of the degree to which these new technological tools can reduce costs and improve access to diabetic retinopathy services in isolated rural communities that face significant barriers to accessing care.

Mission for Vision

Catalyzing Transformative Change Through Enhanced Sight

25

Elizabeth Kurian and Shrikant Ayyangar

Mission for Vision
partners in eye health

Growing up in India, Jagdish Mithu Chanrai was deeply moved by the inequality between the rich and poor; it ignited in him a considerable desire to reduce this gap. He first met St. Teresa (then Mother Theresa) in the 1980s when he was a young man on a quest to help India's poor. Accompanying her as she visited her projects, he was struck by her unswerving belief and dedication. She tended to the poor and sick and learned that it is possible to overcome incredible odds to achieve social change with love, faith, and discipline. As the scion of a family that has been engaging in extensive businesses in Africa and Asia since the 1860s, philanthropy was not new to Mr. Chanrai. However, his approach to giving practices has adapted based on his personal experiences.

After the establishment of Shanti Daan, a shelter for the homeless in Mumbai to house destitute men and boys and various other initiatives along with Mother Teresa's Order, the Missionaries of Charity, he made his foray into eye health in 1990. He was soon joined by some of his close friends and business associates to set up Mission for Vision in the year 2000.

25.1 Setting the Foundation Stone

Mission for Vision is a not-for-profit organization working towards eradicating needless blindness in India, Nigeria, and Bhutan, with the ambitious goal of spreading the effort around the world. It works towards eradicating avoidable blindness by enabling high quality, comprehensive, and equitable eye health systems. The organization's vision is to restore the gift of sight to every visually impaired human being, irrespective of nationality, religion, or socioeconomic status—Mission for Vision's values center on quality, cost-efficiency, sustainability, and service to all.

Mission for Vision is founded on the philosophy of *Caring Capitalism®*, which is rooted in the belief that an individual should give a portion of his/her generated wealth to the communities from which he/she has benefitted. While many philanthropists recognize the power of collective

E. Kurian (✉) · S. Ayyangar
Mission for Vision, Mumbai, India
e-mail: ekurian@missionforvision.org.in;
sayyangar@missionforvision.org.in

T. Das, P. D. Nayar (eds.), *South-East Asia Eye Health*,
https://doi.org/10.1007/978-981-16-3787-2_25

action towards poverty alleviation, only a few can practice it. Mission for Vision is probably the first example of collective "private philanthropy" towards eradicating needless blindness. Ultra-high-net-worth individual philanthropists laid down the organization's foundation with a shared agenda of progressing people out of poverty through improved sight.

25.2 Investing in Equitable Eye Health

Visual impairment limits people's access to opportunities and social participation. The World Report on Vision of the World Health Organization (WHO) reports that at least 2.2 billion people worldwide have vision impairment or blindness, of which over 1 billion cases could have been prevented or are yet to be addressed [1]. The report also highlights that global demand for eye care is set to surge in the coming years due to population growth, aging, and lifestyle changes.

There is evidence of USD 4 of economic gain for every USD 1 spent on eye healthcare in developing countries and that eye health stimulates the broader economy, and brings life-changing benefits to individuals and their families [2].

Mission for Vision's efforts to eradicate avoidable blindness is all towards alleviating poverty and enhancing humanity and quality of life.

25.3 Towards Collaborative Action

With the belief that such transformational change calls for collaboration, all Mission for Vision's work is in partnership with various groups and communities. Today, it partners with 37 leading eye institutes across India to enable delivery of high-quality eye health systems to communities. While these have been established predominantly for marginalized groups, services are accessed by all strata of society, thereby demonstrating that this approach can establish equity, comprehensiveness, and quality of care. Excellence, respect, and empathy are central to its ethos (Fig. 25.1).

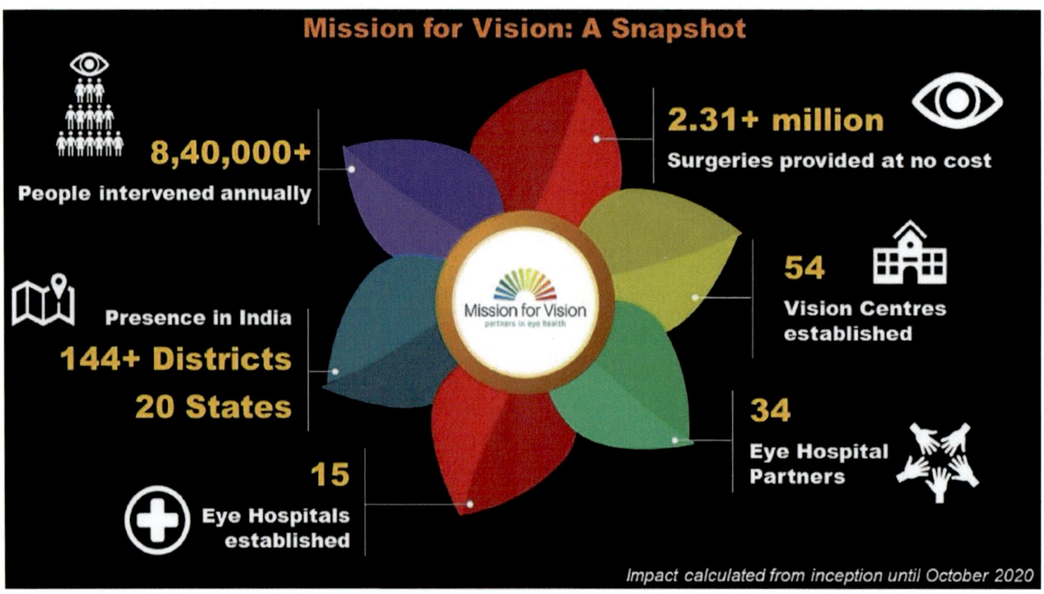

Fig. 25.1 Mission for Vision—Activities in eye care

25.4 Comprehensive and Holistic

Mission for Vision's distinctive approach to reach the vulnerable communities is illustrated below:

1. The *Mission Jyot* program provides primary eye care to the most remote parts of the country. The program aims to establish easily accessible vision centers so that people can seek care earlier; it enables their reintegration into the workforce faster. These sustainable primary eye care clinics offer comprehensive services by trained optometrists or allied ophthalmic personnel (AOP) at affordable cost. Mission for Vision has enabled the establishment of 54 vision centers and has plans for establishing around 500 such centers over the next few years.
2. The *Mission Roshni* initiative provides interventions for the establishment and maintenance of good eye health for children studying in government and government-aided schools.
3. The *Mission Shiksha* promotes math education for visually impaired children through inclusive systems.
4. The *Mission Nayan* program aims to avert blindness among neonates due to retinopathy of prematurity.
5. The *Mission Disha* promotes road safety and good eye health among heavy vehicle drivers, bus drivers, and the skilled workforce such as carpenters.
6. The *Mission Saksham* program focuses on building up the AOP cadre in India. The immense dearth of AOP capacity significantly hampers eye services and prolongs the battle against treatable blindness. This initiative enables rural youth, especially women from socio-economically challenged communities, to undertake training at no cost. The program eventually leads to livelihood opportunities for them, thereby paving the way for such people towards equality and empowerment.

Right from child eye health to enabling eye care for the elderly, Mission for Vision's programs cover the entire spectrum and address the eye health needs of different demographics living in India's most remote locations.

25.5 A PRISM of Possibilities

Apart from enabling access to comprehensive eye care for the most disadvantaged and underserved communities, Mission for Vision's programs are regularly monitored to ensure efficacy and robustness.

Leveraging technological innovations, Mission for Vision developed *PRISM*—"*P*atient-*R*elated *I*mpact *S*tudying *M*echanism," to gather valuable evidence on quality of life and other dimensions of eye health systems. This app is a unique tool that Mission for Vision uses to assess changes in visual acuity and the impact of cataract surgery on personal, social, economic, mobility, and psychological parameters of life in communities accessing Mission for Vision-enabled services.

PRISM demonstrates remarkable, positive post-surgical changes in cataract patients' lives. For instance, during 2016–2017, PRISM recorded data on over 17,000 persons before cataract surgery. Over 8000 were followed up 6 months after surgery to study the impact of the surgery on their lives. Before surgery, 44% of those engaged in livelihood activities mentioned challenges to their ability to earn. That figure decreased to 14% six months after surgery. The visual outcomes after six months also matched with the WHO recommendations.

Utilizing PRISM, Mission for Vision has demonstrated the positive impact of eye health interventions and accountability, which helps partners and other organizations learn from good practice and encourages philanthropists to invest in eye health. Besides this, Mission for Vision also shares these insights with partner hospitals to make timely amendments to their work. PRISM's dynamic functionality can significantly help donors, planners, and policy-makers; Mission for Vision strongly believes that this dynamic functionality can be replicated for other issues impacting universal health coverage.

25.6 Eye Health Research

Mission for Vision is also actively involved in research focusing on workable solutions for appropriate eye healthcare. Mission for Vision's field staff collects data from the ground with the help of PRISM. Some of our research includes an economic analysis of primary eye care centers, effective engagement of community health workers, cataract and mental health outcomes, barriers to surgery uptake, and long-term visual outcomes, to name a few. Some of these have been published in scientific journals. *Repository of featured publications: http://missionforvision.org.in/resources#publications*

25.7 Beyond Boundaries

Other than India, Mission for Vision also supports developmental progress in other countries. For instance, in *Nigeria*, its sister concern, Tulsi Chanrai Foundation, has provided support to 2 million Nigerians; this support includes bringing safe water to 1.4 million people and programs on maternal and child healthcare, immunization, and HIV (Human Immunodeficiency Virus)/AIDS (Acquired Immunodeficiency Syndrome).

Mission for Vision's social change momentum has also led to the identification and diagnosis of uncorrected refractive errors among children in Bhutan. So far, 164,365 school children and 7059 students of monastic bodies in Bhutan (which add up to almost all the children in such institutions in the country) have experienced interventions that will enable then to learn better and provide development opportunities.

25.8 Towards a Better World

Over the years, Mr. Chanrai's philosophy of *Caring Capitalism* has gained much momentum, further widening the scope for private philanthropy for universal eye health. During this period, Mission for Vision has enabled interventions to 16.30+ million people.

Mr. Chanrai firmly believes that one day the world will eliminate needless blindness, and that partnerships are central to this mission. "So long as you have the right intentions and strive for excellence," he says, "others will join you, and if the essence comes from your heart, the forces of nature will be with you."

Case Study (Fig. 25.2)

Mr. Sundaramurthy, aged 66 years, lives in Arani, 45 km from Chennai. He is a painter by profession. His work was hampered when he developed cataract in his right eye. While painting walls, he started leaving uneven, unpainted patches and his co-workers had to point these out to him. Due to his poor eyesight, he was also very accident-prone. He fell on the

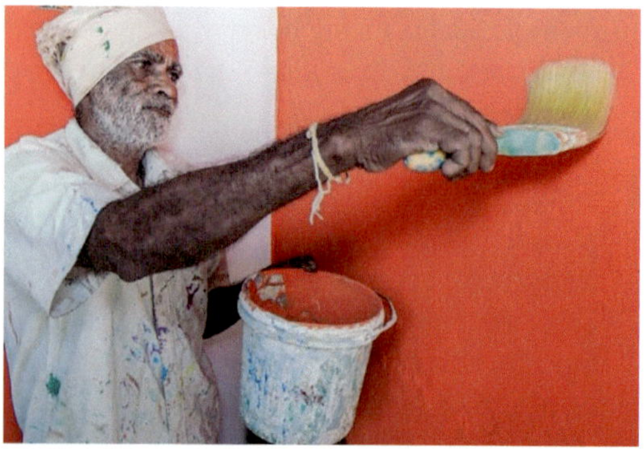

Fig. 25.2 Mr. Sundaramurthy returns to work after cataract surgery enabled by Mission for Vision. © Mission for Vision

road a few times and once he missed a step on the ladder and fell from a height. This also affected his commute, as he had a lot of difficulty in reading bus numbers when he had to go to different locations for his painting contracts.

He heard of an eye-screening camp being held at Arani and visited the camp with the hope of correcting this issue. On examination, he was diagnosed with a cataract in his eye. He was referred to Mission for Vision's Partner Hospital—Sankara Nethralaya—at the Jaslok Community Ophthalmic Centre, where he underwent a cataract surgery at no cost to him. His surgery was successful and he started noticing the positive changes in his daily lifestyle. Mr. Sundaramurthy is back to painting and this intervention has added new colours to his life.

References

1. World report on vision. https://www.who.int/publications/i/item/world-report-on-vision. Accessed 2 Nov 2020.
2. Investing in vision. https://www.hollows.org/au/research/investing-in-vision. Accessed 2 Nov 2020.

26 Operation Eyesight Universal and South-East Asia

Kashinath Bhoosnurmath, Parvez Memon, Harish Kumar, Yashwant Sinha, and Anup Zimba

Operation Eyesight Universal's journey began in 1963 when a businessman from Calgary, Canada, Arthur Jenkyns, met Dr. Ben Gullison, a physician. The latter had worked at a mission hospital in the southern part of India. Mr. Jenkyns was inspired by Dr. Gullison's work and founded Operation Eyesight Universal (Operation Eyesight) to raise funds for people who needed eye care in India. Since then, Operation Eyesight, with its South-East Asia office in Hyderabad, continues to contribute significantly to the cause of the eliminating avoidable blindness. To date, Operation Eyesight's work is guided by the philosophy *"the best for the poorest,"* and the prioritization of local capacity building and sustainability. The organization's mission is *"to prevent blindness and restore sight,"* and it envisions programs to *"eliminate avoidable blindness."* Operation Eyesight has been supporting eye care since 1963 in the South-East Asian countries of Bangladesh, India, Nepal, and Sri Lanka; it later expanded to the African countries of Ethiopia, Ghana, Kenya, Liberia, and Zambia. In all these countries, Operation Eyesight collaborates with the government, non-government organizations (NGOs), and private health care providers to deliver quality eye care services, empower target communities, and eliminate avoidable blindness on a sustainable basis. An overview of Operation Eyesight's work in South-East Asia as of 2020 is shown in Table 26.1.

26.1 Operation Eyesight's Approach to the Elimination of Avoidable Blindness

The foundation for eliminating avoidable blindness revolves around making eye care services available to the unreached individuals and communities. Despite significant strides in making these much-needed services, the numbers of people with avoidable blindness remain a public health issue in many developing countries. The situation and problem analyses conducted

K. Bhoosnurmath (✉) · P. Memon · H. Kumar
Y. Sinha · A. Zimba
OEU, Hyderabad, India
e-mail: bhoosnurmathk@operationeyesight.com; memonp@operationeyesight.com; kumarh@operationeyesight.com; sinhay@operationeyesight.com; zimbaa@operationeyesight.com

T. Das, P. D. Nayar (eds.), *South-East Asia Eye Health*,
https://doi.org/10.1007/978-981-16-3787-2_26

by Operation Eyesight have showed that poor eye health-seeking behavior coupled with a lack of basic water, sanitation, and hygiene (WASH) standards, sub-optimal integration of primary eye care into primary healthcare services, and poor access to quality eye care services are the key factors for poor eye health in most communities. Based on these findings, Operation Eyesight developed an innovative and inclusive approach. The approach includes strengthening eye hospitals to ensure the delivery of quality services, strengthening primary healthcare services that provide primary eye care services, and empowering target communities to implement key strategies. The key contributions made by Operation Eyesight to South-East Asia's eye health sector from 2015 to 2019 are summarized in Fig. 26.1.

Table 26.1 Overview of operation eye sight work in the South-East Asia

Country	Service start year	Nature of Current Intervention (2020)
India	1963	Community eye health, hospital strengthening, disease control, integrated eye health, and research and advocacy
Nepal	1973	Community eye health, hospital strengthening, disease control, and research and advocacy
Bangladesh	1974	Community eye health, hospital strengthening, and disease control
Sri Lanka	1983	Hospital strengthening and disease control

26.1.1 Thematic Areas of Operation Eyesight's Work

Operation Eyesight's five thematic programs are strongly linked with one another and lead to ensuring availability, accessibility, and affordability of eye care services and utilization of these services by empowered target communities. These five thematic programs are: (1) hospital strengthening; (2) community eye health; (3) integrated eye health; (4) disease control; and (5) research and advocacy (Fig. 26.2).

26.1.1.1 Hospital Strengthening

This program is designed to bridge gaps in the availability of quality eye care services. Under this program, Operation Eyesight provides financial and non-financial technical assistance to eye hospitals to establish vision centers, construct new eye hospitals, upgrade infrastructure, and

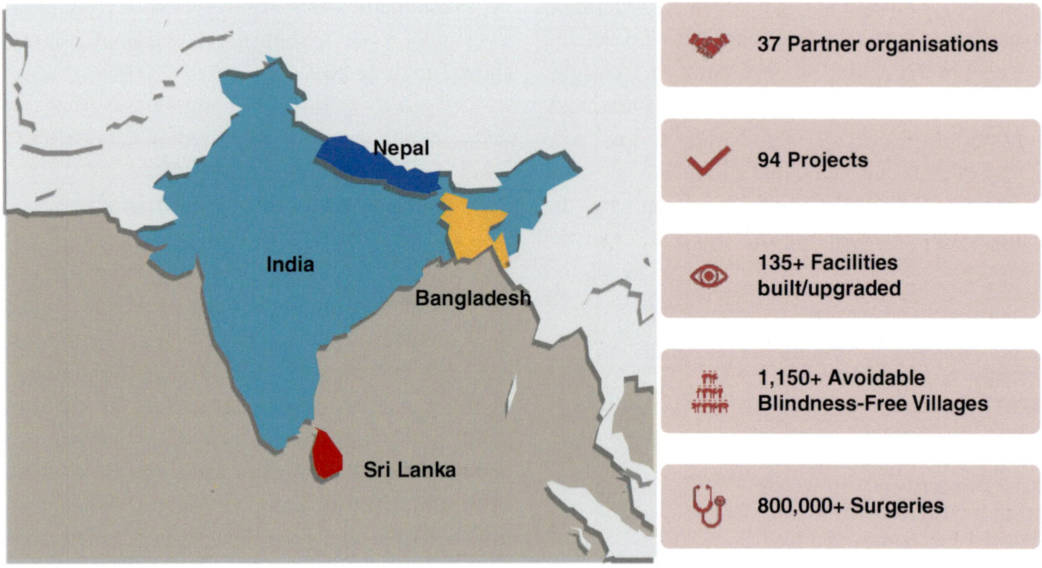

Fig. 26.1 OE's work in South-East Asia (2015–2019)

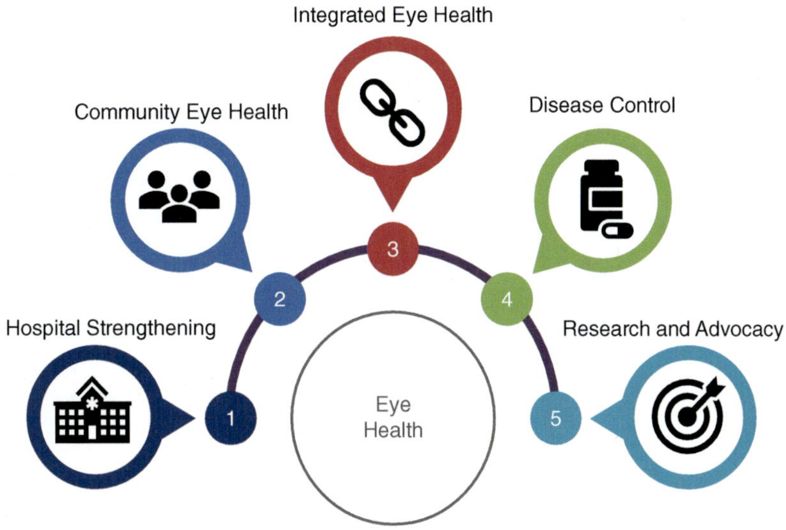

Fig. 26.2 Operation Eyesight's five thematic programs

strengthen the capacities of the partner hospital staff in a structured manner (Fig. 26.3).

26.1.1.2 Community Eye Health

This program is the key focus of Operation Eyesight's interventions. The community eye health program is designed and implemented to empower target communities and eliminate avoidable blindness on a sustainable basis with trained community health workers. Over 85% of these community health workers are women residing in the target areas. The program focuses on instilling health-seeking behavior among the target communities, making them responsible for their eye health. The components of the community eye health program are shown in Figs. 26.4 and 26.5.

26.1.1.3 Integrated Eye Health

Operation Eyesight recognizes the strong linkages between primary eye care and primary healthcare, such as nutrition, drinking water, hygiene, immunization, maternal health, etc. Through this thematic program, Operation Eyesight strives to strengthen the delivery of these health services at the target community levels.

26.1.1.4 Disease Control

Operation Eyesight supports the reduction of cataract backlogs and addresses problems related to untreated refractive errors. Besides these, Operation Eyesight is committed to responding to the increasing prevalence of avoidable blindness caused by emerging eye diseases such as glaucoma, diabetic retinopathy, retinoblastoma, and retinopathy of prematurity in the areas where they operate.

26.1.1.5 Research and Advocacy

Operation Eyesight undertakes and promotes research on community eye health, the impact of eye health initiatives, and sustainability. In partnership with the International Agency for the Prevention of Blindness (IAPB), country-specific chapters of VISION 2020, and other eye health network agencies, Operation Eyesight drives evidence-based advocacy efforts for promoting integrated care models and sustainable eye health initiatives at national and international levels.

26.1.2 Hospital-Based Community Eye Health Program

The Hospital-Based Community Eye Health Program (HBCEHP) is a flagship model of Operation Eyesight that cuts across the five thematic programs and eliminates avoidable blindness on a sustainable basis in the service areas of Operation Eyesight's partner hospitals/geographical areas of intervention. The HBCEHP primarily focuses on quality control, commu-

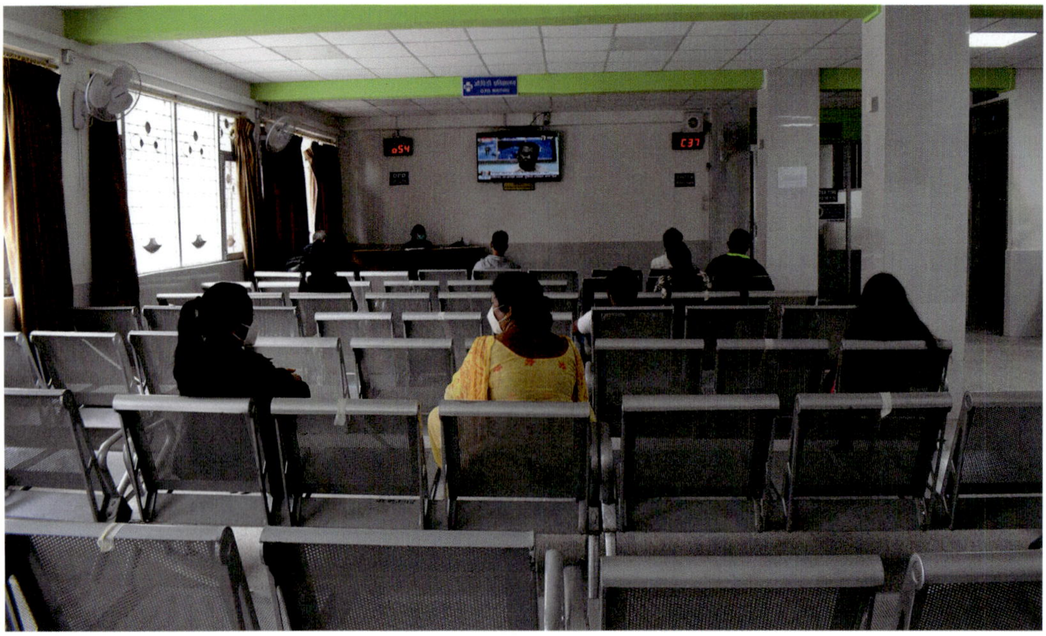

Fig. 26.3 The upgraded out-patient department in Nepal Eye Hospital, Kathmandu. (© Operation Eyesight)

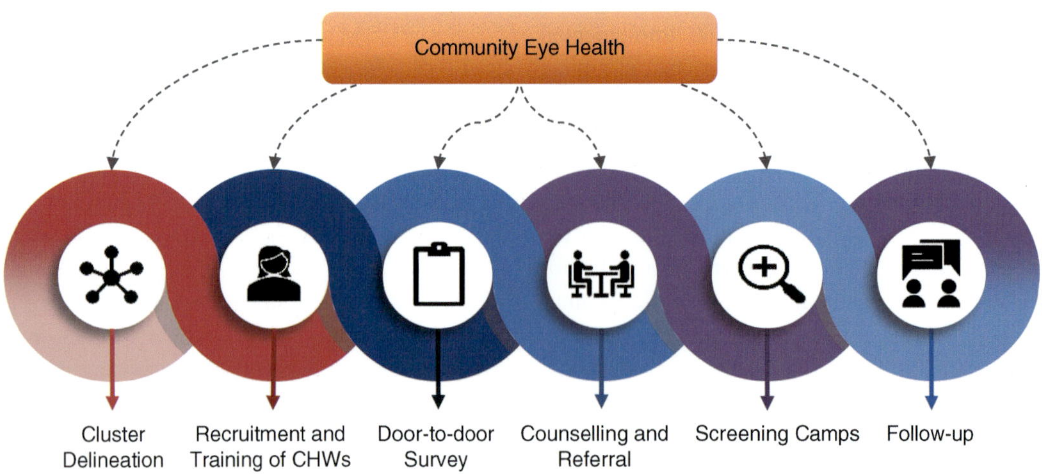

Fig. 26.4 Components of community eye health. (©Operation Eyesight)

nity empowerment, and strengthening primary healthcare (Fig. 26.6).

- *Provision of quality eye care services* is achieved through strategic capacity building of partner hospitals, establishing primary eye care or vision centers in the catchment area, and establishing referral linkage mechanisms.
- *Empowering target communities* is done through a door-to-door survey to identify people with eye ailments, providing health education, counseling, and follow-up.
- *Strengthening primary healthcare services* is achieved by working closely with government primary healthcare centers and workers at the village/community level. Key activities include

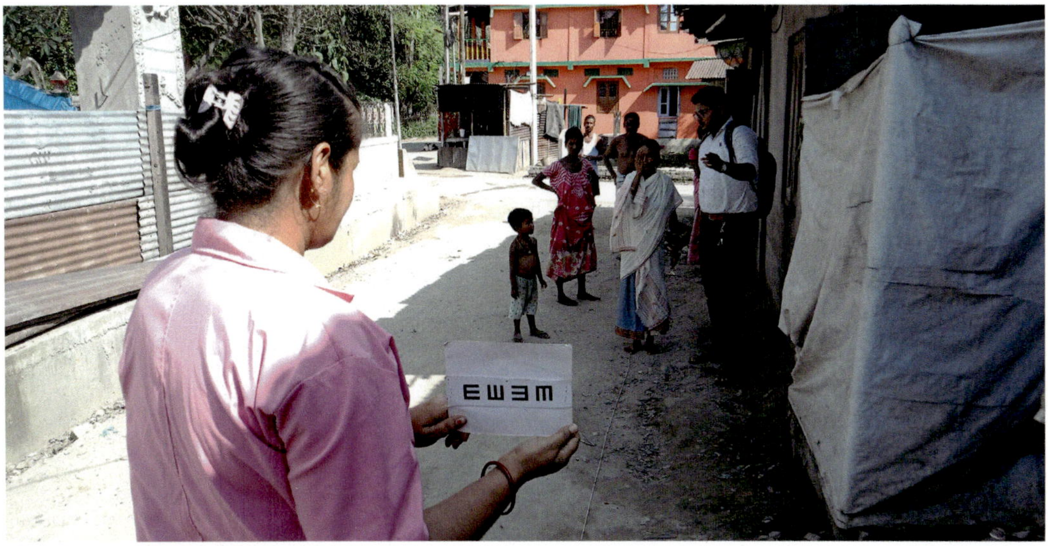

Fig. 26.5 A female community health worker conducting a door-to-door survey in Kaibortotola, Hajo, Kamrup rural district, Assam, India. (© Operation Eyesight)

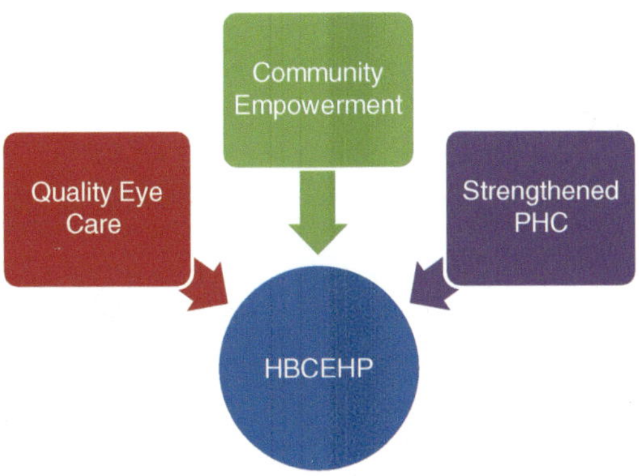

Fig. 26.6 Components of HBCEHP

training the government primary healthcare providers; providing health education to community members; organizing screening camps; promoting health services including immunization, nutrition programs, and antenatal/postnatal care; and appropriate referrals to nearby healthcare centers. Besides, Operation Eyesight partners with relevant community-based organizations (CBOs), NGOs, and the government to strengthen these primary healthcare services' delivery.

26.1.3 Avoidable Blindness-Free Villages

Operation Eyesight has pioneered the concept of avoidable blindness-free villages/communities: *In an avoidable blindness-free village, no patient, regardless of religion, caste, creed, or gender, has a visual acuity less than 6/60 in the better eye due to avoidable or treatable conditions.* This definition has been validated the L V Prasad Eye Institute, Hyderabad, India.

The definition implies that all backlog cases of avoidable blindness have been cleared, the target communities have been adequately empowered to seek eye health on their own, a post-project door-to-door survey has been conducted to verify the same, and the local medical officer has certified those who cannot be treated due to medical or other extenuating circumstances. The declaration of "avoidable blindness-free village" is often marked by a public celebration typically attended by district health authorities, elected representatives, and other agencies operating in the area. In 2014, Operation Eyesight received the prestigious

Innovation Excellence Award from VISION 2020 India for pioneering the concept of avoidable blindness-free villages.

26.1.4 Vision Center-Based Community Eye Health Program (VBCEHP)

VBCEHP is an adaptation of HBCEHP and is implemented in the service areas of the vision centers (primary health centers), and covers a smaller population (up to 100,000 people). The methodology and the activity are the same as those of HBCEHP.

26.1.5 Community-Based Rehabilitation Program (CBRP)

As an integral part of Operation Eyesight's community eye health program, CBRP empowers those who have blindness or vision impairments to lead productive and quality lives. Operation Eyesight operates these programs mainly in India.

26.1.6 World Report on Vision (2019) and Operation Eyesight

All of Operation Eyesight's interventions are in complete alignment with the recommendations of the WHO's World Report on Vision (Table 26.2). Due to its unique presence at the community level, Operation Eyesight is best positioned to contribute to implementing the "integrated people-centered eye care effectively" and "community awareness about eye care needs" recommendations in the report.

Table 26.2 World report on vision recommendations and alignment with operation eyesight's thematic programs

World report on vision recommendation	Operation eyesight's thematic program alignment
Make eye care an integral part of universal health coverage	Research and advocacy
Implement integrated people-centered eye care in health systems	Community eye health, hospital improvement, integrated eye health
Promote high-quality research	Hospital improvement, research and advocacy
Monitor trends and evaluate progress	Hospital improvement, research and advocacy
Raise awareness and engage and empower people and communities	Community eye health, integrated eye health

26.2 Sustainability: A Core Concept in Operation Eyesight's Interventions

Operation Eyesight recognizes that sustainability planning is critical to ensure eye health programs and services are sustained over time. Operation Eyesight's program intervention framework incorporates the following strategies that foster sustainability on a long-term basis.

- *Creating appropriate quality-centric strategies:* Operation Eyesight has incorporated quality as a driver for sustainability and its program strategies to ensure beneficiaries get the best eye care they can receive.
- *Designing financially sustainable approaches:* Operation Eyesight has pioneered cross-subsidization and promotion of optical shops and pharmacies as revenue sources in the partner hospitals to ensure sustainability.
- *Identifying, engaging, and developing leaders:* Operation Eyesight continuously identifies,

engages, and develops leaders and champions from the community and among partners. Capacity building efforts are contextual and relevant for them to keep the program going.

- *Empowering communities to increase demand for quality-assured services:* Operation Eyesight's work supports empowered communities that take care of their health and eye care needs and demand quality-assured health and eye care services as the key to sustainability.
- *Creating strategic partnerships:* Operation Eyesight identifies and engages with appropriate partners to implement and manage impact-oriented eye health programs that benefit communities.

For Operation Eyesight, program sustainability goes beyond financial security. It also provides benefits within the community and target population that may or may not be dependent on the continuation of a single program or service.

26.3 Focus 2020 and Beyond

In the year 2020, Operation Eyesight revised its global and national strategies to bring a holistic approach to health care, with even more agility, efficiency, and comprehensiveness in its operations. Operation Eyesight understands that eye health should be delivered in an integrated manner to be more effective and efficient through both public and private sectors. The COVID-19 pandemic has underscored the urgent need to invest in public health and empower communities to take care of their health. Operation Eyesight is operating from the perspective that the pandemic will change the public health landscape forever across the globe. The optimal use of appropriate technology coupled with evidence-based advocacy will act as drivers for a paradigm shift and a transformational change. Operation Eyesight will continue to work with governments, partners, communities, and other like-minded organizations to advocate and promote integrated, cost-effective, efficient, quality-centric, and sustainable care models that address the primary health care needs communities and other determinants of eye health. Operation Eyesight is fine-tuning its intervention strategies to remain relevant and result-oriented now and into the future.

27 OneSight in South-East Asia

Wayne Tennent

OneSight®

When the world sees better, the world lives better. Yet worldwide, although 1.1 billion people (one in seven) have a clinical need for glasses, they either cannot afford them, access vision care, or both. Since 1988, OneSight has been working toward a world where access to vision care is no longer a barrier to human achievement and possibility. Driven by a mission to improve lives by creating access to quality vision care and eyeglasses in underserved communities worldwide, the goal is to eradicate the global vision care crisis in this century.

Without access to vision care, individuals suffer avoidable impairments to their health, education, livelihood, and dignity. OneSight addresses this solvable need by providing comprehensive vision screenings, eye examinations, and glasses in accessible settings. In partnership with local healthcare and community organizations, school districts, optical professionals, doctors, NGOs, and trained volunteers, the organization works to ensure that services reach those most in need. For 32 years, OneSight has made quality vision care services available to individuals in 54 countries, including extensive work throughout South-East Asia.

27.1 The Strategies

OneSight leverages two proven program strategies, designed to meet the specific needs of each community in need. OneSight's Charitable Vision Clinics deliver same-day vision screening, eye exams, and eyeglasses in underserved communities where an intensive short-term clinic is the best solution. Over a one-to-two-week period, OneSight serves hundreds to thousands of individuals by providing free eye exams and glasses that are manufactured and dispensed on-site, often within a few hours. Clinics are staffed by eye care professionals as well as local volunteers.

W. Tennent (✉)
OneSight, New York, USA
e-mail: WTennent@onesight.org

T. Das, P. D. Nayar (eds.), *South-East Asia Eye Health*,
https://doi.org/10.1007/978-981-16-3787-2_27

In addition to medical staff, OneSight provides all necessary equipment and eyewear materials at no cost for those receiving the services. To date, OneSight has conducted more than 2000 Vision Clinics worldwide, serving communities that include refugee camps, indigenous populations, and low-income families who face barriers in accessing vision care resources.

OneSight's second strategy, Sustainable Vision Centers, delivers a comprehensive, permanent, and scalable solution for communities where the need dramatically overwhelms available services. This approach equips and empowers local partners to establish self-sustaining Vision Centers within existing healthcare systems and infrastructure. Patients of Vision Centers receive a vision screening, an eye exam, and, if needed, affordable eyeglasses that meet their prescription needs. Facilities are staffed by local community members who have been trained by OneSight vision care professionals. In addition to this training, and dependent on the systems and infrastructure already in place, OneSight may provide the hardware (testing equipment, initial eyewear inventory, and future supply-chain, or in some cases, manufacturing equipment to make lenses on-site) and the software (patient and inventory tracking systems, accounting programs) that enable on-going care. Because this model includes selling eyeglasses at an affordable price, the Vision Centers are self-sustaining and do not require on-going philanthropic support. Once a Vision Center is fully operational, management is transitioned to the local government or other local partners for future oversight. OneSight is a pioneer and leader in developing a permanent, self-sustaining solution to the global vision crisis, with 180 Vision Centers providing access to over 37.5 million people in countries in China, India, Timor-Leste, Gambia, Rwanda, Zambia, Liberia, South Africa, and the United States of America.

27.2 South-East Asia

Both programming strategies have been deployed in South-East Asia. While OneSight continues to explore opportunities for development throughout the region, activities have been focused on six countries to date, namely, Bangladesh, India, Indonesia, Nepal, Thailand, and Timor-Leste. The following sections provide an overview of OneSight's work in each of those six countries.

27.2.1 Bangladesh

OneSight's first mission to Bangladesh was in 1998, and since that time, more than 15,000 people have received eye exams through OneSight's Charitable Vision Clinics. The most recent was a visit to Cox's Bazar in early 2020, working in partnership with BRAC (Bangladesh Rural Advancement Committee), LV Prasad Eye Institute (India), and the Better Vision Foundation (Nepal) to bring vision care to the region's vulnerable refugee population (Fig. 27.1). OneSight has also worked as a consultant with BRAC, as the organization opened 20 Vision Centers, creat-

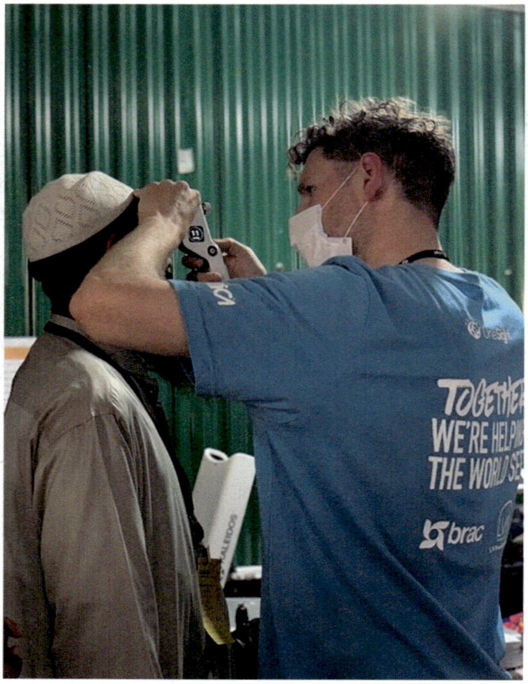

Fig. 27.1 A OneSight volunteer performs an eye exam at the 2020 Vision Clinic in Cox's Bazar. Published with permission from OneSight

ing 80 jobs and providing access to vision care to three million people in rural Bangladesh.

27.2.2 India

OneSight has been holding almost-annual Vision Clinics in India since 2008. From the first visit to Amritsar in the country's north to the most recent 2019 clinic in Ahmedabad, more than 128,000 people have received eye exams across 18 clinics, run in partnership with various local and global organizations.

In recent years, OneSight's focus in India has shifted to the Sustainable Vision Center model, and in 2015, OneSight entered into a multi-phase partnership with LV Prasad Eye Institute (India). During the initial phase, OneSight, along with Luxottica's volunteer support (the world's largest manufacturer of eyewear), conducted a strategic evaluation of LVPEI's existing 129 Vision Centers and made recommendations to maximize their efficiency. Throughout the second phase, OneSight provided recommendations and funding to develop a training program for high school graduates from rural and tribal communities, designed to teach them the skills required to provide vision care in primary care centers, including refraction and dispensing. The third and final phase involved the establishment of 28 OneSight and Luxottica-sponsored Vision Centers in Andhra Pradesh, a project that has resulted in more than 70,000 eye exams, nearly 18,000 pairs of glasses dispensed, approximately 11,000 referrals for further specialist care, almost 5000 telehealth consultations, and access to vision care for the 1.4 million people living in this region (Fig. 27.2).

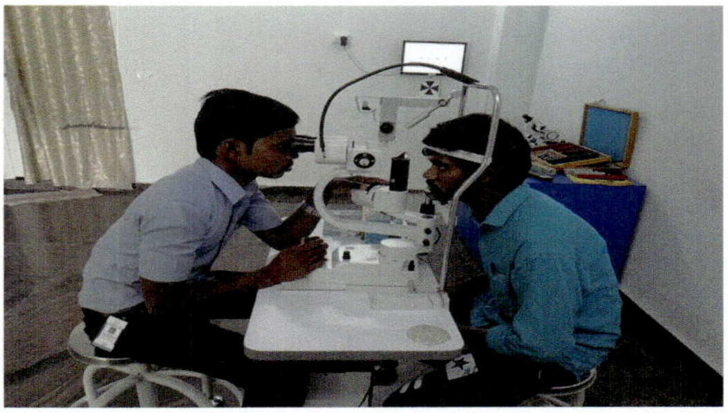

Fig. 27.2 OneSight Vision Centers provide a range of services that previously had not been available to people living in the region, like this patient receiving an eye health assessment at a Vision Center in India (with permission from LV Prasad Eye Institute, Hyderabad, India)

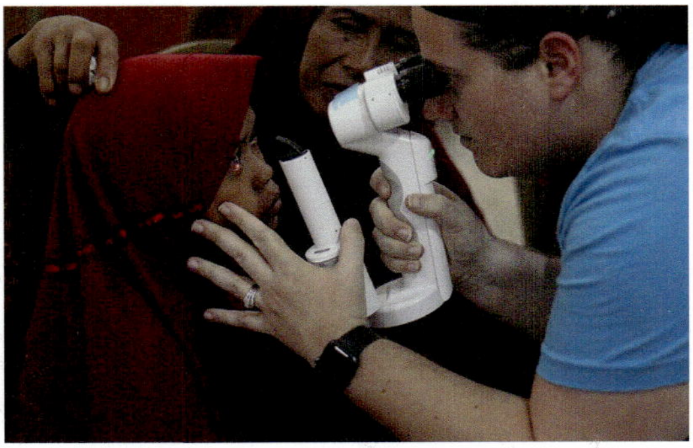

Fig. 27.3 To deliver its programs more efficiently and to more remote areas, whenever possible, OneSight employs lightweight, portable equipment like this handheld slit lamp, in use by a volunteer at the 2019 clinic in Indonesia. (Published with permission from OneSight)

27.2.3 Indonesia

In 2015, OneSight commissioned Deloitte to conduct a study aimed at quantifying the global need for glasses. At that time, Indonesia ranked in the top five countries in need of vision care, with 50 million Indonesians needing but lacking vision and eye care access. To close this gap, OneSight has held several Vision Clinics throughout the country since then, from one-day screening events to the most recent 2019 Vision Clinic in South Sulawesi. A group of OneSight volunteers from around the world visited Makassar for this clinic, working in close partnership with Essilor, a local foundation named Bosowa Peduli, and Perdami SulSel, the local branch of the Indonesian Ophthalmologist Association. Working together, the team performed eye exams for nearly 1600 people and dispensed 1470 pairs of glasses to those in need (Fig. 27.3).

27.2.4 Nepal

OneSight's first visit to Nepal was in late 2019 when a small team visited Kagati, a farming village on Kathmandu's outskirts, whose residents

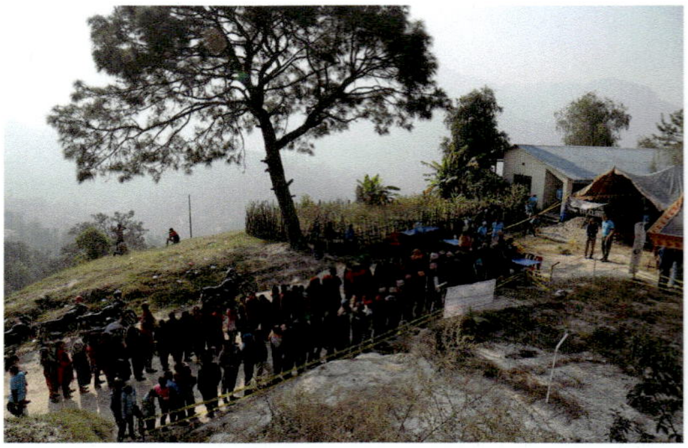

Fig. 27.4 The first group of visitors wait patiently for the 2019 Nepal clinic to open on day one. (Published with permission from OneSight)

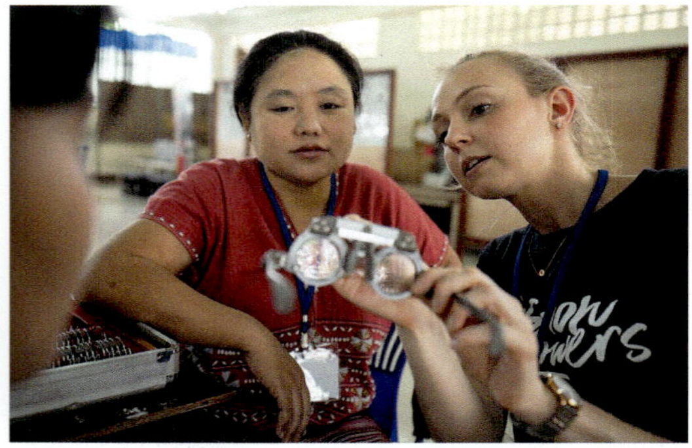

Fig. 27.5 A OneSight volunteer provides coaching to a team member at the Eye Department at Mae Tao Clinic. This health facility provides affordable health care for refugees and migrant workers living along the Thailand–Myanmar border. (Published with permission from OneSight)

were still rebuilding from a 2015 earthquake that left hundreds of thousands of Nepali people homeless. Conducted in partnership with the Better Vision Foundation, a local NGO committed to eliminating avoidable blindness in the country, the Charitable Vision Clinic served nearly 1300 people who trekked through the region's rugged hills and valleys in search of better vision (Fig. 27.4). OneSight continues to seek opportunities to bring permanent access to vision care to Nepal's people through its Sustainable Vision Centers.

27.2.5 Thailand

OneSight started visiting Thailand in 1999 and has conducted 27 Charitable Vision Clinics throughout the country to date. From Chiang Rai in the far north to Ubon Ratchathani in the far east, OneSight has performed nearly 438,000 eye exams for people living in Thailand and has provided tens of thousands of pairs of glasses to those who would not otherwise be able to access or afford vision care.

In 2018, OneSight launched the Thailand Border Project, a three-year plan to deliver vision care to the nearly 200,000 displaced people who are living along the Thailand–Myanmar border. With the support of The International Rescue Committee (IRC), OneSight has held Charitable Vision Clinics in several temporary shelters in the border region, providing much- needed vision care to the residents. The plan also focuses on delivering vision screenings to students in migrant learning centers. This school system has been established along the border region to give all migrant children access to quality education. Finally, a close partnership has been established with the Mae Tao Clinic (MTC). This community-based organization provides and advocates for an equitable and essential health system, education, and protection for vulnerable and displaced people living along the border. In addition to holding a Charitable Vision Clinic at MTC in 2018, OneSight has coordinated the provision of equipment and products through the generous support of Top Charoen, Suwannimit Foundation, Essilor, and Luxottica, and continues to provide on-going administrative expertise and vision care training for MTC health workers (Fig. 27.5). This three-pronged approach will ensure that those living in uncertainty along the border region have access to vision care for years to come.

27.2.6 Timor-Leste

In the 2015 study conducted by Deloitte, the highest acute need for eye care among all the countries in South-East Asia was in Timor-Leste, where over 40% of the population needed glasses but lacked access. As a result, a plan was put in place to open five Vision Centers throughout the country, ensuring that the rural population would have access to vision care. OneSight is currently working with the Timor-Leste Government's Ministry of Health for the advancement of these plans.

At present, there is one Sustainable Vision Center in Oecusse, operated by local health authorities in this Special Administrative Region of Timor-Leste. Since 2018, this center has provided vision care access to the nearly 70,000 people living in the region; one such example is Jacinta, who, at 21 years of age, had never received an eye exam. She visited the clinic on opening day, accompanied by family as she often struggled with her distance vision, and her exam yielded a distance visual acuity of 6/60 (−5.50 D either eye). The team provided Jacinta with a pair of glasses to suit her prescription, assembled on-site, and she left the center that day with clear vision for the first time in her life (Fig. 27.6).

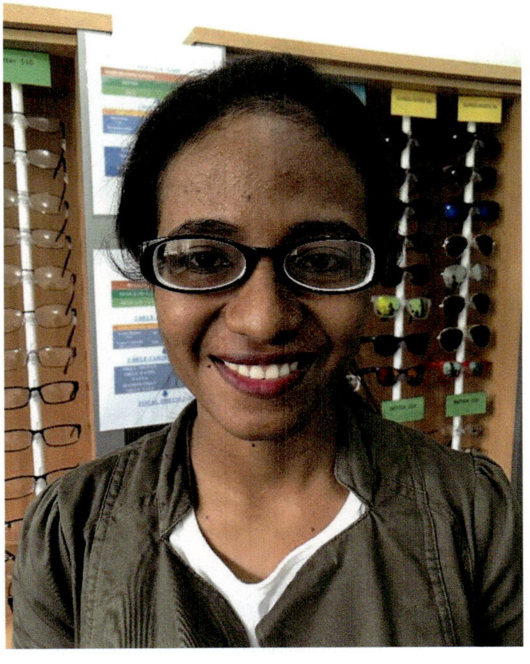

Fig. 27.6 A pair of glasses has the power to increase productivity by 35% and earning potential by up to 20%. This can be life-changing for someone like Jacinta, who at −5.50 D either eye had never received any kind of eye exam or vision correction until she visited OneSight's Vision Center in Oecusse. (Published with permission from OneSight)

27.3 Conclusion

The South-East Asian region has been and will continue to be a focus area for OneSight, with its disproportionate level of need for vision care. While the nearly 600,000 eye exams conducted at the 50 OneSight Charitable Vision Clinics held till now have resulted in clear vision and a better quality of life for many, and the 50 OneSight-supported Vision Centers set up in this region have provided vision care access to 4.4 million people, there is still a great deal of work remining. OneSight is highly committed to working with the International Agency for the Prevention of Blindness (IAPB) and other local stakeholders to close the vision gap for good.

Orbis

28

Rahul Ali

Orbis is an international not-for-profit organization that has been transforming lives by preventing and treating avoidable blindness for nearly four decades. With our network of partners, we mentor, train, and inspire local eye care teams—from health workers in rural clinics to eye surgeons in urban centers—so they can work together to save and restore vision, ensuring no one has to face a life of avoidable blindness.

Founded by leaders of the medical and aviation industries in 1973, Orbis started its work on a plane—a fully equipped mobile teaching hospital, the Flying Eye Hospital. Our expert volunteer faculty taught both on the plane and at hospital-based trainings across the world. Orbis then established long-term country programs across Asia, Africa, Latin America, and the Caribbean. In addition, Orbis's telemedicine platform, "Cybersight," connected these eye care teams with each other and empowered them by enabling easy and free access to global experts and resources across borders. Cybersight has reached 183 of 195 countries globally and is a digital extension of Orbis's mission (Fig. 28.1).

28.1 Orbis and South-East Asia

In South-East Asia, Orbis has long-term programs in Bangladesh, India, Indonesia, and Nepal while the Flying Eye Hospital has visited 12 countries, including those already mentioned (Fig. 28.2).

28.1.1 Bangladesh

Orbis's journey in Bangladesh began in 1985 through a Flying Eye Hospital visit; we celebrated the Flying Eye Hospital's tenth visit in 2017. In 2000, Orbis set up a country office in Dhaka to provide continuous support to our partners there. We focused on pediatric eye disease as at that time, there were no dedicated pediatric eye centers in Bangladesh. Now, there are 13 Children's Eye Centers (CECs) across the country, providing quality eye health services to over 30 million children.

R. Ali (✉)
Orbis, NY, USA

T. Das, P. D. Nayar (eds.), *South-East Asia Eye Health*,
https://doi.org/10.1007/978-981-16-3787-2_28

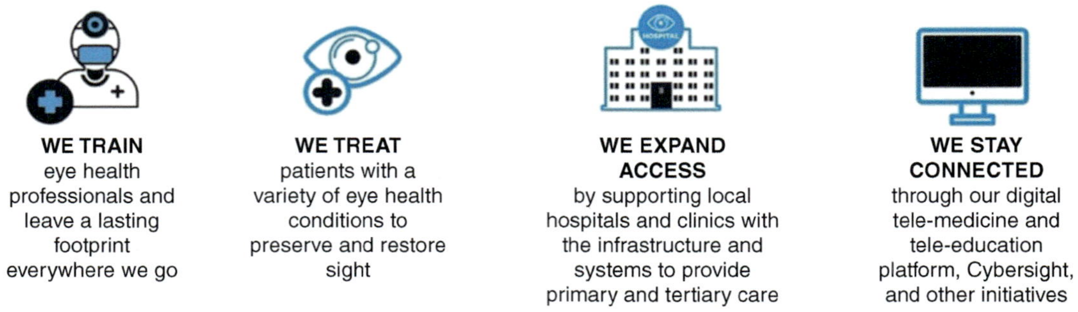

Fig. 28.1 Orbis—Our Work

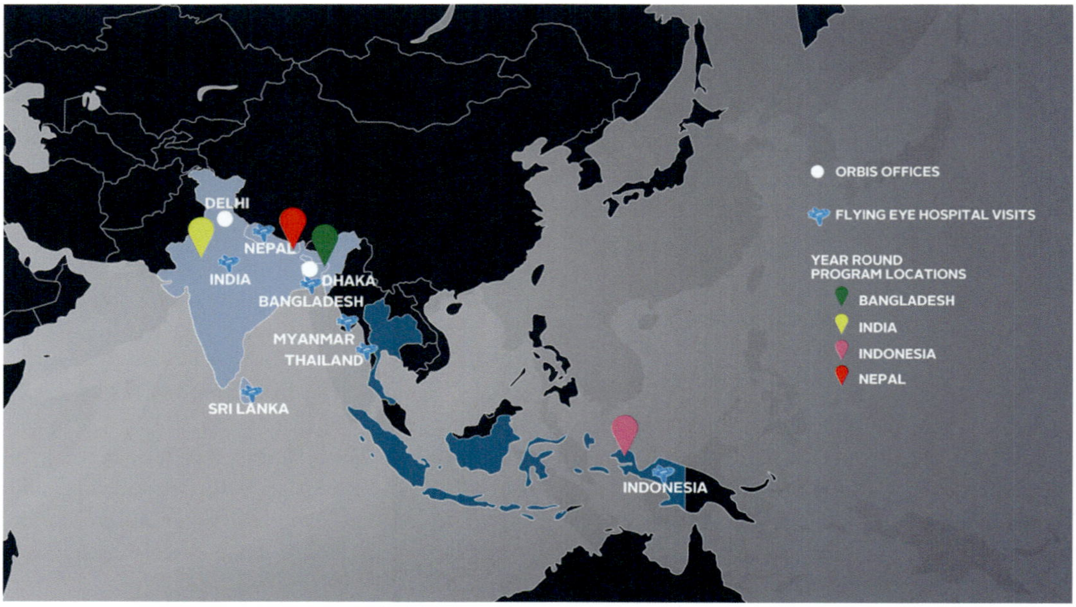

Fig. 28.2 Orbis in South-East Asia

Orbis played a leading role in developing the country's first modern eye bank and in making eye care accessible at the community level by establishing 28 primary eye care centers, 1300 vision points, and 4 Retinopathy of Prematurity (ROP) screening and treatment centers. Orbis also contributed significantly to developing the National Eye Care Plan of the Ministry of Health and Family Welfare. We added a dedicated eye health program for children with diabetes; this is the first such program in the world. Orbis is currently working with 23 partners, including BRAC (Bangladesh Rural Advancement Committee), Grameen, and BADAS (Bangladesh Diabetic Somiti—Diabetic Association of Bangladesh), to cover nearly 50% of the country's districts.

Since February 2018, Orbis has also implemented a program for Rohingya refugees in the Ukhia and Teknaf sub-districts and host communities in south-east Bangladesh. Globally, this is the first such focused effort to provide eye health services to displaced people. Orbis conducted seminal research on eye health issues of the Rohingya, clearly demonstrating the increased burden of eye diseases in this community and reinforcing the global need to prioritize eye health for displaced communities.

28.1.2 India

In 1988, the Flying Eye Hospital first visited India. In the year 2000, Orbis established the country office. India is the second-most populous country in the world and home to over 20% of the world's blind population. Unfortunately, India is also home to the largest number of blind children in any one country. In 2000, the country only had 4 comprehensive tertiary children eye centers (CEC). With a population of 1 billion, India needed at least 100 CECs as per WHO guidelines (one center per ten million population). To this end, Orbis launched the India Childhood Blindness Initiative (ICBI) in 2002. A country-wide survey was undertaken to develop a comprehensive understanding of the current status of human resources and infrastructure for the elimination of avoidable childhood blindness. This led to our work in developing the required cadres of human resources and service delivery infrastructure, including equipping facilities and supporting community work.

After nearly two decades of work and establishing the largest national network of CECs globally, Orbis's significant role in establishing pediatric ophthalmology as a distinct subspecialty in the Indian ophthalmology landscape has been acknowledged. Today, 33 CECs have been developed with Orbis support across 17 Indian states. These centers reach more than a million children annually. Besides, certain centers within the ICBI network also provide training and support the eye care system in India and many neighboring countries. Orbis also pioneered pediatric ophthalmology services in rural India and worked with communities to generate public awareness. Furthermore, this model has been successfully replicated in Nepal and Bangladesh.

A part of prioritizing pediatric ophthalmology as a sub-specialty in India was to enable the Centers of Excellence to ensure pediatric ophthalmology teams were competent and appropriately skilled. Three of the tertiary level pediatric facilities in India that existed in 2000 were developed into Pediatric Ophthalmology Learning and Training Centers (POLTCs). This involved providing infrastructure, technical support, and standardization of curricula for the various cadres of eye health professionals for CECs and related community work. These POLTCs continue to offer fellowships in pediatric ophthalmology and short/long-term training programs. In addition, they also periodically conduct professional development programs to ensure that the teams provide quality care (Fig. 28.3).

In 2016, to build on the strengths of the ICBI network, Orbis launched an innovative school eye health program, REACH (Refractive Error Among Children). REACH is a technology-enabled model for a comprehensive school eye health program that has already touched the lives of millions of school-going children. Orbis, along with its partners, developed teams of ophthalmic personnel and supported them with training as well as digital and clinical equipment to perform vision screening, refraction, prescription and provision of spectacles, and referral of children to fixed facilities for further examination and treatment as needed. REACH also monitors children's compliance with wearing spectacles and encourages good eye health-seeking behavior through evidence-based communication content. To support this very strong focus on data management at all levels and steps of REACH, Orbis developed REACHSoft, a software purpose-built for this program. REACHSoft is designed to support every step of the planning, implementation, and management (including monitoring and evaluation) of the REACH program.

REACH has conducted over 4.5 million screenings across India in the last 3 years. Two sites beyond the initial implementation site have been added in India. REACH was launched in Nepal in June 2018, demonstrating its potential for scalability across the country and beyond.

28.1.3 REACH Model

- Shifting the process from screening to conducting a comprehensive eye examination at school for those children who need it.
- Undertaking all service delivery activities by trained teams while orienting teachers to promote good school eye health practices and liaise effectively with eye health teams.

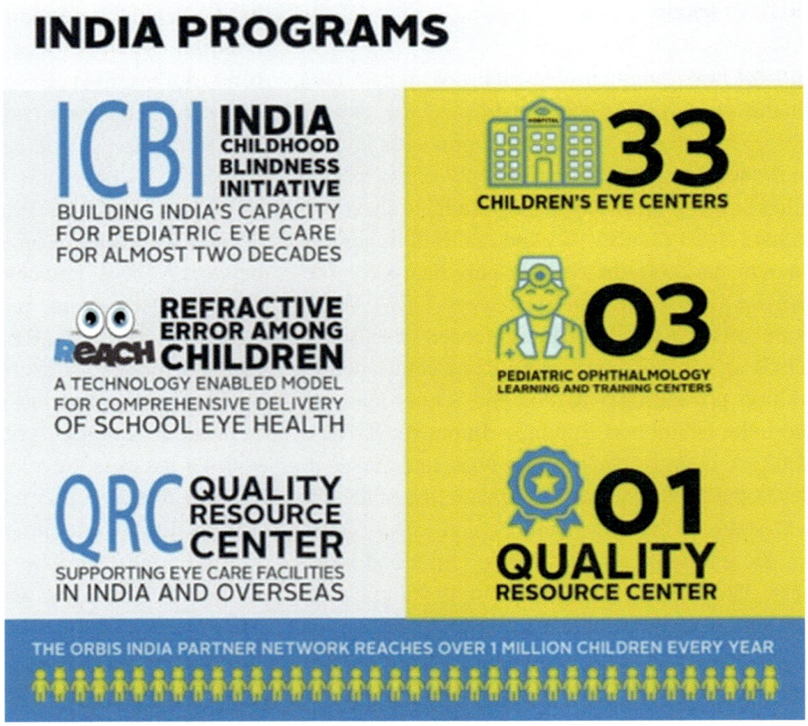

Fig. 28.3 Orbis India programs

- Changing the endpoint of services from spectacle delivery to ensuring that children who are given spectacles are using them (compliance).
- Ensuring school eye health visits is not a one-off event, but to develop an annual follow-up cycle so that children who need care have ongoing access to it.
- Capturing data digitally at all service delivery points to facilitate improved planning, implementation, quality control, and further analysis using REACHSoft.
- Standardization across all key areas of REACH—clinical guidelines, processes, hardware, and software.

Orbis is also a founding member of VISION 2020 India and an active member of this advocacy forum. Over the years, Orbis has also significantly contributed to strengthening eye banks and hospital-based cornea retrieval programs across the country. Building on our work in quality assurance at eye hospitals, Orbis developed the Quality Resource Center, which has supported eye care facilities across India and internationally in countries such as Bangladesh, Indonesia, Nepal, and Vietnam.

28.1.4 Indonesia

Orbis has been supporting eye care in Indonesia since 1982 through multiple visits of the Flying Eye Hospital. In July 2014, Orbis conducted an assessment to understand Indonesia's eye care needs, priorities, and challenges to establish a long-term program in this country. This led to Orbis collaborating with the Hasanuddin University Hospital (or *Universitas Hasanuddin*, UNHAS) in Makassar to build their capacity to provide tertiary level pediatric eye care services. This entailed training doctors, nurses, anesthetists, and other health professionals; equipping the center with necessary diagnostic and surgical equipment; and creating a child-friendly environment.

Working with Helen Keller International (HKI), Orbis developed a model center for ROP screening and treatment in Jakarta by enhancing the capacity of the Dr. Cipto Mangunkusumo National Central General Hospital by training the team, providing equipment, promoting public education, and providing support toward advocacy.

Training is at the core of several Orbis initiatives, and the Sandwich Pediatric Fellowship program initiated in Indonesia is a testament to our constant innovation. This blended one-year pediatric ophthalmology and strabismus training program is delivered through Orbis's award-winning telemedicine platform, Cybersight. It consists of four 3-month rotations; during rotations one and three, the fellow remains at their home institution (UNHAS) and participates in distance learning, remote surgical mentorship, and hospital-based training with visiting Orbis volunteer faculty. Rotations two and four involve hands-on training and skills transfer through wet labs and surgical cases at Dr. Shroff's Charity Eye Hospital, a long-term Orbis partner in India.

28.1.5 Nepal

Orbis began its sight-saving initiative in Nepal in 1985, when the Orbis DC-8 aircraft landed in Kathmandu. The Flying Eye Hospital returned in 1988 to conduct on-board surgical training programs. During these programs, Orbis partnered with the Nepal Netra Jyoti Sangh (NNJS) and the Tilganga Institute of Ophthalmology (TIO) to strengthen Nepal's pediatric eye care services. Besides this, Orbis also sponsored short-term international fellowships for Nepal's ophthalmologists. As a follow-up to these fellowship programs, Orbis conducted several hospital-based training sessions along with continuous e-consultation/telemedicine services through Cybersight.

In July 2004, Shree Rana Ambika Shah Eye Hospital (Lumbini Eye Institute or LEI), one of Nepal's high-volume eye hospitals, was identified as a partner for establishing a dedicated CEC. During the initial 3 year LEI-Orbis partnership, the hospital undertook vision testing for over 270,000 children and performed 2600 pediatric eye surgeries, a 70% increase over past performance. This rapid ascent of the institution highlights how introducing and strengthening pediatric eye care services in an appropriate geographical location can effectively treat avoidable blindness and visual impairment in a substantial number of children.

In 2007, Orbis commissioned a national survey in Nepal to identify gaps in infrastructure and availability of trained human resources for pediatric eye care services. The survey and lessons from the LEI project laid the foundation for the National Program for Control of Childhood Blindness in Nepal. Orbis partnered with TIO and six eye hospitals of NNJS for this program. Through this vital collaboration, 7 more CECs were established across the country, and the CEC at LEI was further strengthened to the level of a Resource Center. This Resource Center at LEI now offers pediatric ophthalmology fellowships for Nepali ophthalmologists in Nepal.

In 2018, Orbis launched REACH in Nepal based on the model developed in India. Orbis is now working with four eye hospitals to provide eye health services to more than 800,000 school children.

28.1.6 The Future

Collaboration is at the heart of all the work we do at Orbis, and our firm belief in it is clear from our organizational mission statement: "With our network of partners, we mentor, train and inspire local teams so they can save sight in their communities." While 75% of all blindness and visual impairment is either treatable or preventable, global blindness and visual impairment are expected to triple over the next three decades. Orbis invests in developing scalable models for service delivery and ensures that appropriate human resources are available to implement these models. Our partnerships span the spectrum—from eye hospitals, governments, and academic institutions, to corporates. It is meaningful collaborations with all these partners that allows us to have true impact. It is only with the spirit of togetherness that we will win this fight against avoidable blindness and visual impairment. And together, we will do it!

29 Seva Foundation

Suzanne Gilbert, Ram Prasad Kandel, Kuldeep Singh, Chundak Tenzing, and Heidi Chase

seva.org
Transforming lives by restoring sight.

Seva is on a mission to end avoidable blindness in our lifetime. Seva is a global nonprofit eye care organization that works with local communities worldwide to develop self-sustaining programs that preserve and restore sight. As many people in the South-East Asian region know, the word "Seva" comes from the Sanskrit word for "service."

Since 1978, the Seva Foundation has been pushing the envelope to bring down the costs of and increase access to eye care for every person, regardless of their ability to pay or their social status. Co-founders, Drs. Larry and Girija Brilliant, who worked with the World Health Organization (WHO) to eradicate smallpox in India in the 1970s, were moved by doctors' and donors' commitment to helping underserved populations in remote parts of the world. Inspired by their generosity and with seed funding from the late Steve Jobs, they, along with a group of colleagues, established Seva. Dr. G Venkataswamy, who had just started the Aravind Eye Hospital, was one of Seva's founders (Fig. 29.1). The Seva Foundation is based in Berkeley, California, USA, with one office in the South-East Asian region in Nepal, and technical staff in India. In 1982, several of Seva Foundation's Canadian founders established Seva Canada, based in Vancouver, British Columbia.

Within the South-East Asian region, Seva works extensively in India, Nepal, and Bangladesh. Throughout 2020, Seva supported training partnerships in Myanmar. Worldwide, Seva serves underserved indigenous communities (including those in the USA) with partners in more than 20 countries. Seva works closely with the WHO, International Agency for the Prevention of Blindness (IAPB), National Eye Institute (NEI), USA, supranational and national ophthalmic societies, and other institutions that promote learning and results.

Seva develops locally designed, run, and sustained programs. Through more than 40 years of partnerships with local eye care providers, Seva's programs have restored sight to more than five million people, provided eye care to more than 40 million patients, and created high-quality jobs

S. Gilbert (✉) · K. Singh · C. Tenzing · H. Chase
Seva Foundation, Berkeley, CA, USA
e-mail: sgilbert@seva.org; ksingh@seva.org; ctenzing@seva.org; hchase@seva.org

R. P. Kandel
Seva Foundation, Nepal Hospital, Nepal Netra Bhavan, Tripureswore, Kathmandu, Nepal
e-mail: rkandel@seva.org

T. Das, P. D. Nayar (eds.), *South-East Asia Eye Health*,
https://doi.org/10.1007/978-981-16-3787-2_29

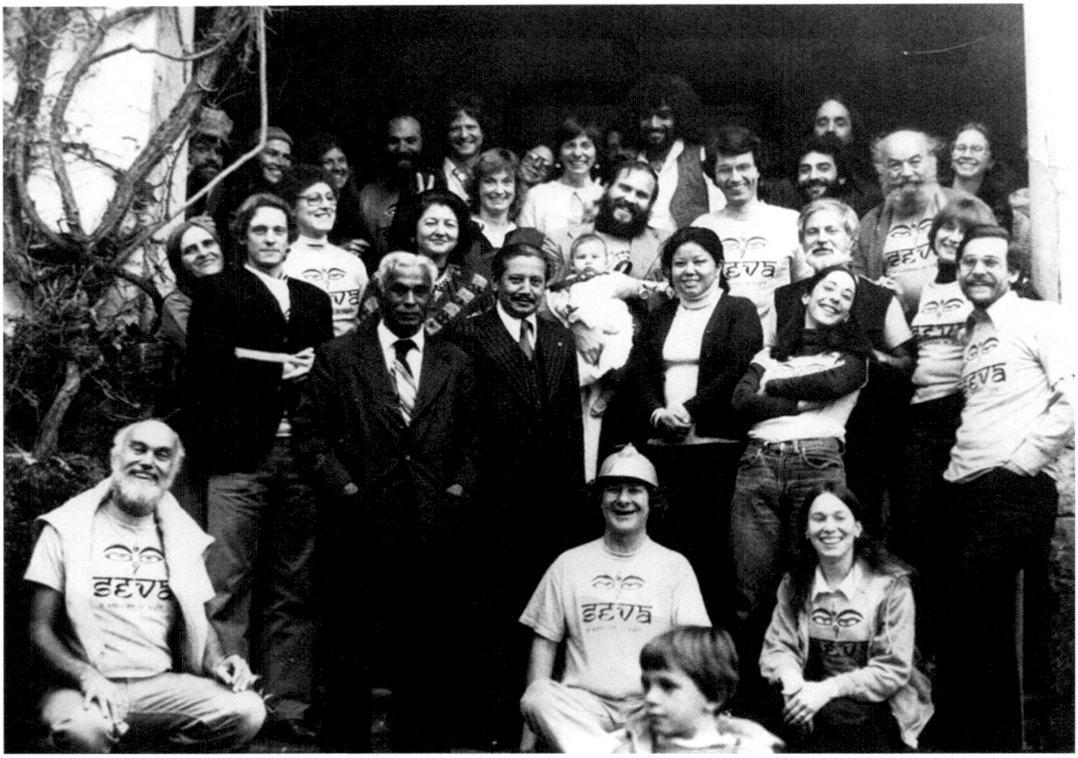

Fig. 29.1 Seva 1979 Board meeting. Participants include Dr. G Venkataswamy from India, Dr. Ram Prasad Pokhrel from Nepal, and Seva founders and friends from the WHO Smallpox Eradication Program and from the worlds of technology, public health, music, art, and service exploration

with essential, supplemental, and dignified wages for thousands. These long-standing relationships with many institutions in South-East Asia have informed and enriched Seva's global approach.

Seva demonstrates the skillful application of community health methods, epidemiology, strategic planning, management, and collaboration relevant to many issues threatening people's vision and well-being [1, 2].

29.1 Breakthroughs

Promoting Gender Equity Seva is dedicated to reaching the most vulnerable members in the communities it serves, particularly women and girls. More than half of the people living with blindness and visual impairment are female. In developing countries, women and girls are far less likely to access eye care services because of cultural and logistical barriers [3–5]. Seva reduces this imbalance by developing systems to collect data, including gender data, and investing in strategies that close this service gap between genders. Seva's practical approach overcomes barriers by supporting supplementary services like transportation to and from eye hospitals [6]. Seva helps communities establish vision centers. Women and girls significantly benefit from these services offered close to the doorstep. Training thousands of female community health volunteers in Nepal every year also addresses the gender gap in eye care.

Human Resources Pipeline for High-Quality, Living-Wage Jobs Seva builds up local talent to help eye care providers to improve systems and efficiency. Seva also uses locally available technology so that these programs can become financially and operationally self-sustaining. Known colloquially as the "human resources pipeline," this approach creates responsible living-wage jobs for many individuals. Seva helped establish ophthalmic residency and specialty training with multiple partners in the South-East Asian region [7].

To rapidly address the global need for allied ophthalmic staff, Seva partnered with the Aravind Eye Care System and the International Council of Ophthalmology to develop the course "*Eyexcel: Excellence in Eye Care Training*" in 2008 [8]. Eyexcel equips eye hospitals to initiate or strengthen staff training, usually young women. This five-day immersion workshop has reached more than 150 eye hospital teams from 33 countries over the past decade. Working with Eyexcel alumni, Seva has adapted the program for delivery in Spanish in Guatemala and Peru. Eyexcel Nepal and Eyexcel Bangladesh are disseminating this effective strategy, which is now online.

Culturally Competent Capacity Building While "capacity building" can be an overused buzzword in philanthropic circles, Seva has been living this approach since the organization's founding. Seva works with local partners to invest in a systems-based approach that makes it possible to see lasting improvement in community vision and well-being. At the core of this process is taking the time upfront to understand the local needs, the motivations and priorities of partners, and to ensure a good fit with what Seva can offer at the time.

An early example is an approach Seva took in 1978 with the Nepal Netra Jyoti Sangh (Nepal Society for Comprehensive Eye Care) and the Government of Nepal. Based on early discussions, Seva recognized Nepal's small ophthalmic community and health planners' concerns in prioritizing the collection and accessing of accurate data on the causes and distribution of blindness in the country. Findings from the Seva-led 1981 Nepal Blindness Survey, the most sophisticated nationwide systematic survey of its kind, were used to design the National Blindness Prevention Program to build Nepal's capacity for training and management of eye care service providers [9]. These baseline results have been used productively to gauge program impact by all institutions working to improve Nepal's eye care services [10–13].

Seva does not own any eye hospital. Seva adopts a partnership model where more mature institutions help develop eye care in communities that are challenged geographically and economically. For example, the Lumbini Eye Care Program helped develop primary eye care centers in Nepal's remote hilly districts.

29.2 Seva in India

Seva started working in India in 1979 and has been consistently invested in developing eye care service strategies, research, and resource institutions over many decades [14]. In the last five years, apart from investing in capacity building of more than 65 partner hospitals and supporting more than 50 vision centers across 15 Indian states and 2 union territories, Seva's partners in the country have provided services to more than ten million patients, completed 1.17 million surgeries, and screened 410,888 children of whom 15,061 received glasses and 1046 had eye surgeries. Seva's investments have resulted in the direct training of thousands of clinical and nonclinical personnel and the development of institutional training and research capabilities in select partners.

29.3 Seva in Bangladesh

In Bangladesh, Seva has applied in-depth analysis and action processes in working with Grameen Health and the Aravind group for over 15 years in the design and launch of four rural eye hospitals. In the last 3 years, with Seva support, our partners have established 9 vision centers (including pediatric intervention centers in 2 divisions) in 4 of the 8 divisions in Bangladesh. Recently, Seva collaborated with the Bangladesh Ministry of Health, leading eye hospitals, international non-government organizations (INGOs), and the IAPB in conducting a situation analysis of eye health needs in the Cox's Bazar district's burgeoning population [15]. This analysis, a subsequent Rapid Assessment of Avoidable Blindness (RAAB), and a planned Rapid Assessment of Refractive Error (RARE) will engage with the host community as well as the migrant community of nearly 900,000 refugees in the district.

In Myanmar and India, Seva pioneered and continues to provide essential sight-saving screening and treatment for HIV (human immunodeficiency virus)/AIDS (acquired immune deficiency syndrome) patients through the AIDS Eye Initiative training program. This compelling combination of compassion and technology reflect Seva's approach to service.

Seva's Response: An International Eye Care Mentoring Network Seva is among the top international organizations working to tackle vision impairment in developing countries. Seva's approach is one of the most multi-faceted in the field.

Seva's strategy for solving the mounting global vision crisis is fundamentally systems-based, data-driven, and results-oriented. The goal is to ascertain barriers to sustainable and comprehensive vision care in each community and how best to overcome them. Seva prioritizes tackling basic factors that are essential to ensuring that eye care facilities treat as many people as possible and deliver high-quality care in a way that such services will remain available for future generations.

Since 2006, Seva has worked closely with long time partners in India (including the Aravind Eye Care System, Dr. Shroff's Charity Eye Hospital, H V Desai Eye Institute, LV Prasad Eye Institute, Sadguru Netra Chikitsalaya, and Vivekananda Mission Asram Netra Niramay Niketan) and Nepal (including Lumbini Eye Institute and Bharatpur Eye Hospital among others) to establish the Global Sight Initiative (GSI).

GSI is a network of eye hospitals in the global south [16]. The initiative matches high performing "mentor" eye hospitals located in developing countries with "mentee" hospitals that seek to improve. This dynamic of "south-south" mentoring cooperation helps hospitals to better utilize staff and facilities to reach more people, enhance service quality, and become financially viable. Worldwide, the GSI network currently works with 11 mentor institutions and more than 100 mentee hospitals [17].

GSI coaching and training initially focuses on improving cataract surgery and refractive error services. However, over time, the coaching expands to cover different aspects of hospital service delivery required for the changing profile of vision-threats, including chronic conditions. These efforts reflect Seva's strategic priorities and the specific drivers which help to achieve them.

In 2019, GSI partner hospitals in India collectively examined over three million patients, completed 400,000 surgeries, and served almost one million patients through outreach activities.

Seva Foundation's work with its partners is guided by the strategic priorities of increasing access to eye care services, building hospital capacity to provide quality services, and supporting promising approaches for effective eye care delivery. Seva propels these priorities by particularly investing in four key program drivers (Box 29.1).

29.4 Building the Future: Scaling Through Partnership

As noted throughout this book and this chapter, the South-East Asian region's eye care needs are growing in number and complexity. Seva strives to provide holistic care by restoring both sight and the dignity of a person. Seva will increase its efforts in introducing effective quality and safety measures, including those for preventing infection, and protecting its allied staff, the patients it serves, and the communities it works for. Seva is committed to continuing its tradition of deep listening, information seeking, and analysis, before designing intervention programs along with partners to ensure that its services are relevant in changing times. By sharing what we are learning and gaining from others' experiences, we will restore sight and transform lives.

Seva's Drivers of Success

Eye Care for Children builds community awareness, provides eye screening, and develops referral networks so that children in need of advanced care can receive the services they need. [1][2][18,19] Findings from India indicate that multiple screening models are needed for school children and that solely screening school-going children can miss a large segment of youth.[3][20][4][21] Seva works with village health representatives to strengthen referral networks and to enhance children's continuity of care.[5][22]

Vision Centers are local permanent establishments that can address up to 80% of all eye care needs. They make basic eye care accessible to a community, no matter how remote. Seva first piloted vision centers in the hills of Nepal in 1989. Since then, Seva's partners in Nepal, India, and Bangladesh have dramatically scaled vision centers, with more than 350 facilities across 10 hospital systems, all in an effort to deliver on WHO's commitment to universal healthcare." [6][23]

Technology helps increase the effectiveness and efficiency of Seva programs and multiplies the efforts of in-demand eye specialists worldwide. In the 1990s, Seva provided critical funding and technical support to Aravind for development of Aurolab. [7][24] This helped make the intraocular lens (IOL) accessible to millions of people. Seva is developing a data platform for easy eye hospital analytics. New frontiers in retina imaging for early diagnosis, monitoring and treatment hold great promise.

Training and Jobs Creation addresses the lack of eye care specialists by scaling up the training and utilization of ophthalmic support staff. By recruiting trainees from the local communities, this program creates jobs and stimulates local economies while expanding access to eye care. Seva aims to increase the availability of online training through the innovative *Eyexcel: Excellence in Eye Care Training*, course.

Box 29.1 Seva's drivers of success

References

1. Gilbert SS, Bassett KL. Building research capacity through global partnerships. Invest Ophthalmol Vis Sci. 2019;60:6487. ARVO Abstract
2. Manandhar L, Rai S, Bajracharya K, et al. Cataract surgical quality and cost in a hill region of Western Nepal: comparing outreach eye camps with base hospital. Asian J Med Sci. 2018;9:10–6.
3. Abou-Gareeb I, Lewallen S, Bassett K, et al. Gender and blindness: a meta-analysis of population-based prevalence surveys. Ophthalmic Epidemiolol. 2001;8:39–56.
4. Joseph S, Ravilla T, Bassett K. Gender issues in a cataract surgical population in South India. Ophthalmic Epidemiolol. 2013;20:96–101.
5. Gilbert SS, Bassett K. Bridging the gender gap. cataract & refractive surgery today. 2007 (January): 65–67.
6. Mercer G, Lyons P, Bassett KL. Interventions to improve gender equity in eye care in low-middle income countries: a systematic review. Ophthalmic Epidemiol. 2019;26:189–99.
7. Ramasamy D, Gilbert SS. How to 'do' CPD with your team (from the organisation's perspective). Community Eye Health. 2017;30:9–10.
8. Gilbert SS, Courtright P, Ramasamy D. Expanding and optimizing human resources for eye care. In: Khanna RC, et al., editors. Innovative approaches in the delivery of primary and secondary eye care. Berlin: Springer; 2018. p. 39–55.
9. Brilliant LB, Pokhrel RP, Grasset NC, et al. Epidemiology of blindness in Nepal. Bull World Health Organ. 1985;62:375–86.
10. Pradhan S, Deshmukh A, Shrestha PG, et al. Prevalence of blindness and cataract surgical coverage in Narayani zone, Nepal – a rapid assessment of avoidable blindness (RAAB) study. Br J Ophthalmol. 2018;102:291–4.
11. Nepal Netra Jyoti Sangh. The epidemiology of blindness in Nepal. 2012.
12. Pokharel GP, Regmi G, Shrestha SK, et al. Prevalence of blindness and cataract surgery in Nepal. Br J Ophthalmol. 1998;82:600–5.
13. Sherchan A, Kandel RP, Sharma MK, et al. Blindness prevalence and cataract surgical coverage in Lumbini zone and Chetwan District of Nepal. Br J Ophthalmol. 2010;94:161–6.
14. Brilliant GE, Lepkowski JM, Zurita B, et al. Social determinants of cataract surgery utilization in South India. Arch Ophthalmol. 1991;109:584–9.
15. Vincent, J, Sapkota, Y. A situational analysis: eye care needs of Rohingya refugees and the affected Bangladeshi host population in Cox's Bazar district Bangladesh. 2018. https://www.iapb.org/news/report-highlights-eye-health-concerns-of-rohingya-refugees/ Accessed 4 October 2020.
16. Herzlinger RE. The global sight initiative. Boston: Harvard Business School Case; 2014. p. 311–44.
17. Judson K, Courtright P, Ravilla T, et al. Impact of systematic capacity building on cataract surgical service development in 25 hospitals. BMC Ophthalmol. 2017;17:96. https://doi.org/10.1186/s12886-017-0492-5.
18. Byanju R, Kandel R, Sharma P, et al. Childhood blindness and visual impairment in the Narayani zone of Nepal: a population-based survey. Ophthalmic Epidemiolol. 2019;26:257–63.
19. Bhandari G, Pradhan S, Shrestha M, et al. Eye glasses compliance among children undergoing school visual acuity screening in Nepal. Adv Ophthalmol Vis Syst. 2016;5:00162. https://doi.org/10.15406/aovs.2016.05.00162.
20. Sabherwal S, Sood I, Siddiqui Z, et al. Out-of-school vision screening in North India: estimating the magnitude of need. Ophthalmic Epidemiolol. 2020;20:1–4.
21. Reddy PA, Kannusamy V, Ravilla T, et al. Visual acuity screening by teachers in southern Indian schools: a non-randomized cluster-controlled trial of alternate screening models. Invest Ophthalmol Vis Sci. 2020;61:827. (ARVO Abstract)
22. Rai SK, Thapa H, Kandel RP, et al. Clinical and cost impact of a pediatric cataract follow-up program in western Nepal and adjacent northern Indian states. JAAPOS. 2014;18:67–70.
23. Khanna RC, Sabherwal S, Sil A, et al. Primary eye care in India – the vision center model. Indian J Ophthalmol. 2020;68:333–9.
24. Brilliant L, Brilliant G. Aravind: partner and social science innovator (innovations case discussion: Aravind eye care system). Innov Technol Gov Globalization. 2007;2:50–2.

30 SightLife and Elimination of Corneal Blindness

Josie Noah, Patrick Emery, Shubhi Sood, Anurag Taneja, Samara Andrade, and Lorraine Misquith

Over the last 50 years, since its start as the Lions Sight Conservation Foundation, SightLife has grown from a local eye bank serving patients and surgeons in Washington State, USA, to become one of the world's largest eye banks and global health organizations dedicated to eliminating corneal blindness by 2040.

More than 12 million people have corneal blindness [1], and an additional 1.5 million people become blind due to corneal problems each year [2]. Over 90% of those with corneal blindness live in low- and middle-income countries (LMICs), where there is limited access to high-quality corneal tissue for transplant. Relying on a corneal tissue supply base from the USA was neither a viable nor appropriate strategy for addressing unmet needs. Hence, SightLife activated a partnership-driven approach to strengthening eye bank capacity globally. The five pillars of this global strategy are: (1) advocacy and policy; (2) prevention and awareness; (3) clinical training; (4) eye bank development; and (5) access and innovation (Fig. 30.1).

30.1 Eye Bank Development in South-East Asia

LMICs carry the highest burden of corneal blindness, and a lack of proper infrastructure for eye banking in these regions often results in a shortage of corneas for transplant. Leveraging decades of experience in the USA and lessons from global partners, the SightLife eye bank development program brings industry's best practices and proven systems to build and strengthen underperforming eye banks. By doing so, high-quality corneas are available for local surgeons to perform sight-restoring transplants. In the past 10 years, SightLife partners have enabled over 100,000 transplants, with an annual growth of over 19% [3]. This transformation has depended on critical paradigm shifts (Fig. 30.2).

J. Noah · S. Andrade
SightLife Seattle, Seattle, WA, USA
e-mail: Samara.andrade@sightlife.org; Samara.andrade@sightlife.org

P. Emery · S. Sood (✉) · A. Taneja · L. Misquith
SightLife, New Delhi, India
e-mail: Patrick.emery@sightlife.org; Shubhi.Sood@sightlife.org; Anurag.taneja@sightlife.org; Lorraine.misquith@sightlife.org

T. Das, P. D. Nayar (eds.), *South-East Asia Eye Health*,
https://doi.org/10.1007/978-981-16-3787-2_30

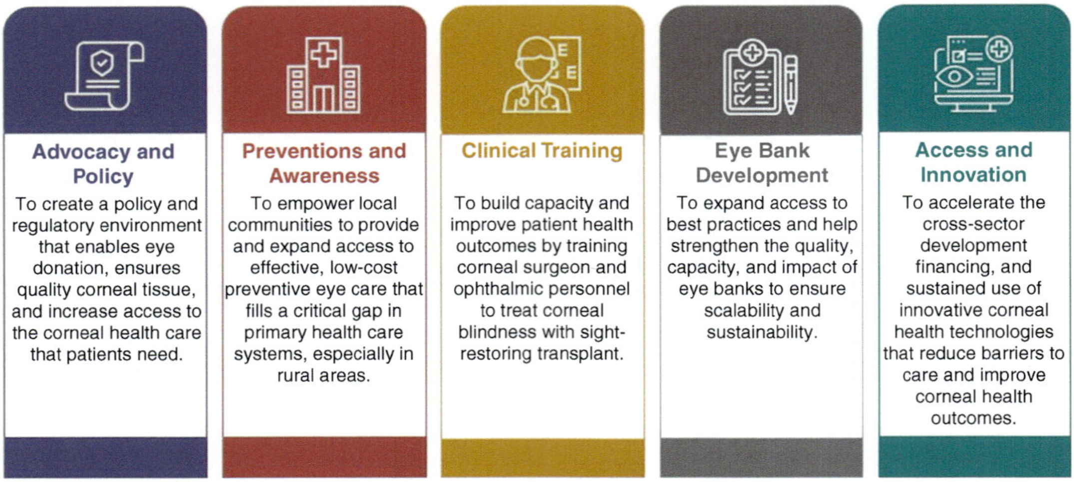

Fig. 30.1 Pillars of SightLife global strategy

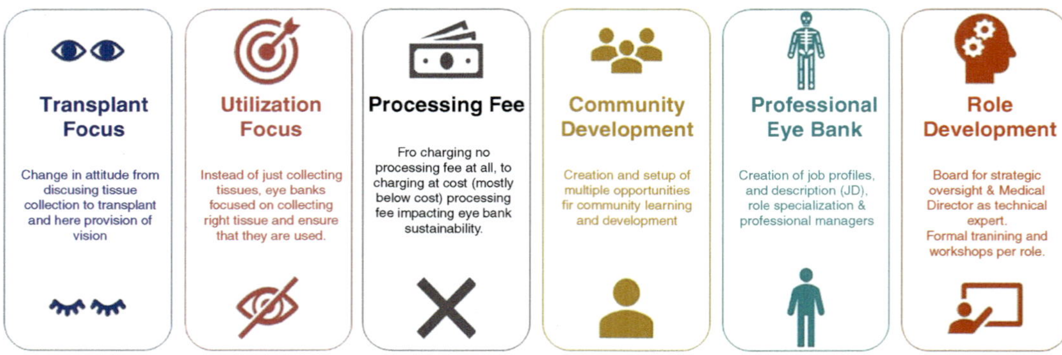
Transplant Focus
Change in attitude from discusing tissue collection to transplant and here provision of vision
Utilization Focus
Instead of just collecting tissues, eye banks focused on collecting right tissue and ensure that they are used.
Processing Fee
Fro charging no processing fee at all, to charging at cost (mostly below cost) processing fee impacting eye bank sustainability.
Community Development
Creation and setup of multiple opportunities fir community learning and development
Professional Eye Bank
Creation of job profiles, and description (JD), role specialization & professional managers
Role Development
Board for strategic oversight & Medical Director as technical expert.
Formal tranining and workshops per role.

Fig. 30.2 Paradigm shifts in eye banking in South-East Asia due to SightLife efforts

30.2 Eye Bank Development: Hospital Cornea Recovery Program

The expansion of the Hospital Cornea Recovery Program (HCRP) has been the most significant shift in South-East Asia eye banking strategy. This model drives quality and scale by ensuring that deaths are referred by hospitals or mortuaries directly to the eye bank on time, along with critical medical history and information; this enables the staff of the eye bank to rapidly determine eligibility. The similarities and differences between the HCRP and voluntary donation are shown in Table 30.1. HCRP best practices from the USA were localized for effective implementation in India, Nepal, and Sri Lanka.

30.3 Eye Bank Development: Quality Development Program

SightLife launched a quality development program in 2013 to overcome the lack of government or independent regulatory agencies to audit against eye banking standards in most countries throughout the South-East Asian region. This program brought consistency and professionalization to the eye banking community by

Table 30.1 Similarities and differences between HCRP and the voluntary donation model

Determinants	Hospital Cornea Recovery Program (HCRP)	Voluntary Donation Model
Notification	Hospital or mortuary notifies eye bank of all deaths	Donor family or community notifies eye bank of the death. This requires the family to have been previously educated about donation
Eligibility confirmation	Determine eligibility through review of medical records and family interview	Determine eligibility based on limited information from the family interview
Modality	Trained eye donation counselors approach families at hospital or mortuary, educate about cornea donation, and request legal consent	Travel to family's home or place of death to complete consent
Donor examination	Perform further medical assessment of potential donor	Perform further medical assessment of potential donor
Harvesting	Recover cornea tissue from the donor	Recover cornea from the donor
Donor age	The average age of donors is 42 years	Mostly age of donors is above 70
Utilization	High utilization of recovered corneas for surgery (>70%)	Low utilization of cornea for surgery (<40%)

implementing an eye bank quality certification methodology.

30.4 Clinical Training: Building Capacity to Improve Surgical Outcomes

Reports suggest that 53% of corneal blind people have no access to the medical care they need, including transplants [4]. Additionally, many surgeons in LMICs utilize only penetrating keratoplasty although newer techniques can offer better patient outcomes [5]. To bridge this gap, SightLife launched a clinical skill-transfer training program on lamellar keratoplasty in 2013. Since then, the clinical training program has expanded to develop the cornea-specific skillsets of various eye health professionals and is continued through a network of global faculty (Fig. 30.3).

30.5 Advocacy and Policy: Enabling Systems and Impact at Scale

Creating a policy environment that enables eye donation ensures availability of quality corneal tissue and increases access to care. SightLife's advocacy and policy program provides guidance on effective laws, policies, and regulations in countries through the Policy Best Practices Guidebook (2018), an advocacy tool targeted at policymakers emphasizing the value of strong donation laws and policies.

30.6 Prevention of Corneal Blindness: A Cost-Effective Intervention

As part of its health systems approach, SightLife's prevention program was launched in 2017 to expand access to corneal care for patients. The program focuses on preventing infectious corneal abrasions from developing into ulcers. Infectious keratitis accounts for approximately 50% of first-time corneal transplants in India and other LMICs. In many rural areas of South-East Asia, abrasions frequently occur during agricultural or factory work, usually due to the people not wearing protective eyewear. The World Health Organization (WHO) recommends reporting to an eye care provider within 7 days of ocular trauma to manage infections effectively. Studies suggest that antibiotic ointment applied soon after a corneal abrasion could dramatically lower the incidence of ulcers, hence avoiding the need for an invasive and expensive corneal transplant

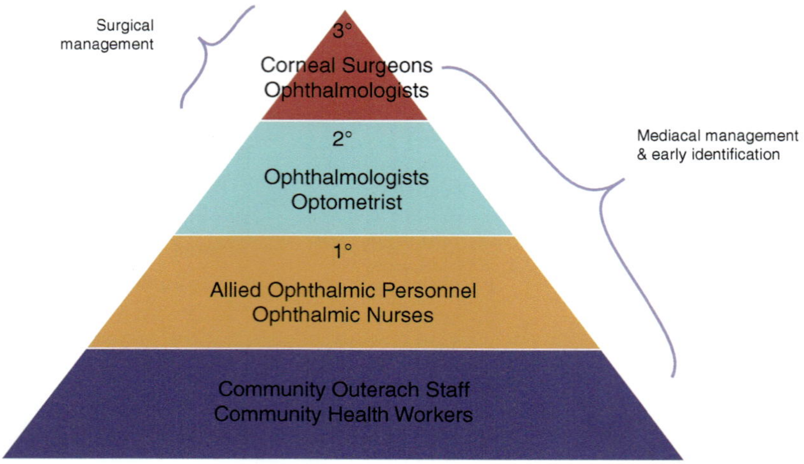

Fig. 30.3 SightLife's "pyramid" approach for training healthcare workers to improve surgical outcomes

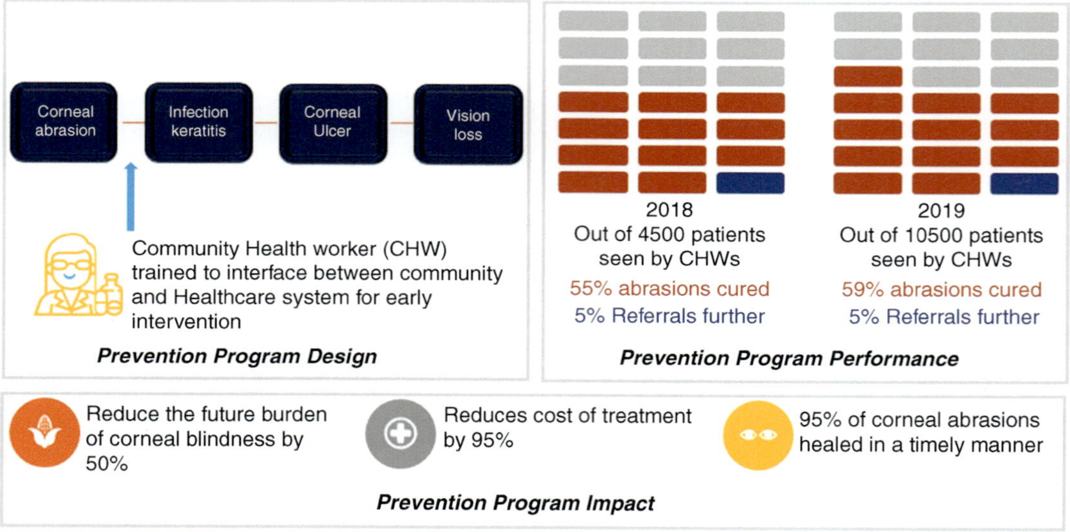

Fig. 30.4 SightLife's preventive program and its impact

[6, 7]. Studies from the Proctor Foundation, University of California, San Francisco, USA, have proven the efficacy of preventing corneal blindness by immediate treatment of corneal abrasions with antibiotic ointment [8]. In 2016, SightLife adopted this methodology and trained community health workers (CHWs) to deliver the first-line treatment (Fig. 30.4). The program, launched in six sites across India and Nepal, is highly cost-effective. The cost of diagnosis and preventive treatment per patient is only INR 70 or USD 1.

30.7 SightLife's Achievements in the WHO South-East Asia Region

30.7.1 India

30.7.1.1 Eye Banking

SightLife's Eye Bank Development Program in India was introduced in 2005 to bring best practices to 5 partner eye banks who had a combined annual transplant volume of just over 3400 (in 2009). SightLife now partners with 23 eye banks with a combined transplant volume of over 19,400 per year (Fig. 30.5). With HCRP, the utilization rate grew from 44% to 67%—even rivaling high-income countries and accounting for over 100,000 sight-restoring corneal transplants in just 9 years [3]. As of 2019, the cornea distribution system jointly developed by the Eye Bank Association of India and SightLife (in 2012) has successfully distributed over 16,000 corneas to more than 300 surgeons in 50 cities. The quality program has grown in parallel with 40 audits conducted across eye banks and 13 eye banks achieving SightLife quality certification (Fig. 30.5).

30.7.2 Clinical Training

Since the program's inception in 2013, nearly 1200 professionals have been trained across India. With 16 graduates from the short-term fellowship, new corneal surgeons can increase their ability to help patients with cornea-related problems.

30.7.3 Advocacy Initiatives

While eye bank capacity has increased, eye banks' sustainability has proved to be a continuous challenge primarily due to the lack of government policies or effective implementation. Despite the amendment of the Transplantations of Human Organs Act (THOA, 1991) there were no specific measures to increase donors' access to eye banks. There is no enabling policy that mandates that hospitals must notify all deaths to eye banks [9]. In a recent favorable policy adoption, the National Program for the Control of Blindness and Visual Impairment (NPCBVI) published the revised "Standards of Eye Banking in India" 2020.

30.7.4 Prevention Program

In the first three years of its prevention program, SightLife has trained 637 CHWs to screen 13,800 low-resource people for whom corneal care would otherwise be unavailable. Of these people, 8600 (62% of screened) were treated and only 162 (1.8% of those treated) people required to visit local hospitals for further care [10].

30.8 Nepal

30.8.1 Eye Banking

Nepal is primarily served by one eye bank that partnered with SightLife and it has become a significant success story. In 9 years, the transplant volumes grew five-fold to over 1100 annually, and the eye bank moved from being a net importer to a net exporter of corneas, supplying corneas to more than 15 countries. Nepal adopted the HCRP with great success [11]. It applied the programmatic structure of the HCRP to its eye banking system, including cornea collections from crematoriums, resulting in a utilization rate of over 80% of the collected tissue; this is comparable and, in many cases, is functioning better than eye banks in high-income countries. The eye bank has been quality certified by SightLife since 2015.

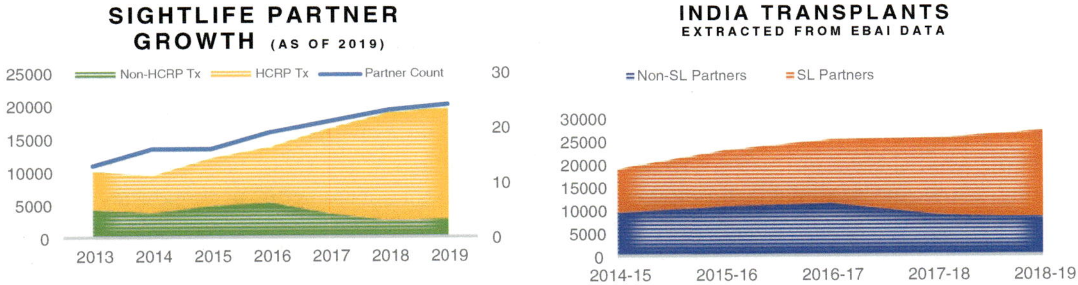

Fig. 30.5 Left: HCRP and corneal transplants in India; Right: Increases in the number of corneal transplants in India

30.8.2 Clinical Training

The SightLife clinical training program began in Nepal in 2015 in partnership with the eye bank by providing surgeons access to training through skills transfer opportunities at the Tilganga Institute of Ophthalmology in Kathmandu. To date, 31 surgeons have been trained.

30.8.3 Advocacy Initiatives

Nepal is one of the few countries in the South-East Asian region to introduce a National Eye Health Strategy while recognizing the right to health for all under its Constitutional and National Health Policy. It also introduced key policies like social insurance to cover costs related to the treatment of corneal ulcers and transplants. If well-implemented, these policies can significantly improve eye health access to thousands and could be a model to emulate.

30.8.4 Prevention Program

In its first three years, the SightLife prevention program has trained 263 CHWs in Nepal to screen 8622 low-resource people, has treated 4500 (53%) of them, and only 260 people (5.7% of those treated) were required to visit a hospital for further care [10].

30.9 Sri Lanka

30.9.1 Eye Bank Development

Effective government policy implementation, international collaboration, HCRP, and cultural norms have set Sri Lanka apart as a global eye banking leader and the number one contributor to international sharing in the region while first meeting 100% of local demand. International sharing allows Sri Lanka eye banks to recover a portion of the costs incurred to prepare corneal tissue, effectively increasing affordability of care for patients in Sri Lanka.

30.10 Bangladesh

30.10.1 Advocacy Initiatives

In 2012, under the Ministry of Health and Family Welfare (MoHFW), Bangladesh launched the National Eye Care plan, prioritizing cataract surgery, childhood blindness prevention, and correction of refractive errors while recognizing the need to focus on the cornea as an emerging priority. Since 2019, SightLife has been working with the MoHFW to develop a comprehensive plan to address the burden of corneal blindness and integrating it into the Operational Plan for 2021. High-level partnerships of this nature have the potential to bring about change at the health systems level in countries, a model which SightLife seeks to scale across the South-East Asian region.

30.11 The Road Ahead

Despite global efforts, health inequities persist. SightLife and partners strive for LMICs to be equipped and empowered to reduce corneal blindness. To address the needs of an estimated 12.7 million people who are blind, and the 1.5 million people who become blind due to cornea-related issues annually, the number of transplants need to increase by more than 500% globally, and continue at an incremental rate of 500% year over year. While transplants remain a critical component of addressing corneal blindness, it is essential to scale preventive care simultaneously. The key steps to achieving the elimination of corneal blindness by the year 2040 include the following:

- Investing in the healthcare workforce's training, including CHWs, eye bank personnel, ophthalmic personnel, and ophthalmologists.
- Ensuring eye care providers in LMICs have access to the latest research, medical technologies, and tools to optimize surgical and patient health outcomes related to corneal disease.
- Advocating for sustained, wide-spread adoption of best practices and favorable eye healthcare policies across geographies.

In high-income countries, many of these interventions are integrated into primary healthcare systems. But these benefits remain out of reach for many individuals and families in LMICs. One needs to upgrade the primary healthcare systems in South-East Asia to eliminate corneal blindness by 2040.

References

1. Gain P, Julienne R, He Z, et al. Global survey of corneal transplantation and eye banking. JAMA Ophthalmol. 2016;134:167–73.
2. Whitcher JP, Srinivasan M, Upadhyay MP. Corneal blindness: a global perspective. Bull World Health Organ. 2001;79:214–21.
3. SightLife Eye Bank development Program Data 2009–2019.
4. NPCB. Managing corneal blindness. India: NPCB; 2012, April–June. www.npcbvi.gov.in. Accessed 18 November 2020.
5. Garg P, Krishna P, Stratis A, et al. The value of corneal transplantation in reducing blindness. Eye. 2005;19:1106–14.
6. Timely Identification and Referral of Potential Organ Donors, NHS Blood and Transplant. A strategy for implementation of best practice. 2014. www.nhsbtde.blob.core.windows.net. Accessed 18 November 2020.
7. Krmpotic K, Payne C, Isenor C, et al. Delayed referral results in missed opportunities for organ donation after circulatory death. Crit Care Med. 2017;45:989–92.
8. O'Brien KS, Lietman TM, Keenan JD, et al. Microbial keratitis: a community eye health approach. Community Eye Health. 2015;28:1–2.
9. The Transplantation of Human Organs and Tissue Rules. 2014. www.notto.gov.in. Accessed 18 November 2020.
10. SightLife Prevention Program Data 2017–2019.
11. Ruit S, Geoffrey T, Gurung R, et al. Temple eye banking in Nepal. Cornea. 2002;21:433–4.

31 Sightsavers International

Rudra N. Mohanty, Sandeep Buttan, Rishibha Gupta, and Amrita R. Rozario

Sightsavers or the Royal Commonwealth Society for the Blind is a global development organization working with partners to reduce avoidable blindness and promote equality of opportunity for people with disabilities. We envision a world where no one is blind due to avoidable causes, as nearly 75% of such blindness can be prevented.

Sightsavers has adopted a health system strengthening approach to promote universal and comprehensive eye health to the most vulnerable communities in the countries that it works in. Primary eye health, disease-specific interventions, human resource development, and eye health advocacy are the pillars of the Sightsavers' program strategies that are delivered by systematically working with local health systems. Globally, Sightsavers is present in 30 countries across sub-Saharan Africa and South-East Asia. In South-East Asia, Sightsavers is present in India and Bangladesh (Sightsavers Pakistan operations are also included in this region).

The Sightsavers program is guided by the principles of universal health coverage (UHC) and health system strengthening based on the World Health Organization's (WHO) six building blocks. Our eye health programs address both supply and demand challenges, ensuring that quality and affordable eye health services are available and accessible for all and that communities proactively seek sight-restoring treatment. Interventions such as training of healthcare workers, community sensitization, encouraging health-seeking behavior, advocating for policy change, and inclusion of the most marginalized people are integral components of our work.

R. N. Mohanty (✉) · S. Buttan · R. Gupta
Sightsavers, New Delhi, India
e-mail: rnmohanty@sightsavers.org; sbuttan@sightsavers.org; rgupta@sightsavers.org

A. R. Rozario
Sightsavers, Dhaka, Bangladesh
e-mail: arozario@sightsavers.org

T. Das, P. D. Nayar (eds.), *South-East Asia Eye Health*,
https://doi.org/10.1007/978-981-16-3787-2_31

31.1 Sightsavers Experiences in India and Bangladesh

Since 1966, Sightsavers has supported the treatment of millions of people with eye disorders and brought eye services to some of the most underserved communities in India. Sightsavers has been working in Bangladesh since 1973; many thousands of irreversibly blind people have received rehabilitation and education support to enable them to lead lives of independence and dignity.

In India and Bangladesh, Sightsavers collaborates with various departments of the governments to scale up operations for social inclusion, inclusive education, and eye health—our three core areas of work. We work in a sustainable way to promote lasting change by strengthening existing health systems, advocating with and influencing governments, and demonstrating best practices.

In the last five decades, Sightsavers has supported more than 5 million sight restoration surgeries and treatment for over 36.5 million people in India. Our priority 100 districts in India are located in 8 states (Bihar, Chhattisgarh, Jharkhand, Madhya Pradesh, Odisha, Rajasthan, Uttar Pradesh, and West Bengal). We also execute multiple programs in another 5 states (Maharashtra, Karnataka, Tamil Nadu, Telangana, Andhra Pradesh), and one Union Territory (Delhi). Sightsavers in Bangladesh have supported 1.8 million sight-restoring cataract surgeries. Our programs have also impacted 30,000 children and 1.5 million people who have benefitted through refractive error corrections. Currently, Sightsavers in Bangladesh is implementing an eye health program in 16 districts of Dhaka, Khulna, Rajshahi, and Rangpur Divisions (Fig. 31.1).

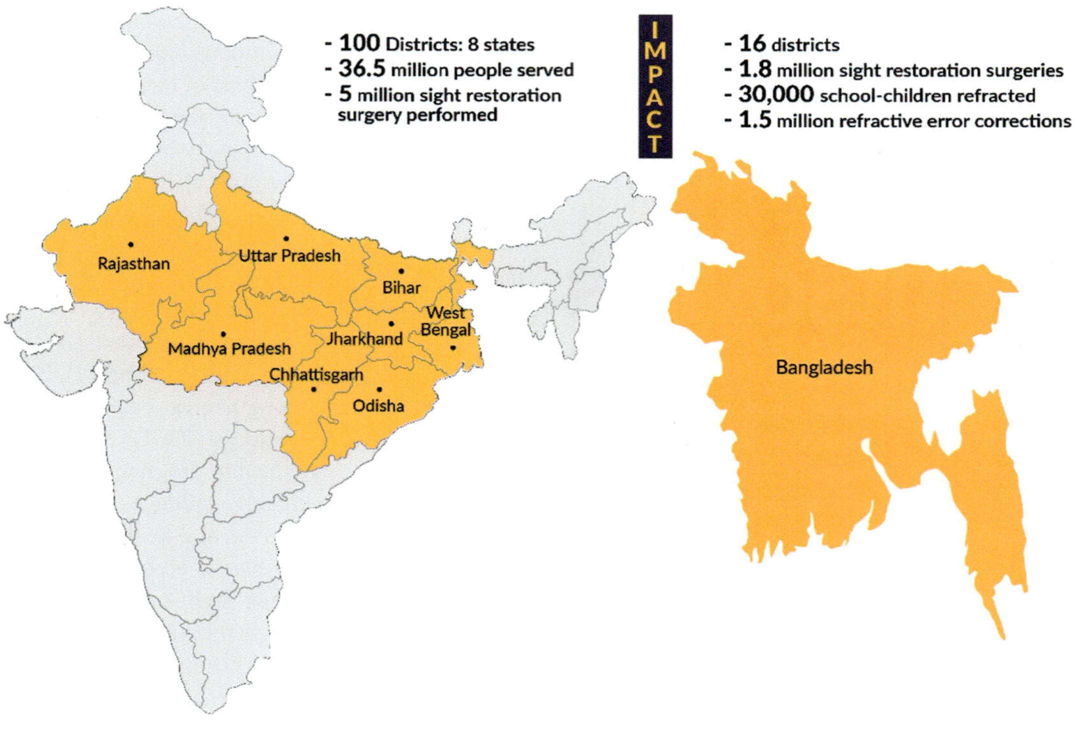

Fig. 31.1 Impact of Sightsavers programs since inception in India and Bangladesh

31.2 India

31.2.1 Eye Health Programs

In India, Sightsavers has four key eye health programs—Rural Eye Health (REH), Urban Eye Health (UEH), School Eye Health (SEH), and National Truckers Eye Health (NTEH). The REH program is designed to transform eye health systems across 100 most vulnerable rural districts by creating awareness and providing quality eye health services. The objective of the Vidyajyoti SEH program is to ensure good eye health of school children in public schools. This essentially includes screening children for vision problems, training teachers on eye health, and provision of quality eyeglasses. Recognizing the importance of eye health for the overworked truckers' community, the Raahi NTEH program aims to improve road safety by correcting truck drivers' refractive errors if any.

We work in some metropolitan cities to ensure comprehensive and sustainable eye health mechanisms for India's urban slums. Simultaneously, Sightsavers is working closely with the Ministry of Health and the National Health Mission (NHM) toward creating systems that provide access to quality eye health to the urban poor.

31.2.2 Taking a Health System Strengthening Approach to District Eye Health Planning and Delivery in Rural India

A "district" is the unit of intervention for Sightsavers in India. This approach ensures greater and more sustainable change for better advocacy with the government. This approach further ensures that joint experiences and recommendations help in improving collaborations, planning, and creation of policies aligned with Sightsavers' objectives.

31.2.3 Methods

We have also developed a structured tool—DEHAT (District Eye Health systems Assessment Tool)—based on the VISION 2020 situation analysis tool, the WHO District health systems assessment guidelines, and the Eye Health Systems Assessment tool (EHSA). DEHAT has qualitative and quantitative components to measure the district health system (context, service delivery, health workforce, infrastructure, financing, and governance). Data collection for DEHAT involved interviewing key stakeholders from state and district health units and on-site evaluations of key health facilities against local health standards. The data is analyzed to provide necessary information about the current status of eye care services and system-level gaps. This is presented to the relevant government authorities and key non-government stakeholders to develop a joint "District action plan" outlining each entity's respective roles and responsibilities. This has paved the way to several successful models of collaborations, namely, the NGO–GO (non-government and government organization) and NGO models; the former model was used in the state of Madhya Pradesh, and the latter was used in the state of Rajasthan (Fig. 31.2).

31.2.4 Sightsavers–Government Collaborations in India

Memorandums of understanding have been entered into with the governments of eight Indian states (Bihar, Madhya Pradesh, Odisha, Rajasthan, Karnataka, Uttar Pradesh, and West Bengal) for implementing eye health programs. Strengthening eye health service units at primary and secondary levels is a core strategy of our programs. Based on negotiations with government departments, special budgetary provisions were made in several states for infrastructure improvement and provision of equipment at primary and secondary level units. Here are a few examples of our successes:

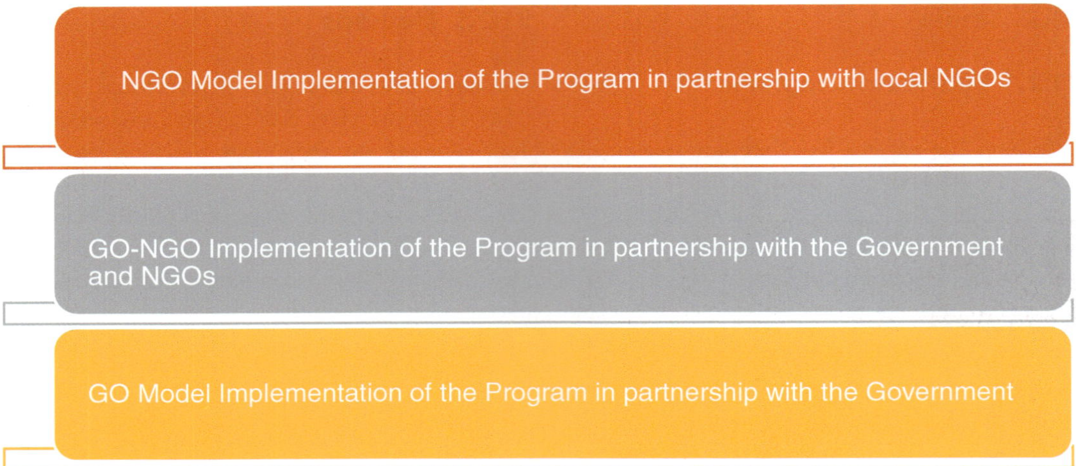

Fig. 31.2 Sightsavers' models of eye care

- Budgetary provision for the establishment of 100 new Vision Centers in Jharkhand.
- Approval for special purchase of equipment in public health units for eye health services in Madhya Pradesh.
- Odisha became the first state in the country to launch the Universal Eye Health program in 2017 that aims to reduce blindness prevalence to 0.3% by 2022. Sightsavers played a significant role in the launching of this program. It is also one of the founding members of the state-level empowered committee formed to implement the program. The state has budgeted INR 6800 million (USD 90 million) to be invested in 5 years to make eye health accessible for all.

31.2.5 Human Resource

As part of the engagement with the NHM, grassroots functionaries such as Mahila Arogya Samiti (MAS) members and Accredited Social Health Activist (ASHAs) were sensitized to the importance of eye health. This led to an increase in the uptake of eye health services by those in need. Through the program, a cadre of MAS members and ASHAs was created and trained to conduct primary screenings and referrals of individuals with symptoms of significant eye problems to vision centers or base hospitals.

Case Story 1. Sightsavers Sundarbans Eye Health Service

Sightsavers India initiated the Sundarbans Eye Health Service Strengthening Project in 2013. The project aimed to address the urgent need for improving eye health in selected blocks in the North 24 Parganas and South 24 Parganas districts in West Bengal, India. The project was financially supported by Standard Chartered Bank under the "Seeing is Believing" initiative. The seven yearlong intervention resulted in reducing blindness prevalence from 1.9% in 2013 to 0.7% in 2019 (Fig. 31.3).

31.2.6 Communication and Outreach Tools

Effective means of communication such as street plays, screening parades using mobile eye clinics, celebrations of important days, etc., were adopted to deliver relevant health messages to communities. Specially designed camps, communication

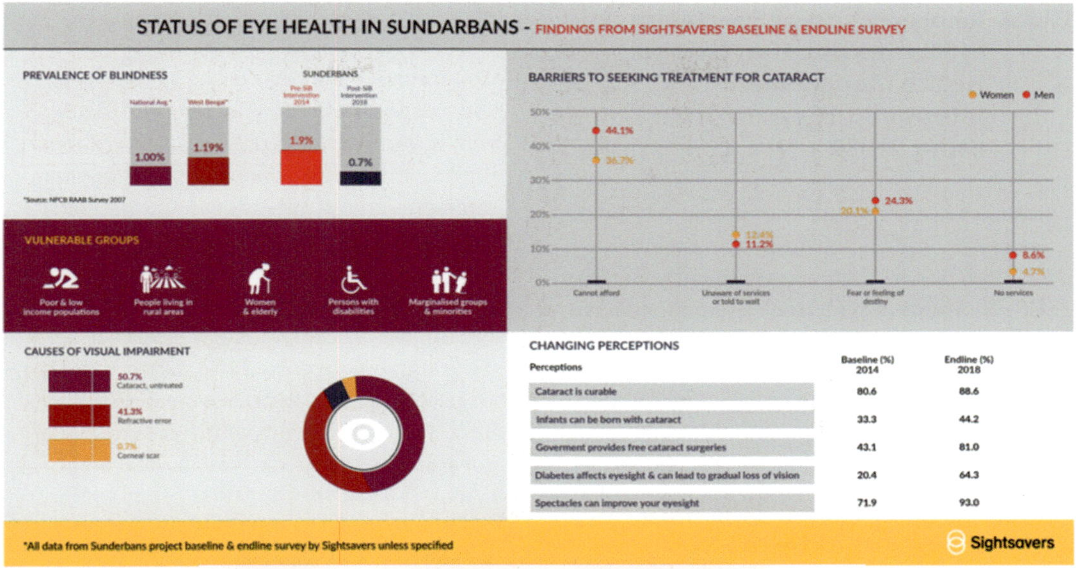

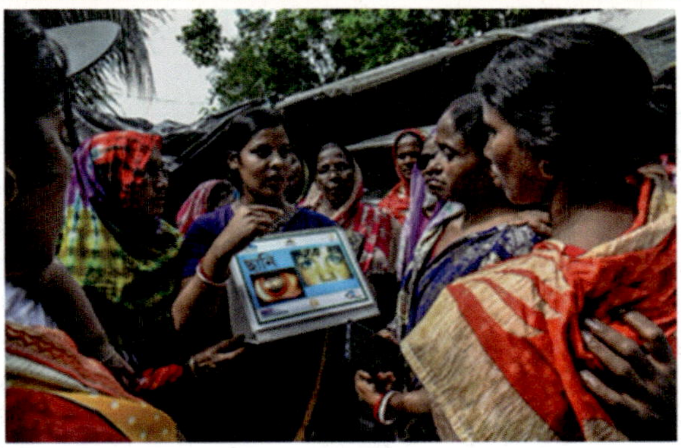

Fig. 31.3 Community Health Worker in Sundarbans explaining eye diseases using a flipchart

materials, etc., for specific groups of people were also adopted to influence these communities. Community leaders and local representatives were looped in to mobilize the community and to assure their participation in program interventions.

31.3 Bangladesh

31.3.1 Strengthening Government District-Level Hospitals as Secondary Eye Care Facilities

Based on lessons learnt from early work in the country, Sightsavers has since supported and contributed towards establishing dedicated operation theaters, necessary eye care equipment, and trained ophthalmologists and nurses to increase the capacity of eye departments of government district hospitals in priority districts. Besides this, Sightsavers provided orientation and awareness to government health workers, local volunteers, and community members on eye care and has linked them to the eye hospital for services. These initiatives contributed to increase in the numbers of cataract surgeries in a district-level hospital. Encouraged by this initial success, Sightsavers supported the establishment of another 15 government hospitals as secondary eye care facilities in collaboration with the Directorate General of Health Services (DGHS) and the National Eye Care (NEC) plan.

31.3.2 Incorporation of Eye Health Indicators into the National Health Management Information System (HMIS) using DHIS2

Sightsavers successfully advocated with the government of Bangladesh to include eye health indicators in the government's existing HMIS. Sightsavers undertook continuous advocacy with the DGHS and successfully included 10 eye health indicators in the national HMIS, DHIS2 (District Health Information Software 2). Besides this, Sightsavers rigorously monitored its implementing partners to incorporate eye health-specific data in the DHIS2 system so that the government could also have comprehensive data about overall eye services in the country.

31.3.3 National Standard Cataract Surgery Protocol

Ensuring quality was one of the main components of our work. Initially, Sightsavers took the initiative to develop a draft protocol for eye care in consultation with 30 ophthalmologists. As a result of Sightsavers' sustained advocacy with the NEC plan, these were endorsed as a national protocol by the Ministry of Health, Bangladesh. This document is currently a holistic guiding document for performing eye surgeries in all eye hospitals operating in Bangladesh. Similarly, the Bangladesh government has endorsed the Pediatric Eye Care Clinical Protocol, Pediatric Eye Care Guideline, and Counseling Manual, all of which received significant support from Sightsavers during their development and endorsement phases.

Case Story 2. Public-Private Partnership (PPP) Model in the Eye Health Sector in Bangladesh

'Vision Bangladesh' was an innovative project implemented as a partnership between Sightsavers, the Ministry of Health (MoH), and BRAC (Building Rural Advancement Committee) Each partner had specific roles and responsibilities (Fig. 31.4). BRAC was responsible for patient mobilization; Sightsavers was responsible for quality cataract surgery with hospital partners; and the MoH was responsible for quality monitoring. This approach was the first of its kind in Bangladesh to demonstrate a PPP model. Through this project, over one million people received eye care services; 109,960 cataract surgeries were performed; 8,862 field-level health workforces from the government and NGOs were trained on primary eye care, identification of, and referral of eye patients. In addition, a total of 44 technical personnel (ophthalmologists, medical officers, nurses and sub-assistant community medical officers) were trained from NGOs and government facilities.

31.4 Disability Disaggregated Data (DDD)

Under the United Kingdom Department for International Development (DFID)-supported "Right to Health" project, Sightsavers conducted a Disability Data Disaggregation (DDD) study to determine the prevalence of disability among men and women who are accessing eye care services at secondary health facilities and Patient Screening Programs (PSPs) in four districts of Bangladesh.

This study generated valuable data on the proportion of people with visual and non-visual disabilities among patients seeking eye health services. Among the patients interviewed, 50% (3568) were considered to have a disability.

An overview of Sightsaver's work in Bangladesh and India is listed in Table 31.1.

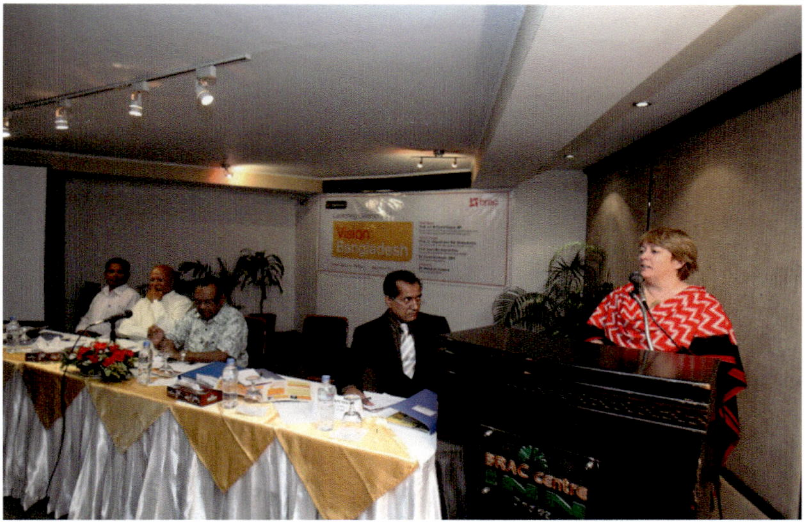

Fig. 31.4 Caroline Harper, Sightsavers, Chief Executive addressing people at the launch ceremony of Vision Bangladesh in 2011

Table 31.1 Snapshot of Sightsavers support in Bangladesh and India

Eye health impact (January 2015–December 2019)				
Indicators	Actual numbers		% of women	
	Bangladesh	India	Bangladesh	India
People examined	45,39,899	1,87,32,241	53	41%
Cataract surgeries performed	2,70,517	10,14,213	52	46%
People refracted	11,23,634	62,50,731	56	42%
Ophthalmologists trained on medical topics	252	286		
Ophthalmic nurses/optometrists trained	24	246		
Primary/community health workers/volunteers trained	21,440	87,018		

Key Lessons

- Engagement with local health systems is the key to sustainable care.
- Focusing on well-defined geographical (and administrative) units such as districts helps refine the approach and increase impact of eye health programs.
- Interventions must be based on systems gaps identified within all health systems components.
- Engaging all major partners (health and non-health) in an area makes interventions more comprehensive and inclusive.
- Inclusion of specific groups, such as women and people with disabilities, is necessary.
- Robust monitoring tools for gender equity and inclusion are essential for universal coverage.
- Health systems strengthening is a slow and deliberate process that requires careful long-term planning to ensure maintenance of the delicate balance between short-term service enhancement and capacity building of systems for a community's future needs.

32 A Powerful Tool for Social and Economic Development: Accelerating the Uptake of Eyeglasses for Working-Age Adults

Ella Gudwin, Anshu Taneja, and Jordan Kassalow

Helena was in her late 30s. She had just been dismissed from her job as a sewing machine operator at a garment factory in Gazipur, Bangladesh. Why? Because she could no longer thread a needle or spot flawed skip-stitches. Helena's future felt precarious. She was a second wife who had had no children of her own, and her familial standing was based significantly on Helena's ability to earn income for the extended household. She took up work as a maid, earning a salary 75% less than what she used to get at the factory.

Several weeks later, upon meeting with a BRAC (Bangladesh Rural Advancement Committee) community health worker in her home village, Helena learned that there might be a simple solution to her problem—a pair of reading glasses. The health worker knew how to conduct a simple vision screening to identify presbyopia and carried a selection of affordable single vision and bifocal readers in her basket of health products. For USD 1.90, Helena bought a pair of +1.5D reading glasses, immediately reacquiring the ability to work as a tailor, earn full wages, and contribute to the financial stability and well-being of her family for many more years, perhaps even decades. Had Helena been suspected of having a more complex eye condition, the health worker would have referred her for higher-level care.

It was because of women like Helena that VisionSpring in partnership with BRAC became the largest single distributor of reading glasses in Bangladesh. In 2017, the *Reading Glasses for Improved Livelihoods (RGIL)* program served its one-millionth customer, with community health workers having screened the vision of 4.6 million people with an average daily income below USD 2.50 across 61 of 64 districts in Bangladesh. BRAC and VisionSpring first joined hands in 2006 to start the RGIL program on the premise that glasses are one of the most underutilized, low-cost, high-impact tools available to boost economic and social outcomes for low-income individuals and their households.

VisionSpring founder Dr. Jordan Kassalow asked why we can buy a pair of reading glasses in

E. Gudwin · J. Kassalow (✉)
VisionSpring, New York, NY, USA
e-mail: ella.gudwin@visionspring.org; Jordan.kassalow@visionspring.org

A. Taneja
VisionSpring India, New Delhi, India
e-mail: Anshu.taneja@visionspring.org

T. Das, P. D. Nayar (eds.), *South-East Asia Eye Health*,
https://doi.org/10.1007/978-981-16-3787-2_32

any pharmacy, book shop, and railway station in the US and Europe, while people in low-income countries have to go to hospitals and optical shops to get simple magnifying lenses? "We don't send people to a dentist to get a toothbrush; why do people need to see an ophthalmologist or optometrist for readers, especially when there are so few specialists per population?," he asked.

Trained as a Doctor of optometry at the New England College of Optometry, with a Master's degree in public health, and a fellowship in preventive ophthalmology from Johns Hopkins University, Dr. Kassalow challenged himself and his peers with a question: "In the name of comprehensive eye care, aren't we denying a billion people the right to see clearly? By insisting that only we can conduct vision screenings and dispense something as simple as reading glasses, are eyecare professionals perpetuating more vision impairment than we are correcting?"

These questions spurred VisionSpring and BRAC to co-create the RGIL program, with 26,500 health workers, mostly women, to bring a 700-year-old technology to working-age adults and elders in their communities in Bangladesh. Through the program, 75% of the customers who acquire glasses are getting their first pair. Of customers, 74% are in their prime working years, ages 35–54 years, and 63% are women.

As the health sector looks to integrate eye care into Universal Health Coverage and eye hospitals and vision centers increasingly include eyeglasses in their outreach activities, lessons from the RGIL program are timely and particularly relevant when considering task shifting and access to vision correction at the primary care level.

First, we have found that health workers, locally called Shasthya Shebikas (SS), with no more than an eighth-grade education, are highly capable and successful in conducting a basic vision assessment, dispensing reading glasses to those who require near distance correction, and referring others on for higher-level care. The vision assessment is conducted only on those aged ≥35 and begins with the SS looking for any symptoms of infection, injury, cataract, or other observable signs of eye disease or damage. If any symptoms or signs are observed, the SS refers the customer to an eye care center for further examination. If the customer does not have any major eye issues, the SS assesses the customer's distance vision, one eye at a time, with an eye chart. If the customer fails the 6/12 line with either eye, the SS will refer the customer for a comprehensive eye exam. Typically, 15% of people examined through the RGIL program are referred for higher-level care.

If the customer passes the distance vision test, s/he is given a near vision assessment with a simple handheld chart. The SS is trained to recognize signs of the customer's straining, such as pulling back the head, furrowing, and extending arms. To guide the SS in determining the correct power lens to choose from, the visual acuity measures on the chart include a corresponding plus-power number. If someone requires near distance correction, the SS provides the customer with one or two spectacles with different powers to try on and offers a newspaper, needle, and thread, or card with symbols, to verify the best power for the customer's typical working distance. The SS may dispense glasses with lenses up to +3D power and offer both single vision and plano bifocals, which are the most popular.

Second, over time, VisionSpring learned several lessons that contribute to the RGIL program's success and are broadly applicable to the provision of reading glasses in primary care and community settings:

1. **Low-income customers will pay 1–2 days' wages for glasses** for the immediate benefit of clear vision, but with limited discretionary income, they are price sensitive. In Bangladesh, RGIL's average customer lives on less than USD 2.50 per day (69%), and 45% live on less than USD 1.75 per day [1]. SS sells the readers for USD 1.90, which includes a USD 0.35 sales commission. Purchase conversation rate, i.e., the percent of people diagnosed with presbyopia who choose to buy glasses on the spot, is 22–32%.
2. **Reading glasses increase worker productivity by 22%**—VisionSpring undertook a randomized control trial in the tea gardens of Assam, India, with the Queens University of

Belfast and Clearly (PROSPER—Productivity Study of Presbyopia Elimination in Rural-dwellers) [2]. The trial aimed to quantify the impact of reading glasses on work productivity. The study found that providing eyeglasses to correct presbyopia among tea workers with age-related near vision problems resulted in a substantial productivity increase of 22%. Moreover, with increasing age, the productivity gain expanded, such that women >50 years demonstrated a 32% increase in productivity. Nearly 95% of trial participants indicated that they were willing to pay for glasses if they lost or broke them.

3. **Purchase priming increases conversion—** People are more likely to buy glasses at a community-based event if they are notified in advance. We found that handing out a simple black and white, quarter-page leaflet served as a kind of invitation to the event and increased footfall by 18%. The inclusion of the price centered on the page and in the largest font results in customers coming with money on the day. When VisionSpring and BRAC tested this strategy in low and medium performing districts, purchase conversion increased from an average of 25% to 32%, resulting in a 28% growth in glasses sales. Giving customers one to three days of advance notification is especially important for women who do not have income and must negotiate a potential purchase with a spouse or other family member in advance.
4. **Style and durability matter—**People, regardless of income, care what they wear on their faces. Because preferences vary by region and gender, we conduct research on focus groups before settling on a limited selection of frames that can be managed with no stock-outs in a "last-mile" supply chain. Regarding quality, the material, finish, and hinges are selected such that they should last at least 12 months with reasonable use and care. In Bangladesh, we have found that gold metal frames in an oval shape are the most commonly selected "entry-level" pair of glasses for both men and women. In Uganda, however, black, plastic, rectangular-shaped frames are preferred.
5. **Sales skills can be taught—**Health workers are often care providers and educators before they are salespeople; but sales skills can be taught. The most important skill to include in sales training is how a health worker can transition from counseling someone about their vision and the benefits of glasses to overcoming the customer's objections and concerns to close a sale. One common customer concern is that glasses will make vision worse. We found 32% of respondents hold this myth in a KAP (knowledge, attitudes, and practices) study undertaken with the Centre for Injury Prevention and Research, Bangladesh (CIPRB) in 2020 (unpublished) [3]. In this instance, the SS must counsel customers about age-related reduced vision and the natural progression of the condition.
6. **Readers are best sold as a margin-positive item in a bundle of goods—**Readers are a slow-moving commodity. Low-income customers are likely to buy just one pair a year or two (if they do not lose or break them). This means that micro-entrepreneurs cannot sustain their livelihoods on readers alone. Readers are a relatively high margin or commissionable item that can be effectively incorporated into bundle of other goods. This makes them especially suitable for inclusion in product offerings by pharmacies and medicine shops, *kirana*-style general stores, and other retail settings.
7. **Reaching those who live on less than USD 4 per day requires some subsidy—**As a social enterprise, for many years, we aspired to break even, but we have concluded that reaching this income segment through the community health worker channel requires some subsidy. At the current scale, screening one million people per year and selling 180,000–200,000 pairs of glasses—the fully loaded cost, inclusive of allocated overheads for both organizations, has plateaued at between USD3.10–3.50 per pair of glasses.
8. **"Readers" is a bad product name for our customer segment—**Most RGIL customers are not very literate. Once a customer declined to purchase glasses, asking, "why do I need

readers? I can't read." Spectacles or near vision glasses appear to be more suitable terms. When raising awareness about spectacles, we have learned to focus our messaging on how glasses help people accomplish up-close tasks such as threading a needle, sorting rice and grain, repairing a bicycle, using a mobile phone, etc.

In addition to being replicated in Uganda, the RGIL program served as an inspiration for three other VisionSpring models that focus on access to vision correction for working-age adults—the "Readers through Pharmacies" program in Bangladesh, the "See to Earn: Vision Access" program in India, and the "Clear Vision Workplaces" program in Bangladesh, India, and Vietnam.

The "Readers Through Pharmacies" Program in Bangladesh To create sustainable access to glasses, VisionSpring developed a new sales channel and model to sell readers through rural medical providers (RMPs), who own independent, bazaar-based pharmacies, and medical shops in Bangladesh. Having piloted the model in 2018, VisionSpring initiated early replication of the program in 2019, enrolling a total of 177 medical shops in the program in Sherpur and Netrakona districts. In 2019, the RMPs corrected the vision of 6000 customers with glasses. Even in its early days, this channel and approach are showing great promise. Of pharmacy customers, 81% are acquiring their first pair of glasses from RMPs. This market-based approach is also advocated for in the eyeglass product narrative prepared by ATscale, the Global Partnership for Assistive Technology [4], in part, based upon VisionSpring's experience, among others [5].

The "See to Earn: Vision Access" Program in India The RGIL program in Bangladesh inspired VisionSpring to develop the "See to Earn: Vision Access" program for weavers in Varanasi, one of India's oldest centers of handloom and traditional textile production. Launched in 2018, the program reached 100,000 weavers and their families in 2019. We found a high refractive error rate (73%) among participants, and 89% received their first pair of eyeglasses through this program. As of now, VisionSpring is replicating the program with another 100,000 weavers in Odisha and Rajasthan, in partnership with state-level Departments of Handlooms and Textiles, and the skill development initiative of the Export Promotion Council for Handicrafts.

The "Clear Vision Workplace" Program in Bangladesh, India, and Vietnam VisionSpring extended its experience in rural communities and the informal sector into workplaces, bringing the "Clear Vision Workplace" program to agricultural estates and garment and home goods factories. Joining with producers and their associations, brands, government ministries, philanthropic funders, and bilateral aid agencies, VisionSpring formed the "Clear Vision Workplace Alliance." Launched in 2020, the Alliance will bring vision correction (both readers and prescription glasses) to an initial half a million workers in factories in India, Bangladesh, and Vietnam.

Beyond productivity gains and increased income-earning potential, interviews with factory workers revealed important well-being benefits. These included workers reporting a 75% decrease in feelings of frustration, an 87% reduction in reports of headaches and fatigue, and greater ease in daily activities such as removing stones and pests from rice [6] (Table 32.1 and Fig. 32.1).

Table 32.1 Comparisons of garment worker's ease with household and daily activities before and after they were provided with spectacles [6]

		Workers reporting "No difficulty"			
		Before glasses		After glasses	
Activity	Improvement with glasses	%	#	%	#
Removing stones and pests from rice or lentils	454%	13%	45	72%	247
Reading newspaper or holy books	364%	14%	47	65%	220
Reading text messages	324%	17%	59	72%	247
Helping child with homework	150%	12%	40	30%	103
Doing home repairs	145%	22%	75	54%	184

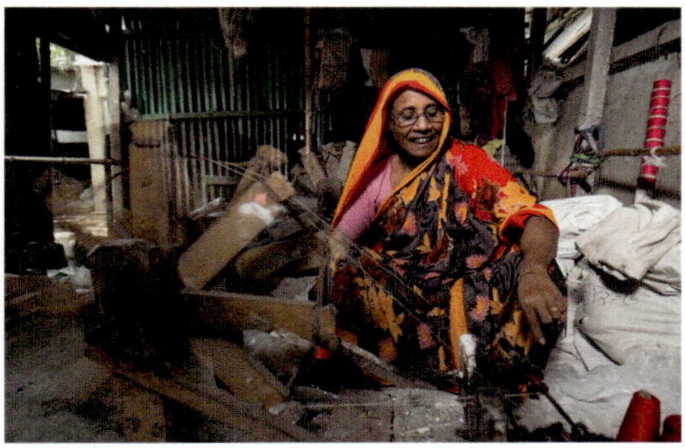

Fig. 32.1 Spinning thread in Narsingdi district after vision correction. She has benefited from a pair of glasses from VisionSpring. © VisionSpring

32.1 Conclusion

We are proud that the World Health Organization (WHO) has recently embraced the concept that task shifting in presbyopia correction is safe and effective, particularly in light of the original skepticism. Thanks to the work of EYElliance, online training to provide ready-made glasses for community health workers and others will be among the first courses to be launched on WHO's new Academy in May 2021. We hope VisionSpring's experience with entrepreneurial models, community health workers, last-mile retail, task shifting, and focusing on livelihoods inspired by customers may inform others looking to increase market-based access to vision correction.

References

1. Customer income levels are measured with the Poverty Probability Index, developed by Innovations for Poverty Action. https://www.povertyindex.org. Accessed 24 Nov 2020.
2. Reddy PA, et al. Effect of providing near glasses on productivity among rural Indian tea workers with presbyopia (PROSPER): a randomized control trial. Lancet Glob Health. 2018;6:E1019–27.
3. Baseline Survey on Prevalence of Refractive Error including Presbyopia and Coverage of Corrective Eyeglasses in Sherpur, conducted by the Centre for Injury Prevention and Research, Bangladesh (CIPRB) on behalf of VisionSpring and the members of the Clear Vision Collective. Data collection 2019. Study manuscript, 2020 (not-yet published).
4. The ATscale Founding Partners are: China Disabled Persons' Federation, Clinton Health Access Initiative, GDI Hub, Government of Kenya, International Disability Alliance, Norwegian Agency for Development Cooperation, Office of the UN Secretary-General's Envoy for Financing the Health Millennium Development Goals and for Malaria, UK Department for International Development, UNICEF, United States Agency for International Development, World Health Organization.
5. ATscale, Product narrative: eyeglasses – a market landscape and strategic approach to increasing access to eyeglasses in low- and middle- income countries. 2020. https://static1.squarespace.com/static/5b3f6ff1710699a7ebb64495/t/5f5f8981cd35d775923e2621/1600096643567/Product_Narrative-Eyeglasses_a11y_rev.pdf Accessed 23 Nov 2020.
6. Program data collected by third-party enumerators in 2018–2019 and evaluated by VisionSpring monitoring and evaluation staff. The sample size consisted of 423 garment factory workers (204 in Bangladesh and 219 in India) ages 35 years and older, diagnosed with presbyopia and with no prior experience wearing glasses.

Part VI

Ophthalmic Industry

Spectacles

33

Saugata Banerjee and Keerti Bhusan Pradhan

Key Points

- Spectacles are the simplest and most effective solution to correcting and protecting one's vision.
- Globally, 2.7 billion people have an uncorrected refractive error, and the demand is increasing (Fig. 33.1).
- Seven of the top ten countries with the largest populations of people with uncorrected refractive errors are in Asia, and three of them (India, 23%; Indonesia, 5%; and Bangladesh, 3%) are in the South-East Asia region.
- By 2050, 3.2 billion people are estimated to suffer from uncorrected refractive errors if the industry maintains its current focus, serving only established markets using similar channels and products.
- The Asia Pacific eyewear market is expected to grow from USD 63.8 billion in 2019 to USD 114.4 billion in 2026 (BlueWeave Consulting).
- The retail volume of India's spectacle lenses is estimated to increase from 210 million units in 2019 to 300 million units in 2025.
- Barriers to use of spectacles are related to access, awareness, supply, affordability, quality, and acceptance.
- ATscale, the global partnership for assistive technologies, suggested five strategies to increasing access to eyeglasses in low- and middle-income countries. These are: mobilize key stakeholders; strengthen global policy of service delivery; support governments to develop comprehensive eye care plans; engage private sectors; and build and drive awareness.

Spectacles are the simplest and most effective solution to correcting and protecting one's vision. First appearing as "roidi da ogli" or "round glass

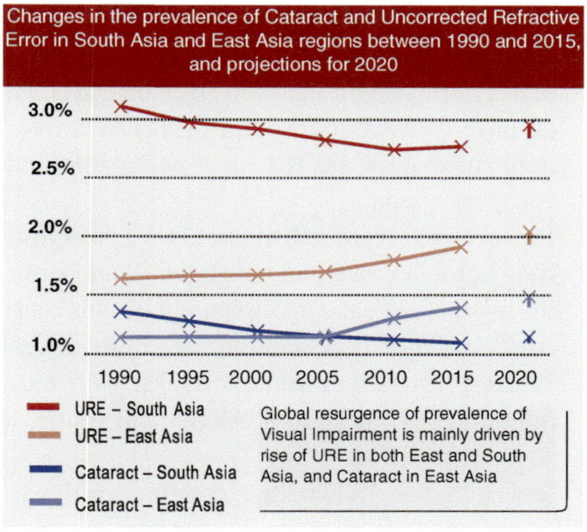

Fig. 33.1 Changes in the prevalence of Cataract and Uncorrected Refractive Error in South Asia and East Asia regions between 1990 and 2015, and projections for 2020. © The International Agency for the Prevention of Blindness (IAPB) 2015. All Rights Reserved

S. Banerjee (✉)
Essilor, Singapore, Singapore
e-mail: saugata@essilor.com.sg

K. B. Pradhan
Global Advisor-Vision Spring, New Delhi, India

T. Das, P. D. Nayar (eds.), *South-East Asia Eye Health*,
https://doi.org/10.1007/978-981-16-3787-2_33

for the eyes" that help all objects be visible clearly, these items were already in routine production in Venice, Italy in the 1200s [1]. It may be thousands of years ago, but the concept remains unchanged, and the joy of seeing clearly has not changed. Innovation and technological changes over the years mean that the correction and protection spectacles can offer is continually evolving.

Spectacles are important for many reasons, and these reasons differ throughout the life stages. As children, we need to be able to see clearly at school to maximize learning; as adults, we need to have good vision to work and live safely; as we get older, our eyesight naturally deteriorates, so we need to correct our vision to be able to maintain a good quality of life.

Put simply; spectacles enable us to:

- **See clearly:** spectacles are needed to correct a range of poor vision conditions such as myopia, hyperopia, presbyopia, and astigmatism. They can also help manage or even relieve vision-related migraines.
- **Read easier**: if we cannot see newspapers or books clearly, then we cannot maximize learning or enjoyment from this activity. Or worse yet, if we cannot read important information such as dosage instructions for medication and, as a result, over-medicate. As we get older, our eyesight naturally worsens, and we all have to wear some form of vision correction. Spectacles are the most accessible and cheapest option.
- **Protect eyes from ultraviolet (UV) rays and blue light**: UV rays and blue light [2] are harmful to our eyes causing digital eye strain, cataracts, macular degeneration, or even cancer. Wearing sunglasses and spectacles with blue light filters is crucial to protecting our vision.

Research has shown that people worldwide will pay up to 3 days' wages [3] for their first pair of spectacles and are willing to pay up to 40% more for their second pair of spectacles [4], having experienced the life-changing benefits of good vision.

33.1 All About Spectacles

There are different types of spectacles available, depending on the condition of the eyes and the level of vision correction needed. These could be corrective or protective.

33.1.1 Corrective

33.1.1.1 Prescription

Prescription lenses are made specifically to match an individual's poor vision and degree of correction needed. They include:

- *Single Vision Lenses*—designed to help people who require correction of farsightedness, nearsightedness, or astigmatism. They have just a single optical prescription correction, and they distribute focus evenly over the entire surface area of the lens.
- *Bifocal Lenses*—Bifocal lenses have been around since the late eighteenth century, and modern-day bifocal lenses are still made up of two parts. The top part of the lens is made for seeing things at a distance, and the bottom part of the lens is made for viewing things at a near object. A visible line usually separates the two sections of the lens. The segment of the lens devoted to correcting near vision can be in several shapes, including a half-moon, a round segment, a narrow rectangular area, or the full bottom half of the bifocal lens.
- With only two zones of vision, bifocal lenses do not account for the intermediate zone of vision, i.e., when you are viewing something between 18 to 24 inches (45–60 cms) away [5]. This means it can be difficult to view things like a computer screen while wearing bifocal lenses.
- *Trifocal Lenses*—To correct the problem of lacking an intermediate viewing area, trifocal lenses were invented. Trifocal lenses offer correction for near and far, and enable a person to see clearly at an intermediate level. Trifocals help correct the intermediate zone

by featuring a second small lens segment directly above the area used to correct near vision. This results in a total of three power zones, thus the name trifocal [5]. This intermediate segment allows the wearer to see things better, like the computer screen or the vehicle instrument panel on the dashboard.

- *Progressive Lenses*—Without any visible lines on the lens, progressive lenses offer a smooth transition from the distance through intermediate vision to near vision. Progressive lenses also provide vision correction for all of the in-between vision zones. Instead of just having two or three different viewing zones, progressive lenses offer vision correction that progresses in power from the bottom to the top of the lens. This progression of correction eases eye strain by providing the most natural vision correction.
- Modern technology has continued to improve the design of progressive lenses. Some progressive lenses on the market today are designed to account for the difference in the prescription for both the right and left eyes. These lenses also help cut down on blurry peripheral vision, which can be apparent in other progressive lenses and cause motion sickness.
- *Photochromic Lenses*—Photochromic lenses look like regular clear lenses when indoors but automatically darken when moving into a brighter area. Ultraviolet (UV) rays from the sun affect the molecules in the photochromic lenses, so they change color. They will darken in the light even on overcast days as UV rays still penetrate clouds. This provides the best possible vision in all lighting through different shades of tint. Photochromic lenses are sometimes called adaptive lenses, auto-tinted lenses, or variable-tint lenses. These are not to be confused with polarized spectacles (sunglasses), which have a set tint that protects from glare but do not adapt to the light in the same way photochromic lenses do.

33.1.1.2 Reading Spectacles

Reading spectacles help compensate for diminished vision related to presbyopia, the normal age-related loss of ability to focus on up-close objects, such as words in a book or a text message on a smartphone.

33.1.2 Protective

33.1.2.1 Blue Light Blocking Spectacles

Blue light is naturally produced by the sun and by computer monitors, smartphone screens, and other digital devices. In addition to these, blue light is produced by LED and fluorescent lights and compact fluorescent light bulbs. Too much blue light exposure can cause digital eye strain and even more serious conditions like macular degeneration and even permanent vision loss. Blue light blocking spectacles have filters in their lenses that block or absorb blue light, and in some cases, prevent UV light from getting through.

33.1.2.2 Sunglasses

Sunglasses help to protect the eyes from prolonged exposure to the sun's UV rays, which can lead to conditions such as cataracts and macular degeneration. The risk of damage to our eyes from UV rays is cumulative, meaning the danger continues to grow as we spend time in the sun throughout our lifetime. Wearing sunglasses that have UV protection can help protect against these conditions, keeping eyes healthier for a more extended period of life.

33.1.2.3 Safety Goggles

Safety goggles are a type of protective eyewear that offers complete protection for the eyes by enclosing the areas surrounding them, so that water, chemicals, particles, and other foreign materials will not touch the eyes.

33.2 An Overview of the Eyewear Industry in the South-East Asia Region

In Asia, research conducted on the eyewear industry is mainly focused on China, India, Japan, South Korea, Australia, and to some extent, also in Indonesia and Thailand. Data on Bangladesh, Bhutan, Maldives, Myanmar, Nepal, Sri Lanka, and Timor Leste are lacking.

Against the COVID-19 pandemic's backdrop, market research firm BlueWeave Consulting forecasted that the Asia Pacific Eyewear market is expected to grow to USD 114.4 billion by 2026 from USD 63.8 billion in 2019, at a compound annual growth rate (CAGR) of 8.7% from 2020 to 2026 [6]. While not entirely representative of the South-East Asia region discussed in this book, this forecast is indicative of the continued growth of the market in this part of the world amidst the pandemic and beyond. According to Euromonitor International, the retail volume of India's spectacle lenses is estimated to increase from 210 million units in 2019 to 300 million units in 2025. In Indonesia, it is estimated to increase from 2.7 million units in 2019 to 3.2 million units in 2025. In Thailand, however, there is an estimated reduction from 3.3 million units in 2019 to 3.0 million units in 2025.

The above trend shows that COVID-19 has impacted the industry due to temporary suspensions of non-essential health services such as eye care and delays in the production and shipping of eyewear. However, COVID-19 has also opened up an avenue of opportunities for the eyewear industry because of more time spent on digital screens and less time outdoors.

According to the same BlueWeave research report [6], the leading players in the Asia Pacific Eyewear market are Prada S.P.A. (Hong Kong), Essilor International S.A. (Singapore), Grand Vision (China), Titan Eyeplus (India), Luxottica Group S.P.A (China), Fielmann AG, Carl Zeiss AG (China), and Johnson & Johnson, Inc. (China and Singapore), and Safilo Group S.P.A (China).

33.3 What is the Magnitude of the Need for Spectacles?

1 in 3 or 2.7 billion people in the world suffer from uncorrected refractive errors [3], 90% of whom live in developing economies at the base of the pyramid [7]. Uncorrected refractive errors impact an individual's ability to learn, work, lead safe, independent lives, and realize their full potential. These also constitute a global public health crisis that costs the global economy USD 272 billion every year in lost productivity [8]. Seven of the top ten countries with the largest populations of people with uncorrected refractive errors are in Asia, and three of them (India, 23%; Indonesia, 5%; and Bangladesh, 3%) are in the South-East Asia region [3]. The need for spectacles is only going to increase—by 2050, 3.2 billion people are estimated to suffer from uncorrected refractive errors if the industry maintains its focus and serves only established markets using similar channels and products [3]. Contributing factors include population growth, an increase in presbyopia due to aging populations, and an increase in myopia due to the rise of modern lifestyles, including children spending less time outdoors and the ever-increasing use of screens. Over 50% of the world's population is expected to suffer from myopia by 2050 [9]. Yet, despite these trends of the growing need for spectacles, demand remains low, especially at the base of the pyramid due to several key barriers preventing people from getting the spectacles they need.

33.4 Barriers Preventing People from Getting the Spectacles They Need

The barriers include:

- *Access*. While vision care and spectacles may be readily available in urban areas, there are limited vision care service access points in developing economies, so people cannot access the care and spectacles they need. Therefore, it is necessary to look at every level of distribution—national/provincial, regional, district, and community. The traditional vision care service delivery model requires high levels of resources in infrastructure and personnel, which most of these economies do not have, making access and affordability difficult. There are currently various delivery models that have been devised to deliver vision care, e.g., the franchise model where potential practitioners are selected, trained, and provided with spectacles to sell.

- *Awareness*. Many people in developing economies are not aware that they have uncorrected refractive errors, and even if they do, they do not necessarily know it is a treatable condition or do not know where to seek help. Finally, there is still low prioritization of vision as a serious public health issue and hence low levels of investment by governments in eye care infrastructure and awareness programs.
- Supply. There is a choice between ready-made and prescription devices in providing the spectacles to patients. Ready-made spectacles are convenient for the refractionists and patients and can be used for spherical distance prescription and for reading glasses when the spherical power difference is less than 0.50D and the cylindrical power less than 0.75D. However, there are issues of cost, availability, quality, and re-supply. Prescription spectacles will be needed for approximately 30% of the patient population, depending on the criteria used. Innovative ways of producing prescription spectacles are being investigated. It is anticipated that with a simple system, there will be minimal need for full laboratory set-up, facilities, and highly trained technicians to provide custom-made prescription spectacles.
- *Affordability*. Spectacles are generally designed and priced for consumers at the top of the pyramid with high disposable income, limiting access for base-of-the-pyramid (BoP) consumers. There are also minimal offerings specifically designed and priced for these BoP consumers. Complex in-country supply chains and high import duties for spectacles (which are categorized as a fashion accessory as opposed to a medical device or assistive technology) can also lead to a higher cost that is passed on to the consumers.
- *Quality*. Spectacles need to be of the highest possible quality, including lenses that adhere to ISO (International Organization for Standardization) ratings of power, prism, and power variation; frames that are sturdy and with a metal hinge, making up a complete pair of spectacles which is lightweight and attractive. The quality of lenses and frames is critical for the effective use of spectacles, especially by children. In recent studies in India of spectacle wearers, comfort and attractiveness were significant factors determining wear patterns [10].
- *Acceptance*. In some developing (and even developed) economies, there is still a stigma about wearing spectacles, simply because it is not a widespread and well-known solution. Even if people have access to spectacles, some may still not wear them when needed due to stigma, not getting into the habit, and many other reasons.

33.5 Approaches and Innovations in Addressing These Barriers

The way to eliminate uncorrected refractive error is to develop all aspects of a self-sustaining eye care delivery system, including the human resource segment and the spectacles themselves. In 2020, ATscale, the global partnership for assistive technologies, published a product narrative on the spectacles market landscape and strategic approach to increasing access to eyeglasses in

LMICs [11]. This report outlined 5 strategic objectives to increase access to spectacles; these are as follows:

- Strategic Objective 1: Mobilize key stakeholders, including donors, multilateral, NGO implementers, and the private sector, around reliable data and scalable, proven models to accelerate efforts against vision impairment caused by refractive errors.
- Strategic Objective 2: Strengthen global policy of service delivery standards for low-resource settings to accelerate the adoption of innovative models, devices, and products that support simplified service delivery.
- Strategic Objective 3: Support governments to develop comprehensive eye care plans, integrating validated models of vision screening and provision within the public health system, and facilitate scale-up of those models.
- Strategic Objective 4: Engage the private sector to expand affordable, quality eyeglasses, and related services in low- and middle-income countries.
- Strategic Objective 5: Build and drive awareness and consumer demand for eyeglasses.

Let us now examine how each strategic objective outlined in ATscale's eyeglasses product narrative can be delivered in real-world conditions by studying the efforts of Essilor International, one of the largest lens-maker in the world, and VisionSpring, a social enterprise in primary eye care.

33.6 Case Study 1: Essilor's Multi-Sectoral Collective Actions

As the leader in ophthalmic optics, Essilor has designed, manufactured, and distributed ophthalmic lenses and equipment for consumers and eye care professionals for the past 170 years.

In 2013, with a global ambition to eliminate uncorrected refractive errors from the world by 2050, the company established a mission division, led by a Chief Mission Officer to drive four areas of social impact action to bring vision care and spectacles to the 2.7 billion people suffering from uncorrected refractive error due to lack of access, awareness, affordability, and acceptance [3]. The division also focuses on forging partnerships to accelerate these actions to create scale and impact. Some of these actions are as follows:

Creating Sustainable Access Points Essilor's flagship inclusive business program Eye Mitra ("Friend of the Eye" in Hindi) seeks to create access to and awareness of vision care for underserved populations and improve local livelihoods. The program has been adapted and expanded to Bangladesh, China, Indonesia, and Kenya. The company also partners governments, hospitals, and NGOs to expand existing access or create new access, e.g., mobile vans, vision centers, and large-scale vision screening events. An example is its collaboration with the Royal Government of Bhutan to help Bhutan become the first country in the world free of uncorrected refractive errors by sustainably strengthening its vision care infrastructure and equipping those in need with spectacles.

Innovating for Affordable Quality Products Essilor's 2.5 New Vision Generation (2.5 NVG) spectacles are designed with base-of-the-pyramid (BoP) consumers' preferences and needs in mind, without compromising quality standards. In rural areas, people travel from far to get their eyes tested, and such a trip usually means a loss in daily wages for them. To save them a return trip, Essilor designed Ready2Clip™ spectacles that enables on-the-spot delivery through pre-cut lenses, which can be popped into frames on the spot. Ready2Clip™ Generation II spectacles enable better customization through adjustable pupillary distance functionality and can equip 92% of the population on the spot. Primary vision care entrepreneurs and NGOs serving BoP communities often rely on Ready2Clip™ spectacles to equip their customers and beneficiaries efficiently (Fig. 33.2).

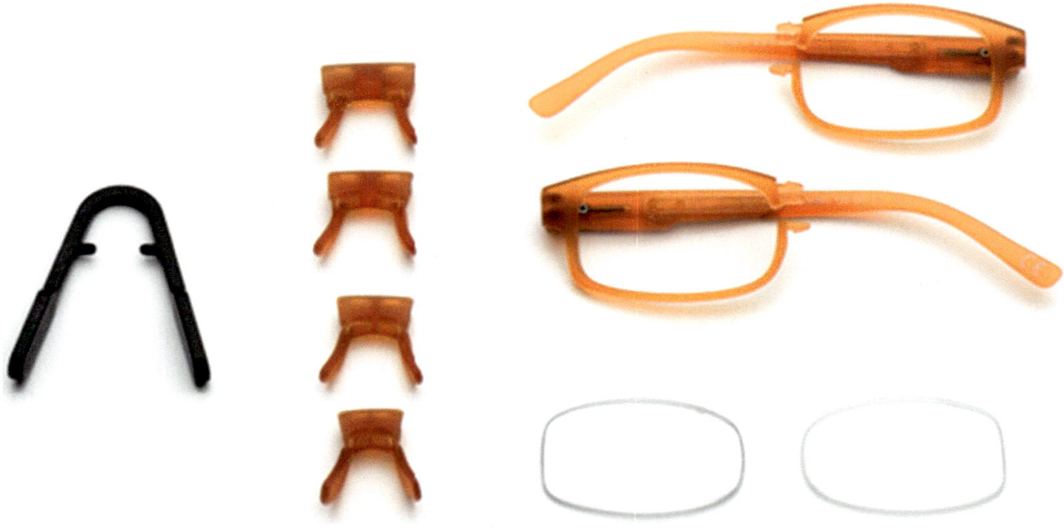

Fig. 33.2 Essilor's Ready2Clip™ Gen II range of spectacles.

Philanthropy Essilor's philanthropic arm, Essilor Vision Foundation, organizes strategic giving programs globally to provide free screening and spectacles to those most in need. Vision For Life, its social impact fund, supports all programs addressing the needs of those with uncorrected poor vision and bringing socio-economic benefits for them and their communities. An example is the Namma Kannu Namma Doddaballapura (NKND) project, which aims to make Doddapallapur, a region in the state of Karnataka (India) with nearly 330,000 residents, the first one in India to be free of uncorrected refractive errors by offering free screening and spectacles. It is a joint initiative by Essilor Vision Foundation India with the Ministry of Health and Family Welfare of the Government of Karnataka; Prerana Trust, a not-for-profit organization, and iDrishti Eye Hospitals, a social impact organization.

Raising Awareness Essilor believes that raising awareness of the importance of good vision needs to happen with individuals and communities, governments, policymakers, and multilateral organizations. This will drive people to access eye care services and spectacles and help stakeholders prioritize vision care and direct more resources toward it. In 2019, Essilor launched the landmark "Eliminating Poor Vision in a Generation" report [3]. Supported by NGOs and governments, the report offers a roadmap to eliminate uncorrected refractive errors from the world by 2050, including how to get spectacles to those who need them. Essilor is a leading partner of See Now, a global campaign by The Fred Hollows Foundation alongside other partners. Fronting the campaign in Uttar Pradesh, India, is celebrity ambassador Amitabh Bachchan who encourages people to get their eyes checked and wear spectacles proudly. The pilot campaign in 2019 was conducted in five districts and reached over 32 million people, with over 9200 people participating in free vision screening programs and those in need receiving either free or subsidized spectacles. In 2020, the campaign was expanded to reach over 49 million people and screened over 87,000 people. Through its social impact fund, Essilor supports the Vision Impact Institute, which raises awareness to make good eyesight a global priority. It has been involved in advocacy work on making eye examinations mandatory for children in the USA before they enter kindergarten.

Forging Partnerships Essilor believes that partnerships are key to accelerating the four areas of action. It is the founding partner of the USD1 billion Vision Catalyst Fund, a multi-stakeholder initiative to bring eye care to everyone around the world. Together with the International Agency for the Prevention of Blindness and other partners, it is forming a coalition focused on addressing uncorrected refractive errors. It is part of the EYElliance, a coalition that collaborates to find solutions to the world's unmet need for spectacles.

33.7 Case Study 2: Capacity-building and Supply Chain in Rural Areas in South-East Asia Region

VisionSpring is a social enterprise in primary eye care with a strong focus in India and Bangladesh. To reach and provide affordable, quality glasses to everyone in the world who needs them, it can dispense and transact two million pairs of glasses per year in these two countries. These two million pairs comprise ready-made reading glasses, prescription glasses, and children's glasses. With a strong focus on capacity-building through various strategies and supply chains in the rural regions of India and Bangladesh, VisionSpring aims to reach ten million pairs per year in terms of the transaction to address the unmet need for glasses in these areas.

One of its key initiatives is the development of Vision Entrepreneurs among the population of one million Accredited Social Health Activists (ASHA) across India [12]. Imagine, if the unmet need for reading glasses in India is 200 million pairs and each ASHA dispenses 10 pairs of reading glasses per month to the communities they serve, it will translate into ten million pairs of reading glasses per month in India, resulting in 120 million pairs reading glasses dispensed per year—an impactful and scalable strategy to bring sustainable vision care and spectacles to underserved communities.

On a similar note, Essilor's Eye Mitra program in India trains under and unemployed youths in rural areas to become primary vision care entrepreneurs for their communities, bringing vision care and spectacles where they were not available before. Today there are over 16,000 primary vision care entrepreneurs globally, making up the world's largest rural optical network and providing more than 360 million people worldwide with sustainable access to vision care spectacles (as of September 2020).

The case studies of Essilor International and VisionSpring have provided examples of the type of multi-sectoral collective and capacity-building work being done in South-East Asia to bring spectacles to everyone who needs them. However, more actions are required to overcome the barriers and drive widespread adoption of spectacles. It is hoped these collaborations will continue to expand and accelerate in the coming years.

References

1. Luxottica, eyeglasses timeline. Luxottica. Page updated 2020. http://www.luxottica.com/en/about-us/museo-dellottica/eyeglasses-timeline. Accessed 23 Nov 2020.
2. Heiting G. Blue light facts: How blue light affects your eyes, AllAboutVision.com. https://www.allaboutvision.com/cvs/blue-light.htm. Accessed 23 Nov 2020.
3. Essilor International, Eliminating uncorrected poor vision in a generation. Essilor International 2019. https://www.essilorseechange.com/wp-content/uploads/2020/02/Eliminating-Poor-Vision-in-a-Generation-Report.pdf
4. An internal study conducted by the Boston Consulting Group for Essilor International.
5. Heiting G. Bifocals and Trifocals: Solutions for "Short Arms", AllAboutVision.com. https://www.allaboutvision.com/lenses/multifocal.htm. Accessed 23 Nov 2020.
6. BlueWeave Consulting, Asia Pacific Eyewear Market Size. By Type (Prescription Glasses, Sunglasses, Contact Lenses, and Others), End-User (Men, Women, and Kids), Distribution Channel (Online Stores and Retail Stores), Countries (China, Japan, India, South Korea and Rest of Asia Pacific); Trend analysis, market competition scenario & outlook, 2016–2026. https://www.blueweaveconsulting.com/asia-pacific-eyewear-market-bwc20121/toc. Accessed 23 Nov 2020.
7. World Health Organization. Universal eye health: a global action plan 2014–2019. World Health Organization. 2013; p 4. https://www.who.int/blind-

ness/AP2014_19_English.pdf. Accessed 23 Nov 2020.
8. Smith TST, Frick KD, Holden BA, et al. Potential lost productivity resulting from the global burden of uncorrected refractive error. Bull World Health Organ. 87(6) (2009, June); 431–437, https://doi.org/10.2471/BLT.08.055673. Accessed 23 Nov 2020. Updated for population and inflation, 2015.
9. Naidoo KS, Fricke TR, Frick KD, et al. "Potential lost productivity resulting from the global burden of myopia: systematic review, meta-analysis, and modeling," Ophthalmology 126, 3 (2019, March); 338–346. https://doi.org/10.1016/j.ophtha.2018.10.029. Accessed 23 Nov 2020.
10. Holden BA, Sulaiman S, Knox K. The challenge of providing spectacles in the developing world. Community Eye Health 2000; 13(33): 9–10. https://www.ncbi.nlm.nih.gov/pmc/articles/PMC1705961/. Accessed 23 Nov 2020.
11. ATscale, A Market Landscape and Strategic Approach to Increasing Access to Eyeglasses in Low- and Middle-Income Countries. ATscale. 2020. https://static1.squarespace.com/static/5b3f6ff1710699a7ebb64495/t/5f5f8981cd35d775923e2621/1600096643567/Product_Narrative-Eyeglasses_a11y_rev.pdf. Accessed 23 Nov 2020.
12. National Health Mission, About Accredited Social Health Activist (ASHA), National Health Mission. https://nhm.gov.in/index1.php?lang=1&level=1&sublinkid=150&lid=226. Accessed 23 Nov 2020.

Ophthalmic Devices and Equipment

34

Ravilla D. Sriram, Nampermulsamy Vishnu Prasad, Alagarajan Soundarrajan, and Kujulva Kannan Rubanbabu

Key Points

- The affordability and accessibility of ophthalmic equipment and devices play an important role in the delivery of eye care in any country.
- The number of cataract surgeries performed in each country directly correlates with the availability of affordable ophthalmic devices such as intraocular lenses (IOLs). High growth of ophthalmic devices is likely to occur ove the coming years (Fig. 34.1).
- Currently, amongst the South-East Asian countries, IOL manufacturing facilities exist in India, Nepal, Indonesia, and Thailand.
- India has manufacturing facilities for both ophthalmic devices and equipment.
- Bhutan and Maldives do not levy taxes on the import of ophthalmic equipment and devices.

South-East Asia accounts for 25.5% of the global population. This translates to around 1.98 billion of the world's 7.8 billion people. The South-East Asian region consists of 11 countries comprising Bangladesh, Bhutan, Democratic People's Republic (DPR) of Korea, India, Indonesia, Maldives, Myanmar, Nepal, Sri Lanka, Thailand, and Timor-Leste. The majority of these are developing nations undergoing rapid advancement in health and infrastructure. However, given the development stage that these countries are currently in, the percentage of GDP (gross domestic product) utilized for health promotion in these countries is relatively low [1].

34.1 Healthcare Challenges

The South-East Asian region is in the middle of an economic, demographic, and epidemiological transition. Those countries with a relatively low healthcare infrastructure [2] carry the burdens of communicable diseases and the increasing burden of non-communicable diseases. The annual number of deaths in the South-East Asian region is 14.6 million; approximately 3.9 million (25%) deaths are due to communicable diseases, and 8.3 million (56.8%) deaths are due to non-communicable diseases (NCDs) such as cardiovascular disease, diabetes, cancer, and substance abuse. Addressing the challenges in healthcare in these countries is possible if greater attention is given to improving the quality of care, financing, and reducing barriers to accessing technology.

R. D. Sriram (✉) · N. V. Prasad · A. Soundarrajan · K. K. Rubanbabu
Aurolab, Madurai, India
e-mail: sriram@aurolab.com; vishnu@aurolab.com; Asia.bde@aurolab.com; Saarc.ba@aurolab.com

T. Das, P. D. Nayar (eds.), *South-East Asia Eye Health*,
https://doi.org/10.1007/978-981-16-3787-2_34

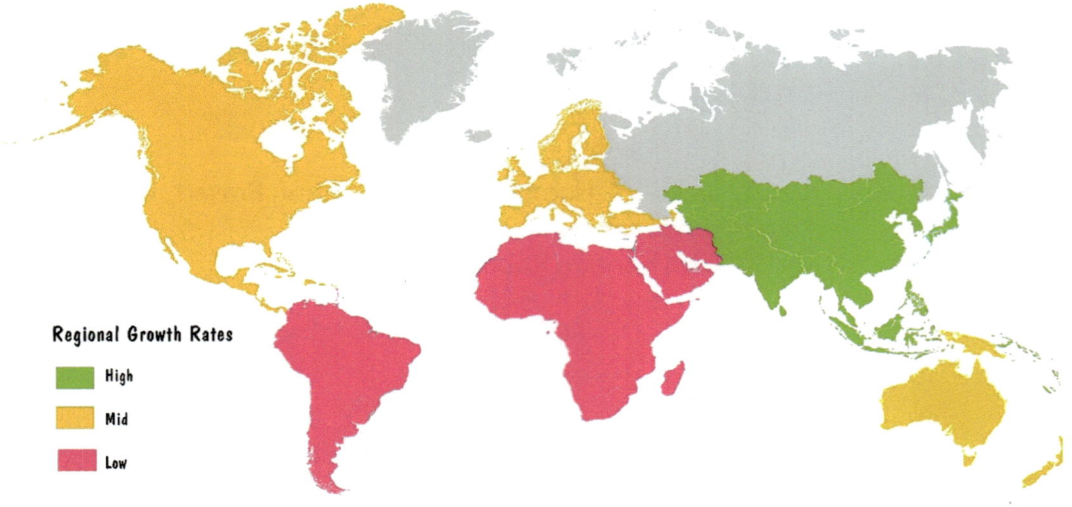

Fig. 34.1 Predicted growth of ophthalmic device market in different regions of the world between 2020 and 2025

34.2 Visual Impairment: Preventive and Non-preventive

According to the International Agency for the Prevention of Blindness (IAPB), there will be an exponential increase in the global need for eye care over the next few years. A lot of progress has been made over the last 30 years, and much yet remains to be done. South-East Asia contributes to one-third of the total number of people with visual impairment globally. Cataract, refractive error, childhood blindness, low vision, glaucoma, and diabetic retinopathy are the leading causes of blindness and visual impairment [3]. On average, there is one ophthalmologist for ~69,000 people and one mid-level eye care personnel for ~27,000 people in this region. Most eye care personnel are located in urban areas, while around 75% of the population lives in rural areas. Since there is an unequal distribution of eye care services, providing access to eye health services is a key challenge. A major factor contributing to this challenge is the non-availability of high quality ophthalmic surgical devices and ophthalmic equipment at an affordable price. Some of the factors that determine the availability and accessibility of such devices and equipment are:

1. Availability of eye care providers.
2. Financing for national eye health.
3. The practice of reimbursement for ophthalmic surgeries.
4. Accessibility to ophthalmic devices and equipment.
5. The regulatory process for consumables and equipment.
6. Import policies and duties related to consumables and equipment.
7. Role of NGOs and other non-government sectors.

This chapter reviews the current availability and indigenous manufacturing facilities of ophthalmic devices and equipment in the South-East Asian region.

34.3 Eye Care in South-East Asia

Blindness prevention is one of the most important healthcare initiatives in all countries in the South-East Asian region. Great importance is given to the process, systems, and resources needed to improve the volume of cataract surgeries in these countries. The number of cataract surgeries in any region largely depends on the accessibility and affordability of ophthalmic surgical equipment and devices in addition to other factors related to human resources for health (HRH) and health finance. The estimated cataract surgical rate (CSR) target in this region by the World Health Organization (WHO) and VISION 2020 is around 3000 per million population/year [4]. The CSR falls short in 6 countries (Timor-Leste, Maldives, Indonesia, Bhutan, Bangladesh, and Myanmar) in South-East Asia region.

The other essential requirements to achieve this target are an adequate number of ophthalmologists (>10/million population), allied ophthalmic personnel (>50/million population), sound public health finance (>5% of country GDP), and reduced out-of-pocket spending (<25%). Currently, 5 countries (Bangladesh, Indonesia, Myanmar, Thailand, Timor-Leste) have a shortage of ophthalmologists; 7 countries (Bangladesh, Indonesia, Maldives, Myanmar, Nepal, Sri Lanka, Timor-Leste) have a shortage of required allied ophthalmic personnel; public finance is <5% of GDP in 8 countries (Bangladesh, Bhutan, India, Indonesia, Myanmar, Sri Lanka, Thailand, Timor-Leste) and out-of-pocket spending >25% in 3 countries (Bangladesh, India, Nepal) in this region [5].

34.4 Accessibility to Ophthalmic Devices and Equipment

Ophthalmic devices are medical equipment designed for diagnosis, surgery, and vision correction. An increase in the prevalence of ophthalmic diseases such as cataract and glaucoma is a key factor that significantly drives growth in the market for ophthalmic devices. However, low awareness about eye diseases and lack of skilled eye care professionals are expected to hamper growth of this market. Emerging countries such as Bangladesh, India, Indonesia, Nepal, Sri Lanka, and Thailand possess high growth potential, owing to their improving healthcare infrastructure, accessibility to cost-effective medical devices/equipment, and therefore, ability to offer eye care services at an affordable cost.

Table 34.1 Country-wise availability of domestic manufacturers of ophthalmic devices and equipment in the South-East Asian region as of 2020

Country	Ophthalmic devices	Ophthalmic equipment
Bangladesh	No manufacturer	No manufacturer
Bhutan	No manufacturer	No manufacturer
India	Aurolab, Appasamy, excellent, biotech, freedom, Omni, excel optics, Mehra eyetech, care group, Nano vision, global Ophthalmics, Truviz, etc.	Appasamy, Aurolab, Optikon, Labomed, akas medical, Reticare, Medisonic, Ascon, Forus health, Remidio, etc.
Indonesia	PT Rohto	No manufacturer
Maldives	No manufacturer	No manufacturer
Myanmar	No manufacturer	No manufacturer
Nepal	The Fred hollows IOL laboratory, Tilganga Institute of Ophthalmology	No manufacturer
Sri Lanka	No manufacturer	No manufacturer
Thailand	HOYA	No manufacturer
Timor-Leste	No manufacturer	No manufacturer

Ophthalmic Devices and Equipment Ophthalmic devices include intraocular lenses (IOL), sutures, blades, etc. Ophthalmic equipment includes a cataract surgical system (phacoemulsification machine), surgical microscope, slit lamps, digital vision chart, ophthalmoscope, refractometers, ultra-sonogram, etc. Domestic manufacture is essential for reduced cost and enhanced servicing (Table 34.1).

34.5 The Regulatory Process for Consumables and Equipment

The regulatory process for importing any product, be it a consumable or ophthalmic equipment, can vary from simple to complex. This depends on the regulatory policies and frameworks set forth by the respective governments. When the regulatory practices are many and complex, many challenges can be expected in the import of ophthalmic equipment and devices, thereby affecting

Table 34.2 Regulatory status for ophthalmic devices and equipment in the South-East Asian region (as of 2020)

	Ophthalmic equipment		Ophthalmic devices	
	Registration		Registration	
Country	Not required	Required	Not required	Required
Bangladesh	X	–	–	X
Bhutan	X	–	–	X
India	–	X[a]	–	X
Indonesia	–	X	–	X
Maldives	X	–	X	–
Myanmar	X	–	–	X
Nepal	X	–	–	X
Sri Lanka	–	X	–	X
Thailand	–	X	–	X
Timor-Leste	X	–	X	–

[a]Non-regulated

quality eye care delivery. On the contrary, simple regulations which conform to specific minimum quality standards will help open the market for many manufacturers, and thereby play a crucial role in ensuring efficient and affordable eye care delivery (Table 34.2).

34.6 Import Policies and Duties Related to Consumables and Equipment

The ophthalmology devices market is highly competitive. The major players focus on developing and launching innovative products to strengthen their foothold in the competitive market. The key players operating in the South-East Asian region ophthalmic devices market are Alcon, Aurolab, Carl Zeiss, HAAG-Streit Holding AG, Johnson & Johnson, Nidek Co., Ltd., TOPCON Corporation, and Ziemer Ophthalmic Systems AG. Others include FCI Ophthalmic, Glaukos Corporation, Gulden Ophthalmics, Hoya group, Sonomed Escalon, and STAAR Surgical [6]. Country-wise import permit status and import duty for ophthalmic devices and equipment in the South-East Asia Region (as of 2020) are shown in Table 34.3.

In general, higher CSR is seen in countries with low import duty. This can be attributed mainly to the lower landing cost of the ophthalmic consumables and equipment in the surgeon's hands as compared to such costs in countries with no domestic manufacturing facilities and high import duties.

34.7 Role of International and National Non-Government Organizations

The role of Non-Government Organizations (NGOs) in making eye care affordable is immense. International NGOs (INGOs) have contributed significantly to eye care service delivery. International NGOs supported the usage of ophthalmic devices and purchase of surgical

Table 34.3 Import permit status in South-East Asian region countries (as of 2020)

Country	Ophthalmic equipment			Ophthalmic devices		
	Import permit			Import permit		
	Required	Not required	Taxation %	Required	Not required	Taxation %
Bangladesh	X	–	15	X	–	15
Bhutan	X	–	Nil	X	–	Nil
India	X	–	27–50	X	–	27
Indonesia	X	–	25–20	X	–	15–20
Maldives	X	–	Nil	X	–	Nil
Myanmar	X	–	5–15	X	–	5 to 15
Nepal	X	–	5	X	–	5–30[a]
Sri Lanka	X	–	18–22	X	–	18–22
Thailand	X	–	0–20	X	–	0–15#
Timor-Leste	–	X	10–12.5	–	X	2.5–10

[a]IOL—30%, others—5%; # IOL—0%, others—15%

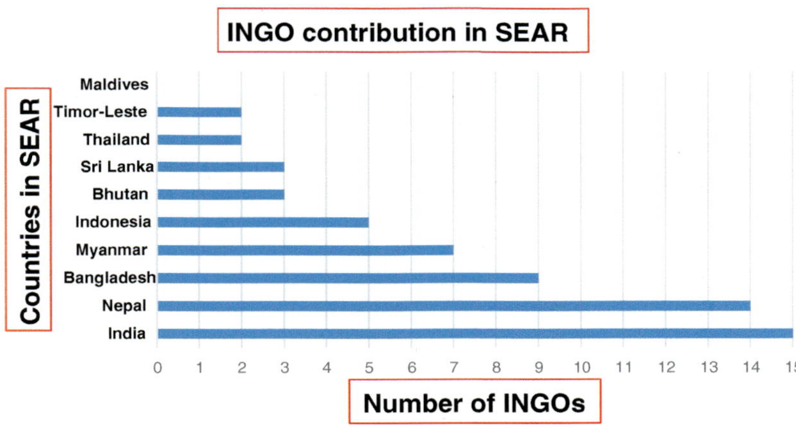

Fig. 34.2 Number of eye care INGOs in the South-East Asian region countries (as of 2020)

and diagnostic equipment. Their presence increased the usage of medical devices and increase of the equipment in the region. Their presence is shown in Figs. 34.2 and 34.3.

The increased consumption of ophthalmic diagnostic and surgical equipment, ophthalmic devices like IOLs and sutures and consumables like blades & instruments has prompted indigenous production of these goods at a reasonable cost in South-East Asia Region. The International NGOs presence has helped to increase the number of cataract surgeries in the region.

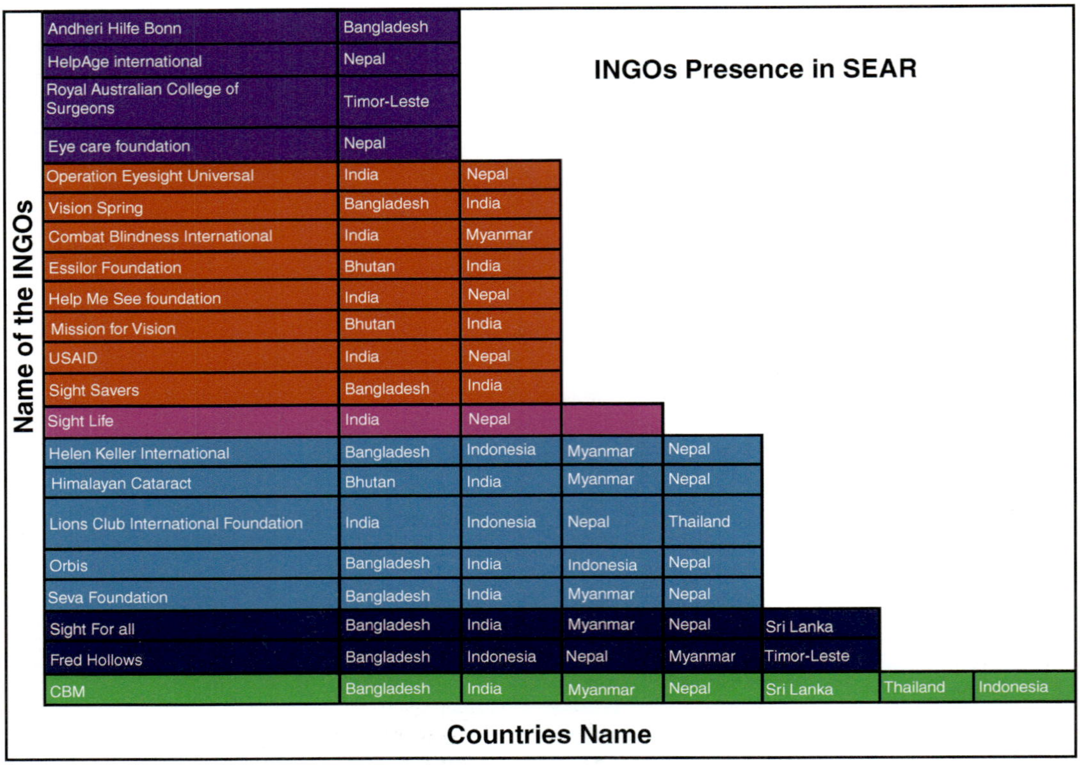

Fig. 34.3 List of eye care INGOs in the South-East Asian region

34.8 Conclusion

The ophthalmic industry plays a crucial role in the delivery of eye care. Very few countries in the South-East Asian region have developed domestic manufacturing facilities for ophthalmic equipment and devices. While importing high-end equipment and devices is inevitable, regulations, including reduced taxation, would make eye care more affordable. Additionally, cooperation between the South-East Asian region countries could also reduce the cost of eye care.

References

1. https://data.worldbank.org/indicator/SH.XPD.CHEX.GD.ZS?locations=BD-NP-LK-BT-MV-IN-ID-TH-MM-KP-TL [Accessed on 17 Dec 2020]
2. https://www.who.int/southeastasia/publications/who-south-east-asia-journal-of-public-health [Accessed on 17 Dec 2020]
3. https://www.iapb.org/connect/regions/south-east-asia/ [Accessed on 17 Dec 2020]
4. https://www.researchgate.net/publication/23442094_Current_status_of_cataract_blindness_and_Vision_2020_The_right_to_sight_initiative_in_India [Accessed on 17 Dec 2020]
5. https://www.researchgate.net/publication/314161083_Is_the_2015_eye_care_service_delivery_profile_in_Southeast_Asia_closer_to_universal_eye_health_need [Accessed on 17 Dec 2020]
6. https://www.alliedmarketresearch.com/ophthalmology-devices-market [Accessed on 17 Dec 2020]

35 Ophthalmic Pharmaceutical Markets South-East Asia Region Perspective 2020

Sandeep Sharma, Varsha Narayanan, Manoj Mahajan, and Y. S. V. S. Naga Mohan

Key Points

- The pharmaceutical industry plays a significant role in quality ophthalmic care through people's access to affordable medicines.
- The global ophthalmology drug market in the Asia Pacific, Latin America-Middle East-Africa (LAMEA), North America, and Europe had a market size value of ~ USD 31.0 billion in 2019. This value is expected to increase to more than USD 38 billion by 2025; the Asia Pacific market is expected to show the highest compound annual growth rate.
- The main drivers of the ophthalmic market are the drugs used for glaucoma, pre-and post-eye surgery (chiefly cataract), dry eye, and retinal conditions such as age-related macular degeneration and diabetic retinopathy.
- Many of the South-East Asian countries procure ophthalmic medicines from local ophthalmic drug industry as well as multinational companies.
- Most generic ophthalmic drugs from companies based in South-East Asia Region countries are accessible and affordable as per the country's economic standards and purchasing power.
- Usually, drugs produced by multinational companies, mainly innovator brands or those based on unique technologies, come at premium prices.
- Promoting affordable and fair prices and cost-effective interventions that can be purchased by patients and/or funded by the public health budgets within a country is central to the achievement of universal health coverage.
- Simultaneously, there should be promotion and policy to sustain research and development, production, and distribution of ophthalmic drugs in the region.

The Vision Loss Expert Group (VLEG) has recently reported that globally, 1.1 billion people live with vision loss and 90% of such people live in low- and middle-income countries (LMICs) [2]. This report further states that with the current strategy of eye care, changing trends in disease profiles, and increased longevity, the number of people with vision loss is likely to increase by 60%, from 1.1 billion to 1.7 billion, by 2050. The numbers of blind people (vision <3/60) will increase from the current 43 million to 61 million (42% increase); those with moderate to severe visual impairment (vision <6/18, but >3/60) will increase from the current 295 million to 474 million (61% increase); people with mild visual impairment (vision <6/12) will increase from the

S. Sharma (✉) · V. Narayanan · M. Mahajan
Y. S. V. S. Naga Mohan
Sun Pharma, Mumbai, India
e-mail: Sandeep.Sharma@sunpharma.com; info@drvarsha.com; Manoj.Mahajan@sunpharma.com; Naga.Mohan@sunpharma.com

T. Das, P. D. Nayar (eds.), *South-East Asia Eye Health*,
https://doi.org/10.1007/978-981-16-3787-2_35

current 258 million to 360 million (39.5% increase), and those with near vision difficulties will increase from the current 510 million to 866 million (70% increase).

The leading causes of vision impairment are untreated cataract, refractive error, age-related macular degeneration (AMD), glaucoma, corneal opacity, and diabetic retinopathy (DR). Other common conditions for which out-patient ophthalmic medical opinion is sought are dry eyes, ocular irritation or allergy, conjunctivitis, and lid infections, in addition to post-surgery eye care. The annual global economic impact of eye diseases on the family and community is estimated to exceed USD3 trillion [3]. Optimal eye health can reduce poverty and promote education, health, well-being, and social and gender equality [4]. All the modern eye care requirements, such as infrastructure, diagnostic equipment, and therapeutic needs, have not yet reached underserved regions in LMICs or underprivileged populations in high-income countries [5].

Eye care medications and the pharmaceutical industry play a significant role in quality ophthalmic care and can help realize one of the stated goals of universal health coverage (UHC): easy access to affordable medicines. In 2020, the global pharmaceutical market was estimated to reach USD 1.3 trillion at a 5% CAGR (compound annual growth rate) [5]. The global market size for ophthalmic drugs was valued at around USD 29 billion in 2016, USD 31.0 billion in 2019, and was expected to be about USD 33 billion in 2020; it is likely to expand at a CAGR 5.2% to USD 43 billion by 2023–25 [6–8]. Although there were an economic slowdown and a 20% decline in CAGR in 2020 due to the COVID-19 (Coronavirus disease-19) pandemic, recovery and expedited growth at a CAGR of 44.6% from 2021 is predicted, and the global market for ophthalmic drugs is expected to reach USD33 billion USD in 2023. The market is expected to grow at a CAGR of 7% to nearly USD 38.3 billion by 2025 and USD 53.7 billion by 2030 [9]. The global market for ophthalmology drugs comprises the Asia Pacific, Latin America-Middle East-Africa (LAMEA), North America, and Europe. The Asia Pacific market is expected to show the highest CAGR of 8.8% in the 2017–23 period [1] (Fig. 35.1).

Global drivers of the ophthalmic drug market include the ones used for glaucoma, pre-and post-cataract surgery, and retinal conditions such as age-related macular degeneration (AMD) and

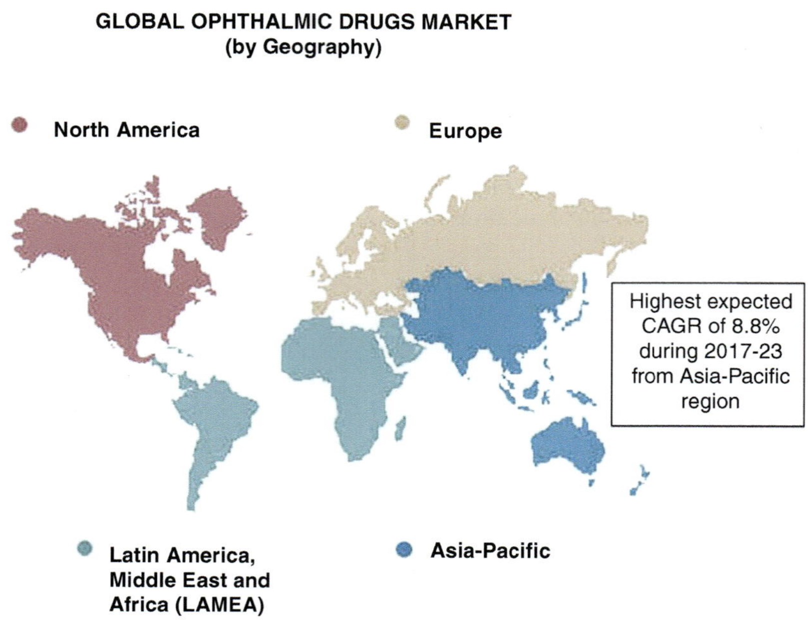

Fig. 35.1 Ophthalmic drug markets according to geography. (Adapted from [1])

diabetic retinopathy (DR). Medications for retinal conditions and glaucoma account for around 20% each of the ophthalmic drug market. The dry eye segment has a prescription share of around 5%, and much of it comes from over the counter (OTC) sales. Retinal disorders have a predicted CAGR of 5.8% from 2017 to 2023, with the AMD segment accounting for the highest share among all current retinal disorders [1]. Glaucoma medications have a high CAGR of 8.0%. There has been a shift towards combination therapies and novel ocular drug delivery with multi-compartment drug delivery systems. The approval of one new drug, *Latanoprostene bunod*, and one new class of drugs, *Rho kinase inhibitors*, has added further impetus to this growing market [10, 11].

The key multinational ophthalmic pharmaceutical companies with a presence in the South-East Asia Region are *Allergan*, *Novartis-Alcon*, *Pfizer*, *Johnson & Johnson*, *Bayer*, and *Santen*.

35.1 South-East Asia Ophthalmic Markets

In 2019, the market for ophthalmic drugs in the Asia Pacific was the fastest-growing regional ophthalmic market, with a value of USD 6.64 billion. It is expected to grow at a CAGR of 7% to reach USD 9.27 billion by 2023–2024 [12]. The Association of South-East Asian Nations (ASEAN) is expected to contribute largely to this market [13]. The International Agency for the Prevention of Blindness (IAPB) South-East Asia Region (SEAR) comprises 11 countries and is home to 26% of the world's population, 30% of the global blind people, and 32% of the global population with visual impairment [14]. The RAAB (rapid assessment of avoidable blindness) survey conducted across 8 countries (Bangladesh, Bhutan, India, Indonesia, the Maldives, Sri Lanka, Thailand, and the Timor-Leste) in this region showed that cataract is the principal cause of blindness and severe visual impairment in all these countries. Refractive error is the principal cause of moderate visual impairment in 4 countries (Bangladesh, India, the Maldives, and Sri Lanka). Cataract continues to be the principal cause of moderate visual impairment in the other 4 countries (Bhutan, Indonesia, Thailand, and Timor-Leste). Although these issues must be addressed, steps must also be made to provide care for other emerging causes of visual impairment and blindness, such as glaucoma and posterior segment disorders, particularly diabetic retinopathy [14].

India has the largest share in value, brands, and players in the SEAR ophthalmic drug market. All countries in the region do not have a pharmaceutical industry. It is at a very rudimentary stage in Bhutan, Maldives, Myanmar, Sri Lanka, and Timor-Leste. All countries in the region also import ophthalmic drugs from other SEAR countries. Besides, all SEAR countries, even those with pharmaceutical manufacturing facilities, import drugs from established multinational companies from Europe, Japan, and the USA. The current pharmaceutical companies producing ophthalmic preparations for use within their own countries and export are listed in Table 35.1 [15].

The prescription ophthalmic drug segment is the regulated market captured by the ophthalmic pharmaceutical industry and the source of most of the market data presented in this chapter. However, several OTCs and herbal topical preparations also form part of the general consumer market and enjoy a certain degree of local popularity. Each country has its regulatory/drug licensing authority for manufacturing, marketing, and import permissions and reviewing clinical trial efficacy and safety, and collecting real-world effectiveness data. Drug pricing is based on manufacturing, technological, and import costs and taxation rates that vary between countries [16]. Most generic ophthalmic drugs from companies based in SEAR countries are easily accessible and affordable as per the country's economic standards and purchasing powers. In general, the drugs from multinational companies, innovator brands, and drugs with unique technologies (such as preservative-free formulations, nano/emulsion forms, polymer-based drug delivery systems, penetration enhancers) are priced at a premium.

The following are brief accounts of the current ophthalmic industry in SEAR countries.

Table 35.1 Key ophthalmic pharmaceutical companies in the South-East asian region

Country	Ophthalmic pharmaceuticals 2019	
	Industry	Market size (USD)
Bangladesh	Acme, Beximco, Drug International, Eskayef, Gaco, General, Healthcare Pharma, IBN-SINA, Incepta Pharma, Navana, Nipa, Opso Saline, Popular, Square	36 million[a]
Bhutan	No local ophthalmic pharma industry	Not available
India	Ajanta, Aristo, Cadila, Cipla, Entod, FDC, Indoco, Intas, Lupin, Micro Labs, Sun, Sunways	360 million^
Indonesia	Cendo, Combiphar, Farenheit, Ferron Par Pharma, Global Multi pharm, Interbat, Konimex, Meiji, Rohto Erela, Sanbe	49 million[a]
Maldives	No local ophthalmic pharma company	Not available
Myanmar	No local ophthalmic pharma company	Not available
Nepal	DCI Pharma, National Healthcare, Nepal Pharma, Sumy Pharma Time Pharma, Yash Pharma	5.75 million[a]
Sri Lanka	No local ophthalmic pharma company	8.3 million[a]
Thailand	Sang Thai Medical, Santen Seiyaku, Pharma Innova, Siam Pharma, Stericon Pharma, Thai Nakorn Patana, Thai PD Chemicals, TRB Chemedica	152.0 million[a]
Timor-Leste	No local ophthalmic pharma company	Not available

[a]IMS MAT June'19, ^ IMS MAT Nov '20 (Intercontinental Medical Statistics Moving Annual Total)

35.2 Industry

35.2.1 Bangladesh

Ophthalmology is a competitive but non-exclusive market in Bangladesh. The total ophthalmic prescription drug market in 2019 was around USD36 million. Although the top ophthalmic pharmaceutical company in Bangladesh is *Aristo* from India (30% market share), local players are equally dominant, such as *General* (16%) and *Popular Pharma* (15%) [15]. In addition to these, a multinational collaboration between *Allergan and Eskayef* also has a share of the ophthalmic drug market [17]. The approval and regulation of drugs are made by the Directorate General of Drug Administration (DGDA) of Bangladesh.

35.2.2 India

India is one of the key pharmaceutical players in South-East Asia by incremental growth, and it is the sixth largest market globally [6, 18]. India is the world's largest provider of generic medicine, accounting for three-fourths of the domestic retail market and one-fifth of global generic drug exports. The export value of Indian pharmaceutical products was nearly USD40 billion in 2020. Currently, India's total ophthalmic market is worth about USD1.3 billion and is expected to grow at a CAGR of 5–6.8% against the global growth of USD 4.06% to USD1.8 billion by 2022 [6]. The ophthalmologic prescription drug market in India was worth roughly USD360 million in 2020 and is growing at a CAGR of about 6%. By market share, the dry eye segment is the largest (28%), followed by anti-glaucoma medications (22%) and anti-infectives (14%) (Fig. 35.2).

35.2.2.1 Key Pharmaceutical Players

In the Indian ophthalmic pharmaceutical market, 73% of the value comes from the Indian pharmaceutical industry growing at a CAGR of around 7.5%. The remaining comes from multinational corporations (MNCs) growing at a CAGR of 3.5% (Fig. 35.3) [15, 19]. The Drugs Controller General of India of the Department of the Central Drugs Standard Control Organization of the Government of India approves and regulates drugs in India.

India is not only self-reliant in manufacturing ophthalmic medicines but also has increased

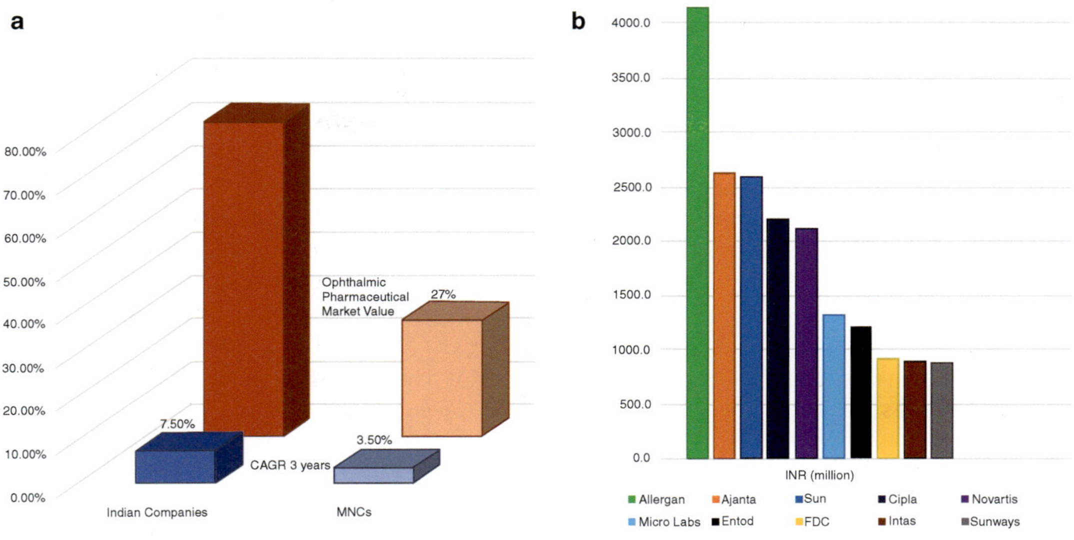

Fig. 35.2 Market share of ophthalmic therapy sub-segments in India (2020)

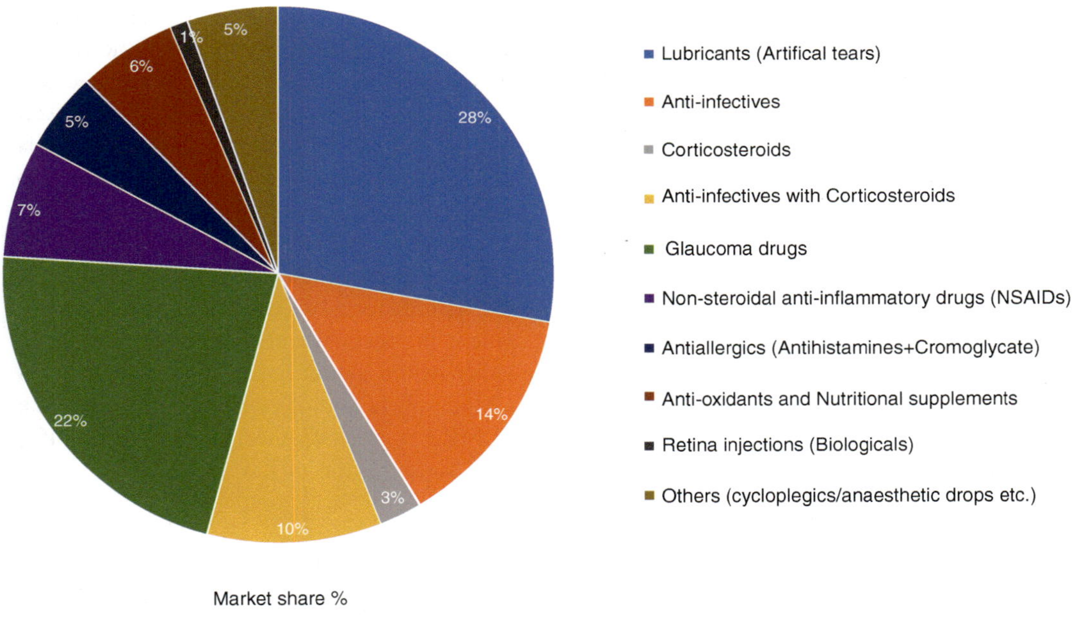

Fig. 35.3 Ophthalmic pharmaceutical companies in India (2020); (**a**) contribution to the ophthalmic pharmaceutical market share by Indian pharmaceutical companies and multinational companies (MNCs); the compound annual growth rate (CAGR) of each segment is also mentioned; (**b**) top 10 ophthalmic pharmaceutical companies by value (in Indian Rupees or INR)

capability and capacity in the research and development of ophthalmic medications. Many Indian pharmaceutical companies are establishing their strong presence in South-East Asia, Europe, and the USA. For example, Sun pharma has recently launched 3 innovative brands in the USA, namely, *BromSite* (0.075% Bromfenac ophthalmic solution), *Xelpros* (0.005% Latanoprost ophthalmic emulsion), and *Cequa* (0.09% cyclosporine ophthalmic solution) [20–22].

35.2.3 Indonesia

The ophthalmic prescription drug market in Indonesia stood at almost USD 49 million in 2019. Ophthalmic pharmaceutical players comprise MNCs and local players, and 50% of the market share rests with the local player, *Cendo* [15]. Drug approvals and drug regulation are handled by the Directorate General of Pharmaceuticals and Medical Devices and the National Agency for Drug and Food Control (NADFC) of Indonesia.

35.2.4 Nepal

Ophthalmic therapy contributes to 2.2% of the total pharmaceutical market in Nepal and is growing at a CAGR of 27%, mostly driven by methylcellulose/CMC brands [23]. The total ophthalmic prescription drug market in Nepal stood at USD5.75 million in 2019. Drug approvals and regulation of drugs are handled by the Nepal Department of Drug Administration at the Ministry of Health and Population.

35.2.5 Thailand

The total ophthalmic prescription drug market stood at USD152 million in 2019. Four international players hold more than 55% of the market share; these are *Novartis* (21–25% with *Alcon*), *Allergan* (16%), *Pfizer* (10.5%), and *Bayer* (9.5%). The local players *Santen Seiyaku* and *TRB Chemedica* hold 10% and 8% of the market shares, respectively [15]. Drug approvals and regulation of drugs are handled by the Food and Drug Administration of Thailand.

35.3 Affordability

Equitable access to essential, high-quality, affordable medicines and other medical technologies depends on affordable and fair pricing and effective financing schemes. Promoting affordable and fair prices and cost-effective interventions is central to the achievement of universal health coverage. An "affordable and fair" price for a commodity is one that can reasonably be paid by patients and health budgets; such a price must simultaneously sustain research and development, production, and distribution of the commodity within a country [24].

Much of the out-of-pocket spending (OOPS) in LMICs is on medicines, as they often constitute a large portion of the total health expenditure. Therefore, affordability of medication should be an important policy goal. While the government must ensure that quality-assured generic medicines are available in the public sector, the pharmaceutical companies also must ensure that their products are not too expensive. The current price variation of common ophthalmic drugs in SEAR countries is listed in Table 35.2.

To promote the concept of affordable medicine, the World Health Organization (WHO) has been publishing a list of "essential medicines" since 1977; this list is revised every 2 years. The list names medications considered to be most effective and safe to meet the most important needs in a health system and are divided into core (75% of all items on the list) and complementary items (25% of all items on the list). The core items are deemed the most cost-effective options for key health problems and are usable with little additional healthcare resources. The complementary items either require additional infrastructures such as specially trained health care providers or diagnostic equipment or have a lower cost–benefit ratio than the core items. While most medications on the list are available as generic products, being under patent does not preclude inclusion. Countries frequently use the list to help develop their local lists of essential medicines. Most countries have created their national lists of essential medicines based on the WHO's model list. Though differences exist, more than 5 billion people live in countries that use essential medicines lists [25]. The current (2019) WHO essential medicines list for ophthalmic preparations are listed in Table 35.3 [26].

Table 35.2 Price variations in ophthalmic drugs in key South-East Asian countries (in USD)

	Tear substitutes (in USD)	Glaucoma# (in USD)	Glaucoma (Timolol) (in USD)	Anti-infectives (in USD)	Anti-allergics (in USD)	Steroids (in USD)	NSAIDs (in USD)
Bangladesh	2.5–3 (**5.5**)	4.5–5.5 (**14.5**)	0.5–1.0	1.1–2.0 (**4**)	1.1–1.8 (**5.5**)	2.0	2.0
India	4.0–6.0 (**8**)* 2–4	250–450 (**500–600**)	0.5–1.0	0.25–3 (**4**)	1.5–4.5	0.25–2.0	1.5–4.0
Indonesia	4.5–5.0*	6–9 (**26**)	1.5–2.5	5–8	(**6.5**)	1.5–2.5	(**6**)
Nepal	1.3–1.5 (**2**)	4.5–5.0 (**6–6.5**)	0.5–0.75	1.0–1.3	1.0–1.2	1.0–1.2	1.0–1.3
Sri Lanka	2.0–3.0	5.0–7.5	1.2–2.0	1.5–2.5 (**3**)	2.0–2.5 (**5.5**)	1.0–1.5 (**2.5**)	2.0–2.5 (**3**)
Thailand	11–14* 2.5–3.0 (**6**)	6.0–7.0 (**20–22**)	1.5–2.8 (**4**)	5.0–7.0	5.0–6.0 (**10**)	(**7.5–8.5**)	(**5**)

Bold values in parentheses () represent innovator brands; *hyaluronic acid tear substitutes; # includes mainly prostaglandin analogs (PGAs), and in India, these include brimonidine, PGAs, and dorzolamides

Table 35.3 WHO list of essential and complementary ophthalmic preparations (2019)

Class		Drug	Preparation
Essential			
Anti-infective	Anti-viral	Acyclovir	3% w/w ointment
	Anti-bacterial	Azithromycin	1.5% solution
		Erythromycin[a,b]	0.5% ointment
		Gentamicin (sulfate)	0.3% solution
		Tetracycline (hydrochloride)	1% ointment
		Ofloxacin	0.3% solution
	Anti-fungal	Natamycin	5% suspension
Anti-inflammatory		Prednisolone (sodium phosphate)	0.5% solution
Diagnostics		Fluorescein (sodium fluorescein)	1% solution
		Tropicamide	0.5% solution
Local anesthetics		Tetracaine[c] (hydrochloride)	0.5% solution
Anti-glaucoma and Miotic		Acetazolamide	250 mg tablet
		Latanoprost	50 µg/ml solution (eye drops)
		Timolol	0.25% solution (eye drops) with 0.5% hydrogen maleate
		Pilocarpine	2% solution (eye drops) with 4% hydrochloride or nitrate
Mydriatics		Atropine	0.1% solution (eye drops) with 0.5% and 1% (sulfate)[d] or homatropine (hydrobromide) or cyclopentolate (hydrochloride)[b]
Complementary			
		Epinephrine/Adrenaline (hydrochloride)	2% solution (eye drops)
Anti-vascular endothelial growth factor (VEGF) preparations		Bevacizumab	25 mg/ml injection

[a]For infections due to *Chlamydia trachomatis* or *Neisseria gonorrhoeae*
[b]There is a specific indication for restricting its use in children
[c]Not to be used for pre-term infants
[d]Only for use in adults and children above 3 months

35.4 Summary

South-East Asia represents a key growing global market in various segments of ophthalmology. The SEAR countries have established regulatory authorities to approve, monitor, and regulate drugs and other pharmaceutical products [27]. The ophthalmic pharmaceutical industry in India and South-East Asia is also an important export center for generic drugs, especially in segments like artificial tears, anti-allergic, anti-infective, and glaucoma medicines. While pricing is high for innovator brands, generics are cheaper and produced in high volumes. Combination brands are gaining popularity, especially with antibiotic-corticosteroid and glaucoma drug combinations. Increasing number of indigenous companies and multinational players are entering the ophthalmic markets in India and the South-East Asia to cater to the large and dense population of the region. In future, contributions from this region will play a significant role in the global growth of the ophthalmic pharmaceutical industry.

References

1. Ophthalmic Drugs Market Expected to Reach $42,663 Million, Globally by 2023: Allied Market Research. https://www.alliedmarketresearch.com/ophthalmic-drugs-market
2. Vision Atlas 2020. www.iapb.org. Accessed 28 Dec 2020.
3. Burton MJ, Faal HB, Ramke J, Ravilla T, Holland P, Wang N, et al. Announcing the Lancet Global Health Commission on Global Eye Health. Lancet. Dec 2019;7(12):E1612–3.
4. The Lancet. A vision for Universal Eye Health. Editorial. Oct 2019;394(10207):1388.
5. Pharma 2020: The vision. Pwc global market report. www.pwc.com. Accessed Nov 2020.
6. Narayanan V. Pharmaceutical ophthalmic market perspectives in India and emerging trends. Clin Exp Vis Eye Res J. 2018;1(1):35–7.
7. Global ophthalmic drugs market size, share, trends and growth analysis report – segmented by therapeutic class, product type, distribution channel, disease, indications, dosage form, technology, region – industry forecast (2020 to 2025). https://www.marketdataforecast.com/market-reports/ophthalmic-drugsmarket. Accessed Oct 2020.
8. Ophthalmic Drug Market Overviews. Allied Market Research. Accessed Dec 2020 https://www.alliedmarketresearch.com/ophthalmic-drugs-market
9. Global Ophthalmology Drugs Market Opportunities and Strategies (2019 to 2030) - COVID-19 Impact and Recovery. www.globenewswire.com/newsrelease/2020/05/28/2040100/0/en/Global-Ophthalmology-Drugs-Market-Opportunitiesand-Strategies-2019-to-2030. Accessed Oct 2020.
10. Serle JB, Katz LJ, McLaurin E, et al. Two Phase 3 Clinical Trials Comparing the Safety and Efficacy of Netarsudil to Timolol in Patients with Elevated Intraocular Pressure: Rho Kinase Elevated IOP treatment trial 1 and 2 (ROCKET-m 1 and ROCKET-2). Am J Ophthalmol. 2018;186:116–27.
11. Weinreb RN, Realine T, Varma R. Latanoprostene bunod, a dual-acting nitric oxide donating prostaglandin analog for lowering of intraocular pressure. US Ophthalmic Rev. 2016;9:80–7. https://doi.org/10.17925/USOR.2016.09.02.80.
12. Asia pacific ophthalmic drugs market research report – segmented therapeutic class, product type, distribution channel, by disease indication, by dosage form, by technology by country – industry analysis, size, share, growth, trends, and forecasts (2019–2024). https://www.marketdataforecast.com/marketreports/asia-pacificophthalmic-drugs-market. Accessed Oct 2020
13. An overview of eye care market in ASEAN. An overview of eye care market in ASEAN. www.hmadvisory.net/assets/pdf/Anoverview-of-Eye care-Market-in-ASEAN-2013-22102013.pdf. Accessed November 2020.
14. Das T. Blindness and visual impairment profile and rapid assessment of avoidable blindness in south east asia: analysis of new data. 2017 APAO Holmes lecture. Asia Pac J Ophthalmol (Phila). 2018;7:312–5.
15. IMS-IQVIA and Country Internal Audit 2020 India and 2019 SEAR countries reports: market share, value and growth of ophthalmic pharmaceuticals data on file: Sun Pharmaceuticals Ltd.
16. Ophthalmic Drug Price India and SEAR countries Data on File: Sun Pharmaceuticals Ltd.
17. Pharmaceutical industry of Bangladesh report. www.arx.cfa/~/media/2A85F9B2CEAB43CFAF325AB54F3EF404.ashx. Accessed Nov 2020.
18. India Pharma 2020 Propelling Access and Acceptance summary: Realizing True Potential: Pharmaceutical and Medical Products Practice. McKinsey report. www.mckinsey.com/~/media/mckinsey/dotcom/client_service/Pharma%20and%2. Accessed Nov 2020.
19. Ophthalmic comprehensive reports: 2020 India ophthalmic market report: A regional analysis for 2019 to 2025, April, 2020. https://www.marketscope.com/pages/reports/177/2020-india-ophthalmicmarket-report-a-regional-analysis-for2019-to-2025-april-2020. Accessed Nov 2020
20. Sun Pharma launches first branded ophthalmic product, BromSite™, in USA. World Pharma Today Apr 2016. www.worldpharmatoday.com/news/sun-pharmalaunches-firstbranded-ophthalmic-product. Accessed Dec 2020.
21. Sun Pharma introduces access program for patients prescribed XELPROS in the U.S. Biospace July 2019. www.biospace.com. Accessed Dec 2020.
22. SunPharmaLaunchesCEQUAforTheTreatmentOfDry Eye Disease in the U.S. Businesswire Oct 2019. www.businesswire.com/news/home/20191013005028/en/Sun-PharmaLaunchesCEQUA-for-the-Treatment-of-Dry-Eye-Disease-in-the-U.S. Accessed Dec 2020.
23. IQVIA Nepal Audit July 2019 Market and Prescription Data on File.
24. Essential medicine. www.who.int. Accessed 28 Dec 2020.
25. Persaud N, Jiang M, Shaikh R, et al. Comparison of essential medicines lists in 137 countries. Bull World Health Organization. 2019;97:394–404C. https://doi.org/10.2471/BLT.18.222448.
26. World Health Organization Model List of Essential Medicines, 21st List, 2019. Geneva: World Health Organization; 2019. Licence: CC BY-NC-SA 3.0 IGO.
27. SEAR-WHO countries, policies, profiles and information worksheet. www.google.com. Accessed Dec 2020.

Index

T. Das, P. D. Nayar (eds.), *South-East Asia Eye Health*,
https://doi.org/10.1007/978-981-16-3787-2